258 Clinical Cases in

Medicine

for MD, DNB and MRCP Examinations

258 Clinical Cases in
Medicine

for MD, DNB and MRCP Examinations

SN Chugh

MD, MNAMS, FICP, FIACM, FICN, FISC, FIMSA

Senior Professor of Medicine
Pt BD Sharma PG Institute of Medical Sciences
and
Pro Vice-Chancellor
Pt BD Sharma University of Health Sciences
Rohtak, Haryana

Eshan Gupta

MD, DM (student)

Senior Resident in Cardiology
GB Pant Hospital
New Delhi

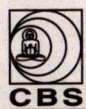

CBS Publishers & Distributors Pvt Ltd

New Delhi • Bengaluru • Chennai • Kochi • Kolkata • Mumbai
Hyderabad • Jharkhand • Nagpur • Patna • Pune • Uttarakhand

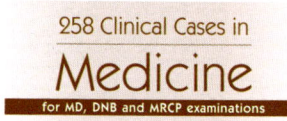

258 Clinical Cases in
Medicine
for MD, DNB and MRCP examinations

ISBN: 978-81-239-2442-7

Copyright © Authors and Publisher

First Edition: 2014

Reprint: 2018

Published by Satish Kumar Jain and produced by Varun Jain for

CBS Publishers & Distributors Pvt Ltd

4819/XI Prahlad Street, 24 Ansari Road, Daryaganj, New Delhi 110 002, India.
Ph: 23289259, 23266861, 23266867   Website: www.cbspd.com
Fax: 011-23243014   e-mail: delhi@cbspd.com; cbspubs@airtelmail.in.
Corporate Office: 204 FIE, Industrial Area, Patparganj, Delhi 110 092

Ph: 4934 4934   Fax: 4934 4935   e-mail: publishing@cbspd.com; publicity@cbspd.com

Branches

- **Bengaluru:** Seema House 2975, 17th Cross, K.R. Road,
  Banasankari 2nd Stage, Bengaluru 560 070, Karnataka
  Ph: +91-80-26771678/79   Fax: +91-80-26771680   e-mail: bangalore@cbspd.com
- **Chennai:** 7, Subbaraya Street, Shenoy Nagar, Chennai 600 030, Tamil Nadu
  Ph: +91-44-26680620, 26681266   Fax: +91-44-42032115   e-mail: chennai@cbspd.com
- **Kochi:** Ashana House, No. 39/1904, AM Thomas Road, Valanjambalam,
  Ernakulam 682 016, Kochi, Kerala
  Ph: +91-484-4059061-65   Fax: +91-484-4059065   e-mail: kochi@cbspd.com
- **Kolkata:** 6/B, Ground Floor, Rameswar Shaw Road, Kolkata-700 014, West Bengal
  Ph: +91-33-22891126, 22891127, 22891128   e-mail: kolkata@cbspd.com
- **Mumbai:** 83-C, Dr E Moses Road, Worli, Mumbai-400018, Maharashtra
  Ph: +91-22-24902340/41   Fax: +91-22-24902342   e-mail: mumbai@cbspd.com

Representatives

- **Hyderabad** 0-9885175004
- **Jharkhand** 0-9811541605
- **Nagpur** 0-9021734563
- **Patna** 0-9334159340
- **Pune** 0-9623451994
- **Uttarakhand** 0-9716462459

Printed at International Print-O-Pac Limited, Noida, UP, India

Preface

It gives me intense pleasure to introduce the first edition of the book entitled *258 Clinical Cases in Medicine* for postgraduate students in medicine (MRCP/MD/DNB) and allied sciences. Over the years, I have realized that the standard of postgraduation in medicine and allied sciences is deteriorating, the reasons are best known to the students and teachers. Postgraduate training in medical colleges is not so much updated because of lack of teachers, privatization of medical education and mushrooming of medical colleges in private sector. The students of medicine do not find much clinical material to learn. The students can read theory of medicine by sitting at residence/hostel but cannot expose themselves to the clinical material which is becoming scanty.

Being an examiner in postgraduate examination, I have found that students lack clinical orientation to medicine. They find difficulty in interpreting clinical signs and their significance. They find difficulty in making differential diagnosis and final diagnosis. The examiner has to struggle hard to get the diagnosis from the students by asking so many questions which not only embarrass the students but also the examiner.

I have picked up courage to discuss 258 cases in medicine for postgraduates. These cases are clinically discussed to make the students oriented to clinical examination and diagnosis. At the end of each case, questions have been answered for making the students updated on the case dicussed. Though these questions may not be sufficient but make the students confident to face any eventuality. To best of my knowledge, there is scarcity of such types of books. Such books on clinical material have now become the need of the hour. Many books written by the foreign authors are not understandable to the Indian students, hence, this book is introduced.

I hereby stress that this book in my opinion will cater to the needs of postgraduates in medicine and allied sciences (pulmonology and dermatology) and make them prepared for postgraduate examination. I have already shown this book to many teachers who have appreciated that each case is discussed with photograph of the patient or an illustration. The important investigations, i.e. radiology/CT scan/MRI, have also been displayed.

At the end, I must say that the book is written single handedly, therefore, any mistake could be inadvertent, hence, I may be excused for that. Suggestion /discussion on any topic will be accepted with thanks.

SN Chugh

Contents

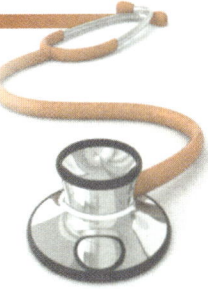

1

Jaundice

INSTRUCTION

Examine the abdomen. Patient has jaundice

SALIENT FEATURES

- Pain abdomen, yellowness of eyes and loss of appetite

HISTORY

Ask for the following:

A complete medical history is perhaps the most important part of evaluation. Ask for the following:
- Duration of jaundice
- *Sore throat* and *rash* (infectious mononucleosis)
- *Occupation:* Weil's disease is common in sewerage workers and farmers
- *Abdominal pain* (cholecystitis, gall-stones, cholangitis, carcinoma of pancreas)
- *Pruritus* (cholestatic hepatitis, primary biliary cirrhosis)
- Triad of *fever*, *rigors* and *upper abdominal pain* (cholangitis)
- Any change in *appetite, taste, weight* and *bowel habits* (hepatitis)
- Any history of *blood transfusions*, IV injections, tattooing, unprotected sexual activity (Hepatitis B)
- Recent travel history
- *Exposure to people with jaundice* either in the family, or locality or outside (hepatitis)
- *Exposure* to possibly *contaminated food*
- *Occupational exposure* to hepatotoxin or chemicals
- Detailed drug history (especially oral contraceptive and phenothiazines), ATT, i.e. taken in the past or are being taken. History of taking herbal or indigenous medicine
- History of alcohol intake
- History of *pregnancy* (pregnancy induced or pregnancy associated jaundice)
- History of *epistaxis*, *hematemesis* or *bleeding tendency* (Bleeding occurs due to vitamin. K dependent coagulation defect in liver disease)
- Family history for congenital hyperbilirubinemia, i.e. Gilbert's, Crigler-Najjar, Dubin-Johnson and Rotor syndromes
- Presence of any accompanying symptoms such as arthralgias, myalgias, weight loss, fever, pain in abdomen, pruritus and change in color of stool or urine (achlouric stools indicate obstructive jaundice)

EXAMINATION

General Physical Examination

- Jaundice (Fig. 1.1)
- Look for stigmatas of chronic liver disease. These are commonly seen in alcoholic cirrhosis;
  - Spider nevi
  - Palmar erythema
  - Gynecomastia
  - Caput medusae
  - Dupuytren's contracture
  - Parotid glands enlargement
  - Testicular atrophy, axillary and pubic hair loss

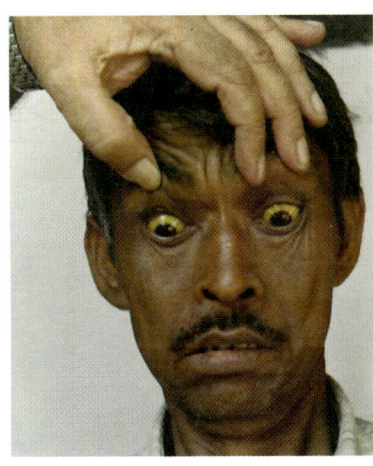

Fig. 1.1: Patient with jaundice

- Look for enlarged lymph nodes
  - An enlarged left supraclavicular node (Virchow's node) or periumbilical nodule (*Sister Mary Joseph's nodule*) suggests an abdominal malignancy
- Look at JVP and other signs of right heart failure
- Look for *pulse rate* (bradycardia in obstructive jaundice), *anemia* and *scratch marks, xanthelasma/xanthomatosis* (occur due to hypercholesterolemia in obstructive jaundice)

Systemic Examination

Abdominal examination for:

- *Hepatomegaly*, e.g. note size, shape, surface, movement with respiration, consistency and whether pulsatile or not. Elicit tenderness
- *Splenomegaly*. Define its characteristic
- *Ascites*. Elicit all the signs for detection of fluid
- Prominent *venous collaterals* or veins must be looked for to determine the flow of blood
- Look at the hernial sites
- Look for scratch marks

Other Systems

- *Cardiovascular*, i.e. valvular heart disease, pericardial effusion
- *Respiratory System for:* Pleural effusion especially right sided
- *Examination of excreta*, e.g.
  - Urine
  - Stool

PROVISIONAL DIAGNOSIS

Patient has acute onset of jaundice with fever and tender hepatomegaly; the provisional diagnosis is hepatitis (lesion) of viral etiology.

QUESTIONS AND ANSWERS

Q. Enumerate the points in favor of your diagnosis?

Ans:
- Febrile onset with GI symptoms and distaste for food
- Jaundice
- Tender moderate hepatomegaly
- Dark colored urine and stool

Q. How do you define jaundice? Where will you look for jaundice?

Ans: Jaundice or icterus refers to yellow discoloration of sclera, conjunctiva, mucous membrane of the tongue and skin due to raised serum bilirubin. Normal serum bilirubin is 0.3 to 1.5 mg%. Scleral staining or jaundice becomes clinically evident when serum bilirubin is at least 3.0 mg/dl. Raised bilirubin in between 1.5 and 3 mg/dl indicates subclinical jaundice.

Sites to be seen for jaundice

Jaundice should be seen in sclera in broad day light (Fig. 1.1) because icterus is difficult to examine in the presence of tube light or fluorescent light because of yellow reflection. The sclera provides white background.

It can be seen underneath the tongue also.

Q. What is differential diagnosis in your case?

Ans: A large number of conditions that produce fever, jaundice and tender hepatomegaly come into differential diagnosis of viral hepatitis such as;

1. *Infectious mononucleosis:* Fever, lymphadenopathy, jaundice and hepatomegaly constitute clinical hallmark. Peripheral blood film will show atypical lymphocytosis. Serology *Paul-Bunnel test* helps in the diagnosis.
2. *Nonviral hepatitis* such as toxoplasmosis and nocardiosis can produce similar picture. Serology can differentiate the non-viral conditions from viral hepatitis.
3. *Autoimmune hepatitis*
4. *Alcoholic and drug induced hepatitis*
5. *Amebic liver abscess.* Acute amebic liver abscess produces, fever, large tender hepatomegaly. Jaundice can occur occasionally. There may or may not be past history of dysentery. USG is diagnostic which reveals an abscess.
6. *Congestive hepatomegaly.* Signs of right ventricular failure, e.g. raised JVP, cyanosis, edema feet and signs of pulmonary hypertension (loud P2, narrow split of S2 and Graham-Steell murmur) separate congestive hepatomegaly from viral hepatitis.
7. *Budd-Chiari syndrome* (occlusion of hepatic vein or inferior vena cava) and *veno-occlusive disease* (involvement of small hepatic veins and venules due to consumption of bush tea) also produce massive hepatomegaly and jaundice, but presence of ascites and signs of portal hypertension differentiate them from viral hepatitis. The absence of signs of congestive heart failure differentiates it from congestive hepatomegaly.
8. *Malignancy liver*
9. *In pregnant women, acute fatty liver of pregnancy*, cholestasis of pregnancy and eclampsia constitute differential diagnosis of viral hepatitis.

Q. To which group of viral hepatitis your case belongs?

Ans: Hepatitis A (short incubation, epidemic form of hepatitis)

Q. How would you confirm the diagnosis?

Ans: The diagnosis of hepatitis A is confirmed during an acute illness by demonstrating anti-HAV of IgM class. After acute illness, anti-HAV of IgG class remains detectable indefinitely indicating past or previous infections.

Q. What is the prophylaxis of hepatitis A?

Ans: Both passive immunization with IG (Immunoglobulin) and active immunization with vaccines are available.

Q. What are the indications of hepatitis A prophylaxis?

Ans: I. *Passive immunization with IG (immunoglobulins)* is indicated in
   i. Pre-exposure prophylaxis or early incubation period prophylaxis.
   ii. For post-exposure hepatitis of intimate contact (household, sexual, institutional).
   Dose is 0.02 ml/kg intramuscular
   II. *Active immunization by vaccine*
   • It is indicated for pre-exposure prophylaxis for travelers to tropical countries, developing countries or other areas
   III. *Both passive and active immunization.* Passive immunization with IG at different site and active immunization with vaccine at another site are indicated during imminent travel or immediate travel
   Two doses of vaccine are given at 0 month and at 6 and 12 months.

Q. What are the other causes of yellow discoloration of tissue? How carotenoderma differs from jaundice?

Ans: Besides jaundice, other causes are:
   • Carotenoderma (hypercarotenemia) due to excessive consumption of fruits and vegetables rich in carotene (e.g. carrots, oranges, squash, peaches)
   • Use of antimalarial drug, e.g. mepacrine, quinacrine. They are not used nowadays.
   • Excessive exposure to phenols.
   Carotenoderma can be distinguished from jaundice by sparing of the sclera and normal colored urine while it stains all other tissues. On the other hand, quinacrine stains the sclera and produces yellow discoloration of urine.

Q. How do you classify jaundice:

Ans: Jaundice is classified in different ways:

1. *Based on coloration of sclera (clinical criteria)*
   • *Medical jaundice* (yellow coloration)
   • *Surgical jaundice* (greenish yellow coloration).
2. *Based on the etiology*
   • *Hemolytic or prehepatic* (excessive destruction of RBCs)
   • *Hepatic* (cause lies inside the liver)
   • *Obstructive or posthepatic* (cause lies outside the liver in extrahepatic biliary system)
3. *Based on chemical nature of bilirubin*
   • *Unconjugated hyperbilirubinemia*
   • *Conjugated hyperbilirubinemia* (conjugated bilirubin is >50% of total bilirubin. The normal conjugated bilirubin is just 15–20%)

Q. What are the common causes of jaundice?

Ans: The common causes depending on the type are as follows:
   I. **Hemolytic jaundice (predominantly unconjugated hyperbilirubinemia)**
   • Hemolytic jaundice due to intracorpuscular/extracorpuscular hemolysis, infections (malaria), drug induced hemolysis in G6PD deficiency, Immune hemolysis and paroxysmal nocturnal hemoglobinuria
   • Congenital jaundice, e.g. Gilbert's syndrome, Crigler-Najjar type I syndrome
   • Hepatitis (viral, drug induced)
   II. **Hepatocellular jaundice (mixed type)**
   • Hepatitis
   • Postoperative
   • Intrahepatic cholestasis
   • Drugs and alcohol
   III. **Obstructive jaundice (conjugated hyperbilirubinemia)**
   • Congenital, e.g. Dubin-Johnson and rotor syndrome
   • Primary biliary cirrhosis
   • Bile duct stone, stricture, cholangitis, worm (round worm),
   • Trauma to bile duct
   • Bile duct obstruction due to tumor (bile duct, pancreas, duodenum)
   • Secondaries in liver or at porta-hepatitis
   • Pancreatitis
   • Choledochal cyst

Q. What are the characteristic features of hemolytic jaundice?

Ans: These are as follows:
   • Anemia with mild jaundice

- Freshly voided urine is not yellow, becomes yellow on standing due to conversion of excessive urobilinogen in the urine to urobilin on oxidation
- Preceding history of fever (malaria, viral), or intake of drugs if patient is G6PD deficient or intake of heavy metals.
- Typical facies, e.g. chipmunk facies seen in thalassemia due to excessive marrow expansion leading to frontal bossing and maxillary marrow hyperplasia
- Mild hepatosplenomegaly. The liver is nontender
- No pruritus or itching. No xanthelasma/ xanthomatosis
- Peripheral blood film examination and other tests for hemolysis will confirm the diagnosis

Q. **Name the familial/congenital causes of jaundice.**
Ans:
- *Gilbert's syndrome* (predominantly unconjugated hyperbilirubinemia)
- Crigler-Najjar syndrome (type I, complete absence of glucuronyl transferase, type II, partial deficiency of enzyme)
- *Dubin-Johnson syndrome* (decreased excretion of bilirubin)
- *Rotor syndrome.* Excretory defect of bilirubin with pigmentation of liver

Q. **What are the clinical characteristics of obstructive jaundice?**
Ans: The clinical characteristics are:
- Deep yellow or greenish yellow jaundice called *surgical jaundice*
- Pruritus or itching present due to retention of bile salts
- Urine is dark colored due to excretion of bile pigments, but stools are clay-colored (acholic)
- There may be associated pain abdomen, severe, colicky with intermittent jaundice, if bile duct stone is the cause
- Gallbladder is palpable if bile duct is obstructed either by an impacted stone or by carcinoma of head of pancreas. A palpable gallbladder in obstructive jaundice is unlikely due to chronic cholecystitis (Courvosier's law)
- Slowing of pulse rate or bradycardia may occur due to retention of bile salts
- In long-standing obstructive jaundice, xanthoma, weight loss, malabsorption or steatorrhea may occur
- Conjugated hyperbilirubinemia with dilatation of intrahepatic or extrahepatic ducts on USG confirm the diagnosis

Q. **What is Charcot's fever?**
- Fever, shaking chills and rigors with jaundice indicating cholangitis and biliary obstruction is called Charcot's fever.

Q. **Name the few causes of postoperative jaundice.**
Ans:
- Hemolysis and reabsorption of hematoma or hemoperitoneum or blood transfusions
- Impaired liver functions due to sepsis, anesthesia, shock
- Extrahepatic biliary obstruction due to biliary stones or unsuspected injury to biliary tree

Q. **What is Gilbert's syndrome?**
Ans: It is a syndrome of congenital unconjugated hyperbilirubinemia due to impaired conjugation of bilirubin due to congenital deficiency or reduced activity of the enzyme glucuronyl transferase in the liver.

Q. **What is Dubin-Johnson syndrome?**
Ans: It is a familial conjugated hyperbilirubinemia in which there is excretory defect of bilirubin excretion and there is pigmentation of liver due to melanin (rotor syndrome) detected on liver biopsy. It is detected by delayed bromosulphthalein excretion test.

Q. **What are the causes of prolonged jaundice (i.e. duration > 6 months)?**
Ans: Read this question in autoimmune hepatitis.

Q. **How would you investigate this patient?**
Ans: 1. Urine examination for urobilinogen, bile salts and bile pigments
2. Complete hemogram and WBC count
3. Liver function tests, e.g. serum bilirubin, serum albumin and liver enzymes
4. Prothrombin time and index
5. Viral serology, i.e. hepatitis antigen and antibodies, EBV antibodies
6. Special investigations
   - Mitochondrial antibodies (AMA)
   - ERCP (endoscopic retrograde cholangiopancreatography)
   - Liver biopsy

Q. **What level of bilirubin do you expect in hemolytic jaundice?**
Ans: Hemolytic jaundice is mild jaundice with serum bilirubin usually < 5 mg% but, does not exceed 10 mg%.

Q. **Which type of jaundice produces highest level of bilirubin?**
Ans: Jaundice produced by cholestasis, i.e. both intrahepatic and extrahepatic obstruction.

Ascites

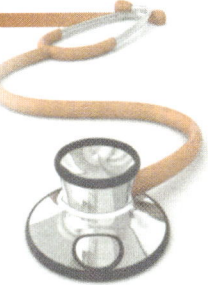

INSTRUCTION

Examine the patient who has distended abdomen

SALIENT FEATURES

- Distension of abdomen

HISTORY

Ask for the following:

- Abdominal distension, e.g. onset, progression
- History of abdominal pain, fever (nephrotic syndrome)
- History of puffiness of face, edema
- History of heart disease, e.g. valvular, ischemic, cardiomyopathies, hypertension (heart failure)
- History of alcoholism (alcoholic cirrhosis)
- Present and past history of jaundice, hematemesis, malena (portal hypertension)
- History of prolonged cough, fever, hemoptysis, night sweats, anorexia and weight loss
- History of rapid loss of appetite and weight and cachexia of malignancy.
- History of prolonged diarrhea >3 months (malabsorption) with weight loss and alteration in bowel habits (malignancy colon)

EXAMINATION

General Physical Examination

- Look for signs of malnutrition and vitamins deficiency
- Anemia and edema feet (present in this case)
- Look for signs of CHF, nephrotic syndrome, cirrhosis of the liver or malignancy
- Look for sacral and abdominal wall edema
- Look for stigmata of alcoholism and signs of hepatic insufficiency, i.e. hepatic encephalopathy.

Abdominal Examination

- The abdomen is distended. The flanks are full
- Umbilicus is bulging look for umbilical hernia
- Look for prominent veins over the abdomen. Determine the flow of blood in the veins.
- Fluid thrill and shifting dullness is present

(read clinical methods in medicine for elicitation of fluid thrill and shifting dullness (Fig. 2.1).
- Feel the liver and spleen by dipping method (Fluid displacement method)
- Auscultate the abdomen for bruit, venous hum or hepatic rub.

PROVISIONAL DIAGNOSIS

The patient has moderate ascites (lesion) probably due to tubercular peritonitis as its cause (etiology).

QUESTIONS AND ANSWERS

Q. **Enumerate the points in favor of diagnosis**
Ans: The points in favor are:
- A middle aged female with slow onset of ascites

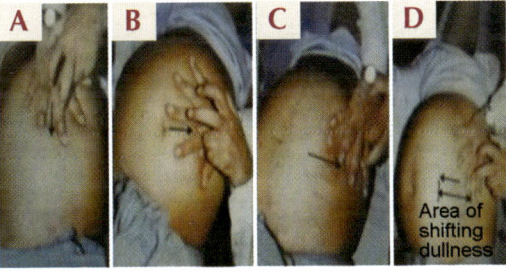

Fig. 2.1: Elicitation of shifting dullness. Start percussing from resonant; (A) area towards dull area; (B) till you reach a dull area; (C) Now while keeping the finger over dull area ask the patient to turn to the other side, now the area which was dull earlier on percussion becomes resonant due to shift of fluid, hence, shifting dullness is present; (D) To further define the area of shifting dullness now start percussion again from this newly found resonant area toward umbilicus to know where the dullness has shifted. Mark the line of demarcation at the start of dull area now. The length of the space between the previous resonant area in D and newly found dull area on change of position indicates the area of shifting dullness, i.e. the space over which fluid has shifted (indicated between arrows by dotted line ⟷ in Fig. 2.1D)

- Distended abdomen with full flank and transverse slit (smiling) umbilicus
- Presence of both fluid thrill and shifting dullness. Edema feet is present
- Flanks are dull with central sparing
- Intestinal sounds are heard in the center of abdomen
- No signs of portal hypertension or liver cell failure

Q. How do you define ascites?

Ans: Normal amount of fluid in the peritoneal cavity is about 50–150 ml of lymph, not detected by any means. Abnormal collection of fluid (>300 ml) in the peritoneum is called *ascites*. This amount is detected on USG abdomen. Significant amount of fluid (>500 ml) produces fullness of flanks on lying down position, is detected clinically. Larger amount of fluid (e.g. 1 liter) produces horse-shoe shape of the abdomen. Tense ascites means the peritoneal cavity is filled with free fluid producing cardiorespiratory embarrassment.

Q. What are the causes of distended abdomen?

Ans: Five "F" denotes distension such as Fat, Fluid, Flatus, Feces and Fetus.

Q. What are the causes of ascites?

Ans: **I. Local Causes (exudative ascites)**
- Tuberculosis
- Malignancy with secondaries in peritoneum, leukemias, lymphoma
- Bacterial peritonitis
- Pancreatitis
- Portal vein thrombosis
- Hepatic vein thrombosis (Budd-Chiari syndrome)
- Chylous ascites

II. Systemic Causes (transudative ascites)
- Nephrotic syndrome
- Cirrhosis of the liver
- Hypoproteinemia, nutritional or following chronic diarrhea or malabsorption
- Congestive heart failure
- Constrictive pericarditis
- Meig's syndrome

Q. What are the differences between transduative and exudative ascites?

Ans: Read Table 2.1.

Q. What are the causes of transudative ascites?

Ans: *Causes are:* Same as systemic causes.

Q. What are the causes of exudative ascites:

Ans: *Causes are:* Same as discussed above as local causes.

Q. What is differential diagnosis of ascites?

Ans: The differential diagnosis of ascites depends on the cause of ascites and whether ascites is a part of generalised *anasarca* (ascites, edema, fluid in serous cavities) or is localized.

The conditions that come into differential diagnosis are:

1. *Ascites of nephrotic syndrome:* There is associated puffiness of face and pitting massive edema of feet.
2. *Ascites due to cirrhosis of the liver with signs of portal hypertension,* e.g caput-medusae splenomegaly, and fetor hepaticus
3. *Ascites due to hypoproteinemia:* There will be signs of anemia and multiple vitamin deficiency.
4. *Ascitic of congestive heart failure:* There will be raised JVP, tender hepatomegaly, edema feet, etc.
5. *Constrictive pericarditis* (Raised JVP, tender hepatomegaly, massive ascites with feeble heart sounds).
6. *Tubercular ascites:* A slow developing ascites with anorexia, low grade fever, common occurrence in females and night sweats.
7. *Malignant ascites:* Acute onset and rapid filling tense ascites in old age with decrease or loss of appetite, marked cachexia.

Q. What is pancreatic ascites?

Ans: *Pancreatic ascites* is due to collection of a large amount of pancreatic secretions either due to disruption of pancreatic duct or pseudocyst formation. It is painless, mild to moderate collection seen in patients with chronic

Table 2.1: Transudative vs exudative ascites	
Transudate (serum ascitic fluid albumin gradient > 1.1 g/dL)	*Exudate (serum/ascitic fluid albumin gradient < 1.1 g/dL)*
• Non-inflammatory fluid, serous or straw colored	• Inflammatory thick, turbid or mucinous, hemorrhage or straw colored fluid
• Fluid protein content <3.0 g/dl (or <50% of serum proteins)	• Protein content >3.0 g/dl (>50% of serum protein)
• Specific gravity low or normal	• Specific gravity is high
• Occasional cell, mostly mesothelial	• Cell count (100–1000 cells/mm^3), mostly either mononuclear or neutrophils

pancreatitis. The ascitic fluid is exudate with low SAAG (<1.1) and high fluid amylase levels (>1, 000 unit/L).

Q. What is chylous ascites? What are its causes?

Ans: Chylous ascites is milky fluid with triglyceride content >100 mg/dl. Turbidity of fluid disappears after extraction with ether.

The causes are:

1. Trauma or penetrating abdominal injury to the thoracic duct
2. Tumors (malignant tumors of lymph nodes or tumors infiltrating the lymphatics)
3. Tuberculosis with lymphadenitis
4. Filariasis (filarial worms obstructing the lymphatics)

Q. What is pseudochylous and chyliform ascites?

Ans: *Pseudochylous ascites* refers to increased amount of proteins and calcium in the fluid leading to turbidity which is not dissolved by ether.

Chyliform ascites means a large number of cells (leukocytes, degenerated epithelial cells or tumor cells) as the cause of turbidity which disappears on extraction with alkali.

Q. What would be the nature of ascites when both fluid thrill and shifting dullness are absent?

Ans: Mucinous ascites.

Q. What is mucinous ascites?

Ans: Rarely, ascitic fluid may be mucinous (gelatinous) in character, giving lobulated (jelly like mass) appearance on palpation of abdomen. The fluid thrill and shifting dullness are absent. It is difficult to aspirate (ascitic tap is dry) the fluid. It may be either due to *pseudomyxoma peritonei* (rupture of mucocele of appendix or mucinous ovarian cyst) or rarely colloid carcinoma of stomach or colon with peritoneal metastases.

Q. What is serum ascitic albumin gradient (SAAG)?

Ans: It is calculated by subtracting the ascitic fluid albumin concentration from serum albumin concentration from samples obtained at the same time. This gradient differentiates transudative from exudative ascites and also correlates directly with portal pressure, i.e. those with gradient >1.1 g/dl have portal hypertension and those with gradient <1.1 g/dl do not. The accuracy of such determination is 97%.

Q. What is refractory ascites?

Ans: Ascites is said to be refractory if it persists in spite of the maximum dose of diuretics (400–600 mg of spironolactone and 120–160 mg of furosemide) and salt restriction. The causes are;

i. Noncompliance of salt restriction
ii. Hepatorenal syndrome
iii. Low serum sodium or failure of diuretic therapy
iv. Infections or subacute bacteria peritonitis
v. Superimposition of hepatoma
vi. GI bleeding
vii. Development of hepatic or portal vein thrombosis

Q. What is genesis of ascites in cirrhosis?

Ans: 1. Increased hydrostatic pressure due to splanchnic vascular dilatation and increased portal venous flow.
2. Sodium retention due to hyperaldosteronism as a result of activation of renin angiotensin aldosterone system.
3. Decreased oncotic pressure due to hypoalbuminemia.
4. Increased formation of lymph due to

Table 2.2: Ascites vs ovarian cyst	
Ascites	*Ovarian cyst*
• Generalized distention to xiphisternum	Localized distention
• Flanks full	Central or iliac fossa swelling
• Umbilicus is transurgery slit or everted	Vertically slit or everted umbilicus
• Umbilicus to symphysis pubis distance is more than xiphisternum to umbilicus	The distances from umbilicus to pubis is smaller than umbilicus
• Swelling does not have well defined demarcation	Swelling is rounded with well defined upper border, i.e. you can reach above the swelling
• Horse-shoe shape dullness on percussion (flanks dull, center spares)	"Dullness is limited to midline or in one or two quadrants (quardrantic dullness)
• Shifting dullness present and characteristic	Shifting dullness absent
• Vaginal examination is negative	Vaginal examination is diagnosis
• USG is diagnostic, detects free fluid and its cause	USG detects localized fluid and confirms the ovarian cyst

vascular dilatation and increased portal venous blood flow.

5. Stimulation of antidiuretic hormone due to hypoperfusion of kidneys.

Q. What are the physical signs of ascites?

Ans: Read "Clinical Methods in Medicine" by Dr. SN Chugh.

Q. What does presence of fluid thrill in the absence of shifting dullness indicate?

Ans: Fluid thrill is present while shifting dullness is absent in following situations in the abdomen:

1. Mild ascites (< 500 ml of fluid)
2. Huge or massive ascites where there is no space for fluid to get shifted
3. Localized ascites
4. Ovarian cyst
5. Distended bladder

Q. How would you differentiate ascites from ovarian cyst?

Ans: Read Table 2.2.

Q. What are the physical signs of mild, moderate and massive ascites?

Ans: The signs are given in Table 2.3.

Table 2.3: Physical signs in various grades of ascites

	Grade	Signs
0	Minimal	Puddle's sign
1	Mild	Shifting dullness present, fluid thrill absent
2	Moderate	Shifting dullness and fluid thrill both present
3	Massive	Fluid thrill present, shifting dullness absent

Q. What are signs of localised ascites?

Ans: Localised ascites will behave like massive ascites, hence, in this also fluid thrill will be present and shifting dullness absent.

Q. What are the causes of rapid filling of ascites?

Ans: • Malignancy (primary and secondary)
• Tuberculosis
• Chylous
• Spontaneous bacterial peritonitis
• Budd-Chiari syndrome

Q. What are the causes of purulent and hemorrhagic ascites?

Ans: They are depicted in Table 2.4.

Q. What are the causes of ascites disproportionate to edema feet (ascites praecox)?

Ans: These are as follows
• Constrictive pericarditis
• Restrictive cardiomyopathy
• Hepatic vein thrombosis
• Cirrhosis of liver

Table 2.4: Purulent vs hemorrhagic ascites

Purulent ascites	Hemorrhagic ascites
• Pyogenic peritonitis	• Abdominal trauma or trauma during tapping of ascites
• Septicemia	• Malignancy of peritoneum (primary or secondary)
• Ruptured amebic liver abscess	• Tubercular peritonitis
• Pelvic inflammatory disease	• Bleeding diathesis
• Penetrating abdominal trauma with introduction of infection	• Acute hemorrhagic pancreatitis

• Tubercular peritonitis
• Intra-abdominal malignancy

Q. How will you investigate a patient with ascites?

Ans: Investigations are done to confirm the diagnosis and to find out its cause. These include:

1. *Blood examination:* Anemia may be present. Presence of neutrophilic leukocytosis indicates infection.
2. *Urine examination:* Massive albuminuria (>3.5 g/day) indicates in nephrotic syndrome. Small amount of proteinuria occurs in pericardial effusion and congestive heart failure.
3. *Stool for occult blood:* If present, may indicate gastrointestinal malignancy.
4. *Ultrasonography:* It is of proven value in detecting ascites, presence of a mass, evaluation of size of liver and spleen, portal vein diameter and presence of collaterals and enlargement of caudate lobe.
5. *Diagnostic paracentesis:* 50–100 ml of ascitic fluid is withdrawn with the help of a needle and biochemically analysed to establish the nature (transudative or exudative), etiology of ascites and to plan its treatment. It is also sent for bacteriological examination.
6. *Serum-ascites albumin gradient:* The gradient >1.1 g/dl indicates transudative ascites and <1.1 g/dl indicates exudative ascites. The fluid protein < 50% of serum protein also indicates transudate; while >50% indicates exudate.
7. *Further investigations:* They are done to find out the cause, e.g. serum proteins, serum cholesterol for nephrotic syndrome, X-ray chest, ECG, echo for congestive heart failure/pericardial effusion, liver function tests and tests for portal hypertension.

Q. What does paracentesis mean? What are its indications?

Ans: Paracentesis means removal of fluid. The indications are:

i. *Diagnostic:* A diagnostic tap of ascitic fluid is done, by putting the needle in the flank in one of the lateral positions. The fluid removed is 50–100 ml for diagnostic purpose, i.e. for biochemical, cytological and bacteriological analysis.

ii. *Therapeutic:* It is done as a part of treatment. Ascitic fluid is rich in proteins, hence should not be routinely tapped. It is removed if patient has cardiorespiratory embarrassment (acute respiratory distress with tachycardia). The amount of fluid removed depends on the relief of symptoms or maximum of 3–5 liters of fluid may be removed in one setting. Repeated tapping should be avoided unless absolutely necessary as this may predispose to secondary infection of peritoneum and also causes protein loss.

iii. *Refractory ascites* (nonresponse to treatment).

iv. *Paracentesis* is attempted before *needle biopsy* of liver, *ultrasonography* and for *better palpation* of *underlying viscera.*

Q. How does ultrasound help in cirrhotic ascites?

Ans: i. To detect presence of ascites (free or loculated) and splenomegaly

ii. To detect portal vein thrombosis or formation of collaterals

iii. To measure the portal vein diameter

iv. To determine the condition of liver and its echotexture

Q. How does ultrasound help in the diagnosis of tubercular ascites?

Ans: It may reveal:

• Enlargement of mesenteric, pre-aortic and para-aortic lymph nodes

• Thick fibrous septa may be seen traversing ascites (septate ascites)

• Thickened mesentery or rolled up omentum

• Tuberculosis of the liver, spleen, etc.

Q. What are the complications of paracentesis?

Ans: Common complications of paracentesis are as follows:

• Sudden withdrawal of a large amount of fluid may lead to dilatation of splanchnic blood vessels with subsequent *development of shock*

• *Introduction of infection (peritonitis)* if sterile precautions are not observed.

• *Hypoproteinemia.* Ascitic fluid is rich in protein, repeated large amount of aspiration may lead to development of hypoproteinemia.

• *Precipitation of hepatic coma.* Sudden withdrawal of ascites in a patient with cirrhotic portal hypertension, any precipitate hepatic encephalopathy.

• *Constant oozing of the ascites* due to the formation of a track (especially in tense ascites).

Q. What are the sequela/complications of ascites?

Ans: These are as follows:

• *Cardiorespiratory embarrassment*

• *Right sided pleural effusion* due to leakage of ascitic fluid through lymphatic channels in the diaphragm

• *Spontaneous bacterial peritonitis*

• *Abdominal hernia* (umbilical, inguinal) and *divertication of recti* due to tense ascites as a result of increased intraabdominal pressure

• *Functional renal failure*

• *Mesenteric venous thrombosis.*

Q. How would you manage a case with ascites?

Ans: 1. Rest in bed

2. *Dietary salt restriction.* In severe ascites, sodium should be strictly restricted to less than 10 meq/l

3. *Diuretics:* A combination of fursemide/torsemide with spironolactone is better than either alone.

4. Fluid restriction in severe ascites

5. *Paracentesis:* It should be done for therapeutic purpose when there is an evidence of cardiorespiratory embarrassment. Repeated tapping should be avoided as far as possible.

6. *Salt free albumin* infusion

7. Treatment of the underlying cause, i.e. ATT for tuberculosis, appropriate treatment of CHF, nephrotic syndrome, pericardial effusion.

8. If cirrhotic portal hypertension is the cause then peritoneocavernous shunting or TIPS may be employed (Read the case discussion on cirrhotic portal hypertension and ascites)

Q. What is the treatment of refractory ascites?

Ans: 1. Dietary sodium restriction plus diuretic.

2. Large volume paracentesis plus albumin.

3. Transjugular intrahepatic portosystemic shunt.

4. Liver transplantation

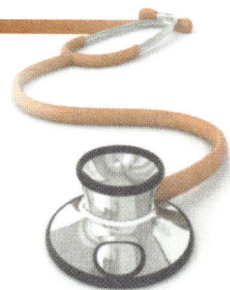

3

Hepatomegaly
(Liver Abscess)

INSTRUCTION

Examine the abdomen of this patient

SALIENT FEATURES
- Mass abdomen

HISTORY

Ask for the following:
- No symptoms (asymptomatic), hepatomegaly is detected during routine examination.
- Pain in right upper quadrant.
- Mass in right hypochondrium.
- Present history of dysentery or GI disorder
- Any history of bleeding from any site.
- History of fever, pigmentation, neck swelling, jaundice, anorexia, weight loss.
- Full drug history.
- Past history of tuberculosis, jaundice, diabetes, RHD (congestive heart failure).
- Personal history, e.g. alcoholism
- Nutritional history
- Family history of polycystic disease.

EXAMINATION

General Physical Examination
- Assess the nutritional status.
- Examine neck for lymph nodes, JVP.
- Look at the skin for purpuric spots, ecchymosis, bruises, pigmentation.
- Note anemia, cyanosis, jaundice, palmar erythema, spider angiomata (hematological cause of hepatomegaly).
- Look for stigmatas of chronic liver disease and hepatic flap (hepatomegaly with chronic liver disease)
- Note pedal edema.
- Examine vitals, e.g. respiration, pulse, temperature and BP.

Abdominal Examination
Inspection
- A right upper quadrantic fullness due to mass

(Fig. 3.1) that moves with respiration (present in this case).
- Umbilicus is normal unless ascites present.
- Normal abdominal movements (present).
- Hernia sites are usually normal.
- Prominent abdominal veins and collateral with flow away from umbilicus suggest portal hypertension (no distended veins in this case).

Palpation
- Define the mass and study its characteristics, e.g. *solid* or *cystic*, *smooth* or *irregular*, *soft*, *firm* or *hard*, *tender* or *nontender*, etc. Note whether it is *pulsatile* or not.
- Elicit intercostal tenderness (*thumbing sign*). It was positive in this case.
- Elicit the signs of ascites if suspected (no ascites in this case).
- Palpate the abdomen for other mass or masses such as spleen or lymph nodes.

Percussion
- Define upper and lower borders of the liver and calculate the liver span. It was 22 cm in this case.
- Hydatid sign if hydatid cyst is suspected.
- Percuss flanks for ascites.

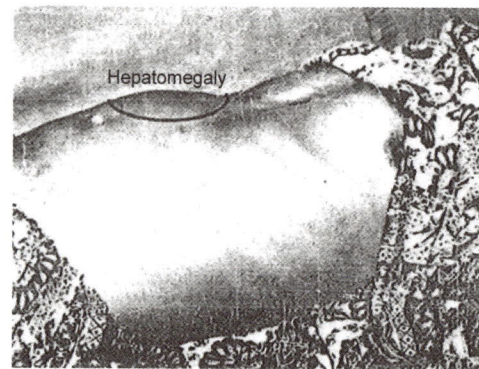

Fig. 3.1: A patient with hepatomegaly due to amebic liver abscess

Auscultation
- A bruit indicates a vascular hepatic tumor or hemangioma
- A rub indicates hepatic infarction or a nodular liver
- A venous hum around umbilicus indicates portal hypertension
- Auscultate for bowel sounds

Other System
- *Cardiovascular system* for heart failure
- *CNS examination* for alcoholism

PROVISIONAL DIAGNOSIS

The presence of fever, tender hepatomegaly of acute onset (lesion) suggest the probable diagnosis of amoebic liver abscess (etiology). Patient has acute pain (functional status).

QUESTIONS AND ANSWERS

Q. **What are the points in favor of your diagnosis?**

Ans: 1. Swinging temperature and chills
2. Positive intercostal tenderness (*positive thumping sign*)
3. Massive (> 8 cm) tender hepatomegaly without jaundice or signs of portal hypertension.
4. Past history of dysentery.

Q. **How do you define hepatomegaly?**

Ans. Liver is placed just below the right dome of diaphragm and its edge is normally palpable on deep inspiration in right hypochondrium in some people and in children. The palpable liver does not mean hepatomegaly because if liver is displaced downwards due to any cause (emphysema, subphrenic abscess) it becomes palpable. Therefore, before commenting on hepatomegaly, the upper border must be defined by percussion in midclavicular line. Upper border of liver dullness is in 5th intercostal space normally.

Hepatomegaly refers to actual enlargement of liver (enlarged liver span) without being displaced downwards, i.e. the upper border of liver dullness stays as normal.

N.B Always tell liver span in case of hepatomegaly instead of commenting palpable liver by so many centimeters.

Q. **What do you understand by the term liver span? What is its significance?**

Ans: The liver span is the vertical distance between the upper and lower borders of the liver which is defined either clinically (on percussion) or on ultrasound. Normal liver span in an adult is variable (10–14 cm), greater in men than in women, greater in tall people than in short.

Significance
- Liver span is actually reduced when liver is small and shrunken (acute fulminant hepatitis) or masked when free air is present below the diaphragm as in a case with a perforated viscus (liver dullness is masked, hence, span appears to be reduced).
- Liver span is increased when liver is enlarged not when liver is displaced.
- Serial observations may show a decreasing span of dullness with resolution of hepatitis, CHF or less commonly with progression of fulminant hepatitis.
- It is used to define actual vs apparent enlargement of liver.
  - Actual or real enlargement means palpable liver with increase in liver span.
  - Apparent enlargement means liver is palpable without being actually enlarged (liver span is normal).

Q. **What are the common causes of hepatomegaly?**

Ans: The causes are:
1. Congestive heart failure/Constrictive pericarditis
2. Leukemias/lymphomas
3. Malaria/kala-azar
4. Fat storage disease (Gaucher's disease), Niemann-Pick's disease
5. Amebic liver abscess
6. Malignancy liver
7. Hemolytic anemia

Q. **List some less common causes of hepatomegaly.**

Ans: 1. Infections, e.g. typhoid fever, bacterial endocarditis, hepatitis (viral)
2. Hemochromatosis
3. Fatty liver, amyloidosis, sarcoidosis
4. Primary biliary cirrhosis
5. Hydatid cyst of the liver
6. Liver hemangioma

Q. **What are the causes of palpable liver without its actual enlargement?**

Ans: This denotes downward displacement of normal liver due to:
- Emphysema
- Thin and lean person
- Subphrenic abscess (right side)

- Visceroptosis (Liver descends down during standing due to weak support)
- Any mass or fluid interposed between liver and the diaphragm will push liver downwards, e.g. subpulmonic effusion. Massive right sided pleural effusion or pneumothorax.

Q.   What are the common causes of mild to moderate hepatomegaly?

Ans:
- Typhoid lever, tuberculosis
- Leukemias
- Congestive splenomegaly (e.g. CHF, pericardial effusion)
- Budd-Chiari syndrome
- Hemolytic anemia
- A hemangioma or congenital cyst
- Fatty liver
- Postnecrotic cirrhosis

Q.   What are the causes of tender hepatomegaly?

Ans: Causes are as below:
- Acute viral hepatitis
- Amebic liver abscess
- Congestive hepatomegaly (e.g. CHF, constrictive pericarditis, pericardial effusion, Budd-Chiari syndrome)
- Pyogenic liver abscess
- Malignancy of the liver
- Perihepatitis, e.g. after biopsy or hepatic infarct)

Q.   What are the causes of massive hepatomegaly?

Ans: Massive hepatomegaly means enlargement > 8 cm below the costal margin. The causes are:
1. Malignancy liver (primary or secondary)
2. Amebic liver abscess
3. Chronic malaria and kala-azar
4. Hepatitis (sometimes)
5. Hodgkin's disease
6. Polycystic liver disease

N.B Acute malaria does not produce hepatomegaly.

Q.   What are the causes of enlargement of left lobe?

Ans: Causes are as below:
- Amebic liver abscess (left lobe abscess)
- Hepatoma
- Metastases in liver.

Q.   What are the different consistencies of liver?

Ans: Table 3.1 explains the answer.

Table 3.1: Differential diagnosis of hepatomegaly depending on consistency of liver

Consistency	Causes
Soft	Congestive heart failure, viral hepatitis, fatty liver, SABE, visceroptosis (drooping of liver)
Firm	Cirrhosis, chronic malaria and kala-azar, hepatic amebiasis, lymphoma
Hard	Hepatocellular carcinoma, metastases in liver, chronic myeloid leukemia, myelofibrosis

Q.   What does the presence of abdominal venous hum indicate?

Ans: It is virtually diagnostic of cirrhotic portal hypertension. When present with hepatic arterial bruit in the same patient, then it suggests cirrhosis with either alcoholic hepatitis or malignancy liver.

Q.   What is Cruveilhier-Baumgarten syndrome?

Ans: It is the presence of abdominal venous hum in portal hypertension secondary to cirrhosis.

Q.   What does a presence of hepatic rub, bruit and venous hum indicate?

Ans.
i. The presence of hepatic rub with bruit indicates cancer of the liver.
ii. The presence of hepatic rub, bruit and venous hum indicates that a patient with cirrhosis has developed a hepatoma.

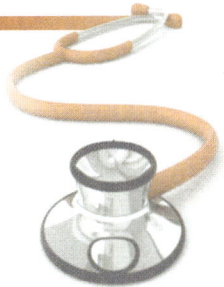

4

Cirrhotic Portal Hypertension

INSTRUCTION

Examine the abdomen of the patient

SALIENT FEATURES

- Hematemesis, distension of abdomen and oedema feet

HISTORY

Ask about the following:

- Progressive distension of abdomen, swelling of legs, hematemesis and malena (e.g. portal hypertension)
- Fatigue, weight loss, flatulent dyspepsia, anorexia, malnutrition, muscle wasting, drowsiness, disturbed sleep pattern (e.g. hepatic encephalopathy)
- History of fever, jaundice, bleeding from any site
- History of disturbance in consciousness, sleep or behavior problem
- Past history of alcoholism (patient is alcoholic), drug intake, jaundice, delivery (in female)
- Family history of jaundice or similar illness
- Nutritional history

EXAMINATION

General Physical Examination

- Look for cirrhotic facies, e.g. earthy look, sunken (hollow) cheeks and malar prominence—present in this case.
- Assess nutritional status—poor in this case.
- Look for stigmatas of cirrhosis (wasting of muscle, palmar erythema, spider angiomatas, testicular atrophy, gynecomastia, bilateral parotid enlargement and Dupuytren's contractures). Few stigmatas are present.
- Look for signs of hepatic insufficiency, i.e. mental features, jaundice, bleeding (purpura, ecchymosis and bruising), clubbing of fingers, flapping tremors.
- Look for signs of portal hypertension, e.g. ascites, collaterals formation, fetor hepaticus and splenomegaly. Ascites and splenomegaly are present in this case.
- Look for anemia, jaundice, Kayser-Feischer's rings.
- Look for signs of malnutrition and vitamins deficiency.
- Look for pedal pitting edema (present in this case)
- Look for signs of CHF or pericardial effusion, e.g. raised JVP, cyanosis, neck pulsations, etc.
- Note the vital signs, e.g. temperature, respiration, BP and pulse.

Abdominal Examination

Inspection

- Skin over the abdomen is thin, shiny due to edema of abdominal wall.
- Abdominal distension with increased abdominal girth—present in this case (Fig. 4.1).
- Prominent veins with flow of blood away from umbilicus (present in this case).
- Hernias (umbilical or inguinal) may or may not be present.
- Umbilicus may be everted or transversely slit (smiling umbilicus) due to ascites (umbilicus was transversely slit in the case).

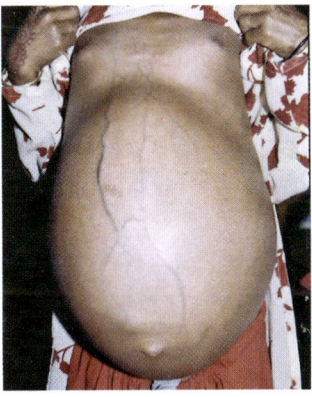

Fig. 4.1: Cirrhotic portal hypertension. Note umbilical hernia, distended veins and bilateral gynecomastia

Palpation
- Liver is palpable, nontender, firm with sharp and irregular margins. Left lobe is enlarged. In some cases, liver may not be palpable.
- Spleen is also palpable, nontender, soft to firm.
- Ascites is detected by fluid thrill.
- Flow of blood in dilated veins was away from umbilicus.

Note: Palpate the liver and spleen by dipping method in presence of ascites.

Percussion
- Shifting dullness is present in this case.
- Flanks are dull with central sparing.
- Liver and splenic areas are dull.

Auscultation
Hear for;
- *Bruit over the liver:* It indicates malignant liver
- *Rub:* It indicates perihepatitis due to infarction or may be heard over a nodule
- *Venus hum* around umbilicus: Its presence indicates portal hypertension (*Curvilinear-Baumgarten syndrome*)

PROVISIONAL DIAGNOSIS

The patient has ascites, splenomegaly and collaterals due to portal hypertension (lesion) caused by alcoholic liver disease (aetiology) without the signs of hepatic encephalopathy (functional status).

QUESTIONS AND ANSWERS

Q.   What are the points in favor of your diagnosis?
Ans: • Long history of alcoholism (chronic alcoholic)
- Past history of jaundice and hematemesis
- Poor nutritional status, e.g. sunken cheeks
- Presence of stigmata of cirrhosis
- Presence of ascites, splenomegaly and collaterals with flow of blood away from umbilicus
- Pitting edema

Q.   What is normal portal venous pressure. What is portal hypertension?
Ans: Normal portal venous pressure is 9–11 mm Hg Portal hypertension is defined as an elevated portal venous pressure more than normal.

Q.   What are the clinical presentations of portal hypertension?
Ans: Patients commonly present with:
- Variceal bleeding, e.g. hematemesis, malena, piles.

- Chronic iron deficiency anemia due to congestive gastropathy and repeated minor gastric bleeding.
- Abdominal distention (ascites), splenomegaly.
- Spontaneous bacterial peritonitis.
- Symptoms and signs of hepatic encephalopathy may be present.
- Oliguria/Anuria due to hepatorenal syndrome.
- Hypersplenism leading to pancytopenia.

Q.   How do you classify portal hypertension?
Ans: Increased portal pressure can occur at three levels relative to hepatic sinusoids (Fig. 4.1)
1. *Presinusoidal:* It means obstruction in the presinusoidal compartment outside the liver (between sinusoids and portal vein)
2. *Sinusoidal:* Obstruction occurs within the liver itself at the level of sinusoids.
3. *Postsinusoidal:* Obstruction is outside the liver at the level of hepatic veins, inferior vena cava or beyond sinusoids within liver (veno-occlusive disease).

Q.   What are the causes of portal hypertension?
Ans: Cirrhosis is the most common cause, accounts for > 90% of cases. The causes are:
1. *Postsinusoidal causes* (Fig. 4.2)
   - Extrahepatic postsinusoidal, e.g. Budd-Chiari syndrome
   - Intrahepatic, postsinusoidal, e.g. veno-occlusive disease.

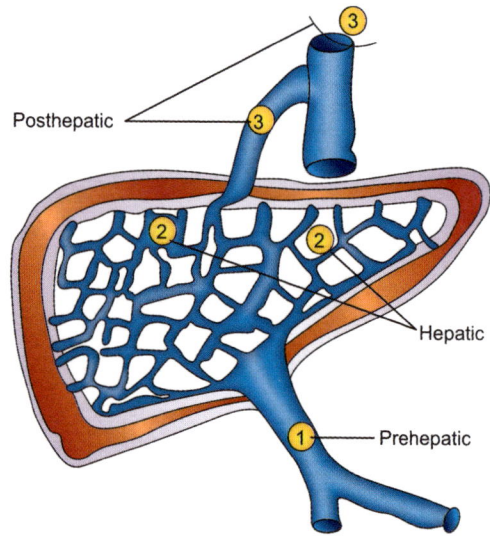

Fig. 4.2: Causes of portal hypertension

2. *Sinusoidal causes* (Fig. 4.2)
   - Cirrhosis of the liver (Fig. 4.2)
   - Cystic liver disease
   - Metastases in the liver
   - Nodular transformation of the liver

3. *Presinusoidal causes* (Fig. 4.2)
   - *Intrahepatic presinusoidal*, e.g. schistosomiasis, sarcoidosis, continental hepatic fibrosis, congenital hepatic fibrosis, drugs and toxins, hematoma, leukemic infiltration, primary biliary cirrhosis.

     Extrahepatic presinusoidal, e.g. portal vein thrombosis, abdominal trauma, compression of portal vein at porta hepatis by malignant nodules or lymph nodes, pancreatitis, etc.

Q. **What is noncirrhotic portal hypertension? What are its causes?**

Ans: As the name suggests, it is defined as portal hypertension without cirrhosis of the liver.

The disorder is usually associated with congenital or acquired hepatic periportal fibrosis. The common causes are:

1. Idiopathic portal fibrosis and phlebosclerosis
2. Portal vein thrombosis
3. Schistosomiasis
4. Congenital hepatic fibrosis
5. Non Hodgkin lymphoma
6. Chronic arsenic poisoning

Q. **What are differences between cirrhotic and noncirrhotic portal hypertension?**

Ans: Differences between cirrhotic and noncirrhotic portal hypertension are given in Table 4.1

Table 4.1: Differentiation between cirrhotic and noncirrhotic portal hypertension

Cirrhotic	Noncirrhotic
• *Slow* insidious onset	• Acute or sudden
• Ascites present	• Ascites absent
• Recurrent hematemesis uncommon	• Recurrent hematemesis is common and presenting feature
• Anemia moderate	• Anemia severe
• Hepatic encephalopathy common	• Hepatic encephalopathy uncommon
• Edema present	• No edema
• Liver biopsy shows cirrhosis	• No evidence of cirrhosis, only portal fibrosis

Q. **Why does ascites absent in noncirrhotic portal hypertension?**

Ans: Ascites is sign of cirrhosis (liver cell dys-

function), hence, is either absent or minimal in non cirrhotic portal hypertension

Q. **What are the causes of cirrhosis?**

Ans:
- Alcoholic cirrhosis
- Posthepatic cirrhosis following viral hepatitis
- Lupoid hepatitis
- Primary biliary cirrhosis
- Metabolic causes, e.g. hemochromatosis, Wilson's disease, α_1-antitrypsin deficiency
- Cryptogenic cirrhosis
- Cardiac cirrhosis (constrictive pericarditis, chronic CHF)

Q. **What are pathological types of cirrhosis?**

Ans:
- Micronodular,
- Macronodular
- Mixed

Q. **Define cirrhosis of the liver. What are its clinical characteristics?**

Ans: Cirrhosis is a pathological term, denotes irreversible destruction of liver cells (necrosis) followed by fibrosis and nodular regeneration of the liver cells in such a way that the normal liver architecture is lost.

The liver in cirrhosis is usually small but may become large due to large nodules transformation. When palpable, it is firm, nodular, nontender with sharp and irregular borders.

Other nonspecific features weakness, fatigue, muscle cramps, weight loss, nausea, vomiting, anorexia and abdominal discomfort. There is muscle wasting and hypotonia. Oedema may be present.

Q. **What are the signs and symptoms of liver cell failure?**

Ans: Signs of liver cell failure are:
- *Hepatomegaly or small shrunken liver*
- *Jaundice, fever*
- *Circulatory changes*, e.g. palmar erythema, spider angiomata, cyanosis (due to AV shunting in lungs). Clubbing of the fingers, tachycardia, bounding pulses, hyperdynamic circulation.
- *Endocrinal changes*, e.g.
  - Loss of libido, hair loss
  - Gynecomastia, testicular atrophy, impotence in males
  - Breast atrophy, irregular menses, amenorrhea in females
- *Haemorrhagic manifestations*, e.g.
  - Bruises, epistaxis, purpura, menorrhagia
- *Miscellaneous*
  - Diffuse pigmentation
  - White nails

– Dupuytren's contractures
– Parotid enlargement
• *Hepatic encephalopathy* — read below

Q. What are the signs of portal hypertension
Ans: Signs of portal hypertension
• *Splenomegaly*
• *Collateral vessels* formation at gastro-esophageal junction, around the umbilicus, behind the liver and in the rectum.
• *Variceal bleeding* (hematemesis and malena)
• *Fetor hepaticus* due to excretion of mercaptans in breaths
• *Ascites*

Q. What are the signs of hepatic encephalopathy?
Ans: It includes *mental features* (e.g. reduced alertness, restlessness, behavioural changes, bizarre handwriting, disturbance in sleep rhythm, drowsiness, confusion, disorientation, yawning, and hiccups). In late stages, convulsions may occur and patient lapses into coma.

Q. What are the precipitating factors for hepatic encephalopathy?
Ans: These are:
• Drugs-like sedatives, hypnotics
• Gastrointestinal bleeding (e.g. varices, peptic ulcer, congestive gastropathy)
• Excessive protein intake
• Diuretics producing hypokalemia and alkalosis
• Rapid removal of large amount of ascitic fluid in one setting (>3 L)
• Acute alcoholic bout
• Constipation
• Infection, septicemia, surgery
• Azotemia (uremia)
• Portosystemic shunts, e.g. spontaneous or surgical

Q. What is the probable pathogenesis of hepatic encephalopathy?
Ans: It is due to retention of following products:
• Increased NH_3 levels in blood
• Increased levels of short-chain fatty acids
• Increase in false neurotransmitters like octopamine and rise in GABA level (true neurotransmitter)
• Rise in methionine levels
• Rise in certain amino acids (ratio of aromatic amino acids to branched chain amino acids is increased) and mercaptans.

Q. How do you stage/grade the hepatic encephalopathy?
Ans: It is divided into 4 stages (Table 4.2).

Q. What are the alcoholic stigmata?
Ans: These stigmata indicate chronic alcoholism proceed to development of cirrhosis, hence, are usually present in alcoholic cirrhosis. They are:
• Red tip of nose and redness of cheeks (malar flush)
• Spider nevi
• Pigmentation of skin; may or may not be present
• Gynecomastia and testicular atrophy in males
• Palmar erythema
• Scanty axillary and public hair in male, breast atrophy in females
• White nails
• Dupuytren's contractures

Q. What are the stages of alcoholic cirrhosis?
Ans: 1. Fatty liver
2. Alcoholic hepatitis/steatohepatitis
3. Alcoholic cirrhosis

Q. What are the complications of cirrhosis?
Ans: Following are the complications:
• Portal hypertension (fatal variceal bleeding)
• Hepatocellular failure and subsequent hepatic encephalopathy

Table 4.2: Clinical staging of hepatic encephalopathy

Stage	Mental features	Tremors	EEG change
I.	Euphoria or depression, confusion, disorientation, disturbance of speech and sleep pattern	+/−	Normal EEG
II.	Lethargy, moderate confusion	+	High voltage triphasic slow waves (abnormal EEG)
III.	Marked confusion incoherent speech, drowsy but arousable	+	High voltage triphasic waves (2–5/sec) (abnormal EEG)
IV.	Coma, initially responsive to noxious stimuli, later unresponsive	−	Delta activity (abnormal EEG)

- Spontaneous bacterial peritonitis
- Septicemia
- Increased incidence of peptic ulcer and hepatocellular carcinoma
- Nutritional debility (e.g. anemia, hypo-proteinemia)
- Hepatorenal and *hepatopulmonary syn-dromes*
- Hemorrhagic tendency

Q. What are the causes of death in cirrhosis?

Ans: Common causes are as follows:
1. Most common cause is fatal septicemia (gram negative)
2. Hepatic encephalopathy
3. Cerebral edema
4. Fatal bleeding
5. Renal failure (hepatorenal syndrome)
6. Hypoglycemia, hypokalemia, etc.

Q. What are the causes of upper GI bleed in cirrhosis of liver?

Ans: The causes are:
1. Esophageal varices
2. Gastric varices/erosions
3. Congestive gastropathy
4. Gastroduodenal ulcerations
5. Mallory-Weiss tear
6. Bleeding tendencies

Q. How will you investigate a case with cirrhosis of the liver?

Ans: Investigations of cirrhosis are as follows:
1. *Complete hemogram for anemia and pancytopenia and ESR:*
2. *Stool for occult blood may be* positive.
3. *Rectal examination* for internal piles
4. *Chest X-ray* for lung pathology or pleural effusion
5. *Hepatic profile*
   - Total serum proteins and albumin may be low. The albumin/globulin ratio is altered.
   - Serum bilirubin is normal or raised
   - Serum transaminases are normal or mildly elevated
   - Alkaline phosphatase is mildly elevated
   - Serum cholesterol is low
   - Prothrombin time is normal or decreased. Low PT is a bad prognostic sign.
   - Viral markers (HbsAg) are negative
   - Serum auroantibodies, antinuclear, anti smooth muscle and antimicrochondrial antibodies level increase in autoimmune hepatitis, cryptogenic cirrhosis and biliary cirrhosis.
   - Serum immunoglobulins, e.g. IgG is increased in autoimmune hepatitis, IgA increased in alcoholic cirrhosis and IgM in primary biliary cirrhosis.
6. *Other blood tests,* e.g. serum copper (Wilson's disease), iron (hemochromatosis), serum alpha-1-antitrypsin (cystic fibrosis) and serum alpha-fetoprotein (hepatocellular carcinoma).
7. *Imaging*
   - Ultrasound for liver may reveal change in size, shape and echo-texture of the liver. Fatty change and fibrosis produce diffuse increased echogenicity. The presence of ascites, portal vein diameter (>14 mm indicates portal hypertension), presence of varices and splenomegaly can be determined on USG.
   - Barium swallow for esophageal varices.
   - CT scan is not better than USG in cirrhosis of liver.
8. *Upper GI endoscopy* for esophageal and gastric varices, peptic ulcer or congestive gastropathy.
9. *Pressure measurement studies*
   - Percutaneous intrasplenic pressure is increased in portal hypertension
   - Wedged hepatic venous pressure is increased
10. *Dynamic flow studies:* These may show distortion of hepatic vasculature or portal vein thrombosis
    - Doppler ultrasound for visualization of portal venous system and duplex Doppler for measurement of portal blood flow and flow reversal in portal and splenic veins.
    - Portal venography by digital subtraction angiography.
11. *Electroencephalogram (EEG)* may show triphasic pattern in hepatic encephalopathy.
12. *Liver biopsy:* It is a gold standard test to confirm the diagnosis of cirrhosis and helps to find out its cause. Special stains can be done for iron and copper.
13. *Ascitic fluid analysis:* Ascites is transudative (serum albumin/ascites albumin gradient >1.1). The fluid should be sent for cytology biochemistry and for culture if bacterial peritonitis is suspected.

Q. **How would you manage cirrhotic portal hypertension?**

Ans: 1. Sodium restriction
2. Diuretics (combination of fursemide and spironolactone is effective)
3. Paracentesis (to remove the ascitic fluid)
4. Infusion of salt free albumin in cases with resistant ascites
5. Transjugular intrahepatic portosystemic shunt to reduce portal pressure and prevent recurrence of ascites
6. Liver transplantation

Q. **What is hepatorenal syndrome?**

Ans: It is functional acute renal failure in a patient with cirrhosis of the liver, develops due to circulatory or hemodynamic changes. Hepatorenal syndrome rarely can develop in hepatitis also. The exact etiology is unknown. The kidneys structurally are normal, but functionally abnormal, hence called functional renal failure. The prognosis is poor.

Q. **What is hepatopulmonary syndrome?**

Ans: *Hepatopulmonary syndrome* is development of cyanosis and clubbing of the fingers due to arteriovenous shunting in the lungs.

Q. **What should be ascitic fluid cell count in spontaneous bacterial peritonitis?**

Ans: Ascitic fluid leukocytes count > 500 cells/μl or > 250 polymorphs/μl indicate spontaneous bacterial peritonitis in cirrhosis of liver.

5

Autoimmune Hepatitis

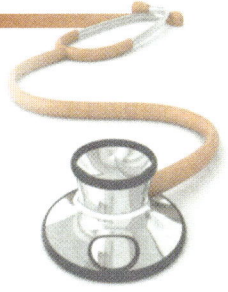

INSTRUCTION

Examine the abdomen of this patient

SALIENT FEATURES

The young female having amenorrhea, fever and jaundice for the last 3 months.

HISTORY

Ask about the following:

- Onset of jaundice with progression (slow onset and slow progression in this case)
- History of fever, arthralgia, sore throat, pain in abdomen, rash
- Exposure to drugs or toxins (nitrofurantoxin, monocycline or infliximab) can produce autoimmune hepatitis
- Ask history of an exacerbation of jaundice during postpartum period
- Occupational exposure to toxins
- History of any associated autoimmune disorder, e.g. Sjögren's syndrome, SLE, thyroiditis, hemolytic anemia, nephritis, ulcerative colitis, etc.
- History of jaundice in the family (Family history)
- History of alcoholism

EXAMINATION

General Physical Examination

- Jaundice is present (Fig. 5.1). Pyrexia also present.
- General appearance for moon-like faces, acne, hirsutism (cushingoid features)
- Look for spider nevi, cutaneous striae and scratch marks
- Eyes for dryness (Sjögren's syndrome)
- Anemia is present
- Look for thyroid enlargement
- Joints; multiple joint tenderness, swelling

Abdominal Examination

- Liver is enlarged, smooth and tender. Spleen is also palpable.

- No ascites
- No other organ palpable

PROVISIONAL DIAGNOSIS

A young female with amenorrhea present with fever and jaundice (lesion) due to an autoimmune hepatitis (etiology). She does not have any evidence of cirrhosis or hepatic encephalopathy (functional status).

QUESTIONS AND ANSWERS

Q. What are the points in favor of your diagnosis?

Ans: 1. A young female
2. Presence of amenorrhea
3. Slow onset of jaundice with fever with slow progression
4. Tender hepatomegaly and splenomegaly
5. Presence of anemia, arthralgia, myalgia

Q. What are the different conditions which come into differential diagnosis?

Ans: All the conditions that produce hepatocellular jaundice comes into differential diagnosis (Table 5.1).

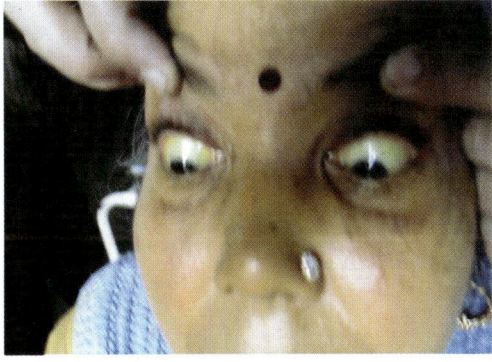

Fig. 5.1: Autoimmune hepatitis

Table 5.1: Differential diagnosis of hepatocellular jaundice

Viral hepatitis	Autoimmune hepatitis	Alcoholic hepatitis	Carcinoma of liver	Drug-induced
• Fever is followed by jaundice. As soon as jaundice appears, fever disappears • Anorexia, nausea, vomiting • Arthralgia, myalgia, headache, pharyngitis, cough, fatigue, malaise • Dark colored urine and clay-colored or normal colored stool • History of exposure to a patient with jaundice or sex contact with a patient of jaundice, etc. • Hepatomegaly. (Liver is moderately enlarged, soft, tender, smooth) • Splenomegaly in 20% cases only	• Insidious onset • Common in females • Fever with jaundice, anorexia, fatigue, arthralgia, vitiligo, epistaxis. • Sometimes a "cushingoid" face with acne, hirsutism, pink cutaneous striae • Bruises may be seen • Hepatosplenomegaly, spider telangiectasis are characteristic • Other autoimmune disorders may be associated • Serological tests confirm the diagnosis	• History of alcoholism • Anorexia, weight loss • Stigmata of chronic liver disease (spider nevi, palmar) erythema, gynecomastia, testicular, atrophy, Dupuytren's contracture, parotid enlargement may be present • Jaundice with enlarged tender liver • May be associated with order manifestations of alcoholism, e.g. cardiomyopathy, peripheral neuropathy	• Common in old age • Progressive jaundice with loss of appetite and weight • Liver enlarged, tender, hard, nodular. Hepatic rub may be heard • Anemia, fever, lymphadenopathy in neck and marked cachexia may be present • Jaundice is deep yellow or greenish • Ascites may be present • Evidence of metastatic spread to lungs, bone, etc. • USG and liver biopsy will confirm the diagnosis	• History of underlying disease, i.e. tuberculosis, diabetes, thyrotoxicosis for which the drug is being taken for a long period • History of intake of hepatotoxic drugs, e.g. INH, rifampicin oral contraceptives • Occasionally rash, fever, arthralgia present • Liver is enlarged and tender • Tests for viral hepatitis are negative

Q. What is the clinical of presentation of auto-immune hepatitis?

Ans: It can present as an acute hepatitis simulating acute viral hepatitis or may progress slowly and mimic a chronic hepatitis (chronic autoimmune hepatitis)

Q. What are the extrahepatic manifestations of autoimmune hepatitis?

Ans: 1. Polyarthritis resembling rheumatic arthritis
2. Coomb's positive hemolytic anemia
3. Autoimmune thyroiditis
4. Autoimmune nephritis
5. Sjögren's syndrome
6. Ulcerative colitis

Q. What are the causes of prolonged jaundice (i.e. duration > 6 months)?

Ans: Causes of prolonged jaundice are as follows:

- Chronic hepatitis or cholestatic viral hepatitis, chronic autoimmune hepatitis
- Cirrhosis of liver
- Malignancy liver
- Hemolytic jaundice (e.g. thalassemia)

- Congenital hyperbilirubinemia
- Drug-induced
- Alcoholic hepatitis
- Primary biliary cirrhosis
- Wilson's disease
- Obstructive jaundice (extrahepatic biliary obstruction)

Q. What is the role of heredity in autoimmune hepatitis?

Ans: The young persons positive for HLA-B8 and HLA-DR3 and older patients positive for HLA-DRY are susceptible to this condition.

Q. What is the risk of this disease?

Ans: Patients with autoimmune hepatitis are at increased risk of developing cirrhosis and hepatocellular carcinoma subsequently

Q. How would you investigate this patient?

Ans: 1. Serum bilirubin will be raised. The liver enzymes (SGOT/SGPT) will also be markedly elevated > 1000 units/L
2. Serum γ-globulins also get raised
3. ANA and smooth muscle antibodies may be detected in serum

4. Other antibodies, e.g. atypical parinuclear antineutrophil cytoplasmic antibodies (pANCA) and antibodies to histone may be found.

5. USG abdomen reveals hepatomegaly. Spleen may also be enlarged.

6. Liver biopsy confirms the diagnosis.

Q. **What are the diagnostic criteria for autoimmune hepatitis.**

Ans: 1. Detection of autoantibodies

2. Elevated IgG levels

3. Characteristic histopathology

4. Exclusion of viral hepatitis

Q. **What is the treatment of autoimmune hepatitis?**

Ans: • Symptomatic relief with analgesic.

• Steroids either alone or with a cytotoxic drug. Cytotoxic drugs (azathioprine) are usually combined to reduce the dose of steroid. The combination is better than single therapy.

• Monitor the blood count while on cytotoxic drug.

• Nonresponder to steroids and azathioprine may be considered for a trial of cyclosporine, tacrolimus, methotrexate or rituximab. Mycophenolate mofetil 1 gm twice a day is an effective alternative.

• Liver transplantation may be required for treatment failures and patients with fulminant hepatitis.

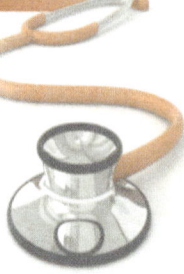

6

Primary Biliary Cirrhosis

INSTRUCTION

Examine the patient's abdomen

SALIENT FEATURES

- Jaundice with pruritus

HISTORY

Ask about the following:

- Onset of jaundice and its progression
- Pruritus, fatigue, lethargy, weakness (present)
- Pain in right hypochondrium, distension of abdomen
- Variceal bleed
- Steatorrhea, malabsorption, bone pain (osteomalacia)
- History of other autoimmune diseases, e.g arthritis, dryness of mouth (Sjögren's syndrome), thyroiditis
- History of proximal muscles weakness

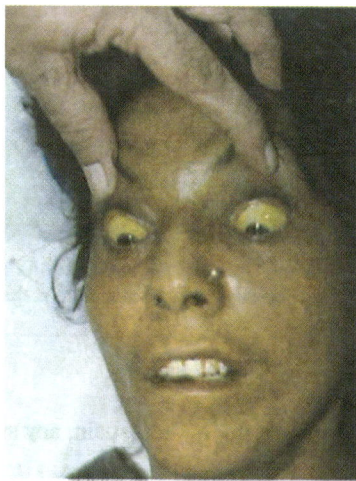

Fig. 6.1: Primary biliary cirrhosis with deep jaundice and pruritus

EXAMINATION

General Physical Examination

- Look for generalized pigmentation
- Clubbing of fingers
- Xanthelasma, xanthomatosis (over joints, skin folds and site of trauma)
- Jaundice
- Scratch marks due to pruritus
- Glossitis, ecchymoses
- Bone tenderness

Abdominal Examination

- Abdomen is distended
- Liver and spleen are palpable
- No ascites

Other Systems

- *Nervous system examination* for peripheral neuropathy
- *Rheumatological examination* for polyarthritis
- *Endocrinal examination* for thyroiditis

PROVISIONAL DIAGNOSIS

The middle aged women presenting with pigmentation, jaundice and pruritus was found to have hepatosplenomegaly (lesion), the provisional diagnosis is primary biliary cirrhosis (etiology). There is no evidence of liver cell failure (functional status).

QUESTIONS AND ANSWERS

Q. **Enumerates the points in favor of your diagnosis?**

Ans: • Middle aged female
- Slow onset of jaundice with pruritus and presence of scratch marks
- Hepatosplenomegaly

Q. **What are the clinical presentations of primary biliary cirrhosis?**

Ans: 1. Asymptomatic patients (Jaundice detected on examination)

2. Symptomatic with jaundice, pruritus and hepatosplenomegaly (in this case)
3. Symptomatic with abnormal liver function tests
4. Decompensated primary biliary cirrhosis

Q. What is the mechanism of pruritus in these patients?

Ans: There are two mechanisms:
1. Retention of bile acids/salts with cholestasis.
2. Increase in the concentration of endogenous opioid receptors and their up-regulation. This mechanism led to the use of opioid antagonists in the treatment of pruritus in these patients.

Q. What are the diseases associated with primary biliary cirrhosis?

Ans: The diseases are same those associated with autoimmune hepatitis (read autoimmune hepatitis).

Q. Is primary biliary cirrhosis predispose to cancer?

Ans: Yes. It is estimated that patients with primary biliary cirrhosis have a 20 fold increased risk of developing liver cancer (hepatocellular carcinoma).

Q. How would you investigate this case?

Ans: I. *Liver function tests*, i.e.
- *Bilirubin* is raised (conjugated hyperbilirubinemia) due to cholestasis.
- *Enzymes,* e.g. alkaline phosphatase, 5-nucleotidase and γ-glutamyl transferase are raised due to cholestasis and serum aminotransferase may be sharply raised due to hepatocellular damage.
- *PT and PTI* are normal; if raised indicate vitamin K deficiency due to steatorrhea.
- *Immunological testing.* IgM and IgG are elevated.
  – Antimitochondrial antibodies (AMA) are elevated.
II. *Serum lipids* reveal hypercholestrolemia
III. *USG of abdomen* will reveal hepatosplenomegaly. Biliary system is normal. Which excludes secondary biliary cirrhosis in which biliary ductal system is dilated
IV. *Liver biopsy* will show nonsuppurative cholangitis or granulomatous cholangitis.

Q. What are the histological stages of primary biliary cirrhosis?

Ans: There are four histological stages:

Stage 1: Inflammation is limited to portal triads.

Stage 2: Inflammation extends beyond portal triads into liver parenchyma. The number of normal bile ducts is reduced.

Stage 3: Fibrous septa connects the portal triads.

Stage 4: End-stage liver disease with cirrhosis, fibrosis and regenerating nodules.

Q. Name the drugs used for pruritus.

Ans: First line drug is cholestyramine.
Second line drugs include; rifampicin and ursodeoxycholic acid.
Third line drugs, are naloxone, nalmefene and propofol.

Q. What is the rationale for bile salt therapy in primary biliary cirrhosis?

Ans: Accumulation of endogenous bile acids such as chenodeoxycholic acid and cholic acid may also injure the liver cells affected by autoimmune process, hence their partial replacement with water soluble bile acids (ursodeoxycholic acid) may reduce pruritus and liver damage.

Q. Is liver biopsy necessary for confirmation of the diagnosis of primary biliary cirrhosis?

Ans: Although liver biopsy is being used routinely for confirmation of the diagnosis, but need for this procedure for either diagnosis and prognosis is questionable. The close association between liver histology and E2AMA in primary biliary cirrhosis means liver histology is not required.

Q. What is the indication of liver transplantation in primary biliary cirrhosis?

Ans: 1. Primary biliary cirrhosis with intractable symptoms.
2. Primary biliary cirrhosis with end-stage liver disease, e.g. intractable ascites, encephalopathy, spontaneous bacterial peritonitis.

Q. What is the cause of peripheral neuropathy in this disease?

Ans: It is nutritional neuropathy due to vitamins deficiency as a result of steatorrhea.

Q. What is the cause of osteomalacia?

Ans: Vit. D deficiency due to malabsorption induced by cholestasis.

Q. What is the treatment of primary biliary cirrhosis?

Ans: I. *Immunosuppressive drugs*, e.g. steroids, azathioprine, cyclosporine, penicillamine, etc.

II. *Colchicine* and *ursodeoxycholic acid* to improve liver functions and may slow histological progression.

III. *Treatment of pruritus.* It has been discussed as a separate question.

IV. *Treatment of symptoms of malabsorption* by vitamins and calcium supplementation Bisphosphonates are required for osteoporosis.

V. *Liver transplantation* is the last option.

Q.   What are the prognostic factors in primary biliary cirrhosis?

Ans: Bad prognostic factors are:

- Presence of ascites, encephalopathy
- Raised blood urea (hepatorenal syndrome)
- Low serum albumin
- Recurrence of symptoms
- Treatment failure

Q.   What is secondary biliary cirrhosis?

Ans: Biliary cirrhosis secondary to extrahepatic bile duct obstruction (due to stricture, stones, sclerosing cholangitis) resulting in dilatation of biliary system leading to liver cell damage is called secondary biliary cirrhosis. The USG of liver differentiates secondary biliary cirrhosis from primary.

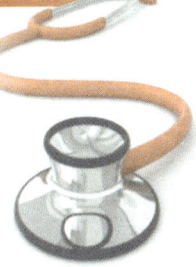

7

Budd-Chiari Syndrome

INSTRUCTION

Examine the abdomen of this patient

SALIENT FEATURES

- Distended abdomen with prominent veins

HISTORY

Ask about the following:

- Onset of jaundice and its progression (acute or chronic Budd-Chiari syndrome)
- Abdominal pain, nausea, vomiting, distension of abdomen (present)
- Symptoms of polycythemia (suffusion of face, headache, vertigo, lack of concentration, bruising or bleeding)
- Symptoms of leukemia
- Paroxysmal noctural hemoglobinuria
- Pregnancy or history of intake of oral contraceptive
- Symptoms of malignancy (cachexia, anorexia, weakness)
- History of radiotherapy to abdomen
- History of abdominal trauma or surgery

EXAMINATION

General Physical Examination

- Anemia or polycythemia
- Jaundice (present, Fig. 7.1)
- Lymph nodes enlargement (leukemia)
- Bruises, ecchymotic patches, epistaxis
- Gynecomastia, spider nevi, palmar erythema, parotid enlargement
- Hepatic flaps

Abdominal Examination

- Distended veins over the abdomen and chest present (Fig. 7.1)
- Tender hepatomegaly (massive) and splenomegaly
- Ascites present

- Demonstrate the direction of flow through these veins. In inferior vena cava obstruction, the venous drainage is from below upward (in this case)

PROVISIONAL DIAGNOSIS

The onset of jaundice with ascites and distended veins over the abdomen and chest with direction of flow from below upwards indicate inferior vena cava obstruction with cirrhosis (lesion) due to Budd-Chiari Syndrome (etiology) without signs of liver cell decompensation (functional status).

QUESTIONS AND ANSWERS

Q. What is Budd-Chiari syndrome?
Ans: Budd-Chiari syndrome is an uncommon acute, subacute or chronic condition characterized by occlusion of the hepatic veins or hepatic portion of inferior vena cava by thrombotic and nonthrombotic causes.

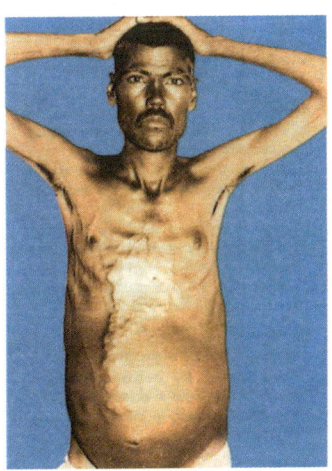

Fig. 7.1: Budd-Chiari syndrome secondary to cancer of the liver

Q. What are the causes of Budd-Chiari syndrome?

Ans: I. Congenital or acquired hypercoagulable states, e.g.
- Polycythemia
- Myeloproliferative disorders
- Activated protein C or S (resistance), factor V Leiden mutation
- Protein C or S or antithrombotic deficiency
- Antiphospholipid syndrome
- Hyperprothrombinemia

II. Congenital hepatic or caval webs

III. Paroxysmal nocturnal hemoglobinuria

IV. Pregnancy and use of oral contraceptive

V. Obstruction of hepatic veins by tumors (Fig. 7.2) and secondaries in the liver

VII. Veno-occlusive disease caused by drugs pyrrolizidine alkaloids

VIII. Radiotherapy

IX. Abdominal trauma

X. Idiopathic

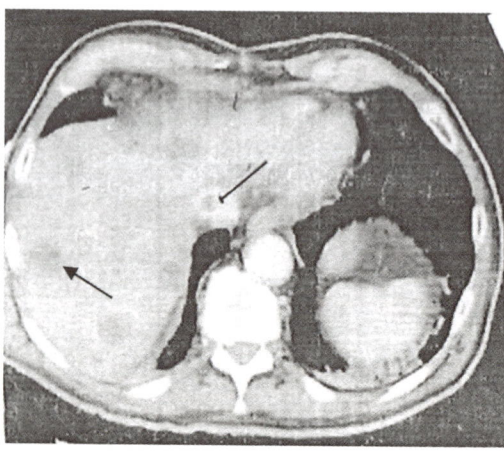

Fig. 7.2: CT scan shows a clot in the inferior vena cava and the metastasis in the liver (arrows)

Q. What is clinical triad of Budd-Chiari syndrome?

Ans: The clinical triad of abdominal pain, ascites and tender hepatomegaly suggests Budd-Chiari syndrome.

Q. What is nutmeg liver?

Ans: In chronic Budd-Chiari syndrome, there is centrilobular necrosis and peripheral lobule fatty change called 'nutmeg liver'.

Q. How would you investigate this patient?

Ans:
- Bilirubin and liver enzymes may be raised.
- Ascitic fluid examination. It is transudative ascites.
- USG abdomen shows altered echotexture and enlargement of caudate lobe Doppler ultrasound may demonstrate the obliteration of hepatic veins and reversed flow through them (present in this case).
- CT scan and MRI may show enlargement of caudate lobe. There may be vena cava obstruction or occlusion of hepatic vein (Fig. 7.2) with diffuse abnormal liver parenchyma on contrast enhancement.
- Liver biopsy demonstrates centrilobular congestion and fibrosis.
- Blood tests and coagulation profile studies for hypercoaguable state.

Q. What are the complications of Budd-Chiari syndrome?

Ans:
- Severe variceal bleed
- Intractable ascites
- Hepatic encephalopathy
- Cirrhosis of liver
- Hepatocellular carcinoma
- Hepatopulmonary syndrome

Q. How would you treat it?

Ans:
1. Find out the underlying cause and treat it accordingly.
2. Thrombolytic therapy for recent venous thrombosis.
3. Ascites is managed medically. For intractable cases, TIPS, may be recommended.
4. Liver cell transplantation for progressive liver cell failure.

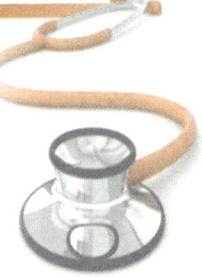

8

Wilson's Disease

INSTRUCTION

- Look at the eye
- Examine the abdomen of this patient

SALIENT FEATURES

- Jaundice in a young patient

HISTORY

Ask about the following:

- Age and sex
- History of consanguinity
- Ask history of hepatitis, hypersplenism, hemolytic anemia, portal hypertension and neuropsychiatric manifestations in young adults and children.
- History of chronic hepatitis (>6 months) or fulminant hepatitis in persons under the age of 40 years.
- In adolescents, it presents with chronic hepatitis or chronic liver disease (cirrhosis).

EXAMINATION

General Physical Examination

- Anemia may be present
- Jaundice may be seen
- Eyes: Greenish yellow to golden brown pigmentation at the limbus of the cornea [Kayser-Fleischer ring (Fig. 8.1)]
- Look for cataract (Sunflower)
- Look for the signs of liver cell failure

Abdominal Examination

- Liver is enlarged, non tender
- Spleen may be palpable

Other Systems

Neurological Examination

- Look for parkinsonism (tremors), chorea (involuntary dancing movements), ataxia, dystonic spasms, dysarthria, incoordination and rigidity.

Psychiatric Examination

- Behavioral and personality changes and emotional lability.

PROVISIONAL DIAGNOSIS

The young patient has jaundice, Kayser-Fleischer ring and hepatomegaly (lesion) caused by Wilson's disease (cause) and does not have signs of liver cell failure (functional status).

QUESTIONS AND ANSWERS

Q. **What is Wilson's disease?**

Ans: It is a hereditary disorder of copper metabolism characterised by deposition of copper in the liver and brain.

Q. **What is the genetic defect in Wilson's disease?**

Ans: It is an autosomal recessive disorder due to genetic defect located on chromosome 13,

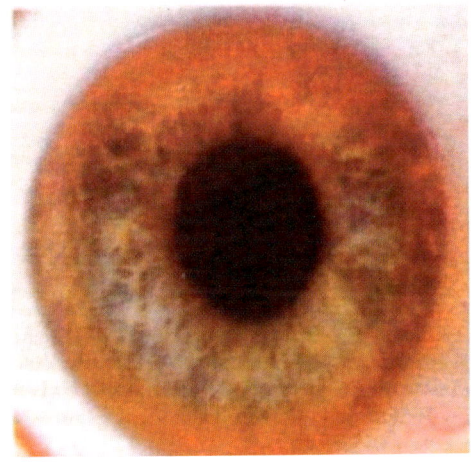

Fig. 8.1: A Kayser-Fleischer ring. It is seen in Wilson's disease

affects a copper-transporting adenosine triphosphatase (ATP7B) and is often associated with a family history of consanguinity. It results due to mutation in encoding of a copper-transporting ATPase, i.e. Wilson's disease protein (WNDP). A large number of mutations have been reported in this disease, but the most common leading to substitution HIO69Q is present in one-third of the patient.

Q. What is Kayser-Fleischer ring?

Ans: It is present as fine pigmented granular deposits in descemet membrane in the cornea. The ring is usually most marked at superior and inferior poles of the cornea. It is readily detected on slit lamp examination, but can occasionally be seen by naked eye. It may be absent in patients with hepatic manifestations, but is usually present in those with neuropsychiatry manifestations.

Q. Is Kayser-Fleischer ring pathognomonic of Wilson's disease?

Ans: No. This ring is seen in many other conditions such as
- Primary biliary cirrhosis
- Chronic active hepatitis with cirrhosis
- Cryptogenic cirrhosis
- Long-standing intrahepatic cholestasis

Q. When do neurological manifestations appear in Wilson's disease?

Ans: They appear during childhood and adulthood, i.e. between 12 and 30 years of age. The most common early neurological feature is difficulty in speaking and/or writing in school.

Q. What is the pathophysiology of this disease?

Ans: Excessive absorption of copper from the gut with decreased clearance/excretion of copper by the liver result in an increase in deposition of copper in tissues particularly in the cornea, brain, liver and kidneys.

Q. What are the biochemical changes in Wilson's disease?

Ans: 1. Low level of copper-binding protein called ceruloplasmin
2. Serum copper concentration may be high, low or normal
3. Increased urinary excretion of copper
4. Radiolabelled copper if given orally gets incorporated into ceruloplasmin

Q. What are the renal manifestations of Wilson's disease?

Ans 1. Renal calculi
2. Aminoaciduria
3. Renal tubular acidosis

Q. What are the clinical stages of Wilson's disease?

Ans: 1. Asymptomatic disease when child is born
2. Patient remains either asymptomatic or manifests with hemolytic anemia or liver failure as he/she grows
3. Copper accumulates slowly and consistently in the brain
4. Progressive neurological features

Q. How would you confirm your diagnosis?

Ans: The diagnosis will be confirmed by demonstration of one of the following:
1. Low serum ceruloplasmin level (<20 mg/L) and Kayser-Fleischer rings
2. Serum ceruloplasmin concentration <200 mg/L and copper content in liver biopsy specimen greater than 250 mg/gm in dry weight basis
3. Increased urinary copper excretion (>40 μg/day and usually <100 μg/day and low ceruloplasmin level).

Q. What are the radiological features in this disease?

Ans 1. Osteopenia seen in radiology of hands and feet
2. Arthropathy
3. Articular abnormalities, i.e. subchondral bone fragmentation, cyst formation commonly seen in wrist, hand, foot, hip, shoulder, elbow and knee
   There may be irregularity and in distinctness of subchondral bone resulting in a characteristic 'paintbrush' appearance.
4. Radiological changes of osteomalacia and rickets
5. Periosteal bone formation and chondrocalcinosis

Q. How would you treat this case?

Ans 1. Restriction of dietary copper (shell fish, organ food, nuts, mushrooms and chocolate).
2. **Oral D-penicillamine:** A copper chelating agent removes and detoxifies deposits of copper. Treatment is lifelong.
   - D-Penicillamine should not be given as initial therapy to those with neurological features.
   - Trientine is another copper-chelating agent that can be used in those patients who are intolerant to penicillamine.
3. Zinc salts can be given.
4. Tetrathiomolybdate with zinc salts is the treatment of choice in those with neurological manifestations.

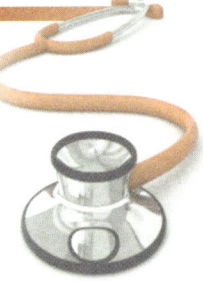

9

Hemochromatosis

INSTRUCTION

- Look at the patient
- Examine the abdomen including genitalia

SALIENT FEATURES

- Patient complains of hyperpigmentation of the body

HISTORY

Ask for the following:

- Jaundice, malena, hematemesis, distension of abdomen
- History of pigmentation
- Age of onset (usually after 30 years)
- History of dyspnea (for cardiac failure)
- Fatigue, joint pains (polyarthritis)
- History of amenorrhea
- Impotence
- History of diabetes (polyuria, polydipsia, polyphagia, weakness)
- Family history

EXAMINATION

General Physical Examination

- Jaundice
- Pigmentation (bronze color due to combination of iron and melanin (Fig. 9.1)
- Palmar erythema, spider nevi
- Signs of liver cell failure may be present (present in this case)
- Signs of cardiac failure may be present, i.e. edema feet, raised JVP

Systemic Examination

I. *Abdominal examination*
- Hepatomegaly (present)
- Ascites (present)

II. *Cardiovascular system examination*
- For cardiomegaly with or without heart failure (dilated cardiomyopathy)
- Arrhythmia and conduction defect

III. *Diabetic status and its complications*

IV. Examination of genitalia for hypogonadism, i.e. small testes due to atrophy

V. Examination of joints for arthritis

PROVISIONAL DIAGNOSIS

A 40-year male patient has generalized hyper-pigmentation, liver enlargement and signs of liver cell disease (lesion) caused by hemochromatosis which is a hereditary disorder (etiology). There is no evidence of cirrhosis or diabetes (functional status).

QUESTIONS AND ANSWERS

Q. **What is hemochromatosis?**

Ans: It is an autosomal recessive disorder caused by gene mutation encoding protein involved in iron metabolism resulting in an increased iron absorption and its subsequent deposition in liver, heart, skin, pancreas, joints, testes, pituitary, abdomen and kidneys.

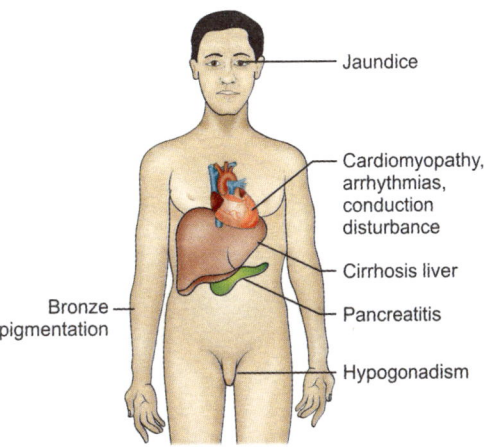

Fig. 9.1: Hemochromatosis (clinical features)

Q. Is hemochromatosis a familial disease?

Ans: **Yes.** At least four different gene mutations are involved in 90% cases.

1. HFE is common gene mutation involving chromosome 6 in addition to HJV, HAMP and TIR1.
2. However 10% patients with severe hereditary hemochromatosis do not have these mutations and this limit the role of diagnostic DNA testing.

Q. What is the cause of increased iron absorption in hemochromatosis?

Ans: The iron absorption is mediated by the duodenal metal transporter DMT-I also called NRAMP-2, the increased expression of mRNA for NRAMP-2 in the duodenal mucosa of patients with hemochromatosis causes increased duodenal uptake of iron resulting in iron overloading.

Q. What is the importance of its early detection?

Ans: Early detection is beneficial in many ways, i.e. early detection and early venesection in patients who have not developed DM or cirrhosis prevent progression of the hepatic disease and may consequently prevent complications of hepatocellular carcinoma.

Q. What investigations would you like to perform to confirm the diagnosis?

Ans:
1. Serum ferritin levels. They are raised.
2. Transferrin saturation is also increased.
3. Liver biopsy is done to measure iron stores in liver.
4. MRI is noninvasive method to quantify the iron stores in the liver. It allows repeated measurements and reduces sampling error.

Q. Enumerate some causes of pigmentation.

Ans:
1. Sun exposure and racial cause
2. Hemochromatosis (in males)
3. Primary biliary cirrhosis
4. Addison's disease
5. Pellagra
6. Uremia
7. Chronic debilitating disease and malignancy

Q. How would you treat this case?

Ans:
- Avoidance of food cooked in iron utensils
- Avoidance of alcohol
- Avoidance of uncooked shellfish and marine fish since these patients are susceptible to fatal septicemia from the marine bacterium *Vibrio vulnificus*
- **Phlebotomy/venesection:** It protects and reverses tissue damage. Initially weekly venesection (500 ml of blood) is done for 2 years followed by once every 3 months
- *Deferoxamine,* an iron chelating agent is used when venesection is not permitted
- Screening of the family members by measuring fasting transferrin saturation and ferritin levels
- Screen the patient for diabetes and treat it accordingly

Q. What is the cause of death in such patients?

Ans: The commonest cause of death is development of hepatocellular carcinoma.

10 Hepatocellular Carcinoma

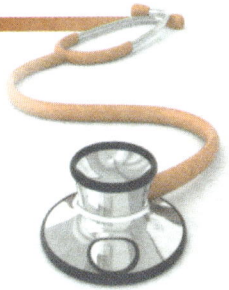

INSTRUCTION

Examine the abdomen

SALIENT FEATURES

- A mass in the abdomen

HISTORY

Ask for the following:

- Age of the patient
- Pain abdomen, jaundice, ascites, pruritus
- Weakness, anorexia, weight loss
- History of cirrhosis of the liver
- History of hemochromatosis (hyperpigmentation, diabetes, neuropsychiatric manifestations and cirrhosis)
- Exposure to aflatoxins and drug, i.e. oral contraceptive

EXAMINATION

General Physical Examination

- Jaundice (present)
- Palmar erythema, spider nevi, scratch marks
- Edema feet
- Finger clubbing
- Anemia

Abdominal Examination

1. Liver is enlarged, firm to hard, nodular (in this case) and tender. On auscultation over the liver may reveal a bruit over the tumor or a friction rub
2. Splenomegaly if portal hypertension present (present)
3. Ascites

PROVISIONAL DIAGNOSIS

The 60-year-old male patient has nodular hard hepatomegaly with jaundice with portal hypertension (lesion) due to malignancy of liver (etiology). There is no evidence of liver cell failure (functional status).

QUESTIONS AND ANSWERS

Q. **What are the causes of irregular surface of liver?**
Ans. Following are causes:
- Cirrhosis (micronodular or macronodular)
- Secondaries in the liver
- Hepatocellular carcinoma
- Hepatic abscesses (pyogenic, amebic)
- Multiple hepatic cysts

Q. **What are the causes of hepatic bruit and a rub?**
Ans: Following are the causes:
Bruit
- Hepatocellular carcinoma
- Hemangioma liver
- Alcoholic hepatitis/liver disease

Rub
- Infections of liver
- Following liver biopsy
- Hepatic infarction (embolic)
- Perihepatitis due to any cause (gonococcal perihepatitis in women)
- Carcinoma of liver

Q. **What factors protect the individuals from carcinoma of liver?**
Ans: - Consumption of coffee
- Statins especially in diabetics

Q. **What are the complications of carcinoma liver?**
Ans: 1. Portal hypertension
2. Hepatic vein thrombosis (Budd-Chiari syndrome)
3. Dissemination to other organs
4. Hepatocellular failure

Q. **How would you investigate this patient?**
Ans: - Blood tests, including hematocrit (elevated due to erythropoietin production)
- Alkaline phosphatase raised

- Serum levels of α-fetoproteins are raised
- Serum levels of des-gamma-carboxy-prothrombin are elevated
- Viral serology for hepatitis B and C
- Ascitic fluid examination for malignant cells
- USG of liver will detect hepatic nodules from which biopsy can be taken
- Multiphase helical CT scanning (Fig. 10.1) and MRI with contrast enhancement are preferred imaging studies for determination of the location and vascularity of the tumor
- In selected cases, endoscopic USG may be useful
- The role of PET is under study
- *Liver biopsy:* It is diagnostic. Biopsy can be deferred if imaging studies and α-fetoprotein levels are diagnostic

Q.   **How would you stage the liver carcinoma?**
Ans: TNM classification is used to stage the tumor;

    T0: No evidence of primary tumor
    T1: Solitary tumor without vascular invasion

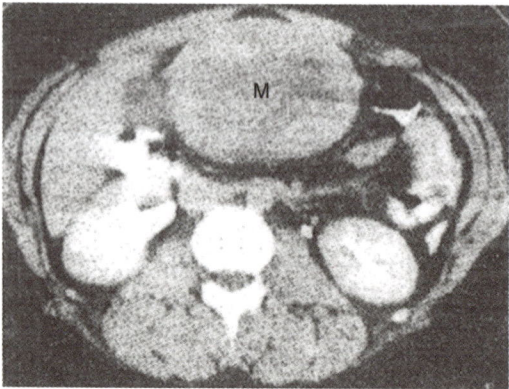

Fig. 10.1: Hepatocellular carcinoma: Contrast enhanced CT scan demonstrates a large mass in the upper abdomen

    T2: Solitary tumor with vascular invasion or multiple tumors not more than 5 cm
    T3: Multiple tumors more than 5 cm (3a) or tumor involving a major branch of portal or hepatic vein (3b)
    T4: Tumor(s) with direct invasion of adjacent organs other than gallbladder or with perforation of the visceral peritoneum.
    N1: Regional lymph node metastases
    M1: Distant metastases
    F0: Nil to moderate fibrosis of liver
    F1: Severe hepatic fibrosis to cirrhosis

Q.   **How would you treat this patient?**
Ans: 1. Surgical resection of solitary hepatocellular carcinoma if liver function is preserved and portal vein thrombosis is not present.
2. Treatment of underlying chronic hepatitis. Adjuvant chemotherapy and adaptive immunotherapy may lower postsurgical recurrence rates.
3. In patients with large tumors, high serum α-fetoprotein levels and MELD score (Model for end-stage liver disease score). ≥20 should be treated by palliative therapy combining chemotherapy, hormonal therapy with transarterial chemoembolisation, transarterial chemoperfusion and transarterial radioembolisation to prolong survival in patients with large or multifocal tumor without extrahepatic spread.
4. Patients with non-resectable growth can be treated with injection of alcohol into the tumor or radiofrequency ablation or, cryotherapy or microwave ablation of small tumors.
5. New chemotherapy and radiation therapy, novel biological approaches (a proteosome inhibitor, anti-angiogenesis agents, inhibitors of growth factors signalling and gene therapy) and multimodel approaches are under study.

11

Abdominal Aortic Aneurysms

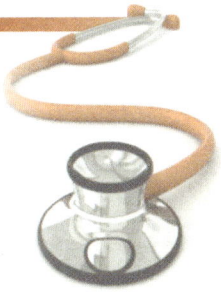

INSTRUCTION

Examine the abdomen

SALIENT FEATURES

- Low back pain and palpitations

HISTORY

Ask for the following:

- Age and gender of the patient
- Abdominal pain and its radiation to back
- History of embolisation
- History of smoking (aneurysm common in elderly male smokers)
- Family history of rupture of abdominal aneurysm
- 75% patient may not have any symptom
- History of diabetes, hypertension, hyperlipidemia

EXAMINATION

General Physical Examination

- Pulse and BP (hypertension)
- Look for signs and symptoms of diabetes with vascular disease (peripheral vascular disease)
- Look for signs of hyperlipidemia (xanthelasma or xanthomatosis)
- Eyes for arcus senalis
- Carotid pulsations are weak due to atherosclerosis. Palpate all other vessels
- Trash foot, e.g. digital infarcts of foot due to embolisation

Abdominal Examination

Inspection

- Pulsations are visible in mid-abdomen especially in epigastrium (in this case)

Palpation

- Expansile pulsation over the abdominal aorta are felt with both hands placed on either side of the aorta [bimanual palpation (Fig. 11.1)].

Auscultation

- Auscultate for the bruit over the area of pulsations and over the femoral artery.

PROVISIONAL DIAGNOSIS

A 60-year male smoker has a large expansile palpable mass in the epigastrium (lesion) caused by an aneurysm of the abdominal aorta (etiology). The mass is tender suggesting inflammation and impending rupture (functional status).

QUESTIONS AND ANSWERS

Q. **What do you mean by an aneurysm?**
Ans: Transverse dilatation of a segment of vessel is called *aneurysm*. It contains all the three layers.

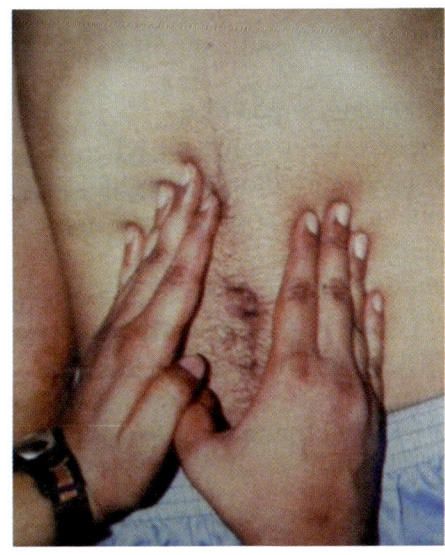

Fig. 11.1: Abdominal aortic aneurysm: On palpation of abdomen expansile pulsations over the abdomen are felt

Q. When would you say that aortic aneurysm is present?

Ans: Normally the infra-renal aorta of healthy young man measures approximately 2 cm. Aneurysm is said to be present if aortic diameter exceeds 3 cm.

Q. What is the common site of abdominal aortic aneurysm?

Ans: The aneurysm usually involves the aortic bifurcation and often involves the common iliac arteries.

Q. What are the common causes of abdominal aortic aneurysm?

Ans:
1. About 90% abdominal aneurysms are due to atherosclerosis
2. Inflammatory aneurysms are less common

Q. How would you palpate for aortic aneurysm?

Ans: Read the Clinical Method in Medicine by Prof SN Chugh

Q. What are the signs of impending rupture of an aneurysm?

Ans: Severe abdominal pain, a palpable abdominal mass and hypotension indicate the rupture.

Q. What are the factors that govern rupture of aneurysm?

Ans:
1. Diameter of the aneurysm. Aneurysm rarely rupture until their diameter exceeds 5 cm
2. Smoking predispose to rupture
3. High diastolic BP
4. CAD
5. Family history of rupture of aneurysm
6. Inflammatory aneurysms easily rupture

Q. What do you mean by rupture? Where does an abdominal aneurysm rupture?

Ans: Rupture of an abdominal aneurysm means leakage of blood into retroperitoneal space which is usually contained by the formation of thrombus and palpable mass (contained rupture) which may arrest the blood loss long enough for the patient to undergo urgent operation.

The abdominal aneurysm rupture:
1. Into retroperitoneal space
2. Into the duodenum
3. Into the ureters
4. Into the inferior vena cava

Q. What are the types of aneurysms?

Ans: Aneurysms are usually of three types, i.e. *true, false* and *dissecting aneurysm.*

Q. How would you classify abdominal aortic aneurysm?

Ans: Based on anatomical site and extent of involvement *Clawford* classified it into 4 types.

Type I: Involves all or most of the descending thoracic aorta and the upper abdominal aorta

Type II: Involves all or most of the descending thoracic aorta and all or most of the abdominal aorta

Type III: Involves lower part of the descending thoracic aorta and most of the abdominal aorta

Type IV: Involves all or most of the abdominal aorta including the visceral aorta

Q. What is the pathogenesis of abdominal aortic aneurysm?

Ans: The pathogenic mechanisms that play some part are:
1. Degradation of the elastic media of atherosclerotic aorta
2. Inflammatory cell infiltration, neovascularisation, and production and activation of proteases and cytokines
3. Elastic fragmentation and attenuation of tunica media.
4. Collagen degradation by the proteolytic enzymes and plasmin generated by the plasminogen activators have been shown to take part in aneurysm formation and rupture (animal studies)

Q. How would you investigate this patient?

Ans:
1. Plain X-ray abdomen for calcification of aneurysmal wall
2. Ultrasonography of the abdomen for localisation and size of aneurysm
3. CT scan abdomen
4. MRI angiography

Q. How would you manage this case?

Ans:
1. Aneurysm <5 cm requires follow up by ultrasonography at an interval of 3 to 6 months depending on the size.
2. Aneurysm up to 5.5 cm may require surgery or follow up.
3. Aneurysm >5.5 cm should be subjected to surgery (endovascular repair or open surgical resection).
4. Anticoagulation for thrombus in aneurysm.

Q. What are the complications of aneurysmal surgery?

Ans:
• Increased incidence of myocardial infarction following open surgical resection
• Renal injury for repair in intrarenal aneurysm
• Respiratory complication
• GI hemorrhage may occur years after surgery due to graft-enteric fistula

N.B: Mortality rates are low with endovascular than open surgical repair.

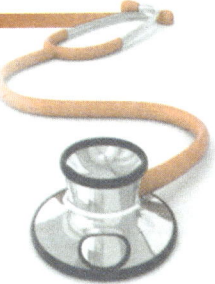

12

Splenomegaly

INSTRUCTION

Examine the abdomen of the patient

SALIENT FEATURES

- Mass abdomen

HISTORY

Ask for the following:

- History of abdominal distention
- History of fever, sore throat, bleeding from nose, mouth, rectum, etc.
- History of piles and/or hematemesis, jaundice
- History of palpitation, dyspnea, orthopnea and PND
- Any history of weight loss, fatigue, bone pain, night sweats (CML)
- Is the area endemic for malaria or kala-azar?
- Family history of Gaucher's disease
- Past history of jaundice, hematemesis, RHD, tuberculosis, malignancy

EXAMINATION

General Physical Examination

- *Face* for puffiness or edema

- *Mouth* for any evidence of infection, ulceration or excoriation or thrush
- *Tongue and mucous membranes* — look for anemia
- *Neck* for lymphadenopathy, JVP, thyroid enlargement
- *Pulse*, BP, *respiration* and *temperature*
- *Hands* for clubbing, splinter hemorrhage, Roth's spots, gangrene
- *Feet* for edema

Abdominal Examination

Examination of Abdomen

- Look for any swelling or protuberance of abdomen especially in left hypochondriac region (Fig. 12.1A). It is present in this case.
- Palpate the abdomen for enlargement of spleen (Fig. 12.1B), liver and lymph nodes. In case spleen or liver is enlarged, note the details of characteristics of liver or splenic mass.
- Method of palpation for spleen (Fig. 12.1B). Start low while examining the spleen and be gentle during palpation. Even if you are certain it is spleen, you must follow the rules of palpation of

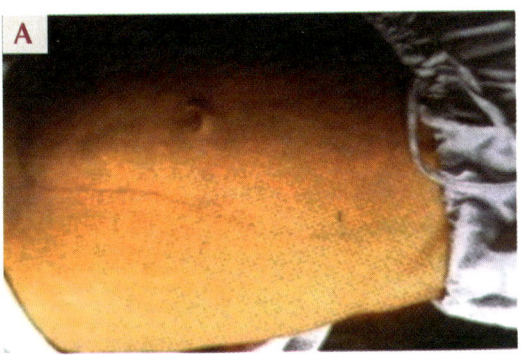
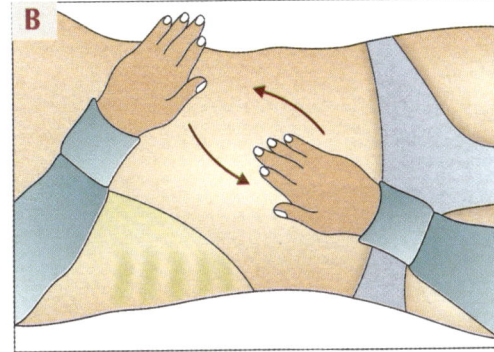

Fig. 12.1: (A) A patient with massive (>8 cm) splenomegaly producing left hypochondriac protrusion; (B) Method of palpation for splenomegaly (diagram)

spleen to rule out renal mass. Do not forget to do a bimanual palpation (spleen is bimanually palpable and kidney is ballottable). Feel for the splenic notch and auscultate for the splenic rub.

- Normally the spleen is neither palpable nor becomes palpable unless enlarged by two and half times, hence, spleen may be enlarged but not palpable. Therefore, percussion of 9th, 10th and 11th space (*Traube's area*) is a useful diagnostic technique.
- Percussion over the mass. In a case with splenomegaly percuss for Traube's area for dullness.
- Auscultate over the mass for any rub, bruit, etc.

Examination of Respiratory System

- Examine for signs of hilar lymphadenopathy (e.g. superior mediastinal syndrome — read case discussion on it)
- Auscultate for crackles

Examination of CVS

- Inspect the precordium for any precordial bulge or cardiac enlargement
- Palpate the apex for any evidence of deviation/shift or thrill
- Auscultate the heart for sounds, murmurs or rub and for evidence of LVF or pericardial disease especially pericardial effusion or rheumatic valvular disease

Examination of Blood

- Look for signs of hemorrhage or bleeding into the skin or an organ
- Elicit sternal tenderness

PROVISIONAL DIAGNOSIS

The patient has massive splenomegaly (lesion) caused by chronic myeloid leukemia (cause). Patient is dyspnoeic due to severe anemia (functional status).

QUESTIONS AND ANSWERS

Q. **What are the points in favor of your diagnosis?**

Ans: 1. A young female patient.
2. History of fever, bone pains, night sweats, dyspnea, dragging pain abdomen due to mass.
3. Presence of anemia and sternal tenderness.
4. Massive non-tender splenomegaly (>8 cm).

Q. **Which bed side investigations would you carry out to confirm the diagnosis?**

Ans: Peripheral blood film examination for total leucocyte count and immature cells. High TLC (in lacs), immature cells >30% and myeloblasts >5 % will clinch the diagnosis.

Q. **How do you define splenomegaly?**

Ans: Splenomegaly literally means enlargement of spleen. Palpable spleen means its enlargement 2 to 3 times than normal. Normal spleen measures 12 × 7 cm on ultrasonography, radionuclide scan and CT scan. Spleen is palpable in 1–3% normal individuals without any cause. Its incidence in normal population in New Guinea has been reported to be very high (up to 60%). Spleen is said to be enlarged if its span on USG is > 14 cm.

Q. **What is differential diagnosis of massive splenomegaly (> 8 cm)?**

Ans: The following conditions must be considered:
- Chronic malaria
- Kala-azar
- Chronic myeloid leukemia/hairy cell leukemia
- Myelofibrosis/myelosclerosis
- Gaucher's disease
- Chronic lymphatic leukemia

Q. **What are the causes of mild and moderate splenomegaly?**

Ans: The causes are tabulated (Table 12.1).

Table 12.1: Causes of mild and moderate splenomegaly	
Mild (< 3 cm)	*Moderate (3–8 cm)*
• Congestive heart failure • Bacterial endocarditis • Typhoid fever • SLE • Acute malaria (Remember chronic malaria produces massive splenomegaly) • Rheumatoid arthritis, sarcoidosis • Glandular fever (infectious mononucleosis) • Idiopathic thrombocytopenia purpura • Polycythemia	• Cirrhosis of liver with portal hypertension • Lymphomas • Hemolytic anemia • Infectious mononucleosis • Amyloidosis • Chronic lymphatic leukemia • Hairy cell leukemia • Splenic abscess or cyst • Idiopathic thrombocytopenic purpura

Q. What are the causes of palpable spleen without enlargement?

Ans: Normally spleen may be palpable without being enlarged in:
- Some children below 10 years of age
- Thin lean persons
- COPD (spleen is pushed down by hyper-inflated lung)
- Visceroptosis (drooping of viscera including spleen)

Q. What are the causes of splenomegaly with fever?

Ans: Spleen enlarges within few days to few weeks of fever. Causes are:
- Bacterial endocarditis
- Acute malaria
- Kala-azar
- Tuberculosis
- Infectious mononucleosis
- Histoplasmosis
- Typhoid fever
- Acute leukemia
- Lymphoma
- SLE
- Hemolytic crisis

Q. What are the causes of splenomegaly with anemia?

Ans: The causes are:
- Bacterial endocarditis
- Hemolytic anemia
- Cirrhotic portal hypertension with repeated hematemesis
- Myeloproliferative syndromes
- Malaria (hemolysis)
- Felty's syndrome
- SLE
- Rheumatoid arthritis

Q. What are the causes of splenomegaly with jaundice?

Ans: Jaundice may be hemolytic or hepatic. Causes are:
- Cirrhosis of liver
- Acute viral hepatitis (rare)
- Acute malaria (P. falciparum) due to hemolysis
- Hepatic vein thrombosis (Budd-Chiari syndrome)
- Hemolytic anemia
- Lymphoma
- Miliary tuberculosis

Q. What are the common causes of fever, lymphadenopathy, splenomegaly with or without rash?

Ans: The conditions are:
- Infectious mononucleosis

- Sarcoidosis
- Acute leukemia or blast crisis in chronic leukemia
- SLE
- Lymphoma, Felty's syndrome

Q. What are the causes of splenomegaly with ascites?

Ans: The causes are:
- Portal hypertension
- Budd-Chiari syndrome
- Lymphoma
- CML
- Hepatocellular carcinoma with portal vein thrombosis

Q. What are the causes of splenic rub? Where do you hear it? What does it indicate?

Ans: Splenic rub can be heard over the enlarged spleen or lower chest during respiration with stethoscope in conditions associated with splenic infarction (perisplenitis) due to vascular occlusion of spleen. The patient complains of acute left upper quadrantic pain abdomen which may radiate to tip of left shoulder. The spleen is enlarged and tender. The causes are:
- Subacute bacterial endocarditis
- Chronic myeloid leukemia
- Sickle cell anemia
- Following splenic puncture for diagnosis of kala-azar

Q. What is hypersplenism? What are its causes?

Ans: Hypersplenism refers to overactivity of the splenic function, has nothing to do with the size of the spleen. It is characterized by a tetrad consisting of:
- Splenomegaly of any size
- Cytopenias/pancytopenia (anemia, leukopenia and/or thrombocytopenia)
- Normal or hypercellular marrow
- Reversibility following splenectomy

Causes of hypersplenism are:
- Lymphoma
- Cirrhosis of the liver
- Myeloproliferative disorders
- Connective tissue disorders

Q. What is bone marrow picture in hypersplenism?

Ans: Hypercellular

Q. What are the causes of hyposplenism?

Ans: It refers to virtual absence of spleen (asplenia) or malfunctioning spleen (hyposplenism). It is usually associated with:
- Dextrocardia

- Sickle cell disease leading to multiple infarcts
- Coeliac disease
- Fanconi's anemia (aplastic anemia with hypoplasia of spleen, kidney, thymus, etc.)
- Surgical removal of the spleen
- Splenic irradiation for autoimmune or neoplastic disease

Q. **How will you investigate a patient with splenomegaly?**

Ans: The investigations to be done are:

- *Hemoglobin and RBCs count.* Hemoglobin is *low* in thalassemia major, SLE, cirrhotic portal hypertension and *increased* in polycythemia rubra vera.
- *WBC count.* Granulocyte counts may be *normal, decreased* (Felty's syndrome, congestive splenomegaly, aleukemic leukemia) or *increased* (infections, or inflammatory disease, myeloproliferative disorders).
- *Other investigations* are same as discussed under hepatosplenomegaly (read them there).

Q. **What are the indications of splenectomy (removal or spleen)?**

Ans: Indications are:

1. For correction of cytopenia in immune thrombocytopenia and hypersplenism.
2. For sickle cell crises (splenic sequestration) in young children.
3. Hereditary spherocytosis.
4. For disease control in patients with splenic rupture.
5. More often splenectomy is performed in stage III and IV of Hodgkin's disease. Splenectomy is necessary for routine staging of Hodgkin's disease (stage I and II in whom radiation therapy is done).
6. For symptom control in patients with rarely painful massive splenomegaly in CML unresponsive to chemotherapy.

Q. **What are the clinical manifestations of splenectomy?**

Ans: These will be:

- The immediate manifestation within 2 – 3 weeks is leukocytosis and thrombocytosis.

- *Marked variations in size and shape of RBCs* (anisocytosis, poikilocytosis).
- *Presence of Howell-Jolly bodies* (nuclear remnants), *Heinz bodies* (denatured Hb), *basophilic stippling* and an occasional *nucleated RBC* in the peripheral blood.

Q. **What will be the consequences of splenectomy?**

Ans: The consequences will be:

1. The most serious consequence of splenectomy is predisposition to bacterial infections, particularly with S. *pneumoniae, H. influenzae, pneumococci and* some gram-negative enteric organisms. They should be immunized against these organisms.
2. The splenectomized patients are more susceptible to a parasitic disease *babesiosis,* hence, they should avoid visit to areas where the parasite Babesia is endemic.
3. The vaccination against N. *meningitidis* should also be given to patients in whom elective splenectomy is planned.

Q. **What is abscopal effect?**

Ans: Tumor regression or regression of systemic illness following splenectomy or splenic irradiation in patients with CML and prolymphocytic leukemia is known as abscopal effect.

Q. **What is Traube's area? What is its significance?**

Ans: Read the Clinical Methods in Medicine by Prof SN Chugh.

Q. **What are the differences between a splenic and left renal mass?**

Ans: Read clinical method by Prof SN Chugh.

Q. **How will you palpate spleen in the presence of ascites?**

Ans: For method of palpation of spleen (Fig. 12.1B), read clinical methods. However, in the presence of ascites, spleen is palpated by dipping method.

Q. **What are the characteristics of a splenic mass?**

Ans: Read Clinical Method in Medicine by Prof SN Chugh.

Q. **What are the other causes of mass in left hypochondrium?**

Ans: Read Clinical Method in Medicine.

13 Hepatosplenomegaly
(Chronic Myeloid Leukemia)

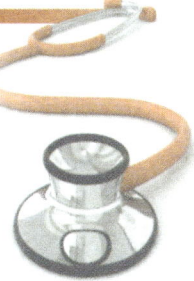

INSTRUCTION

Examine the abdomen of the patient

SALIENT FEATURES

- Pain and masses in abdomen, palpitation

HISTORY

Ask for the following:

- History of fever or sore throat, jaundice, bleeding from any site
- History of palpitation, breathlessness, orthopnea, PND (for anemia)
- Any history of infection, mouth ulcerations, mouth thrush, excoriation, etc. (for infections)
- Any history of lump/masses in abdomen

EXAMINATION

General Physical Examination

Look at:

- *Face* for puffiness, edema
- *Mouth* for ulceration, excoriation or thrush
- *Tongue* for anemia (present). Look at other sites for anemia
- *Gums* for hypertrophy and bleeding
- *Neck* for lymph node enlargement, JVP and thyroid enlargement
- *Pulse, BP, temperature* and *respiration*
- *Hands* for koilonychia, platynychia, splinter hemorrhage, clubbing
- *Feet* for edema
- *Sternal bone tenderness* present

Systemic Examination

Abdominal Examination

- Look for any swelling or bulge
- Palpate the masses in the abdomen and describe their characteristic. Both liver and spleen are palpable (Fig. 13.1)
- Percuss for Traube's area for splenic dullness and define the upper borer of the liver for its enlargement and liver span measurement
- Auscultate over the mass(es) for any bruit or rub

CVS Examination

- Examine the heart for any enlargement, murmur, sounds or rub
- Look for the signs of valvular heart disease, LVF, SABE and pericardial disease especially pericardial effusion

Examination of Blood

- Look for any hemorrhage into the skin or joint or organ
- Examine ocular fundi for hemorrhage

PROVISIONAL DIAGNOSIS

The patient has hepatosplenomegaly with anemia (lesion) the cause of which has to be found out.

QUESTIONS AND ANSWERS

Q. **What are common causes of hepatospleno-megaly?**

Ans: 1. *Infections,* e.g. malaria, kala-azar, brucellosis, typhoid, disseminated tuberculosis

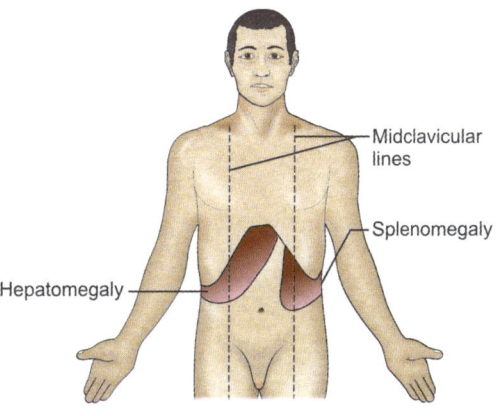

Fig. 13.1: Hepatosplenomegaly

2. *Blood disorders*
- Leukemias (acute and chronic)
- Lymphomas
- Hemolytic anemias
- Polycythemias
3. *Myelofibrosis/myelosclerosis*
4. *Budd-Chiari syndrome*
5. *Congestive hepatosplenomegaly*
- Constrictive pericarditis/pericardial effusion
- Congestive heart failure (cardiomyopathy)
6. *Amyloidosis*
7. *Sarcoidosis*

Q. Could your case be a case of miliary tuberculosis?

Ans: No. The points against are:
1. No history of fever, anorexia, weight loss and night sweats
2. No cough, breathlessness, hemoptysis
3. No chest signs e.g. crackles/wheezes
4. No neck rigidity/Kernig's sign
5. No evidence of choroid tubercles on fundus examination

Q. What are the characteristics of myelofibrosis/myelosclerosis?

Ans:
- It may be primary or secondary to toxins, malignant infiltration of bone marrow, lymphoma or irradiation.
- Massive splenomegaly with moderate hepatomegaly occur due to extramedullary hematopoiesis. Splenic rub may be present occasionally.
- Leucoerythroblastic blood picture with high platelet count
- Ground glass appearance of bone on X-ray
- Bone marrow examination may yield a "dry tap", hence, trephine biopsy is needed to confirm the diagnosis (Fig. 13.2).

Q. What are the clinical characteristics of amyloidosis?

Ans:
- It is secondary to suppurative lung disease (lung abscess, bronchiectasis), Crohn's disease, multiple myeloma, rheumatoid arthritis, leprosy
- Macroglossia may be present
- Mild to moderate hepatosplenomegaly
- Evidence of renal involvement, i.e. massive proteinuria (nephrotic syndrome)
- Other associated involvements include malabsorption, lymphadenopathy, peripheral neuropathy, cardiomyopathy

- The diagnosis is confirmed on liver, gingival or rectal biopsy

Q. What are the causes of fever with hepatosplenomegaly?

Ans: The presence of fever indicates infection or inflammation, hence, may be associated with leukocytosis or leukopenia. The causes are:
- Parasitic infections, e.g. malaria, kala-azar
- Bacterial infection, e.g. enteric fever, brucellosis, miliary tuberculosis
- Viral infection, e.g. acute lupoid hepatitis
- Acute leukemia and lymphoma
- Hemolytic crisis

Q. What are the causes of hepatosplenomegaly with jaundice?

Ans: Jaundice in presence of hepatosplenomegaly occurs either due to decompensation of liver or infection of the liver or due to hemolysis. The causes are:

- Cirrhosis of liver with decompensation
- Budd-Chiari syndrome (hepatic vein thrombosis)
- Lupoid hepatitis
- Malaria (falciparum infection producing hemolysis)
- Lymphoma (especially non-Hodgkin's)
- Miliary tuberculosis

Q. What are the conditions that produce hepatosplenomegaly with ascites?

Ans: Ascites in the presence of hepatosplenomegaly may be a sign of portal hypertension or hepatocellular failure or may be due to malignant infiltration of the peritoneum. The causes are:
- Malignancy liver (primary or secondary) with portal hypertension
- Cirrhosis of liver with portal hypertension
- Budd-Chiari syndrome with portal hypertension
- Chronic myeloid leukemia
- Lymphoma (non-Hodgkin's)
- Subacute or lupoid hepatitis with or without hepatocellular failure
- Congestive hepatosplenomegaly (CHF, pericardial effusion)

Q. What are the clinical characteristics of kala-azar?

Ans:
- Hepatosplenomegaly in which spleen is massively enlarged while liver enlargement is moderate. Both are firm and nontender.

- Fever and hyperpigmentation. Fever is nocturnal.
- The diagnosis is confirmed by demonstration of LD bodies in buffy coat preparations of blood or from the bone marrow smear or lymph node, liver or spleen aspirates (splenic puncture).
- Patient belongs to an endemic area
- Double rise or peak in temperature (biphasic pattern) in 24 hours may be present.

Q. How would you investigate this case?

Ans: The investigations to be done are:

1. TLC and DLC. Leukocytosis indicates pyogenic infections, polycythemia and leukemia while leukopenia occurs in malaria, enteric fever, kala-azar. Pancytopenia indicates hypersplenism.

2. *Peripheral blood film* for MP, kala-azar (LD bodies) and hemolytic anemia (abnormal type of cells) or other types of anemia. Reticulocytosis indicates hemolytic anemia. Presence of premature WBCs indicates leukemia (acute or chronic).

3. *Blood culture* for enteric

4. *Special tests*
   - Paul-Bunnell test for infectious mononucleosis
   - Widal test for typhoid and brucella
   - Serum bilirubin for jaundice
   - Aldehyde test for kala-azar
   - Tests for hemolysis, e.g. osmotic fragility, Coombs' test

5. *Radiology*
   - Chest X-ray for:
     - miliary tuberculosis (miliary mottling)
     - lymphoma and sarcoidosis (mediastinal widening due to mediastinal lymphadenopathy)
   - X-ray bones
     - Skull ('Hair on end' appearance in thalassemia)
     - Long bones, e.g. expansion of lower ends of the bone in Gaucher's disease. Increased density of the bones in myelofibrosis or myelosclerosis

6. USG *of abdomen*
   - To confirm hepatosplenomegaly
   - To detect the presence of ascites, portal hypertension (portal vein diameter >14 mm) and dilated venous collaterals
   - To detect echogenic pattern of the liver (heterogenous pattern indicates cirrhosis)

7. *Biopsy*
   - Lymph node biopsy for tuberculosis, sarcoidosis and lymphoma
   - Liver biopsy for cirrhosis of the liver and amyloidosis
   - Bone marrow biopsy (trephine) for myelofibrosis
   - Bone marrow aspiration for leukemia, lymphoma, Gaucher's disease, hypersplenism (pancytopenia with hypercellular marrow), and splenic aspirate for kala-azar.

8. *Skin tests*
   - Mantoux test for tuberculosis
   - Kveim test for sarcoidosis (not done now a days)

9. *CT scan abdomen*
   - To detect lymph node enlargement
   - To confirm the findings on USG
   - To stage the lymphoma

14 Hepatosplenomegaly with Lymphadenopathy

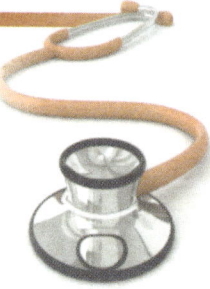

INSTRUCTION

- Perform general physical examination
- Examine the abdomen

SALIENT FEATURES

- Swelling neck and masses abdomen

HISTORY

Ask for the following:

- Site(s), duration and extent
- Any history of swelling in the axilla or groin
- Any history of pain abdomen or mass abdomen (e.g. spleen and/or liver)
- Any history of cough, dyspnea or hoarseness of voice (for hilar lymphadenopathy)
- Any history of injury or infection of neck or extremity
- History of fever, drenching night sweats and weight loss ('B' symptoms of lymphoma)
- Past history of fever, tuberculosis, malignancy or injury/infection (HIV)
- Personal history including occupation

EXAMINATION

General Physical Examination

- *Face* for puffiness or edema
- *Mouth* for anemia (present) or evidence of infection (ulceration) petechiae and pharyngitis (glandular fever)
- *Skin* for evidence of bleeding or infection
- *Neck.* There is a visible swelling in the right side of neck. Examine the swelling for groups of cervical lymph nodes (Fig. 14.1) and describe the number, consistency, tenderness, matting, adherence to underlying structures or overlying skin. Note the temperature over the mass. Look for JVP and thyroid. Examine also the pre-auricular, post-auricular, submental lymph nodes, etc.
- Examine *axillae* and *inguinal regions* in addition to all other sites of lymph node.

- Look for *engorgement of neck/chest veins, suffusion of the face* and *cyanosis* (e.g. superior mediastinal compression).
- Record pulse, BP, respiration and temperature
- Look for *anemia, jaundice, edema*, etc.

Systemic Examination

Examination of Abdomen

- Inspect the abdomen for any swelling or protuberance
- Palpate the abdomen for liver, spleen or lymph node enlargement. They are enlarged (Fig. 14.1)
- Look for the presence of ascites (absent in this case)

Examination of Respiratory System

- Inspect the chest for any retraction or deformity
- Palpate the trachea for any deviation
- Look for any evidence of mediastinal shift due to lung collapse
- Look for signs of superior mediastinal compression, e.g. periorbital edema, chemosis, conjunctival suffusion, prominence of neck veins and veins over the chest, absent venous pulsations in the neck (not present in this case)

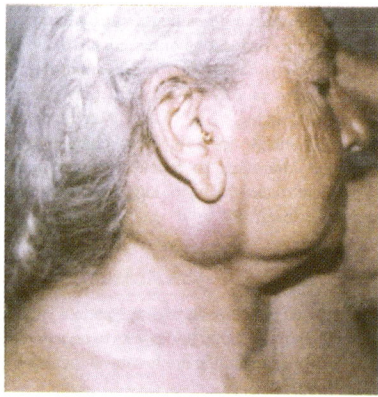

Fig. 14.1: A patient with cervical lymphadenopathy with hepatosplenomegaly due to lymphoma

Examination of Hematopoietic System
- Look for any evidence of purpuric or ecchymotic patches
- Elicit sternal tenderness
- Any evidence of infection
- Ocular fundus examination

PROVISIONAL DIAGNOSIS

The patient has non-tender lymphadenopathy neck with hepatosplenomegaly (lesion) caused by non-Hodgkin's lymphoma (etiology). There are no B symptoms (functional status).

QUESTIONS AND ANSWERS

Q. What are the points in favor of your diagnosis?

Ans: • Painless progressive lymphadenopathy in a middle aged female
- The lymph nodes enlargement is diffuse, involves all groups of lymph nodes in the neck. The nodes are firm, isolated and non-tender

- Liver and spleen are enlarged
- Presence of anemia
- B symptoms, i.e. low grade fever, sweating, weight loss, fatigue not present

Q. Why your case is not a case of Hodgkin's lymphoma?

Ans: The characteristics of Hodgkin's lymphoma are given in Table 14.1.

Q. Why your case is not of lymphatic leukemia?

Ans: Read Table 14.1.

Q. What is non-Hodgkin's lymphoma?

Ans: They are heterogenous group of malignant disorder of lymphoid tissue involving chiefly the B cells (85%) and to some extent T cells and NK cells (15%). They vary in their presentation and natural history varying from slow indolent course (low grade) to a rapidly progressive disease (intermediate and high grade).

Q. What are the causes of hepatosplenomegaly with lymphadenopathy?

Ans: The liver, spleen and lymph nodes constitute the lymphoreticular system, hence, the

Features	Lymphoblastic leukemia	Non-Hodgkin's lymphoma	Hodgkin's lymphoma
1. Cellular derivation	80% B, 20% T cells	90% B, 10% T	Unresolved
2. Age	Children	Young age	Middle age around 30–40 years
3. Site of the disease			
• Localised	Uncommon	Uncommon	Common
• Nodal spread	Common, non-contiguous lymph nodes involved	Discontiguous nodes involved	Contiguous nodes involved
• Nodal characteristics	Discrete, painful, soft	Painless, discrete lymph nodes, soft to firm	Rubbery consistency, discrete nodes
– Common groups involved	Cervical and axillary groups	Involvement of Waldeyer's ring, Epitrochlear node	Cervical group is involved early, but later all groups may be involved
– Mediastinal (pressure symptoms, e.g. superior vena cava, bronchus, spinal cord compression)	Common	Common	Common
– Abdominal	Uncommon	Common	Uncommon
4. Extranodal involvement	Common	Common	Uncommon
5. Bone marrow involvement	Always	Common	Uncommon
6. B symptoms (e.g. fever, weight loss, night sweats)	Common	Uncommon	Common
7. Chromosomal defects	Common (translocations, deletion)	Common (translocations, deletion)	Common (aneuploidy)
8. Curability	40–60%	30–40%	75–85%

Table 14.1: Lymphoid leukemia and lymphomas

disorders involving this system will produce their enlargement such as:

- Acute leukemia especially ALL in children
- Lymphoma (Hodgkin's and non-Hodgkin's)
- Miliary tuberculosis
- Sarcoidosis
- AIDS
- Infectious mononucleosis
- Collagen vascular disorder, e.g. SLE

Q. What is HIV-AIDS related lymphoma?

Ans: It is aggressive lymphoma and accounts for 20% cases of NHL (non-Hodgkin's lymphoma). This lymphoma is identical to Burkitt's lymphoma most of the times and carries a poor prognosis.

Q. What is MALT lymphoma?

Ans: It is B-cell gastric lymphoma called *maltoma* (mucosa associated lymphoid tissue lymphoma). It is induced by *H. pylori* infection of the stomach.

Q. What is the mode of presentation of Hodgkin's disease?

Ans: • Usually as a painless lymph node enlargement in young age
- Other presenting symptoms include systemic features such as pyrexia, drenching night sweats, weight loss, pain in the affected lymph nodes after ingestion of alcohol and generalized itching.

Q. How do you classify non-Hodgkin's lymphoma?

Ans: Previous classification of non-Hodgkin's lymphoma into low grade (slow, indolent and favorable prognosis) and high grade (aggressive, unfavorable) has been replaced by WHO (2001). The proposed WHO classification of non-Hodgkin's lymphoma is as follows:

1. *Precursor B-cell lymphoblastic lymphoma Mature B*
   - Diffuse large B-cell lymphoma
   - Mediastinal large B-cell lymphoma
   - Follicular central cell lymphoma
   - Small lymphocytic lymphoma
   - Lymphoplasmacytic lymphoma (Waldenstrom macroglobulinemia)
   - Mantle cell lymphoma
   - Burkitt lymphoma

- Marginal zone lymphoma
  — Malt type
  — Nodal type
  — Splenic type
2. *Precursor T-cell lymphoblastic lymphoma*
3. *Mature T (and NK cell)*
   - Anaplastic T-cell lymphoma
   - Peripheral T-cell lymphoma
   - Cutaneous T-cell lymphoma (mycosis fungoids)
   - T/NK cell lymphoma

Q. How do you stage Hodgkin's disease?

Ans: Stage I: Only one lymph node site involved

Stage II: More than 2 lymph nodes sites involved on one side of the diaphragm

Stage III: Lymph nodes involved on both sides of the diaphragm

Stage IV: Disseminated disease with extranodal involvement (e.g. bone marrow, liver)

A means absence of systemic symptoms and **B** means presence of systemic symptoms, e.g. fever, sweating, weakness and weight loss.

Q. What do you understand by the term Hodgkin's disease?

Ans: It is an abnormal proliferation of lymphoid tissue (neoplasm of lymphoid tissue), characterized by development of lymphadenopathy at single or multiple sites. The pathological hallmark is *Reed-Sternberg cells* derived from germinal center B cells, rarely peripheral T cells.

Q. What are the histological subtypes of Hodgkin's disease?

Ans: The 4 subtypes are:
- Lymphocyte predominance
- Nodular sclerosis
- Mixed cellularity
- Lymphocyte depletion

Q. How would you treat Hodgkin's lymphoma?

Ans: • Localized disease (stage IA, IIA) is treated by radiotherapy.
- Disseminated disease (IIIB and IV stages) is treated with combination chemotherapy (e.g. A B V D and M O P P regimen).
- Stages IIB and IIIA are nowadays treated with combination chemotherapy.

15

Lymphadenopathy

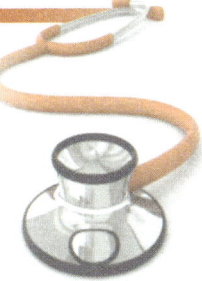

INSTRUCTION

- Perform general physical and relevant systemic examination

SALIENT FEATURES

- Patient complains of multiple swellings in the neck

HISTORY

Ask about the following:

- Age of onset and progression of masses
- Occupation (sarcoidosis)
- Site of involvement
- Duration of swellings
- Ask about associated symptoms of tuberculosis (anorexia weight loss, evening rise of temperature, drenching sweats), and 'B symptoms' of lymphomas (unexplained weight loss, profuse night sweats, fever)
- Ask about any abdominal mass, pain, etc.
- Any history of cough, dyspnea, hoarseness of voice, suffusion of face, periorbital puffiness (superior mediastinal compression)
- Any history of trauma or infection of extremities (regional lymphadenopathy)
- History of HIV (sexual history)
- Past history of tuberculosis, malignancy, injury

EXAMINATION

General Physical Examination

1. *Neck*
   - Inspect the neck and describe the location of the mass(es) and their surface and condition of the skin over the mass(es), e.g. sinuses, pigmentation or scrofuloderma.
   - Palpate the lymph nodes and comment on their size, shape, locations (groups involved), texture, tenderness, consistency, matting/adhesiveness, margins and fixa-

tion to overlying/underlying structures. The *sites of lymph nodes* to be examined are:

1. Pre-auricular in front of ear
2. Posterior auricular superficial to mastoid process behind the ear
3. Occipital below the occiput
4. Tonsillar at the angle of mandible
5. Submandibular below the mandible
6. Submental below the chin
7. Superficial cervical superficial to sternomastoid
8. Posterior cervical along the anterior edge of trapezius
9. Deep cervical chain deeper to the sternomastoid. To palpate them, hook your thumb and fingers around either side of sternomastoid to find them.
10. Supraclavicular. Palpate them deep in the angle formed by the clavicle and sternomastoid
11. Axillary lymph nodes in the axillary pit
12. Epitrochlear lymph nodes at elbow
13. Inguinal lymph nodes in the inguinal region
14. Popliteal lymph nodes in the popliteal fossa

    Depending on the lymph nodes enlargement, proceed further as follows:

    a. For enlargement of inguinal lymph nodes:
       - *Examine the lower extremities and external genital for any lesion.*

    b. When axillary lymph nodes are palpable and enlarged:
       - *Examine chest, breast and upper limbs.*

c. When upper cervical lymph nodes are enlarged:

- *Examine the chest, breast and upper limbs.*
- *Examine ear, nose and throat for nasopharyngeal carcinoma.*

d. When lower cervical and supraclavicular lymph nodes are enlarged:

- *Examine thyroid, chest, abdomen for gastric carcinoma (Virchow's nodes) and testis.*

2. *Mouth:* Examine the mouth for:

- Tonsillar enlargement/peritonsillar abscess
- Palate for petechiae
- Pharynx for infection (glandular fever)
- Neoplasms of mouth (tongue)

Systemic Examination

a. *Abdomen:* Examine abdomen for lymph nodes enlargement (pre and para-aortic lymph nodes), liver and spleen.
b. *Chest:* Examine the chest for evidence of tuberculosis, malignancy, sarcoidosis, etc.

PROVISIONAL DIAGNOSIS

The patient has a mass of lymph nodes in the neck with skin changes of sacrofuloderma (lesion) caused by tubercular lymphadenitis (cause) without any evidence of pulmonary tuberculosis (functional status).

QUESTIONS AND ANSWERS

Q. What are the points in favor of your diagnosis?

Ans: The presence of a lobulated, irregular mass in cervical region with irregular surface, firm in consistency, non mobile, fixed to the skin with formation of a sinus and skin pigmentation indicate this lymph node mass due to tuberculosis, e.g. tubercular lymphadenitis with sacrofuloderma (Fig. 15.1).

Q. What is differential diagnosis?

Ans: The following conditions come into differential diagnosis of cervical lymphadenopathy:
- Tubercular lymphadenitis, HIV infections
- Infectious mononucleosis
- Hodgkin's and non-Hodgkin's lymphoma, leukemia (ALL)
- Lung carcinoma
- Infection in the draining area, i.e. face, neck
- Sarcoidosis

Q. What are the causes of regional lymphadenopathy?

Ans: The sites of lymph nodes enlargement and their causes are given in Table 15.1.

Q. How do you define lymphadenopathy? What is significant lymphadenopathy?

Ans. Lymphadenopathy literally means enlargement of lymph nodes whether significant or insignificant.
Significant lymphadenopathy means enlargement that needs further evaluation. Lymph

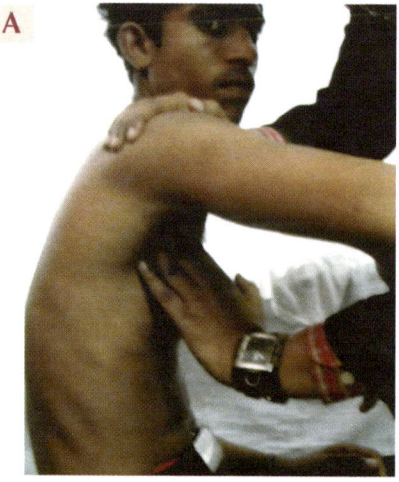
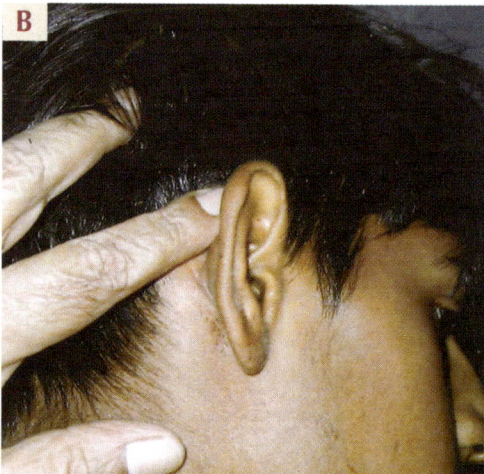

Fig. 15.1: A palpation of lymph nodes; (A) Axillary; (B) Posterior auricular

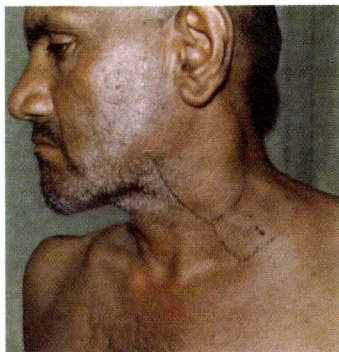

Fig. 15.2: Cervical lymphadenopathy (encircled)

nodes enlargement >1 cm in size anywhere in the body is considered as significant except the groin where >2 cm size of the lymph node is considered significant. Insignificant enlargement means nonspecific, small lymph nodes usually <0.5 cm in diameter, may be palpable due to past infection.

Q. **What is generalized lymphadenopathy? What are its causes?**

Ans: A generalized adenopathy has been defined as involvement of three or more noncontiguous lymph node areas. The causes are:

- Tuberculosis, syphilis
- Infectious mononucleosis
- Toxoplasmosis, histoplasmosis
- AIDS and other viral infections
- Collagen vascular disorders

- Leukemias, e.g. acute and chronic lymphocytic leukemia
- Lymphomas (Hodgkin's and non-Hodgkin's)
- Sarcoidosis
- Drugs, e.g. phenytoin, hydralazine, gold

Q. **What are the causes of painful tender enlarged lymph nodes?**

Ans: Tenderness or pain in lymphadenopathy is due to stretching of the capsule as a result of rapid or sudden enlargement of lymph node. The causes are:

1. *Acute inflammation or infection*
   - Viral (infectious mononucleosis)
   - Bacterial (pyogenic infections, tuberculosis, brucellosis, plague, diphtheria, leprosy)
   - Parasitic (toxoplasmosis)
   - Fungal infections
2. *Immunological causes*
   - SLE and other collagen vascular disorders
   - Rheumatoid arthritis
3. *Neoplastic*
   - Acute leukemia (lymphoblastic)
   - Metastases in the lymph node

Q. **What is the cause of egg-shelled calcification in hilar lymph nodes?**

Ans: Silicosis.

Table 15.1: Site of involvement of lymph node as a clue to the diagnosis

Site	Cause(s)
Occipital adenopathy	Scalp infection
Pre-auricular adenopathy	Conjunctival infection
Left supraclavicular lymph node (*Virchow's gland*) and other supraclavicular nodes enlargement	Metastasis from gastric or gastrointestinal cancer • Tuberculosis, sarcoidosis, toxoplasmosis • Metastases from lung, breast, testis or ovary • Injuries of upper limb
Axillary lymphadenopathy	• Localized infection of ipsilateral upper extremity • Malignancies, e.g. melanoma, lymphoma and breast carcinoma
Inguinal lymphadenopathy	• Infections or trauma of lower extremity, plague • Sexually transmitted diseases, e.g. lymphogranuloma venereum, primary syphilis, genital herpes or chancroid • Lymphomas and metastases from rectum and genitalia
Thoracic lymph nodes (hilar lymphadenopathy)	• Tuberculosis, sarcoidosis, fungal infection • Lymphoma, malignancy lung with metastases in lymph node
Abdominal lymphadenopathy (retroperitoneal, para-aortic)	• Tuberculosis (mesenteric lymphadenitis) • Lymphoma • Metastases from the abdominal viscera

Q.   **What do you know of Sister Joseph's nodule?**

Ans: It refers to a nodule around umbilicus seen in gastric adenocarcinoma, represents either a metastatic deposit or an enlarged anterior abdominal wall lymph node.

Q.   **What are the causes of fixation of the lymph nodes to surrounding structures?**

Ans: The causes are:
- Tuberculosis
- Malignancy or metastases in the lymph nodes

Q.   **What are the causes of lymphadenopathy with splenomegaly?**

Ans: The causes are:
- Infectious mononucleosis
- Lymphoma, lymphatic leukemia
- Sarcoidosis
- Collagen vascular disorders, e.g. SLE, RA
- Toxoplasmosis
- Cat-scratch disease
- Disseminated or miliary tuberculosis.

Q.   **How will you investigate a case with lymphadenopathy?**

Ans: The investigations are done to find out the cause. They are planned depending on the site and type of involvement.

1. *Complete hemogram.* Presence of anemia with lymphadenopathy indicates chronic infections, chronic disorders (e.g. rheumatoid arthritis, or Felty's syndrome, SLE) or malignant disease (e.g. leukemias, lymphomas, metastasis).

    Complete blood count can provide useful data for diagnosis of acute or chronic leukemia (leukocytosis with immature cells), infectious mononucleosis (leukopenia), lymphoma, pyogenic infections (leukocytosis) or immune cytopenia in illness like SLE.

    Raised ESR suggests tuberculosis, rheumatoid arthritis, SLE, acute infections.

2. *Serological tests*
    - To demonstrate antibodies specific to components of EBV, CMV, HIV and other viruses, *Toxoplasma gondii, brucella*
    - VDRL test for syphilis
    - Antinuclear antibodies, LE cell phenomenon and anti-DNA antibodies for SLE and other collagen vascular disorders
    - Rheumatoid factor for rheumatoid arthritis

3. *Blood culture* for acute infections

4. *Chest X-ray.* For hilar or mediastinal lymph node enlargement, if any. Unilateral hilar lymph node enlargement usually suggests malignancy lung or tuberculosis; bilateral enlargement indicates sarcoidosis, histoplasmosis or lymphoma.

    The chest X-ray will also confirm the involvement of lung in acute infections, tuberculosis, and primary or metastatic lung tumours.

5. *Imaging techniques* (ultrasound, color Doppler ultrasonography, CT scan, MRI) have been employed to differentiate benign from malignant lymph nodes especially in head and neck cancer. These techniques especially USG have been used to demonstrate the ratio of long (L) axis to short (S) axis in cervical nodes. An L/S ratio of <2.0 is used to distinguish between benign and malignant lymph nodes in head and neck cancer and has sensitivity and specificity of 95%. This ratio has greater sensitivity and specificity than palpation or measurement of either the long or short axis alone.

    Ultrasonography or CT scan abdomen will also reveal lymph node enlargement in the chest and abdomen (mesenteric, para-aortic) which are not palpable on per abdomen examination. These imaging techniques are used for staging lymphomas and to detect enlargement of spleen before it becomes palpable.

6. *Lymph node biopsy.* The indications for lymph node biopsy are impressive in spite of so many studies done in this regard, yet it remains a valuable diagnostic tool. It is useful to carry out lymph node biopsy:
    - If history and physical findings suggest a malignancy, i.e. a solitary, hard, nontender cervical node in an older patient who is chronic smoker.
    - Supraclavicular lymphadenopathy.
    - Generalized or solitary lymphadenopathy with splenomegaly suggestive of lymphoma.

Find needle aspiration should not be performed as the first diagnostic procedure. Most diagnoses require more tissue than obtained on FNAC.

- A young patient with peripheral lymphadenopathy (lymph node size >2 cm in diameter with abnormal chest X-ray).

Generally, any lymph node >2 cm in diameter should be biopsied for etiological diagnosis.

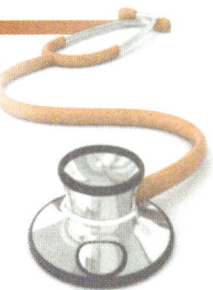

16

Abdominal Masses

INSTRUCTION

Examine the abdomen of the patient

SALIENT FEATURES

- Mass(es) in the abdomen

HISTORY

Ask about the following:

- Age of the patient (old patient), anorexia, nausea, vomiting fullness of epigastrium after meals (present in this case), hematemesis, malena (black color stools)
- Alcohol intake, spicy food, salted or pickled food, smoking
- History of dysphagia
- Family history of gastric carcinoma
- History of long duration of dyspeptic symptoms (*H. pylori infection*)
- History of painless progressive jaundice (*pancreatic cancer*)
- History of fullness and abnormal pulsations (*aneurysm of the aorta*)
- History of abdominal discomfort and pain (*lymphoma*)

EXAMINATION

General Physical Examination

Neck: No lymphadenopathy, skin is pale and patient is anemic

Systemic Examination

Examination of Abdomen

Inspection

- There is fullness in the epigastrium
- No visible peristalsis (pyloric stenosis)
- A skin nodule is present around the umbilicus (Fig. 16.1C)

Palpation

- There is ill-defined masses in the epigastrium which is mobile from side to side, tender, firm in consistency, becomes less prominent when patient raises his head against resistance.
- There is no hepatomegaly, ascites
- A firm nodule about 1 cm in diameter is felt around the umbilicus (Fig. 16.1C)

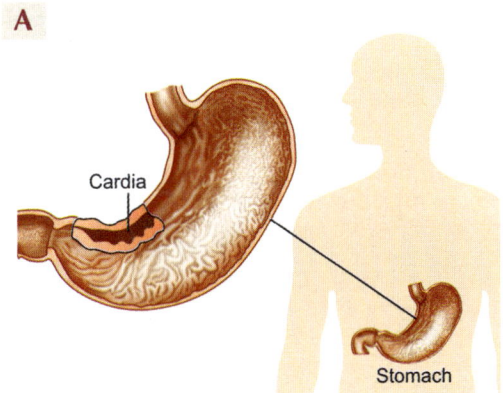

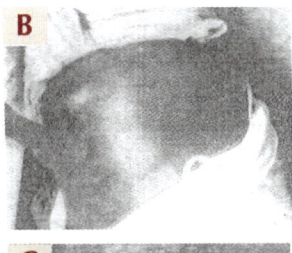

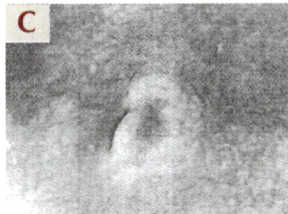

Fig. 16.1: (A) Adenocarcinoma of stomach; (B) Patient with abdominal swelling; (C) Sister Mary Joseph nodule around umbilicus

Percussion

Mass is dull on percussion

Auscultation

- Abnormal borborygmi sounds (peristaltic movements from left to right are increased after water drinking)
- Succession splash is present

Other Systems

- Lung and bone are not involved.

PROVISIONAL DIAGNOSIS

The old person presenting with anorexia and dyspeptic symptoms, has an ill-defined mass in the epigastrium (lesion) due to gastric malignancy (aetiology) which has not spread to distant organs (functional status).

QUESTIONS AND ANSWERS

Q. What are the points in favour of diagnosis?
Ans: • Old person
- Anorexia, nausea and dyspeptic symptoms
- Anemia and asthenia
- Ill-defined mass in the epigastrium
- Visible peristalsis from left to right indicating pyloric obstruction

Q. What is differential diagnosis of this mass?
Ans: The causes of mass in this region are:
1. Gastric carcinoma
2. Pancreatic carcinoma or pseudopancreatic cyst
3. Abdominal aortic aneurysm
4. Retroperitoneal lymphoma (lymphadenopathy)
5. Epigastric ventral hernia

Q. What are the characteristics of pancreatic carcinoma?
Ans: 1. Painless progressive jaundice
2. Pruritus
3. An abdominal lump in a male patient
4. A palpable gall bladder

Q. What are the characteristics of abdominal aortic aneurysm?
Ans: This has been discussed as a separate case.

Q. What are the characteristics of lymphoma?
Ans: • An ill defined mass in the epigastrium
- Mass is retroperitoneal
- Mass is irregular, non tender and firm, non mobile
- There many be lympadenopathy, splenomegaly and hepatomegaly

Q. What are the characteristics of a gallbladder mass?
Ans: The gallbladder mass is palpable either due to impacted cystic duct stone or carcinoma of head of pancreas or malignancy of gall bladder. The characteristic features are:
1. The mass is globular in shape, firm in consistency, palpable in right hypochondrium
2. Firm in consistency, moves with respiration
3. Dull on percussion
4. Jaundice with pruritus is usually present
5. Common in females
6. CT scan (Fig. 16.2) is diagnostic

Q. What are the characteristics of para-aortic lymph nodes mass?
Ans: Lymph node mass is common in para-aortic region either due to tuberculosis or lymphoma. The characteristic features are:
1. A lobulated intra-abdominal mass around the umbilicus.
2. It is firm to hard in consistency.
3. It is immobile, dull on percussion.
4. CT scan is diagnostic (Fig. 16.3).

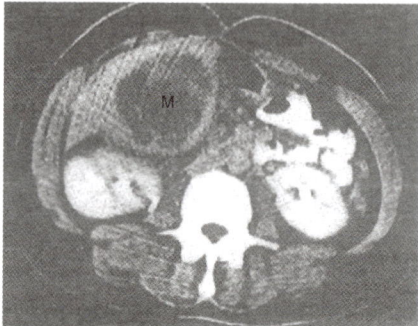

Fig. 16.2: Gall bladder carcinoma. CT scan shows squamous cell carcinoma

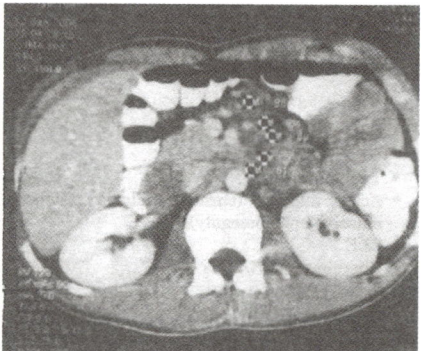

Fig. 16.3: Abdominal lymphadenopathy. CT scan shows enlarged para-aortic group of lymph nodes (indicated by XXXX)

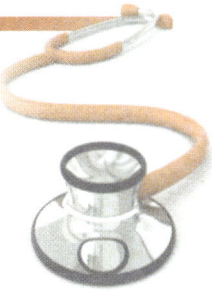

17

Dysphagia

INSTRUCTION

Examine the abdomen of the patient

SALIENT FEATURES

• A malnourished patient

HISTORY

Ask about the following:

• Onset and duration of symptom(s)
• Is difficulty in deglutition progressive or stationary (progressive dysphagia indicates an organic cause)?
• Is difficulty in swallowing is limited to liquids, solids or both?

  Dysphagia to liquids suggest motility disorders, while to solids indicates esophageal stricture

• Nasal regurgitation
• Does swallowing provoke cough?
• Is the swallowing painful (odynophagia)?
• Is dysphagia intermittent?

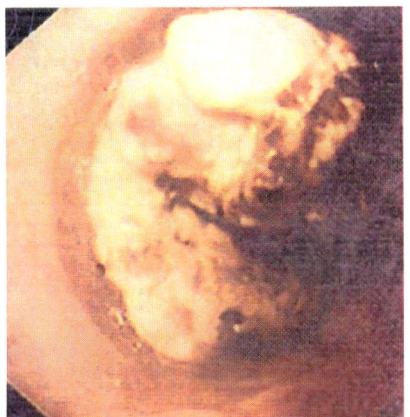

Fig. 17.1: Dysphagia; upper gastrointestinal endoscopy showing polypoidal, ulcerated growth suggestive of esophageal cancer

• Where does the bolus of food stick, i.e. suprasternal notch or midsternal region?
• Does the neck distend or gurgle during swallowing (pharyngeal pouch)?
• Is there any associated symptoms, e.g. nausea, vomiting, heart burn, sour erectation?
• History of stroke or myasthenia gravis or any other neurological disorders (motor neuron disease)

EXAMINATION

General Physical Examination

• Person is emaciated, malnourished
• Mouth for ulcer, thrush, pallor, angular stomatitis, cheilosis, bald tongue (present)
• Neck for lymph nodes, goitre, raised JVP (superior mediastinal compression, mitral valve disease)
• Examine skin for scleroderma
• Elicit gag reflex and jaw jerk for bulbar or pseudobulbar palsy

Other System Examination

1. *Abdominal examination* for any mass or organomegaly
2. *Neurological examination* for cranial nerves or neurological cause of dysphagia
3. *Cardiovascular system examination* for mitral valve disease or aortic arch aneurysm

PROVISIONAL DIAGNOSIS

The patient has dysphagia to solids (lesion) due to esophageal growth (etiology). He is anemic, emaciated and malnourished (functional status).

QUESTIONS AND ANSWERS

Q. What is odynophagia?
Ans: Painful swallowing is called *odynophagia*. It is caused by oesophageal ulcer, esophagitis, oesophageal spasm and oesophageal cancer,

Q.   What is photophobia?

Ans: Photophobia means fear about swallowing, occurs in hysteria, rabies, tetanus and pharyngeal paralysis.

Q.   What do you mean by the term sensation of globus?

Ans: Globus means persistent or intermittent sensation of a lump or a foreign body in the throat in between meals. It is a symptom of psychiatric disorder or hysteria, hence called globus hystericus.

Q.   What are the common causes of dysphagia?

Ans: The cause are:

I. Mechanical causes

   A. *Intrinsic obstruction within esophagus*
   - Foreign body in esophagus
   - Congenital atresia
   - Esophagitis, glossitis
   - Esophageal/pharyngeal web (Plummer-Vinson's syndrome)
   - Esophageal stricture and neoplasm

   B. *Extrinsic compressions of esophagus*
   - Retropharyngeal mass or abscess
   - Retrosternal goitre
   - Enlargement left atrium (mitral valve disease)
   - Aortic aneurysm
   - Posterior mediastinal mass

II. Neuromuscular causes (motor dysphagia)
   - Bulbar and pseudobulbar paralysis
   - Myasthenia gravis
   - Oculopharyngeal myopathy
   - Achalasia cardia
   - Diffuse esophageal spasms
   - Chagas' disease
   - Scleroderma
   - Diabetes mellitus
   - Presbyoesophagus

Q.   What is Plummer-Vinson's syndrome?

Ans: It has already been answered in case discussion on anemia. However, it comprises iron deficiency anemia, koilonychia, dysphagia with or without splenomegaly.

Q.   What do you understand by term presbyoesophagus?

Ans: It is a condition seen in elderly in which there is impaired motility of the esophagus due to ageing.

Q.   How would you investigate a case of dysphagia?

Ans: 1. Complete hemogram for anemia
   2. Chest X-ray for cardiac enlargement, mediastinal enlargement, tuberculosis and aspiration pneumonia.
   3. Endoscopy of esophagus to localize the obstruction or to find out the cause.
   4. Barium swallow and videofluoroscopy.
   5. Esophageal manometry for esophageal spasm, achalasia cardia, and systemic sclerosis.

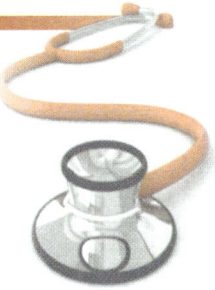

18

Ulcerative Colitis

INSTRUCTION

Examine the abdomen of the patient

SALIENT FEATURES

- Blood and mucus in stools

HISTORY

Ask about the following:

- Age and sex
- Onset of symptoms
- History of chronic diarrhea with blood and mucus
- Abdominal pain, tenesmus and discomfort
- Anorexia, weight loss, malaise
- Symptoms of anemia (fatigue, weakness palpitation, breathlessness, headache) present
- Perianal symptoms if any, i.e. pain
- Extraintestinal manifestations, i.e. iritis, episcleritis, skin changes, heart valve involvement

EXAMINATION

General Physical Examination

- General pallor (anemia) is present in this case
- Mouth for ulcer, cheilosis, angular stomatitis, aphthous ulceration
- Eye for uveitis, iridocyclitis
- Joints are arthropathy
- Skin for erythema nodosum, pyoderma gangrenosa
- Jaundice (sclerosing cholangitis, hepatitis)

Abdominal Examination

- Abdomen is soft and diffusely tender (in this case)
- Tenderness can be elicited on the left side of the colon (Fig. 18.1)
- There is no mass palpable
- Perianal examination shows no hemorrhoids/skin, stricture, fissure or fistula
- Rectal examination shows staining of the finger with blood and mucus (in this case). No mass palpable per rectum

PROVISIONAL DIAGNOSIS

The patient has fever, loose motions with blood and mucus for >3 months, has developed anemia and diffusely tender distended abdomen (lesion) probably due to inflammatory bowel disease, i.e. ulcerative colitis (etiology). Patient is depressed (functional status).

QUESTIONS AND ANSWERS

Q. **What are the characteristic features of ulcerative colitis?**

Ans: Read Table 18.1.

Q. **How does ulcerative colitis differ from Crohn's disease?**

Ans: Read Table 18.1.

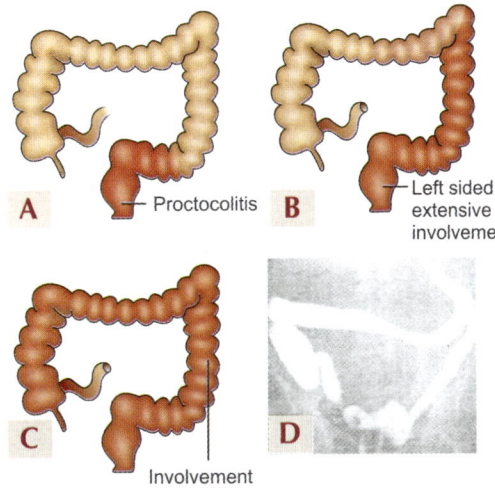

Fig. 18.1: Colonic involvement in ulcerative colitis. (A) Proctocolitis; (B) Extensive left side colitis; (C) Pancolitis; (D) Barium enema showing stem-pipe colon

Table 18.1: Clinical features of inflammatory bowel disease

Features	Crohn's disease	Ulcerative colitis
Presenting symptoms	Diarrhea and pain abdomen in right lower quadrant with tenderness and guarding.	Diarrhea with blood, mucus and pus. Pain abdomen and fever may be present. There is tenderness in left side of abdomen or left iliac fossa.
Palpation	A mass may be palpable on abdominal or rectal examination. It is an inflammatory mass.	No mass palpable.
Colics/diffuse pain	Recurrent abdominal colics are common due to obstruction.	No colicky pain. Toxic megacolon may produce diffuse pain associated with distension of abdomen and stoppage of loose motions.
Signs and symptoms	• Moderate diarrhea and fever. • Stools are loose but well formed. • Features of malabsorption of fat, carbohydrate, protein and vit. D and vit. B_{12} are common. • Anemia, weight loss, growth retardation in children.	• Patients have severe diarrhea with tenesmus. • Stools are passed with blood and mucus. • Malabsorptive features are less common but dehydration is common. • Anemia, weight loss present.
Complications		
Relpases or remissions	Common	Common
Hemorrhoids/skin tag	Common	Uncommon
Stricture/fissure	Common	Less common
Abscess and fistulas	Common	Less common
Carcinoma *in situ*	Less common	More common in long standing diseases.
Extraintestinal features		
• Eye (Uveitis, episcleritis, conjuctivitis)	Less common	Common
• Joints (arthritis, arthralgia and ankylosing spondylitis)	Less common	Common
• Skin (erythema nodosum, pyoderma gangrenosa)	Common	Less common
• Liver (sclerosing cholangitis, hepatitis, fatty liver)	Common	Uncommon
• Heart (AR, mitral valve prolapse)	Less common	Common

Note: These distinctions in clinical features are arbitrary and should not be interpreted in absolute sense.

Q. What is the differential diagnosis?

Ans: Following conditions have to be differentiated

1. Amebic colitis
2. Nonspecific colitis
3. Irritable bowel syndrome
4. Tuberculosis of the intestine
5. Carcinoma of colon
6. Diverticulitis

Q. What are the extraintestinal manifestations of this condition?

Ans:
1. Iritis, conjunctivitis, anterior uveitis, keratitis, keratoconjunctivitis sicca, choroiditis.
2. Arthritis
3. Erythema nodosum, pyoderma gangrenosa
4. Sclerosing pericholangitis, hepatitis
5. Aortic regurgitation, mitral valve prolapse

Q. **Name few conditions which are associated with it.**

Ans: 1. Ankylosing spondylitis

2. Sacrolitis

3. Cholangitis, hepatitis

Q. **What are the complications of ulcerative colitis?**

Ans: 1. Intestinal hemorrhage

2. Toxic megacolon

3. Carcinoma colon

4. Pericholangitis and pyogenic liver abscesses

5. Intestinal perforation (rare)

Q. **How would you investigate this patient?**

Ans: • Complete hemogram, ESR and C-reactive protein

• Stool examination for blood and pus cells

• Stool and blood culture

• Testes for malabsorption especially serum iron, B_{12} and folate level

• Liver function tests

• Sigmoidoscopy, colonoscopy and rectal biopsy

• Small bowel enema

• Capsule endoscopy to determine the extent of small bowel involvement

• Barium enema (Fig. 18.2) shows polyps and pseudopolyps, superficial colonic ulceration with no skip areas. In advan-

ced disease, there is loss of haustrations with 'stem-pipe' appearance of colon (Fig. 18.1D).

• Colonoscopy (Fig. 18.3) may show ulceration and pseudopolyposis

• MRI of small bowel as well as of pelvis to determine pelvic involvement, strictures and fistulae.

Q. **How would you treat it?**

Ans: 1. *5-aminosalicylic acid (5-ASA) compounds* (sulphasalazine, balsalizide, alsalazine).

2. Oral steroids to induce remissions.

3. Azathroprine may be used in severe cases.

4. Rectal steroids (suppository or enema) for local colonic disease.

5. Surgery is reserved for acute ulcerative colitis not responding to medical therapy or chronic disease with stricture formation.

Q. **How would you diagnose toxic megacolon?**

Ans: It is a dreadful complications of acute ulcerative colitis in which the colon especially the transverse colon dilates due to loss of mucosal folds. Patient looks toxic, dehydrated and abdomen becomes distended. Loose motions stop and fever, tachycardia and tachypnea appear. On radiology, the transverse colonic diameter > 5 cm confirms the diagnosis.

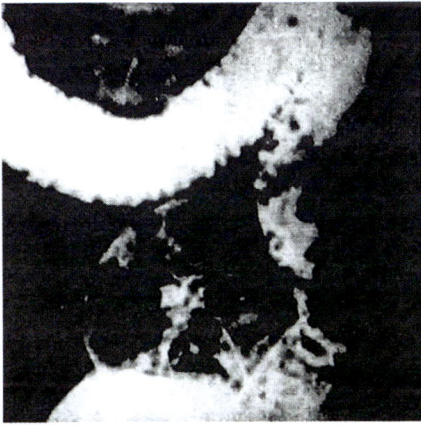

Fig. 18.2: Barium enema (double contrast study) shows multiple polyposis of colon in a patient with ulcerative colitis

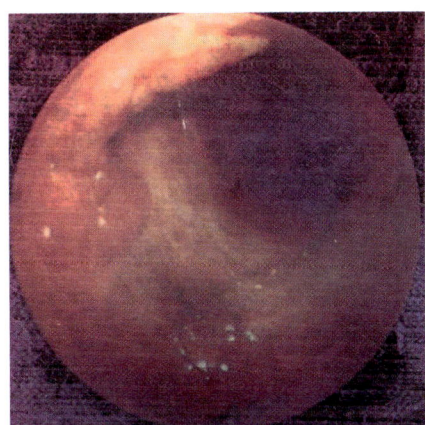

Fig. 18.3: Colonoscopy showing ulcerations and pseudopolyps in a patient with ulcerative colitis

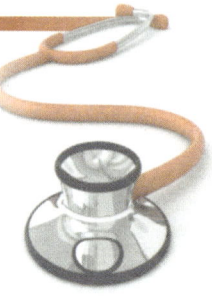

INSTRUCTION

Examine the abdomen

SALIENT FEATURES

- Diarrhea more than 3 months.

HISTORY

Ask about the following:

- Onset of symptoms
- Duration of diarrhea (> 6 month in this case)
- Frequency of stools
- Nocturnal frequency
- Whether stool contains any blood, mucus
- Does stools stick to the toilet sheet?
- Nature and character of the stools (pale, frothy, difficult to flush away indicate steatorrhea)
- Associated diseases, i.e. type I DM, thyroiditis
- Associated pain in the abdomen or tenesmus
- Bone pains, tetany, paresthesias
- Appetite decreased or increased
- Weight loss, muscle wasting, mouth ulcers
- Drug history (laxatives, antibiotics)
- Foreign travel (Traveler's diarrhea)
- Nocutria, menstrual irregularity, loss of libido
- Edema legs

EXAMINATION

General Examination

- Stunted growth (Fig. 19.1) and under developed sexual characters
- Anemia is present (in this case)
- Glossitis, aphthous ulcer, cheilosis, angular stomatitis
- Rickety rosary present

Abdominal Examination

- Abdomen is proturbant, nontender (in this case)
- No mass is palpable
- Rectal examination is normal

PROVISIONAL DIAGNOSIS

A young adolescent has chronic diarrhea, anemia, multiple vitamin deficiency, muscle weakness (lesion) due to malabsorption caused by coeliac disease (etiology). Patient develops intermittent diarrhea (functional status).

QUESTIONS AND ANSWERS

Q. How would you define diarrhea?

Ans: It implies passing of increased amount of loose stool (Stool weight > 250 g/day).

Q. How do you define malabsorption syndrome?

Ans: Malabsorption syndrome refers to defective absorption of one or more essential nutrients through the intestine. It includes maldigestion also. The malabsorption is usually nonspecific (involves more than 2 nutrients),

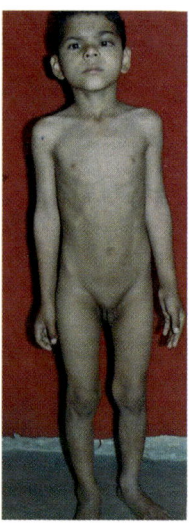

Fig. 19.1: A patient with chronic diarrhoea and multiple deficiencies, e.g. coeliac disease

but can be specific such as lactose intolerance, vit. B$_{12}$ malabsorption.

Q. What is coeliac disease?

Ans: It is a permanent dietary disorder characterised by malabsorption, small bowel abnormality and intolerance to gluten related substance gliadin.

Q. Name few causes of malabsorption syndrome.

Ans:
1. Pancreatic disorders, e.g. cystic fibrosis chronic pancreatitis, Zollinger-Ellison's syndrome
2. Inflammatory bowel disease
3. Blind loop (stagnant loop) syndrome
4. Tropical sprue and nontropical sprue (*coeliac disease*)
5. Parasitic infestation (giardiasis)
6. Strictures, fistula or ileal resection
7. Endocrinal causes, e.g. thyrotoxicosis, diabetes mellitus
8. Lactose intolerance/food allergy

Q. What are the diagnostic criteria for coeliac disease?

Ans:
1. *Clinical:* Chronic diarrhea of long duration
2. *Biochemical:* Evidence of fat, proteins, carbohydrate, vit. B$_{12}$ and folate malabsorption
3. *Immunological:* Endomysial antibodies and anti-tissue transglutamase (anti-Tg) antibodies
4. *Histopathology:* Villous or subvillous atrophy with mononuclear cells infiltration of lamina propria
5. *Therapeutic response:* Clinical, biochemical and histopathological improvement on gluten free diet

Q. What are the other autoimmune disorders which can be associated with it?

Ans:
1. Hashimoto's thyroiditis
2. Type I DM
3. Primary biliary cirrhosis
4. Sjögren's syndrome
5. Chronic active hepatitis
6. Fibrosing allergic alveolitis

Q. How would you investigate this case?

Ans:
1. *Blood tests*
   - Hemoglobin for anemia
   - Serum albumin for hypoalbuminemia
   - Serum calcium for hypocalcemia
2. *Malabsorption tests*
3. *Endomysial and tissue transglutamase antibodies (anti-Tg)*
4. *Barium study* of small intestine which may show coarsening, thickness of mucosal folds resulting in the flocculations of barium
5. *Small intestinal biopsy* for histopathology which shows villous or subvillous atrophy and long lymphocytic infiltration of lamina propria

Q. How would you treat it?

Ans:
1. Gluten free diet: Removal of all gluten from the diet is the main stay of management. All wheat, rye, and barley must be excluded although oats appear safe.
2. Vitamins (vit. B$_{12}$, folate, A, D, E), iron and calcium must be supplemented.
3. Dietary counselling regarding exclusion of gluten-free diet and replacement with nongluten diets. Prepared booklets on nongluten diets are available.
4. Corticosteroids to suppress immune response.
5. First degree relative must be screened for coeliac disease.
6. Pneumococcal vaccine every 5 years.

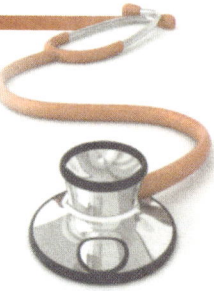

20

Peptic Ulcer

INSTRUCTION

Examine the abdomen

SALIENT FEATURES

- Episodic nocturnal abdominal pain relieved by food

HISTORY

Ask about the following:

- Age of the patient (20–40 years), onset of symptoms
- Abdominal pain and its characteristics, i.e. nature, location, periodicity, relation to food, etc.
- Aggravating and relieving factors for pain
- Is nausea, vomiting associated with pain?
- History of hematemesis and malena
- History of relapses and remissions
- Intake of alcohol and history of smoking
- Drug history (NSAIDs)

EXAMINATION

Abdominal Examination

- The abdomen is normal in shape. No distension. There is tenderness in the epigastrium
- No mass palpable
- Anemia is present

PROVISIONAL DIAGNOSIS

The patient has typical epigastric pain, worst at night or fasting, relieved by food and antacid (lesion) and anemia caused by peptic ulcer disease (etiology). Patient is at risk of recurrences (functional status).

QUESTIONS AND ANSWERS

Q. What is the relation of *H. pylori* with duodenal ulcer?

Ans: *H. pylori* infection appears to be necessary cofactor for majority of the patients with duodenal and gastric ulcers not associated with NSAIDs. Ulcer disease develops in 10% of infected patients. The prevalence of *H. pylori* infection in duodenal ulcer is 75–90%.

Q. How does *H. pylori* lead to duodenal ulcer?

Ans: *H. pylori* causes antral gastritis associated with depletion of somatostatin from D cells and gastrin release from G cells leading to hypersecretion of acid by hypergastrinemia and formation of small islands of gastric metaplasia in duodenal bulbs. Colonisation of these islands with *H. pylori* leads to duodenal ulcer.

Q. What are *H. pylori* associated gastric conditions?

Ans: 1. *H. pylori* gastritis
2. Chronic duodenal and gastric ulcerations
3. Gastric carcinoma
4. Maltoma (mucosa associated lymphoid tissue lymphoma)

Q. What is aggravating and relieving factor for peptic duodenal ulcer?

Ans:

Aggravating factors	Relieving factors
• Hypersecretion of acid and pepsin	• Prostaglandin secretion
• Increased bile acids	• Bicarbonate secretion in the gastric mucosa
• Excessive consumption of tea, coffee	• Mucosal secretion
• Alcohol, smoking	• Antacids
• Drugs (NSAIDs, etc.)	• Food
• Anxiety and stress	• Plenty of cold water
• Diet, i.e. high spicy food	

Q. What are the complications of duodenal ulcer?

Ans: 1. Gastric outlet obstruction (pyloric stenosis)

2. Gastric hemorrhage
3. Gastric perforation
4. Paralytic ileus
5. Pancreatitis due to ulcer penetration (posteriorly situated gastric ulcer)
6. Gastric malignancy
7. Recurrence of ulcer

Q. **How would you investigate this case?**
Ans: 1. Complete hemogram for anemia
2. Stool for occult blood
3. Upper GI tract endoscopy (Fig. 20.1)
4. Barium-meal double contrast study
5. Serum gastrin levels
6. Detection of *H. pylori* in gastric biopsy specimen

Q. **How would you treat it?**
Ans: 1. General measures include avoidance of tea, coffee, alcohol and smoking. Take adequate mental and physical rest. Do not eat the food in haste. (Avoid hurry and worry)
2. Relief of pain and neutralisation of acid by
   - Antacids and H_2 receptor antagonists
   - Proton pump inhibitor
   - Demulsants (mucosal defendants)

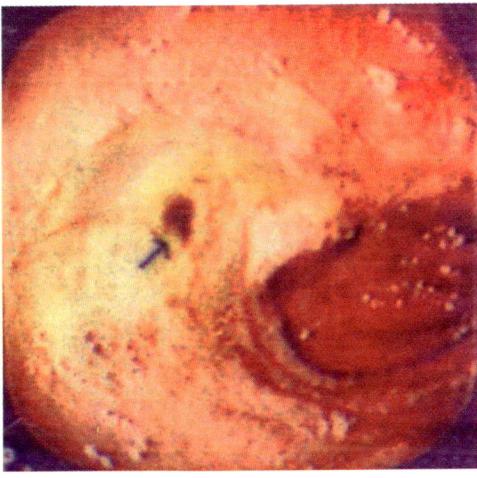

Fig. 20.1: Duodenal ulcer with a feeding vessel (↑) was a cause of upper GI bleed in a patient

3. Eradication of *H. pylori* with anti *H. pylori* regimen for 10 – 14 days

   I. Standard Triple therapy
   - Proton pump inhibitor orally twice daily
   - Clarithromycin 500 mg orally twice daily
   - Amoxicillin 1 g orally twice daily or metronidazole 500 mg orally twice daily, if penicillin allergy

   II. Standard Quadruple therapy
   - Proton pump inhibitor twice daily
   - Bismuth subsalicylate two tablets orally four times daily
   - Tetracycline 500 mg orally four times daily
   - Metronidazole 250 mg four times or 500 mg three times daily

   After completion of the course, continue treatment with proton pump inhibitor for 4 – 6 weeks. Confirm the eradication by various tests.

4. Surgical treatment for recurrent ulceration and upper GI bleeding or perforation.

Q. **What are the complications of surgery?**
Ans: Most surgical procedures done include vagotomy and a drainage procedure (pyloroplasty, gastroenterostomy) with or without enterectomy.
The complications are:
- Recurrent ulcer
- Dumping syndrome
- Malabsorption
- Weight loss
- Anemia
- Development of malignancy

Q. **What are the causes of recurrence of ulcer?**
Ans:
- Failure to eradicate *H. pylori* successfully
- *H. pylori* reinfection (rare)
- NSAIDs induced recurrence
- Hypergastrinemia (Zollinger-Ellison syndrome)
- Malignant ulcers

Q. **Name the drug used for prophylaxis of NSAIDs induced ulcer.**
Ans: Misoprostol 200 mg orally four times a day.

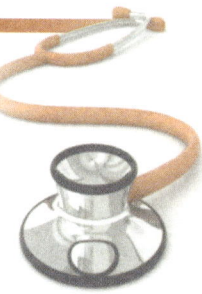

21

Aortic Stenosis

INSTRUCTION

Examine the cardiovascular system (CVS)

SALIENT FEATURES
- Breathlessness on exertion

HISTORY

Ask for the following:
- No symptom. It may be asymptomatic, detected on examination as an incidental finding. Congenital or mild AS remains asymptomatic throughout life.
- History of exertional dyspnea, fatigue.
- History of cough, hemoptysis, dyspnea, orthopnea, PND due to left heart failure.
- History of exertional syncope due to low cardiac output.
- Past history of sore throat, rheumatic fever, skin infection, fleeting joint pains.
- History of sudden death.

EXAMINATION

General Physical Examination
- Pulse is low volume, anacrotic, slow rising in moderate severe stenosis (in this case). Pulse may be normal in mild AS.
- Pulse pressure is low (mostly < 20 mm Hg).
- Jugular venous pressure is raised (in this case) if right heart failure develops. Prominent 'a' wave may be seen.
- Ankle edema may be present if heart failure develops (present in this case).

Systemic Examination

I. Cardiovascular system

Inspection
- Apex beat may be normally placed or displaced down beyond left 5th intercostal space outside the mid-clavicular line due to left ventricular hypertrophy. It is forceful and sustained (heaving).

Palpation

It is done to confirm findings of inspection.
- Apex beat may be normally placed or displaced downwards and outwards due to left ventricular hypertrophy. It is forceful and sustained in this case.
- Left ventricular thrust may be palpable (palpable in this case).
- P_2 may become palpable if pulmonary hypertension develops (P_2 palpable in this case).
- Palpable systolic thrill over the aortic area and carotids. It is best felt with the patient in the sitting position during full expiration and leaning forward (present in this case).

Percussion
- Cardiac dullness is within normal limits.

Auscultation
- A mid-systolic ejection murmur which is diamond-shaped [crescendo-decrescendo (Fig. 21.1)] often with thrill, best heard at right 2nd space (A_1 area) or left 3rd space (A_2 area). It radiates to carotid vessels and downwards to apex (Gallavardin phenomenon). Murmur is best heard in sitting position with patient bending forward in forced expiration (present in this case).
- An ejection click (EC) is heard in valvular aortic stenosis (Fig. 21.1).
- Second heart sound is short and feeble (in this case), normal or paradoxically split.
- An atrial sound (S_4) may be heard.

II. Other systems examination

1. *Respiratory system*
   - Basal rales at both the bases of the lungs.

2. *Abdomen*
   - Tender hepatomegaly may be present (present in this case).
   - No ascites, no splenomegaly.

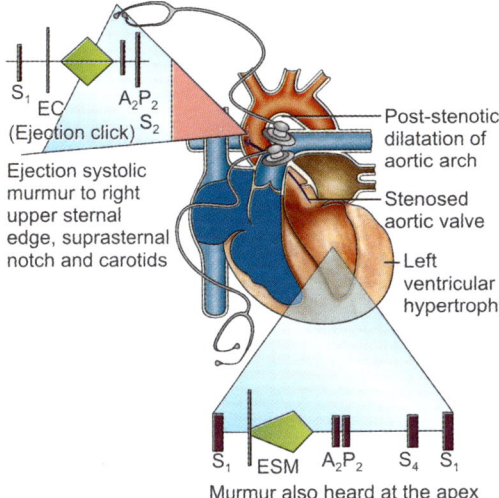

S_1
EC
(Ejection click) A_2P_2
S_2

Ejection systolic
murmur to right
upper sternal
edge, suprasternal
notch and carotids

Post-stenotic
dilatation of
aortic arch

Stenosed
aortic valve

Left
ventricular
hypertrophy

S_1 ESM A_2P_2 S_4 S_1

Murmur also heard at the apex

Fig. 21.1: Aortic stenosis. The radiation of the murmur in aortic stenosis with left ventricular hypertrophy and enlargement of the ventricle on pressure trace there was systolic gradient (>50 mmHg) between LV and aorta

PROVISIONAL DIAGNOSIS

The patient has pure aortic stenosis either rheumatic or congenital (aetiology) in origin. It is moderate in severity with CHF with sinus rhythm without SABE (functional status).

QUESTIONS AND ANSWERS

Q. **What are the points in favor of your diagnosis?**
Ans: 1. History of exertional dyspnea, syncope, chest discomfort.
2. Signs of CHF, e.g. raised JVP, cyanosis, edema and tender hepatomegaly.
3. Displaced apex beat (down and out) with heaving character.
4. Signs of pulmonary hypertension, e.g. loud P_2 with narrow splitting.
5. An ejection click and ejection systolic murmur over A_1 and A_2, best heard in sitting position and leaning forward. It radiates to carotid. A_2 is soft.
6. Systolic thrill over aorta and carotids.

Q. **What are the various types of congenital aortic stenosis?**
Ans: 1. *Valvular aortic stenosis* (bicuspid aortic valve). It is congenital and commonest in young age.
2. *Congenital subvalvular AS*. This congenital anomaly is produced by either a membra-

nous diaphragm or a fibrous ridge just below the aortic valve, or asymmetrical hypertrophy of the interventricular septum called idiopathic hypertrophic subaortic stenosis (IHSS).
3. *Supravalvular AS.* This uncommon congenital anomaly is produced by narrowing of the ascending aorta or by a fibrous diaphragm with a small opening just above the aortic valve. It is commonly seen in William's syndrome.

Q. **What is William's syndrome?**
Ans: It is characterised by
- *Elfin facies*, e.g. broad forehead, pointed chin, upturned nose, hypertelorism, peg-shaped incisors, low set ears.
- Supravalvular aortic stenosis
- Mental retardation
- Hypercalcemia

Q. **What are the causes of aortic stenosis?**
Ans: The likely etiology varies with the age of the patient. The causes are:
1. **Infants, children, adolescents**
   - Congenital aortic stenosis (valvular)
   - Congenital subvalvular aortic stenosis
   - Congenital supravalvular aortic stenosis
2. **Young adults and middle aged persons**
   - Calcification and fibrosis of congenitally bicuspid aortic valve
   - Rheumatic aortic stenosis
3. **Old age**
   - Senile degenerative aortic stenosis
   - Calcification of bicuspid valve
   - Rheumatic aortic stenosis

Q. **What does second heart sound tell us in AS?**
Ans: - A soft and muffled S_2 indicates valvular stenosis
- A single S_2 indicates fibrosed/fused cusps or fenestrated valve
- Reverse splitting of S_2 indicate mechanical or electrical prolongation of ventricular systole
- A normal S_2 rules out the possibility of critical aortic stenosis

Q. **How would you grade AS on echocardiography?**
Ans: It is graded as mild (valve area >1.5 cm^2), moderate (valve area 1–1.5 cm^2) and severe (valve area <1 cm^2).

Q. **Is there any relation of the murmur with severity of AS?**

Ans: 1. Loudness of murmur does not have any relation.

2. Duration of murmur reflects a long aortic gradient, hence, duration of murmur increases with severity of AS.

Q. **What are the causes of systolic murmur in aortic area (A_1 and A_2 e.g. left 3rd space)?**

Ans: • AS
• Systemic hypertension
• Coarctation of the aorta
• Aneurysm of the ascending aorta
• Atherosclerosis of the aorta (old age)
• Functional flow murmur in AR

Q. **What are the clinical features of idiopathic hypertrophic subaortic stenosis (IHSS)?**

Ans: The features are:
• Dyspnea, angina pectoris, fatigue and syncope
• Double apical impulse (apex beat)
• A rapidly rising carotid arterial pulse
• Pulsus bisference (double upstroke)
• A harsh, diamond-shape ejection systolic murmur without ejection click is best heard at lower left sternal border as well as at the apex. It does not radiate to neck vessels. It becomes louder with valsalva maneuver.
• Early diastolic murmur of aortic regurgitation may also be heard in some patients
• No post-stenotic dilation
• Second heart sound is normal, single

Q. **What are the characteristic features of supra-valvular AS?**

Ans: • Unequal BP in both arms (right > left)
• May be associated with other features of William's syndrome
• No ejection click, only ejection systolic murmur
• Systolic thrill is more pronounced and radiates to the neck vessels but not to the apex

• A_2 is accentuated
• No post-stenotic dilation

Q. **What is genetic defect in William's syndrome?**

Ans: 1. Mutation in the gene for elastin.
2. Microdeletion in chromosome.

Q. **How will you differentiate between aortic stenosis and pulmonary stenosis?**

Ans: The differences are:

Features	AS	PS
Pulse	Small amplitude, anacrotic, parvus et tardus	Normal
BP	Low systolic	Normal
Apex beat	Heaving	Normal
Second heart sound	A_2 soft	P_2 soft
Splitting of S_2	Reverse	Wide
Location of systolic murmur	Aortic area, conducted to carotids	Pulmonary area No conduction
Relation to respiration	No change	Increases on inspiration
Associated ventricular hypertrophy	LVH	RVH

Q. **What are the characteristics of severe aortic stenosis?**

Ans: Aortic stenosis is said to be severe when:
• Pulse character is slowly rising plateau
• Pulse pressure is narrow (Low systolic pressure)
• Signs of LVF present
• S_2 is soft, single or paradoxically split
• Presence of S_4

Q. **How would you differentiate valvular aortic stenosis from degenerative aortic sclerosis?**

Ans: The differences are:

Feature	Valvular AS	Degenerative aortic sclerosis
Age	Young age	Old age
Pulse	Anacrotic, slow rising	Normal
Apex beat	Shifted down and outwards	Normally localised
Murmur	Radiates to carotids and lower down to apex	Localised
Other changes	Not present	Changes of old age, i.e. palpable vessels, arcus senalis, thin lax skin
Calcification	Uncommon	Common
Hypertension	Uncommon	Systolic hypertension common

Q. How will you investigate a patient with AS?

Ans: Following investigations are done:

1. *Electrocardiogram (ECG)* may show left atrial and left ventricular hypertrophy with strain, i.e. ST-T wave changes due to myocardial ischemia may be present. Heart blocks and bundle branch block in calcific aortic stenosis may occur sometimes.

2. *Chest X-ray:* It may be normal. Sometimes, heart is enlarged due to left ventricular hypertrophy. Post-stenotic dilatation of aorta may be seen in some cases. Lateral view may show calcification of aortic valve.

3. *Echocardiography:* It will show left ventricular enlargement and hypertrophy, severity of AS, calcification of valve and decreased left ventricular function.

4. *Doppler echocardiography* (Fig. 21.2): Demonstrates systolic gradient across the valve.

5. Cardiac catheterization reveals transvalvular gradient > 60 mmHg

Q. What are the complications of AS?

Ans: Common complications are as follows:
- Left ventricular failure

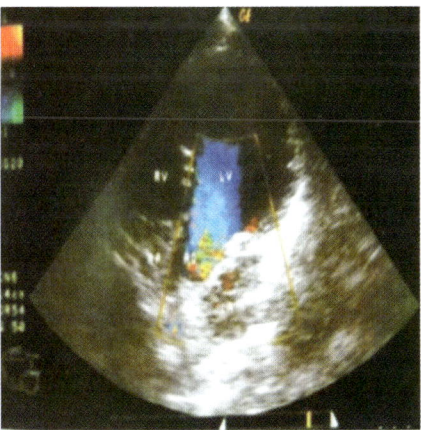

Fig. 21.2: Aortic stenosis. Color Doppler Echocardiogram showing aortic stenosis with gradient of 50 mm across the valve

- Hemolytic anemia
- Systemic embolization
- Congestive cardiac failure
- Infective endocarditis
- Arrhythmias (ventricular) and conduction disturbances (heart blocks)
- Precipitation of angina
- Sudden death. It is more common in hypertrophic obstructive cardiomyopathy (HOCM)

Q. How would you manage this condition?

Ans: Mild asymptomatic AS with valvular gradient < 50 mmHg needs observation only. Moderate AS with symptoms needs medical management of LVF with salt restriction, diuretics and vasodilators. Digoxin should not be used. The patients with moderate to severe AS need valve replacement.

Q. What are the indications of valve replacement?

Ans:
- Symptomatic AS with valvular gradient > 50 mmHg. It is an absolute indication.
- Asymptomatic patients with severe AS (gradient > 50 mm Hg. LVH, left ventricular systolic dysfunction and valve area < 0.6 cm^2)
- Asymptomatic moderate AS in patients who are undergoing mitral or aortic root surgery or coronary artery bypass surgery.

Q Which valve would you prefer for replacement?

Ans: Mechanical prosthetic valve in young age and tissue valve (bioprosthetic valve) in old age.

Q. What is the cause of GI tract bleeding in AS?

Ans: Associated angiodysplasia of colon.

Q. What is Gallavardin phenomenon?

Ans: The radiation of ejection systolic murmur of AS to the apex is called Gallavardin phenomenon. This can falsely suggests mitral regurgitation.

Q. Could it be a case of severe anemia?

Ans: Anemia is associated with hyperdynamic circulation, i.e. good volume, pulse, wide pulse pressure similar to AR. Hemic murmur (an ejection systolic murmur heard at aortic area can be confused with AS).

22

Aortic Regurgitation

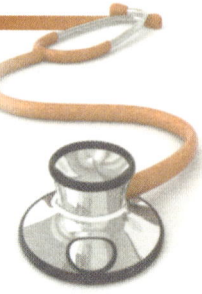

INSTRUCTION

Examine the cardiovascular system

SALIENT FEATURES

- Palpitation and breathlessness

HISTORY

Ask for the following:

- Onset of symptoms and their course.
- Ask the history of cough, dyspnea, orthopnea, PND.
- Ask for history of hemoptysis, anginal pain, headache.
- History of fever, chills and rigors.
- History of edema feet and legs.
- History of loss of function of any part, i.e. paralysis (monoplegia, hemiplegia).
- Past history of sore throat, skin infection or arthralgia (fleeting pains) or fixed joint pain (arthritis).

EXAMINATION

General Physical Examination

- *Face* for appearance, i.e. dyspneic or orthopneic, ill-look. Note puffiness.
- Look for *Argyll-Robertson pupils of syphilis* (Read A–R pupil in separate case discussion).
- *Mouth.* Look for anemia or bleeding or evidence of infection, high-arch palate (*Marfan's syndrome*).
- *Neck* examination for arterial pulsations, JVP and lymph nodes.
- Record pulse, BP, respiration and temperature.
- Note the following other peripheral signs in a case with AR, if suspected:
    - i. Collapsing or good volume pulse (wide pulse pressure > 40 mmHg).
    - ii. Bounding peripheral pulses.
    - iii. Dancing carotids (*Corrigan's sign*).
    - iv. Capillary pulsations in nailbeds (*Quincke's sign*).

- v. Pistol shots sound and *Duroziez's sign/ murmur* (to and fro systolic and diastolic murmur) produced by compression of femoral artery by stethoscope.
- vi. Head nodding with carotid pulse—*de Musset's sign*.
- vii. *Hill's sign* (BP in lower limb > upper limbs).
- Cyanosis (peripheral, central or both) may be present.
- Pitting ankle edema may be present.
- Tender hepatomegaly if right heart failure present.
- Look for stigmatas of Marfan's syndrome, e.g. tall stature, arachnodactyly, high-arched palate, ectopia lentis.
- Look for joint deformity for rheumatoid arthritis and ankylosing spondylitis.

All these peripheral signs may not be evident in mild AR. In our case, they were present indicating severe AR.

Cardiovascular System

Inspection

- Apex beat is displaced down and outside the midclavicular line and is forceful in this case
- Left ventricular thrust (present in this case)
- Pulsations in suprasternal notch and epigastrium are usually seen (seen in this case)

Palpation

- Apex beat is forceful and sustained (present)
- No thrill is palpable
- Tender hepatomegaly if right heart failure present (present in this case)

Percussion

- Cardiac dullness is within normal limits

Auscultation

- An *early diastolic murmur* is best heard in A_2 area (3rd left intercostal space) or A_1 area (2nd right intercostal space) in sitting position with patient leaning forward and during held expiration (characteristic in this case).

- An *ejection systolic murmur* in the same area. It is due to increased stroke volume (functional murmur). It may also radiate to neck vessels.
- An ejection click suggests bicuspid aortic valve.
- *Austin flint murmur* (soft, mid-diastolic) at apex in severe AR (present).
- Second heart sound is soft and feeble.
- Loud pulmonary component in second left space indicates pulmonary hypertension (present).
- Signs of left heart failure (fine end-inspiratory crackles at bases of lungs).
- A 3rd heart sound at apex may be present in severe AR (present).

PROVISIONAL DIAGNOSIS

In view of clinical features and auscultatory findings, the provisional diagnosis is isolated aortic regurgitation with congestive cardiac failure (lesion) probably non rheumatic in origin (etiology) without any evidence of endocarditis or thromboembolic complication (functional status).

QUESTIONS AND ANSWERS

Q.   What are the causes of chronic AR?
Ans: The causes are:
   I. *Congenital*
   - Bicuspid valve
   II. *Acquired*
   - Rheumatic heart disease
   - Infective endocarditis (acute regurgitation)
   - Trauma leading to valve rupture

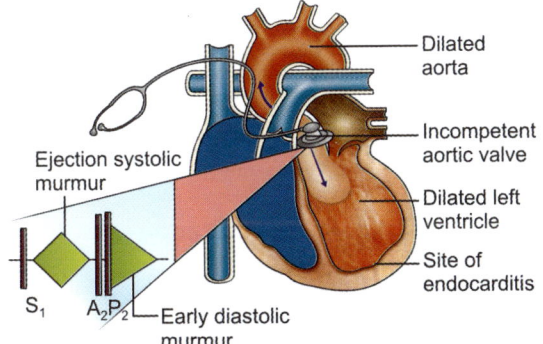

N.B. Lean the patient forward with breath held in expiration to hear the murmur best

Fig. 22.1: Aortic regurgitation. The early diastolic murmur is best heard at the left sternal edge and may be accompanied by an ejection systolic murmur (functional). The murmur is best heard with the patient leaning forward and during expiration.

- Atherosclerosis, hypertension
- Marfan's syndrome (aortic dilatation)
- Syphilitic aortitis
- Ankylosing spondylitis, rheumatoid arthritis
- Dissecting aneurysm of ascending aorta

N.B. Non rheumatic causes dominate over rheumatic cause in isolated AR.

Q.   What are the causes of acute AR?
Ans: Causes of acute AR
   - Acute bacterial endocarditis
   - Rupture of sinus of valsalva
   - Failure of prosthetic valve
   - Trauma to the chest
   - Acute dissection of the aorta

Q.   What are functional murmur?
Ans: These murmurs occur in the absence of organic heart disease, are due to turbulence produced by rapid flow of blood across a normal valve (flow murmurs). These may be systolic and diastolic (Table 22.1). These murmurs are not loud, are localized in nature, and usually not associated with thrill. They are hemodynamically insignificant, do not produce cardiomegaly.

Table 22.1: Functional murmurs	
Systolic	*Diastolic*
• Systolic murmur occurs across pulmonary valve in left to right shunt, e.g. ASD, VSD	• Graham-Steell murmur (early diastolic) due to pulmonary regurgitation in pulmonary hypertension
• Functional systolic murmur in aortic area is heard in patients with severe AR	• Apical mid-diastolic murmur (*Austin-Flint murmur*) in severe AR

Q.   Is AR moderate or severe in your case?
Ans: The presence of all the signs of wide pulse pressure indicates severe AR in this patient. However, the signs of severity are described in Table 22.2 (Remember the signs of moderate and severe AR).

Q.   What are the clinical features of acute AR?
Ans: The clinical features of acute AR will be:
   - An acutely ill patient with severe breathlessness, chest discomfort
   - Acute left ventricular failure (LVF)
   - Peripheral signs of AR will be absent
   - An early diastolic murmur is diagnostic

Q.   What is differential diagnosis of AR?
Ans: The common causes of AR are compared clinically in the Table 22.3 for differential diagnosis.

Table 22.2: Signs of aortic regurgitation (AR) and its severity.

Signs of moderate AR
Peripheral signs*

- Collapsing or good volume pulse (wide pulse pressure)
- Bounding peripheral pulses
- Dancing carotids (*Corrigan's sign*)
- Capillary pulsations in nailbeds (*Quincke's sign*)
- Pistol shot sound and *Duroziez's sign/murmur*
- Head nodding with carotid pulse de *Musset's sign*
- *Hill's sign* (BP in lower limb > upper limbs)
- Cyanosis (peripheral, central or both) may be present
- Fundus examination will reveal capillary pulsations
- Pitting ankle edema may be present
- Tender hepatomegaly if right heart failure present

Sign of severe AR

- All signs of moderate AR
- Wider pulse pressure (normal 20–40 mm). Wider the pulse pressure, severe is AR (> 60 mmHg).
- Soft second heart sound
- Signs of left heart failure
- Duration of the decrescendo diastolic murmur, longer the murmur, severe is AR
- Hill's sign (normal difference in BP of LL and UL is < 20 mm Hg). Larger the difference, severe is the AR. A difference of 20–40 mm indicates moderate AR and > 60 mm difference suggests severe AR.
- Presence of third heart sound. It indicates severe AR.
- *Austin flint murmur*—a low pitched, soft mid-diastolic murmur caused by vibration of the anterior mitral cusp by the regurgitant jet and is heard at the apex. It indicates severe AR.

* All these peripheral signs may not be evident in mild AR because these indicates wide pulse pressure due to significant aortic run-off into the heart.

Q.   How will you decide whether it is AR or PR?
Ans: Read the Table 22.4.

Q.   How will you decide whether MDM in mitral area is due to severe AR or due to associated MS?
Ans: The mid-diastolic murmur in AR may be confused with MDM of MS though both lesions may coexist. The differentiation is given in Table 22.5.

Q.   How will you investigate a patient with AR?
Ans: Following investigations are done:

1. *Chest X-ray (PA view) may show:*
   - Cardiomegaly (LV enlargement-boot shaped heart)
   - Dilatation of ascending aorta, valvular calcification
   - Aortic knuckle prominent

2. *ECG may show*
   - LVH and left atrial hypertrophy in moderate to severe AR (Fig. 22.2)
   - ST segment depression and T wave inversion due to left ventricular strain

3. *Echocardiogram.* It detects:
   - Left ventricular enlargement, hyper-dynamic left ventricle and assessment of severity of AR
   - Fluttering of anterior mitral leaflet in severe AR
   - Aortic root dilatation and valve morphology
   - Vegetations may be detected in a case with endocarditis
   - Assessment of LV (dimension, size and systolic function)

4. *Color Doppler flow studies* detect the reflux through aortic valve and its magnitude

Table 22.3: Differential diagnosis of AR		
Rheumatic AR	*Syphilitic AR*	*Aortic dilatation (Marfan's syndrome)*
Young age group	Older age group	Young age
History of rheumatic fever in the past	History of sexual exposure	Eunuchoidism (lower segment > upper segment, arachnodactyly)
Other valves may be involved	Usually an isolated lesion	Mitral valve may be involved (floppy mitral valve syndrome)
Diastolic thrill absent	Thrill may be present	Aortic pulsation in suprasternal notch. No thrill
A$_2$ diminished or absent	A$_2$ may be loud (tambour like)	A$_2$ normal
Murmur best heard in left 3rd space (A$_2$ area)	Murmur best heard in right second or 3rd space along right sternal border	Murmur heard in second right and third left intercostal space
Peripheral signs present	Peripheral signs are marked, Austin-Flint murmur may be present	Peripheral signs are usually absent

Table 22.4: Differentiation between AR and PR

Feature	AR	PR
Peripheral signs of wide pulse pressure	Present	Absent
Apex beat	Hyperdynamic	Normal
Site of early diastolic murmur	Best heard in aortic area	Best heard in pulmonary area
Relation of murmur to respiration	None	Increases with inspiration
Ventricular enlargement	LVH	RVH

Table 22.5: Differential diagnosis of MDM in AR

Feature	Severe AR (Austin-Flint murmur)	AR with MS
Peripheral sign of AR	Florid	Masked
Character of murmur	Soft	Rough and rumble
First heart sound (S_1)	Normal	Loud
Opening snap (OS)	Absent	Present
LA enlargement	Absent	Present
Calcification of mitral valve	Absent	May be present
Echocardiogram	Normal	Suggestive of MS

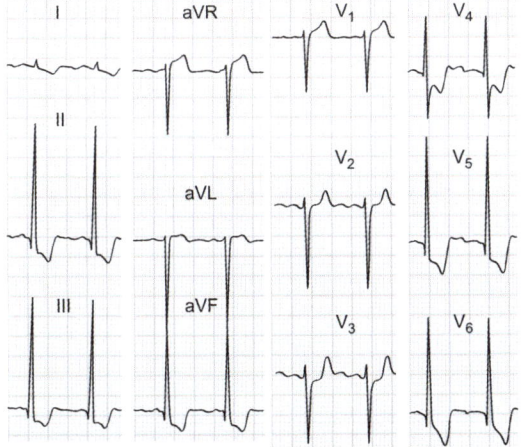

Fig. 22.2: Left ventricular hypertrophy in a patient with aortic regurgitation

The ECG shows:
- R Wave in avf > 21 mm.
- RVS + SV1 ≥ 41 mm
- Associated ST – T the wave changes with accentuated Q waves

5. *Radionuclide imaging* in asymptomatic patients where echocardiographic images are of poor quality
6. *Cardiac catheterization* is necessary when coronary artery disease is suspected
7. *MRI* and *spiral CT scan* for assessment of aortic root size

Q. What are the complications of AR?

Ans: Following are the common complications:
- Acute LVF
- Infective endocarditis
- CHF
- Cardiac arrhythmias
- Heart blocks (calcific aortic valve)
- Precipitation of angina

Q. What are the causes of an ejection systolic murmur in aortic area? How would you differentiate them?

Ans: The ejection systolic murmur in aortic area occurs either in severe AR (functional) or when AR is associated with AS or an isolated AS. The AS has already been discussed. The differences between severe AR or AR with AS are discussed in case no 23.

Q. How would you treat AR?

Ans:
- *Mild asymptomatic* disease does not require treatment.
- *Moderate to severe disease* is treated by salt restriction, diuretics, digitalis and vasodilators (ACE inhibitors). Surgery is the final answer.
- *Severe AR* needs surgery (valve reconstruction or replacement) in addition to medical management.

Q. What are the indications of surgery in AR?

Ans:
- Severe AR with concomitant angina
- Severe AR with heart failure and reduced ejection fraction (e.g. between 30 and 50%).
- A reduction in exercise ejection fraction by 50% or more even in the absence of symptoms
- When end-systolic dimension of aorta or aortic root diameter is > 55 mm

Q. Which prosthetic valve would you prefer for replacement in AR?

Ans:
- If patient is young, mechanical prosthetic valve would be preferred as they are more durable.
- Bioprosthetic (tissue valve) valve is used in elderly because they are prone to degeneration and calcification may need re-operation after 7–10 years.

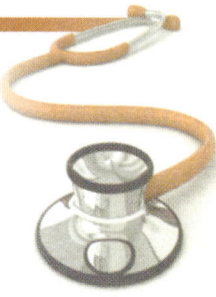

INSTRUCTION

Examine the cardiovascular system

SALIENT FEATURES

- Cough, dyspnea and chest discomfort, edema feet

HISTORY

Ask for the following:

- Onset of symptoms and their course.
- Ask history of cough, dyspnea, PND, orthopnea.
- History of palpitation, pain chest, syncope.
- History of hemoptysis, fever.
- History of edema feet and legs.
- History of paralysis of a limb/limbs.
- Past history of sore throat, skin infection or arthralgia (fleeting joint pain) or arthritis.

EXAMINATION

General Physical Examination

- *Bisferiens pulse* (double peak pulse). It may be low volume (if AS is dominant) or good volume (AR dominant)
- *Pulse pressure:* Pulse pressure is narrow (AS dominant) or wide (AR dominant)
- *JVP* raised if right heart failure present
- *Ankle edema* present if heart failure develops

Systemic Examination

CVS

Inspection

- Apex beat may be normally placed, displaced down and outside the mid-clavicular line due to left ventricular hypertrophy/dilatation

Palpation

- Apex beat is palpable, forceful and sustained or hyperdynamic depending on the dominance of aortic lesion. It is displaced down and outside the mid-clavicular line.

- Palpable left ventricular heave/thrust (present in this case)
- Systolic or diastolic thrill over the aortic area depending or the dominance of the lesion (systolic thrill present in this case)

Percussion

- Cardiac dullness increased. Left border on percussion corresponds with the apex beat.

Auscultation

- A diamond shaped ejection systolic murmur often with thrill heard in aortic area (A_1 area, i.e. 2nd right intercostal space) which radiates to neck vessels (present in this case). Murmur has all characteristics of aortic stenosis (Fig. 23.1)
- An early diastolic murmur best heard in A_2 area having all characters of aortic regurgitation murmur (present)
- Ejection click (present in this case) may be heard if AS dominant (Fig. 23.1)

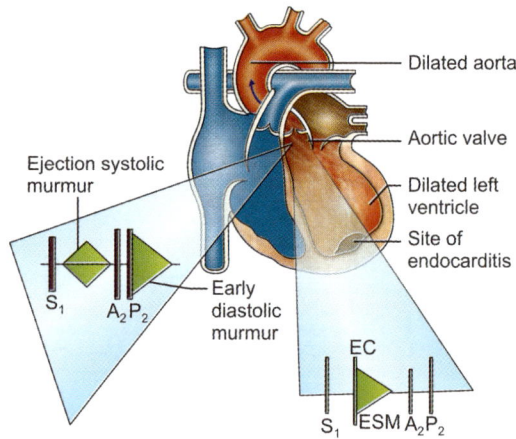

Fig. 23.1: Combined aortic stenosis and aortic regurgitation

- An Austin flint (soft, mid-diastolic) murmur at the apex may be sometimes heard if AR is dominant and regurgitant jet is large.
- P_2 may be loud and single if pulmonary hypertension develops
- A_2 is soft and not audible usually
- A 3rd heart sound present if LVF present.

Other System Examination

1. *Respiratory system:* There will be fine crackles at both the bases of lungs with wheezes if LVF presents.
2. *Abdomen:* A tender hepatomegaly and ascites may be present if right heart failure presents.

PROVISIONAL DIAGNOSIS

The patient on history and examination has AS and AR (lesion) caused by rheumatic heart disease (etiology). He has dominant aortic stenosis and at present is in congestive heart failure (functional status).

QUESTIONS AND ANSWERS

Q. **What are the common causes of combined aortic valve lesions, i.e. AS and AR?**

Ans: 1. Rheumatic aortic valve disease
2. Bicuspid aortic valve
3. Degenerative (atherosclerotic) aortic valve disease

Q. **Could it be only aortic regurgitation with functional AS rather than organic AS and AR?**

Ans: The differences are discussed below

Feature	Severe AR with functional AS	AR with AS (organic)
Signs of wide pulse pressure (water-hammer pulse, Corrigan's sign, dancing carotids and pistol shot sounds, etc.)	Present	May (if AR dominant) or may not (if AS dominant) be present
Systolic BP	High systolic	Normal or low systolic
Ejection click	Absent	Present widely
Radiation of murmur	Usually localized, may radiate to neck vessels	Radiates to neck vessels as well as to apex
Systolic thrill	Absent	Present
Calcification of valve	Common	Uncommon
Cause	Non rheumatic	Rheumatic

Q. **How would you decide the dominance of AS or AR in combined aortic lesions**

Ans: Read Table 23.1.

Q. **How would you confirm the diagnosis?**

Ans: 1. *Electrocardiography:* It will show left ventricular hypertrophy with strain/ischemic pattern.

Table 23.1: Dominant aortic stenosis vs aortic regurgitation in combined AS and AR

Features	Dominant AS	Dominant AR
I. Symptoms • Exertional angina • Dyspnea on effort • Fatigue • Syncope • Palpitation	All are marked	Chest pain, dyspnea, palpitation common
II. Signs Pulse	• Low volume • Pulsus bisferiens (tidal wave prominent than percussion wave)	• High volume collapsing pulse • Pulsus bisferiens (percussion wave prominent than tidal wave)
BP	• Low systolic BP • Low pulse pressure	• High systolic BP • Wide pulse pressure
Peripheral signs of AR	Marked	Marked
Apex beat	Heaving	Hyperdynamic
Thrill	Systolic	No thrill
S_3	Absent	Present
S_4	May be present	Absent
Ejection click	Present	Absent
Diastolic murmur	Short early diastolic	Prominent early diastolic
Systolic murmur	Marked, radiating to neck vessels	Present, does not radiate to neck vessels

2. *Chest X-ray may* show lung congestion if AR if dominant.
3. *Echocardiography* will reveal aortic pressure gradient, aortic root area and LV dimension and presence of vegetations.
4. *Color Doppler Studies:* It will accurately measure the valve area and magnitude of reflux through it.
5. *Cardiac Catheterization* is necessary when coronary artery disease is suspected.
6. *MRI and CT scan* for assessment of aortic root size and calcification of valve.

Q.   How would you manage such a case?

Ans: I. Medical treatment with diuretics, salt restriction and vasodilators

II. Surgical management:
- Surgical management (valve replacement) for moderate to severe disease.
- If aortic valve stenosis is dominant, surgical correction should be attempted early if symptoms are present and severe.
- If aortic regurgitation is dominant, the surgery can be delayed until symptoms or LV dysfunction develop.

24

Mitral Stenosis

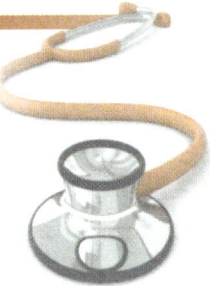

INSTRUCTION

Examine cardiovascular system

SALIENT FEATURES

- Breathlessness and hemoptysis, edema feet

HISTORY

Ask for the following:

- History of exertional dyspnea, orthopnea, and PND
- Any history of pain chest, hemoptysis, hoarseness of voice
- History of fever, joint pain (fleeting) or urinary disturbance
- History of pain abdomen (hepatomegaly)
- History of puffiness of face, edema feet or legs, distention of abdomen (ascites)
- History of any paralysis (motor or sensory deficit)
- History of missing of heart beats or palpitations (AF)

Past history

- History of sore throat, joint pain, rash or abnormal movement or skin infection
- History of recurrent chest pain or hemoptysis

EXAMINATION

General Physical Signs

- *Mitral facies* — A characteristic bilateral, cyanotic or dusky pink hue (malar flush) on cheeks.
- *Low volume pulse*, which may be irregularly irregular if atrial fibrillation is present.
- *Low pulse pressure*
- *Raised jugular venous pressure* and 'a' wave on jugular venous pulse will be absent in atrial fibrillation
- *Cold extremities:* Extremities are usually warm but may be cold in severe mitral stenosis or due to embolization.
- Pitting ankle edema
- Look for the signs of bacterial endocarditis and rheumatic activity

Note: Always look for the signs of bacterial endocarditis (Read Case 31) or acute rheumatic activity in case of MS, if complicated.

Systemic Examination

1. Estimation of Heart (CVS)

Inspection

- Apex beat is normally situated or apex beat is displaced outwards but not downwards
- Pulsation of pulmonary artery may be visible in 2nd left intercostal space.
- Epigastric pulsations may be visible due to right ventricular hypertrophy.
- Left parasternal lift may be visible.

Palpation

- Apex beat is palpable and tapping in character (in this case).
- An apical diastolic thrill may be palpable in left lateral position (present in this case).
- 1st heart sound at apex (mitral area) may become palpable, best demonstrated in left lateral position.
- Parasternal heave is usually present (present in this case).
- Second sound (pulmonary component) may become palpable at left 2nd intercostal space (palpable).
- Right ventricular pulsations may be palpable in epigastrium (palpable).

Percussion

- Left border of heart corresponds with apex beat
- 2nd and 3rd left intercostal spaces may become dull due to pulmonary hypertension.

Auscultation

1. *Mitral area (apex)*
   - *Heart beats* may be irregular due to atrial fibrillation
   - *First heart sound* is loud and banging, short and snappy

- A *mid-diastolic murmur* (Fig 24.1) best heard in left lateral position with the bell of stethoscope. It is rough and rumble. It is accentuated during late diastole called 'presystolic accentuation' (present in this case). A presystolic murmur without middiastolic murmur is an early sign of mitral stenosis, and in mild mitral stenosis this may be the only finding.
- *Opening snap (OS)* is present in this case (Fig. 24.1). It is snapping sound heard after 2nd heart sound. Its proximity of S$_2$ determines the severity of mitral stenosis. Nearer the opening snap to 2nd heart sound, more severe is the mitral stenosis. It is absent if valve becomes calcified.

2. *Pulmonary area* (left 2nd intercostal space)
   - Loud 2nd heart sound due to pulmonary arterial hypertension
   - There may be an ejection systolic or an early diastolic murmur (*Graham-Steell murmur*) due to pulmonary regurgitation
   - Splitting of 2nd heart sound becomes narrow

3. *Tricuspid area* (lower left parasternal border). There may be a pansystolic murmur due to functional tricuspid regurgitation which may develop in cases with severe mitral stenosis.

4. *Aortic area* (right 2nd intercostal space) Normal 2nd heart sound heard. No abnormality detected in this area.

II. Examination of Other Systems

i. *Examination of lungs*
   There may be fine crepitations (end-inspiratory crackles) at both the bases of lungs due to LHF. There may be hydrothorax (pleural effusion)

ii. *Examination of abdomen*
   Liver is enlarged, soft and tender. Ascites may be present. Spleen gets enlarged in presence of subacute bacterial endocarditis.

iii. *Examination of nervous system*
   - Monoplegia/hemiplegia due to embolism
   - Sydenham's chorea (Rheumatic activity)
   - Optic fundi for Roth's spots (bacterial)

PROVISIONAL DIAGNOSIS

The provisional diagnosis is mitral stenosis (lesion) probably rheumatic in origin (etiology) with atrial fibrillation and congestive heart failure (functional status) without bacterial endocarditis, thrombo-embolism and acute rheumatic activity.

QUESTIONS AND ANSWERS

Q. **What are points that favor your diagnosis of MS?**

Ans: *Points in favor of mitral stenosis are:*
   1. *History* of cough, dyspnea, orthopnea and PND. Hemoptysis was present.

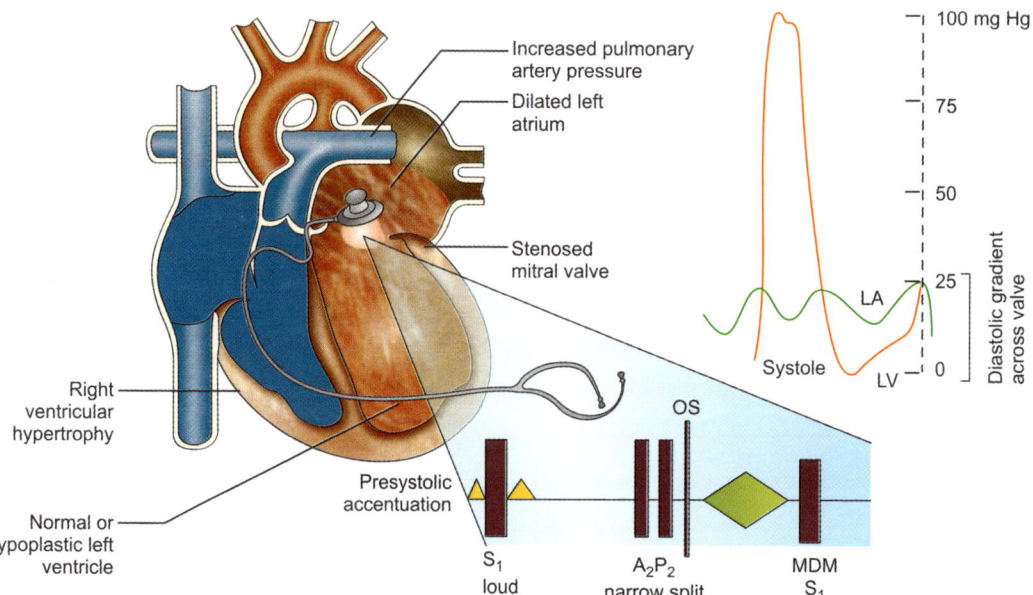

Fig. 24.1: Mitral stenosis: Genesis and conduction of the murmur and illustration of the diastolic gradient

2. *Palpable apex beat*. Apex beat is palpable and tapping in character (tapping character is due to palpable first heart sound)

3. *Loud first heart sound (S_1)*.

4. *Mid-diastolic murmur (MDM) with presystolic accentuation*. The murmur is rough, rumbling, low pitched, low frequency, of variable duration, best heard at the apex in left lateral position with bell of the stethoscope.

5. Opening snap (OS).

Q. What conditions simulate MS?

Ans: 1. *Atrial myxoma*—The murmur appears with position, i.e. appears in sitting position, disappears on lying down

2. *Ball valve thrombus* in left atrium

3. *Cortriatum*—a rare congenital heart condition

4. Acute rheumatic carditis

N.B. These conditions constitute the differential diagnosis of MS.

Q. What do you understand by opening snap?

Ans: This is a snappy sound produced due to sudden forceful opening of the mitral valve during diastole due elevated left atrial pressure. It is heard in expiration with diaphragm of stethoscope at or just medial to cardiac apex. This sound follows aortic component of second heart sound (A_2) by 0.05 to 0.1 sec.

Q. What is significance of OS?

Ans: • The presence of OS indicates organic MS

• The OS indicates that mitral valve is still pliable (i.e. not calcified). It disappears if valve is calcified

• It also decides the severity of MS. Diminishing A2–OS gap (gap between second heart sound and OS) indicates increasing severity of the MS.

• It disappears following valvotomy.

Q. How would you explain loud first heart sound in MS?

Ans: Due to persistent rise in left atrial pressure, the diastolic gradient across the mitral valve is increased that keeps the valve cusps wide open at the end of diastole with the result when ventricular systole starts, the widely opened mitral valve cusps close rapidly like a thud producing a loud S_1.

Q. What are the common causes of mitral stenosis?

Ans: The causes are:

1. *Rheumatic*: MS is invariably rheumatic.

2. *Congenital*, e.g. parachute mitral valve

where all chordae tendinae are inserted into a single papillary muscle.

3. *Rarely-carcinoid syndrome, SLE, endomyocardial fibrosis, Hurler's syndrome, RA* (rheumatoid arthritis) and *calcification of mitral annulus and leaflets*.

Q. What is normal cross-sectional area of mitral valve? When do symptoms and signs of MS appears? What is tight MS?

Ans: The normal mitral valve orifice is 4–6 cm^2 (average 5 cm^2) in diastole in adults. Narrowing of the mitral valve is called *mitral stenosis*. The symptoms arise due to hemodynamic disturbances such as rise in left atrial pressures, pulmonary arterial pressure when valve orifice is reduced to half of its original size (2.0 cm^2 approx). Mitral stenosis is severe when orifice is 1 cm^2 or less and said to be critical (≤ 0.5 cm^2). The hemodynamic consequences in severe stenosis include rise in left atrial, pulmonary venous pressure and pulmonary edema (LVF) followed by pulmonary arterial hypertension and right heart failure. This is called backward failure theory of heart failure.

Q. What are the causes of loud S_1?

Ans: Following are the causes:

• Mitral stenosis

• Tricuspid stenosis

• In tachycardia. S_1 is loud due to short P–R interval.

• Hyperkinetic circulation (exercise, anemia, thyrotoxicosis, fever, pregnancy, etc.)

• *Short P–R interval (WPW syndrome)*. The P–R interval influences the heart rate, short P–R causes loud S_1 while long P–R causes muffling of S_1.

• Children or young adults (physiological)

Q. What are the causes of muffing of S_1 in MS?

Ans: 1. Mitral regurgitation or aortic regurgitation

2. Mitral valve calcification

3. Acute rheumatic carditis and digitalis toxicity or overdosages

4. Myocardial infarction with dilated heart (gross CHF)

5. Emphysema, pericardial effusion, obesity, rotation of the heart (loud sound is not heard)

Q. What are causes of mid-diastolic murmur (MDM) at the apex?

Ans: In addition to MS, the other conditions are:

1. *Active rheumatic carditis (valvulitis)*. It produces a soft mid-diastolic (*Carey-Coombs' murmur*) without loud S_1, opening snap and diastolic thrill. It is due to

edema of valve cusps just producing obstruction. The murmur disappears as soon as the acute condition is over.

2. *Severe aortic regurgitation (Austin-Flint murmur)*. It is due to functional MS produced by the aortic regurgitant jet striking against the anterior mitral leaflet forcing its partial closure. The murmur has following characteristics.

   - It is neither associated with loud S_1 or presystolic accentuation
   - Opening snap is absent
   - No thrill
   - The patient has florid signs of severe AR (read aortic regurgitation)

3. *Functional mid-diastolic murmur* (increased flow through a normal valve). This is seen in left to right shunts (VSD, ASD, PDA) or in hyperdynamic circulation. The murmur is soft, not associated with thrill and opening snap. The third heart sound (S_3) may be present.

4. *Severe mitral regurgitation*
   - A soft mid-diastolic murmur with a pansystolic murmur and S_3 in patients with MR indicates severe MR

5. *Left atrial myxoma*. A pedunculated myxoma may strike against the valve in diastole producing signs of MS with mid-diastolic murmur. The characteristic features of atrial myxoma are:
   - *Tumor plop* — a sound produced by striking of myxoma against the valve.
   - *Disappearance or change in the intensity* and *character* of the murmur during lying down. The murmur is best heard in sitting position.
   - No associated thrill or opening snap.
   - Constitutional symptoms (fever, weight loss, arthralgia, rash) or embolic episodes may occur

6. *Tricuspid stenosis*. The murmur has similar characteristics as in MS, but is heard at left sternal edge.

7. *Ball valve thrombus*. It floats in the left atrium and produce functional MS similar to atrial myxoma.

Q. What are the causes of split S_1?
Ans: Normally the two components of first heart sound (e.g. mitral and tricuspid) cannot be heard separately. However, the S_1 gets split under following conditions.

   i. RBBB
   ii. Mitral or tricuspid stenosis
   iii. Ventricular pacing.

Q. What are the causes of opening snap?
Ans: Following are the causes:
   - Mitral stenosis
   - Tricuspid stenosis
   - Left to right shunt (VSD, ASD, PDA)
   - Sometimes in severe MR.

Q. What is Lutembacher's syndrome?
Ans: It comprises:
   - Atrial septal defect (ASD)
   - MS (rheumatic in origin)

Q. What does presystolic murmur in MS indicate? What do you mean by presystolic accentuation of MDM in MS?
Ans: The presystolic murmur is due to forceful atrial contractions against the stenotic mitral valve. The presystolic murmur without other auscultatory findings of MS, indicates mild MS; on the other hand in sinus rhythm presystolic accentuation of the middiastolic murmur indicates severe mitral stenosis. Presystolic accentuation of MDM disappears in AF and big atrial thrombus.

Q. How do you decide the severity of mitral stenosis?
Ans: The auscultatory findings that determine the severity of MS are:
   - Lower volume pulse and low pulse pressure
   - Cold peripheral extremities
   - Longer duration of the mid-diastolic murmur with the presystolic accentuation.
   - Proximity of the OS to second heart sound. More near is the OS to the aortic component of second heart sound, more severe is the MS.

Q. What is Juvenile MS?
Ans: In the West, MS is seen usually in 4th or 5th decade, but in India, it develops early and may be seen in children commonly. The criteria for juvenile MS are:
   - Occurs below 18 years of age
   - It is usually severe (pin-point mitral valve)
   - Atrial fibrillation is uncommon.
   - Calcification of valve uncommon
   - Needs immediate surgical correction.

Q. What is Ortner's syndrome?
Ans: It is hoarseness of voice due to compression of recurrent laryngeal nerve by an enlarged left atrium in MS.

Q. How will you investigate a case with MS?
Ans: The investigations are as follows:
   1. *ECG:* It may show left atrial hypertrophy (P mitrale), right ventricular hypertrophy and atrial fibrillation.

2. *Chest X-ray:* Mitralised heart (Fig. 24.2), Left atrium is conspicuously prominent on left border of heart which is straightened. There is double atrial shadow (→). Signs of pulmonary congestion present. Pulmonary conus is prominent (←).

3. *Echocardiogram shows:*
   - Thickened immobile mitral cusps.
   - Reduced rate of diastolic filling (EF slope is flattened)

4. *Cardiac catheterization*
   Pressure gradient between I.A. and I.V. is present

Q. **In which trimester of pregnancy do the patients of MS usually become symptomatic and why?**

Ans: Patients usually become symptomatic in second trimester of pregnancy. This is due to an increase in blood volume which increases pulmonary pressure. The symptoms improve late in the 3rd trimester due to decrease in blood volume.

Q. **What are the complications of mitral stenosis?**

Ans: Common complications are as follows:
1. *Acute pulmonary edema* (left heart failure). In patients with MS, the left ventricle is hypoplastic (under-filled) hence, pulmonary edema is due pulmonary venous hypertension resulting in transudation.
2. *Pulmonary hypertension and right heart failure*
3. *Arrhythmias*, e.g. atrial fibrillation, atrial flutter, VPCs

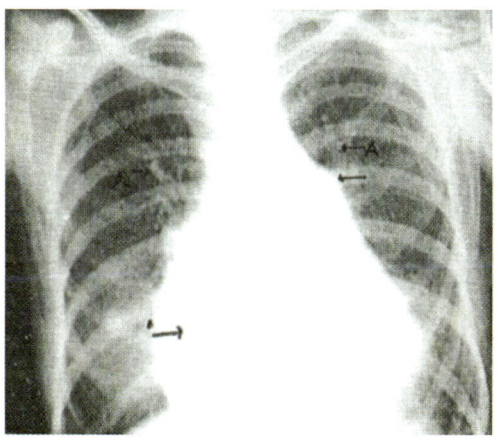

Fig. 24.2: Chest X-ray (PA view) showing mitralised heart

4. *Left atrial thrombus* with systemic embolization leading to stroke, Lerische's syndrome—occulsion of bifurcation of aorta

5. *Recurrent massive hemoptysis* leading to hemosiderosis

6. *Infective endocarditis*—rare. It is common in mitral regurgitation than stenosis

7. *Recurrent pulmonary infection* due to chronic passive venous lung congestion

8. *Complications produced by enlarged left atrium*
   - *Ortner's syndrome.*
   - Dysphagia (compression of esophagus)
   - Clot in the left atrium gives rise to embolization in sinus rhythm
   - Collapse of the lung due to pressure on left bronchus

9. Sudden death due to *ball valve thrombus*—a big thrombus fits like a ball into mitral valve.

10. Interlobar effusion (*phantom tumor*) or hydrothorax (*pleural effusion*).

Q. **What are clinical signs of acute pulmonary edema?**

Ans: Read mitral regurgitation.

Q. **How would manage the patient?**

Ans:
- If the patient is in acute LVF, then it is an emergency requiring parenteral diuretics, bronchodilators, vasodilators along with oral digoxin (0.5 mg stat) or I.V. digoxin (not preferred now a days). In addition, patient needs prop up position and O_2 inhalation
- Mild stenosis is treated with salt restriction and diuretics.
- Moderate to severe MS needs, propped up position, O_2 inhalation, oral digoxin and diuretics. Vasodilators are needed to reduce afterload. As patient improves, he/she is prepared for surgery.
- Treatment of atrial fibrillation if present, by digitalis or calcium channel blocker or beta blocker. Anticoagulant is also needed to prevent thromboembolism.
- Prophylaxis against bacterial endocarditis by penicillin, benzathine penicillin 12.5 lac units/every 3–4 weeks for 5 years or up to 25 years of age depending on the age of onset of MS.
- Surgery

Q. **What are indications for surgery?**

Ans:
- Severe or significant symptomatic MS with pliable valve

- Patient with recurrent hemoptysis and pulmonary hypertension.
- Recurrent thromboembolism despite anticoagulation.

Q. Name the surgical procedures for MS.

Ans: 1. *Closed commissurotomy* (closed mitral valvotomy by mechanical dilators or valvuloplasty by balloon dilation of the mitral valve)

2. *Open commissurotomy:* It requires cardiopulmonary bypass and allows surgical repair of valve under direct vision.

3. *Valve replacement:* It is done when valve is fibrosed, disorganized, calcified or when there is an associated mitral regurgitation.

Q. What are complications of surgery?

Ans:
- Mitral regurgitation may occur
- Risk of thromboembolic event
- Restenosis

Q. What factors determine the success of balloon valvuloplasty?

Ans:
- Pliable valve cusps
- Absence of or little calcification
- Good left ventricular function

25

Mitral Regurgitation

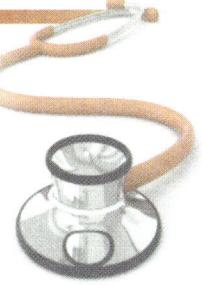

INSTRUCTION

Examine cardiovascular system.

SALIENT FEATURES

- Palpitation and dyspnea on exertion

HISTORY

Ask for the following:

- Exertional dyspnea, nocturnal dyspnea, palpitation
- Symptoms of acute pulmonary edema, e.g. cough, frothy sputum, dyspnea at rest and hemoptysis
- Fatigue, weakness, tiredness due to reduced cardiac output
- Puffiness of face, ankle or leg swelling, ascites due to right heart failure
- History of trauma to chest or cardiac surgery, MI, connective tissue disease, infective endocarditis.

Past History

- Ask for history of sore throat, skin infection, rheumatic fever (joint pain)
- History of recurrent chest infections, fever, paralysis.

EXAMINATION

General Physical Examination

- Pulse may be good volume or normal volume or jerky. It is usually regular but becomes irregular in presence of atrial fibrillation or ventricular ectopics
- Pulse pressure may be wide or normal. Note BP, temperature and respiration
- Cyanosis (peripheral or central or both) may be present
- Raised jugular venous pressure with prominent 'a' wave in severe pulmonary hypertension (present in this case) and 'v' wave if TR develops
- Pitting pedal edema (present)

- Look for signs of bacterial endocarditis
- Look for signs of acute rheumatic activity, e.g. arthritis, fever, erythema marginatum, subcutaneous nodules, etc.

Cardiovascular System

Inspection

- Apex beat is displaced down beyond 5th intercostal space outside the midclavicular line and is diffuse but forceful.
- Pulmonary artery pulsations in 2nd left intercostal space may be seen.
- Left parasternal heave may be visible.

Palpation

- Left parasternal heave may be palpable (present).
- Displaced down and out forceful apex beat (present).
- Systolic thrill at apex may be palpable
- P_2 may be palpable in pulmonary area in pulmonary hypertension (palpable in this case).

Percussion

- Left border of heart corresponds to apex beat, i.e. dullness does not extend beyond apex beat.

Auscultation

- First heart sound soft or muffled and buried in the pansystolic murmur (present in this case)
- Pansystolic murmur at apex (Fig. 25.1), high pitched, soft and radiates to left axilla, heard with diaphragm of the stethoscope in expiration (present)
- Third heart sound (S_3) may be present, is caused by rapid flow of blood causing tensing of papillary muscle, chordae tendinae and valve leaflets
- P_2 may be loud and narrowly split. An ejection systolic and/or diastolic murmur (Graham Steell) may be heard at 2nd left space.

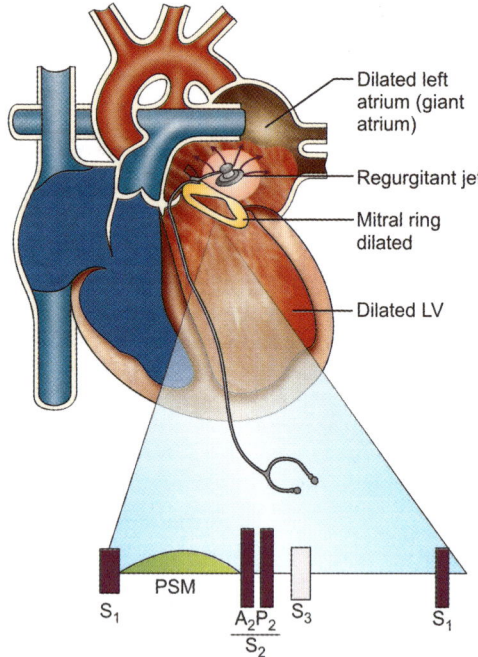

Dilated left atrium (giant atrium)

Regurgitant jet

Mitral ring dilated

Dilated LV

PSM

S_1 $\dfrac{A_2P_2}{S_2}$ S_3 S_1

Fig. 25.1: Mitral regurgitation, Hemodynamic effects and auscultatory findings, S_3: Third heart sound, PSM: Pansystolic murmur

Examination of Other Systems

1. *Respiratory system*
   - Tachypnea may be present
   - Crackles and rales at bases of lungs

2. *Abdominal examination*
   - Mild tender hepatomegaly
   - No ascites, no splenomegaly.

PROVISIONAL DIAGNOSIS

In view of patient's symptoms and signs, the provisional diagnosis is mitral regurgitation, the cause of which could be rheumatic or ischemic. Patient is in congestive cardiac failure (functional cardiac status) without any evidence of infective endocarditis or thromboembolic phenomenon.

QUESTIONS AND ANSWERS

Q.   **What are points in favour of your diagnosis?**
Ans: 1. History of dyspnea, orthopnea and PND.
      2. Signs of MR, i.e. down and out apex beat, parasternal heave, a pansystolic murmur radiating to axilla, muffled S_1 and presence of S_3.

3. Signs of pulmonary hypertension, e.g. loud P_2, narrow split S_2.
4. Signs of CHF, e.g. raised JVP, tender hepatomegaly and edema feet.

Q.   **What are the causes of mitral regurgitations?**
Ans: 1. *Rheumatic (less common)*
         - Rheumatic heart disease, acute rheumatic fever
      2. *Non-rheumatic (common)*
         - Mitral valve prolapse
         - Myocarditis
         - Acute MI (due to papillary muscle dysfunction or rupture of chordae tendinea producing acute mitral regurgitation)
         - Infective endocarditis
         - Dilated cardiomyopathy
         - Trauma during valvotomy
         - Marfan's syndrome
         - SLE (Libman-Sack's endocarditis)
         - Rarely congenital
      3. *Left ventricular dilatation (valve ring dilatation) secondary to:*
         - Aortic valve disease, e.g. AS, AR or both
         - Systemic hypertension

Note: Isolated mitral regurgitation is commonly non-rheumatic in origin.

Q.   **What is the sequence of valvular involvement in rheumatic heart disease?**
Ans: - Mitral valve disease (80%). MS is the commonest lesion followed by combined MS and MR
      - Aortic valve (50%)
      - Combined mitral and aortic valve lesion (20%)
      - Tricuspid valve involvement (10%)
      - Pulmonary valve involvement rare (<1%)

Q.   **What are congenital causes of MR?**
Ans: - Ostium primum atrial septal defect (cleft mitral valve)
      - Endocardial cushion defect (partial atrioventricular canal)
      - Corrected transposition of great vessels

Q.   **What are clinical characteristic features of severe MR?**
Ans: Characteristic features of severe MR are;
      i. A good volume pulse with wide pulse pressure
      ii. Raised JVP with prominent 'a' wave due to severe pulmonary hypertension, and prominent 'v' wave if there is associated TR

iii. Signs of severe pulmonary hypertension (Read signs of pulmonary hypertension in MS).

iv. *Auscultatory signs of severe mitral regurgitation*
   - The S_1 is generally muffled, soft or buried within pansystolic murmur
   - A pansystolic murmur radiating to left axilla
   - S3 may be audible
   - A short-soft diastolic murmur even in the absence of MS (functional MS) may be heard
   - An S_4 is audible in acute severe MR
   - An OS may be heard in the absence of MS. Usually OS indicates associated MS but can be heard in severe MR.

Q. How would you grade systolic murmurs?

Ans: Read Clinical Methods in Medicine by Prof SN Chugh.

Q. What is pansystolic murmur and what are its causes?

Ans: *Definition:* A pansystolic or holosystolic murmur starts with the first heart sound (S_1) and continues throughout the systolic and embraces S_2. It has uniform intensity hence called holosystolic.

Causes

1. MR due to any cause
2. Mitral valve prolapse
3. *TR:* The pansystolic murmur is best audible in the tricuspid area (left parasternal), increases in intensity with inspiration (Carvallo's sign) and does not radiate to axilla. There may be prominent 'v' waves in JVP and liver may be pulsatile.
4. Ventricular septal defect (*mala de Roger*): The murmur is rough, pansystolic, best heard across the chest (on both sides of sternum). Very often there is an associated thrill.
5. Dilated cardiomyopathy, and sometimes myocarditis
6. Functional murmur (Left ventricular dilatation): These murmurs are usually soft, mostly midsystolic, may be pansystolic and do not radiate to the axilla. No change with posture and respiration.
7. Papillary muscle dysfunction.
8. Redundant or rupture chordae tendinae

Q. What does mid-diastolic murmur in MR indicate?

Ans. 1. Associated MS (i.e. MR with MS)
2. Severe MR with functional MS.

Q. What are causes of acute MR?

Ans: Causes of acute MR are:
- Acute myocardial infarction with either rupture of papillary muscle or chordae tendinae.
- Acute bacterial endocarditis with rupture/perforation of valve cusps or chordae tendinae.
- Traumatic rupture of chordae tendinae.
- Myxomatous degeneration of the valve

Q. What are the complications or MR?

Ans: • Complications of MR are:
- *Acute LVF (acute pulmonary edema).* It is characterized by persistent coughing with bringing out of small amount of frothy pink colored sputum with increasing breathlessness, orthopnea, PND, tachypnea, tachycardia and central cyanosis The chest shows diffuse bilateral crackle and rales throughout both lungs. The X-ray is diagnostic.
- *Infection endocarditis.*
- *Arrhythmias,* e.g. ventricular ectopics, atrial fibrillation common.
- *Giant left atrium* may produce pressure symptoms, e.g. hoarseness, dysphagia.
- *Thromboembolism*
- *Atypical chest pain*

Q. What is cooing or 'Seagull' murmur?

Ans: When a patient of MR either develops SABE or rupture of chorade tendinae, a systolic murmur appears that has either a cooing or musical or seagull quality — here the chordae tendinae act like strings of a musical instrument. This type of murmur is also found in acute myocardial infarction and in acute rheumatic carditis.

Q. How will you investigate a patient with MR?

Ans: Investigations required are as follows:
1. *Chest X-ray.* It may show:
   - Cardiac shadow is enlarged and occupies > 50% of transthoracic diameter.
   - The left atrium may be massively enlarged and forms the right border of the heart.
   - The left ventricle is also enlarged producing a boot-shaped heart.
   - There may be pulmonary venous congestion (e.g. upper lobar veins prominent producing increased bronchovascular markings or there may be diffuse haze from hilum to periphery — pulmonary edema), interstitial edema (Kerley's B lines) and sometimes interlobar fissure effusion or hydrothorax.

- Mitral valve calcification may occur, seen in penetrating films.
2. *ECG.* It may show:
   - Right atrial, left atrial or biatrial hypertrophy
   - LV or biventricular hypertrophy
   - AF
   - Inferior or posterior wall ischemia/infarction if CAD is the cause.
3. *Echocardiogram and Doppler imaging:* The 2D-echocardiogram is useful for assessing the cause of MR, displacement of one or both cups into left atrium during systole in MVP and for estimating the LV function and ejection fractions. Left atrium and left ventricle enlarged. Vegetations may be seen in infective endocarditis. The echocardiogram M-mode shows characteristic feature of MVPS (incomplete coaptation of anterior and posterior leaflets during mid and late systole).
4. *Color Doppler flow study* (Fig. 25.2) is most accurate diagnostic technique for detection and quantification of MR. It shows a characteristic regurgitant jet.
5. *Trans-esophageal echocardiography* is useful in those in whom transthoracic echocardiography provides non-diagnostic images.
6. *Cardiac catheterization:* It is useful to determine coronary artery disease or aortic valve disease, done prior to surgery.

Q. How will you treat a patient with MR?
Ans: 1. Medical treatment
   - Asymptomatic disease (e.g. MVP) does not require treatment except penicillin prophylaxis.
   - Salt restriction, digitalis and diuretics
   - Bronchodilatation if there is severe bronchospasm
   - Vasodilators (ACE-inhibitors) to reduce the regurgitant flow in severe cases.
   - *Prophylaxis:* Penicillin prophylaxis is must for symptomatic cases
2. Surgical treatment is valve replacement

Q. What is indication of surgery in MR?
Ans: Moderate to severe symptomatic disease with good left ventricular function.

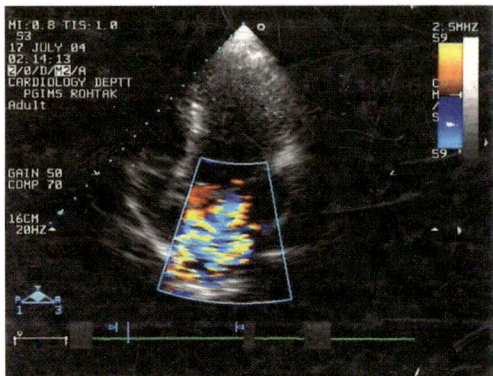

Fig. 25.2: Colour Doppler study showing regurgitant Jet through the mitral valve

Q. How will you decide the dominance of mitral valve lesion in a patient with combined mitral valve disease?
Ans: Read mixed mitral valve lesion as a Case 27.

Q. What does 3rd heart sound in MR indicate?
Ans: The presence of 3rd heart sound in MR indicates rapid ventricular filling due to free flow of blood through mitral valve. It signifies moderate to severe MR and in combined mitral valve lesion (MS with MR), it indicates dominance of MR over MS.

Q. What are signs of digitalis toxicity?
Ans: The signs are as follows:
1. *GI manifestations*, e.g. anorexia, nausea, vomiting. These are earliest to appear.
2. *Cardiac arrhythmias* and conduction disturbances.
   - Premature ventricular complexes (VPCs) usually ventricular bigeminy or multiforme.
   - Nonparoxysmal atrial tachycardia with block
   - Varying degrees of AV block
   - Sinoatrial block (SA block)
   - Ventricular tachycardia; bidirectional ventricular tachycardia is mainly due to digitalis
   - Ventricular fibrillation
3. *Miscellaneous effects*
   - Weight loss
   - Cardiac cachexia
   - Gynecomastia
   - Yellow vision (xanthopsia)
   - Mental features, e.g. agitation

26

Mitral Valve Prolapse (MVP)

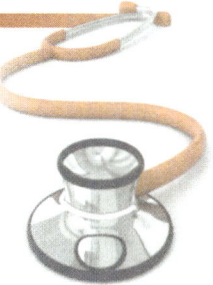

INSTRUCTION

Examine the cardiovascular system.

SALIENT FEATURES

- Palpitation

HISTORY

Ask for the following:

- Age and sex
- History of palpitation, dyspnea on exertion
- Atypical chest pain, fatigue
- Symptoms of hyperadrenergic syndrome
- Anxiety

EXAMINATION

General Physical Examination

- Look for height and signs of Marfan's syndrome (high arched palate, arm span > height, long slender fingers)
- Pulse may be normal or good volume depending on severity of MR
- Pulse pressure is normal, sometimes may be wide
- Look for the signs of endocarditis, i.e. fever, splinter hemorrhage, palmar erythema, Janeway's lesion, clubbing of fingers, cold extremities, high color urine and painful fingertips
- Look for signs of acute rheumatic activity (use John's criteria)

CVS Examination

- On inspection, palpation, percussion and auscultation, findings of MR will be present
- The murmur on auscultation has following characteristics
  - Murmur is midsystolic with a click (mid systolic click murmur syndrome), occasionally may be pansystolic, soft, blowing and radiating to the axilla.
- Valsalva maneuver and standing increase the murmur of MVP while squatting decreases the murmur

PROVISIONAL DIAGNOSIS

The young female complaining of palpitation has mitral valve prolapse (lesion) the cause of which is idiopathic (etiology). She does not have LHF or endocarditis (functional status).

QUESTIONS AND ANSWERS

Q. **What are the points in favour of your diagnosis?**

Ans: 1. A young female with complaint of palpitation.
2. A midsystolic click and hollow-systolic murmur not radiating to axilla.
3. Murmur increases on Valsalva maneuver and exercise and decreases with squatting.

Q. **What are the causes of mitral valve prolapse?**

Ans: Following are the causes:
- Marfan's syndrome
- Ehlers-Danlos syndrome
- Collagen vascular disorders (genetically determined)
- Straight-back syndrome (a thoracic cage abnormality)
- As a sequal of acute rheumatic fever
- Ischemic heart disease
- Cardiomyopathy.

Q. **What is prevalence of MVP in general population?**

Ans: About 9–10%. It is more common in young females (15–35 years).

Q. **What is mechanism of click in MVP?**

Ans: It is due to sudden tensing of mitral valve apparatus as the leaflet prolapses into the left atrium during systole.

Q. **What is effect of Valsalva maneuver on MR?**

Ans: The systolic murmur of MR is increased by isometric strain (hand–grip) but is reduced during the Valsalva maneuver.

Q. What is mitral valve prolapse syndrome?
Ans: Mitral valve prolapse syndrome (*Barlow's syndrome, midsystolic click murmur syndrome, floppy mitral valve syndrome*) is characterised by:
1. It is common in young females
2. Mostly asymptomatic, but common symptoms include palpitations, fatigue, etc.
3. Midsystolic murmur with a click (click-murmur syndrome) increasing on standing and Valsalva maneuver and decreasing on squatting is characteristic
4. It is commonly associated with Marfan's syndrome or marfanoid habitus.

Q. Where does the murmur of MVP radiate?
Ans: • In prolapse of anterior cusp of mitral valve, murmur radiates to the axillary region
   • In posterior leaflet prolapse, murmur radiates anteriorly to the chest

Q. How would you confirm the diagnosis?
Ans: The diagnosis is confirmed on echocardiography. *M-mode echocardiography* shows incomplete coaptation of anterior and posterior leaflets during mid and late systole. *2D-Echocardiogram* (Fig. 26.1) reveals displacement of one or both cusps into left atrium and the left ventricle is enlarged.
Vegetations can also be detected if present. *Color Doppler* flow studies detect the regurgitant jet and its magnitude.

Q. What are the complications of MVP?
Ans: • Tachyarrhythmias
   • Infective endocarditis
   • Left heart failure (LHF)

Q. Do the patients of MVP require prophylaxis against endocarditis?
Ans: Yes. Prophylaxis with benzathine penicillin is indicated as usual.

Q. How would you treat this patient?
Ans: The patient has only mild MVP without left heart failure and endocarditis, hence, she needs only prophylaxis against bacterial endocarditis and a small dose of betablocker to control palpitation.

Q. Name the drug which helps to reduce the prolapse.
Ans: Betablockers.

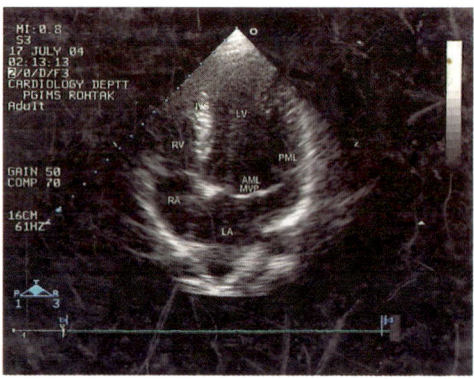

Fig. 26.1: Echocardiogram (4 chamber view) shows mitral regurgitation due to mitral valve prolapse of anterior leaflet (AML – MVP)

27 Combined Mitral Valve Disease (Mitral Stenosis with Mitral Regurgitation)

INSTRUCTION

Examine the cardiovascular system

SALIENT FEATURES

- Breathlessness, cough, palpitation, edema feet

HISTORY

Ask for the following:

- History of dyspnea, orthopnea, PND
- History of cough, sputum mostly on winter seasons
- History of swelling legs, pain abdomen (hepatomegaly) and distension of abdomen (ascites)
- Past history of acute rheumatic fever
- History of fever, focal neurological deficit, flank pain (hematuria) for infective endocarditis
- History of mitral valvotomy

EXAMINATION

General Physical Examination

- It is same as discussed in case discussion on MS and MR
- Extremities for cyanosis, edema, coldness tender spots and gangrenous fingers.
- Look always for the peripheral signs of infective endocarditis and rheumatic activity.

Cardiovascular Examination

- On examination, patient will have signs of mitral stenosis (mid-diastolic murmur) and signs of mitral regurgitation (a pansystolic murmur). The other signs depend on the dominance of the lesion (Fig. 27.1)
- Always look for scar of mitral valvotomy under the left nipple (Remember, the scar can be missed in females with pendulous breast)
- Hear always for the cardiac signs of infective endocarditis (Read infective endocarditis as a case)

Other Systems

- *Respiratory system examination* for basal crackles for LVF

- *Abdominal examination* for tender hepatomegaly and ascites

PROVISIONAL DIAGNOSIS

The symptoms and signs in this patient suggest the diagnosis of combined mitral stenosis and mitral regurgitation (lesion) due to rheumatic heart disease (etiology). Patient has congestive cardiac failure (NHYA class III or IV functional status), sinus rhythm without infective endocarditis, and without any acute rheumatic activity.

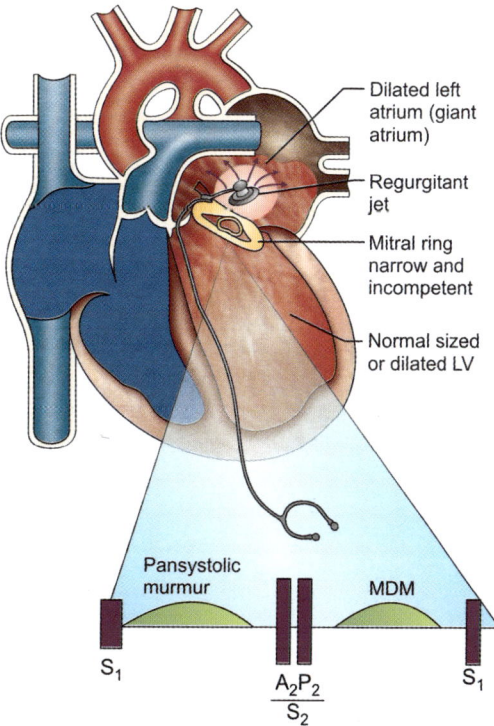

Fig. 27.1: Mitral stenosis with mitral regurgitation. Hemodynamic effects and auscultatory findings. S3: Third heart sound not shown was present in this case

QUESTIONS AND ANSWERS

Q. **Which is the dominant lesion out of the two?**

Ans: The dominant lesion is mitral regurgitation. The points in favor are:
1. Cardiomegaly (apex beat is down and outside the midclavicular line)
2. Heaving apex beat
3. Soft first heart sound
4. Presence of third heart sound (S_3)
5. A systolic thrill.

Q. **What signs of MS get masked by coexistence of MR?**

Ans:
- Loud first heart sound of MS gets muffled.
- Instead of opening snap, third heart sound becomes audible
- Tapping apex beat is masked.
- Murmur of MS gets shorter and louder but rumbling character is masked.

Q. **How would decide dominance of one lesion over the other?**

Ans: The dominance of the lesion is decided on clinical feature, physical signs and investigations (Table 27.1)

Q. **Could he/she be a case of MS with tricuspid regurgitation instead of MR?**

Ans: No, because of following points favour MR.
1. Good volume pulse and left parasternal heave
2. Raised JVP without 'VY' Collapse (VY collapse is a sign of TR)
3. Pansystolic murmur at the apex, radiating to the axilla
4. Ist sound is muffled while in MS and TR, it will remain loud, rough and rumbling
5. Presence of 3rd heart sound (in TR, there will be 4th heart sound)
6. Liver is tender but nonpulsatile (pulsatile liver indicates TR)

Q. **What does giant atrium indicate in combined mitral lesion?**

Ans: Giant atrium in combined mitral lesion indicates insignificant mitral stenosis.

Q. **What are the causes of organic combined mitral lesions?**

Ans: 1. Chronic Rheumatic heart disease alone is the cause of organic combined mitral lesions?

Q. **What is Jet mitral incompetence in MS?**

Ans: A soft midsystolic or pansystolic murmur in presence of significant mitral stenosis indi-

Table 27.1: Features of dominant MS or MR in combined valvular lesion

Feature	Dominant MS	Dominant MR
1. Clinical presentations	Dyspnea on exertion, orthopnea and PND, palpitation is uncommon occurs if AF present	Palpitations common, followed by dyspnea, orthopnea and PND
2. Symptoms	Marked	Mild
• Hemoptysis and PND		
• Symptoms of CHF	Marked	Present
• Systemic embolization		
• Lung congestion		
3. Signs		
Pulse	Low volume	Normal volume
BP	Low systolic	Within normal limits
Apex	Tapping, not displaced	Heaving and displaced down and out
Left parasternal heave	Grade III	Grade I
First heart sound	Short, loud and snappy	Soft or muffled
Opening snap	Present	Absent
Third heart sound (S_3)	Absent	Present
Murmur and thrill	• Rough and rumbling diastolic murmur • Pansystolic murmur present, does not radiate to axilla	• Soft pansystolic murmur radiating to axilla with a systolic thrill • Soft mid-diastolic murmur of MS present
4. Chest X-ray	Mitralized heart	Cardiomegaly with giant left atrium forming right heart border
5. ECG	RVH with left axis deviation	LVH with right axis deviation

cates Jet incompetence. It is due to fixed narrow lumen of mitral valve which allows mild regurgitation to occur.

Q. **How would you decide whether MDM in your case is organic (due to MS) not functional due to dominant MR?**

Ans: Remember. Inhalation of amyl nitrate will differentiate between the organic and functional MS in a patient with MR. It will increase both the duration and intensity of the murmur in organic MS but functional murmur will decrease.

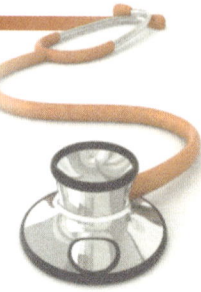

28

Mixed Mitral and Aortic Valve Disease

INSTRUCTION

Examine the cardiovascular system

SALIENT FEATURES

- Palpitation and dyspnea and edema feet

HISTORY

Ask for the following:
- History of dyspnea, orthopnea, PND (LVF)
- History of palpitation, fatigue, weakness (LVF)
- History cough, sputum, hemoptysis (pulmonary edema)
- History of pain abdomen (hepatomegaly), puffiness of face, swelling of legs (right heart failure)
- Symptoms suggestive of infective endocarditis or acute rheumatic activity (*Jone's Criteria*)
- History of paralysis of a limb/limb's, flank pain, gangrene of fingers (embolization)
- Past history of acute rheumatic fever/skin infection

EXAMINATION

General Physical Examination
- Note the pulse and its characteristics
- Pulse is good volume and regular (in this case)
- JVP is raised. No prominent wave
- No cyanosis. Puffiness over the face present
- Pitting edema over the ankles (present)
- No peripheral signs of infective endocarditis or acute rheumatic activity

Cardiovascular System
- *Apex beat*. It is down and outside the midclavicular line.
- Left ventricular heave—present (palpable)
- A diastolic thrill is palpable at apex and at 3rd left intercostal space.
- P_2 is also palpable (pulmonary hypertension)
- *Murmurs:*
  - i. Mid-diastolic murmur at apex (Fig. 28.1), heard in left lateral position with bell of

stethoscope during expiration. It indicates mitral stenosis. P_2 is loud and narrowly split (pulmonary hypertension)
  - ii. A pansystolic murmur (Fig. 28.1) is heard at apex, grade IV/VI radiates to the axilla, soft and blowing. It indicates mitral regurgitation.
  - iii. An early diastolic murmur heard at 2nd right space (A_1 area) and left third space (A_2 area), in held expiration when patient leans forward.

Other System Examination
- Examination of respiratory system shows bilateral basal crackles indicating congested lungs due to LVF
- *Examination of abdomen* for tender hepatomegaly and ascites

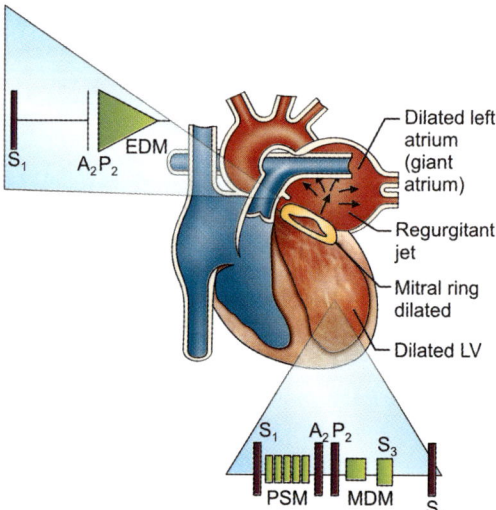

Fig. 28.1: Mitral regurgitation, mitral stenosis and aortic regurgitation. Hemodynamic effects and auscultatory findings

PROVISIONAL DIAGNOSIS

The patient has symptoms and signs suggestive of mitral stenosis, mitral regurgitation and aortic regurgitation (lesion) caused by chronic rheumatic heart disease. Patient has congestive heart failure (NHYA functional cardiac status III or IV), normal sinus rhythm without evidence of infective endocarditis or acute rheumatic activity.

QUESTIONS AND ANSWERS

Q.   What are the common causes of combined mitral and aortic valve lesions?
Ans: 1. Rheumatic heart disease
      2. Infective endocarditis (acute/subacute)
      3. Marfan's syndrome
      4. Idiopathic calcification of aortic and mitral valve apparatus

Q.   How would you diagnose aortic stenosis in presence of mitral stenosis?
Ans: Both lesions are stenotic and produce low cardiac output. The severe mitral stenosis may mask the symptoms and signs of aortic stenosis because both produce low cardiac output. However, a history of angina, syncope, ECG evidence of left ventricular hypertrophy, presence of an ejection systolic murmur with click at aortic outflow tract (A_1 area) suggest the diagnosis of aortic stenosis in combined aortic and mitral stenosis.

Q.   What will happen to signs of MS when aortic stenosis is dominant
Ans: In combined mitral stenosis and aortic stenosis, if physical findings of aortic stenosis are dominant, then physical findings of mitral stenosis are masked except a mid-diastolic rough and rumble murmur of mitral stenosis

Q.   What will be the physical signs of aortic regurgitation in combined lesion of mitral stenosis and aortic regurgitation?
Ans: The combination of mitral stenosis and aortic regurgitation has confusing pathophysiology and often leads to misdiagnosis.

Remember mitral stenosis being inflow obstruction to left ventricle, restricts left ventricular filling while aortic regurgitation produces left ventricular volume overload, but in the combined lesions if mitral stenosis is dominant, the peripheral signs of aortic regurgitation (Read signs of AR) will be masked with the result severe aortic regurgitation may fail to produce signs of hyperdynamic circulation.

Q.   What will happen if mitral and aortic regurgitation are present?
Ans: Both the lesions produce left ventricular burden/overload, therefore, the symptoms and signs of left ventricular failure will appear early and will be florid. The ECG will show left ventricular hypertrophy with strain pattern.
      The signs of hyperdynamic circulation will be present and florid as both lesions produce hyperdynamic circulation and supplement each other's effects.

Q.   What are the causes of aortic stenosis and mitral regurgitation?
Ans: 1. Rheumatic heart disease
      2. Congenital aortic stenosis with mitral valve prolapse (MVP)
      3. Atherosclerotic/aortic stenosis and mitral regurgitation

Q.   How would you investigate such a case?
Ans: The investigations are same as discussed under individual mitral or aortic valve lesion.

Q.   How would you treat?
Ans: I. Treatment of CHF by salt restriction, diuretics, ACE inhibitors, digoxin, etc.
      II. Surgery (Valve replacement)

Q.   What are indications of surgery?
Ans: I. NYHA class III status
      NYHA class II status with LV dysfunction, i.e. volume overload, for example severe aortic regurgitation with moderate mitral valve disease.

29

Prosthetic Heart Valve

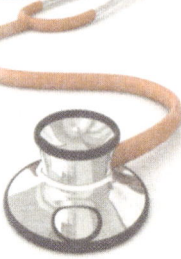

INSTRUCTION

Examine the Cardiovascular (Heart) System.

SALIENT FEATURES

• Patient had undergone valve replacement

HISTORY

Ask for the following:

• History of valvular heart disease (rheumatic or non-rheumatic)
• History of valve replacement (type of valve and duration)
• Present history of cough, dyspnea, palpitation, etc.
• History of irregular heart beats

EXAMINATION

General Physical Examination

• Perform physical examination in same fashion as in a patient of RHD. Look for cyanosis, clubbing edema feet, JVP (neck veins), gangrenous fingers, etc.
• Look for signs of acute rheumatic activity

Cardiovascular System Examination

• Look for scar of valve replacement
• Hear the heart sounds, murmurs or any other sound (metallic sound is heard in this case)

Q. How would you recognise prosthetic valve.
Ans: I. *Clinical recognition of mitral valve prosthesis is recognised;*
  i. By the site and horizontal thoracotomy scar
  ii. Metallic first heart sound
  iii. Normal second heart sound
  iv. Metallic opening snap
  v. *Murmurs.* Systolic as well as diastolic flow murmur can be heard normally over the disc valves

II. *Recognition of aortic prosthesis.*
  It is recognised by:
  i. Site
  ii. Normal first heart sound at apex
  iii. Metallic second heart sound
  iv. Midsternal thoracotomy scar

III. *Recognition of both mitral and aortic valve prostheses*
  • Both the heart sounds will be metallic in character
  • The presence of systolic murmur does not indicate valve dysfunction but presence of an early diastolic murmur across aortic valve indicate its dysfunction.

Note: Porcine and cadaveric heterografts do not produce metallic sounds

PROVISIONAL DIAGNOSIS

In view of first heart sound being metallic in character and second being normal, the patient has replaced prosthetic mitral valve (lesion). The patient is not in left heart failure (functional status) and there is no complication of mechanical valve.

QUESTIONS AND ANSWERS

Q. What was the indication for valve replacement in your case?
Ans: Patient has undergone valve replacement for mitral valve disease, i.e. MS, MR or MS and MR (Read the indications in separate cases discussion).

Q. How would you confirm your diagnosis?
Ans: By radiology (Fig. 29.2). Metabolic valves can be seen on radiology but not the tissue valve.

Q. What are various types of prosthetic valves?
Ans: I. *Mechanical valves* (Fig. 29.1)
  • Ball and cage (Starr-Edwards)

- Tilting disc valve, i.e. Single tilting disc (Bjork-Shiley) and double tilting disc (bileaflet *valve St Jude*)

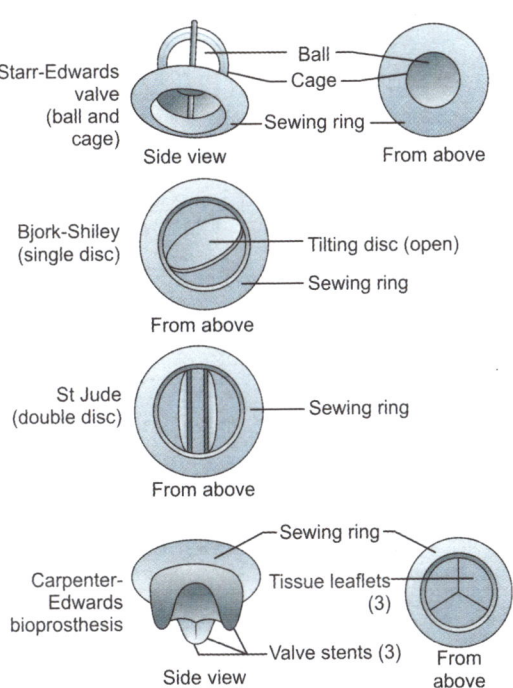

Starr-Edwards valve (ball and cage)
— Ball
— Cage
— Sewing ring
Side view   From above

Bjork-Shiley (single disc)
— Tilting disc (open)
— Sewing ring
From above

St Jude (double disc)
— Sewing ring
From above

Carpenter-Edwards bioprosthesis
— Sewing ring
— Tissue leaflets (3)
— Valve stents (3)
Side view   From above

Fig. 29.1: Types of valves (metallic and bioprosthetic)

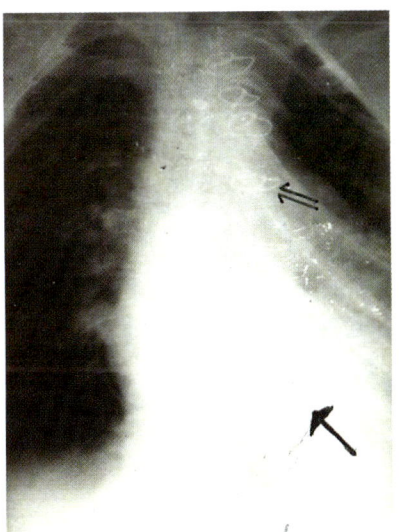

Fig. 29.2: Prosthetic mitral valve in position chest X-ray showing mechanical valve apparatus supported by hooks as indicated by an arrow

II. *Tissue (biological valves)*
  - Xenografts (porcine valves and pericardial valve derived from animal tissue)

  Homograft (Fig. 29.1)
  - Cadaveric aortic or pulmonary valve (human valve)

Q. **What are indications of various valves replacement?**

Ans:
- Severe calcified mitral stenosis
- Calcific aortic stenosis
- Severe mitral regurgitation
- Severe aortic regurgitation
- Severe combined lesions, i.e. MS and MR or AS and AR

Q. **What kind of valve would you use to replace mitral valve? and why?**

Ans: Mechanical valve because of durability. Anticoagulation is to be used to protect them.

Q. **Why mechanical valves are preferred over bioprosthesis?**

Ans: Mechanical valves are preferred because of two reasons:
- Lower rate of reoperation
- Lower chances of anticoagulant related bleeding

Q. **Which bioprosthesis is commonly used?**
Ans: Porcine heart valve.

Q. **What are complications of porcine heart valve?**
Ans:
- Degeneration with time
- Calcification

Q. **What are the complications of mechanical valves?**

Ans:
- High incidence of hemolysis leading to *anemia*
- *Thromboembolism*
- *Bleeding* due to anticoagulants use
- Endocarditis
- *Valve dysfunction*, e.g. valve leak, valve dehiscence and valve obstruction by a thrombus or clogging of valve
- *Structural dysfunction*, e.g. fracture, cuspal tear and calcification.
- *Nonstructural dysfunction*, e.g. perivalvular leak, suture entrapment.

Q. **Which patients should receive bioprosthetic valve?**

Ans:
- Those unable to take anticoagulants.
- Those not expected to live longer than predicted lifespan of prosthesis (7–10 yrs).
- Patients over the age of 70 years who require aortic valve replacement as the rate of degeneration is slow in these patients.

Q. **In women of child bearing age, which valve would you prefer?**

Ans: Until recently bioprosthetic valves were being preferred to avoid risk of anticoagulation on the fetus and spontaneous abortion but the major disadvantage of these valves is degeneration requiring reoperation. Nowadays mechanical valves are preferred because studies have now shown low risk of warfarin and spontaneous abortion in women.

Q. **Which valve would you use in presence of AF?**

Ans: Mechanical valve as these patients need warfarin treatment.

Q. **What are the causes of anemia in a patient with prosthetic valve?**

Ans: 1. Patient with mechanical valves being on anticoagulants, hence, bleeding can cause anaemia.

2. Mechanical destruction of RBCs (hemolytic anemia) by mechanical valves.

Q. **What kind of valve would you use to replace the aortic valve?**

Ans: • Mechanical valves in young persons because of durability and less chances of failure

• Porcine valves for elderly patients because there is no need of anticoagulation and there is limited life expectancy of the old persons.

Q. **What is life span of porcine valve?**

Ans: Porcine valve life span is limited. Mitral prosthetic valve has about 7 yrs span while aortic valve has about 10 yrs span in younger persons.

30

Pulmonary Stenosis

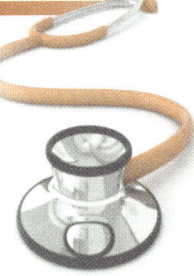

INSTRUCTION

Examine the Cardiovascular (Heart) System.

SALIENT FEATURES

- Edema feet, distension of abdomen

HISTORY

Note the following:

- Patients may be symptomatic or asymptomatic
- Ask about maternal rubella during pregnancy, atypical chest pain
- History of abdominal pain, puffiness of face and swelling (ascites)

EXAMINATION

General Physical Examination

- Puffy, bloated round facies
- Normal or low volume pulse
- Raised JVP with prominent 'a' wave (present)
- BP is normal.
- Cyanosis will be present in severe pulmonary stenosis due to patent formen ovale.
- Edema feet (present)
- Clubbing of fingers may occur if patent formen ovale present

Systemic Examination

- Apex beat may be normal on inspection and palpation.
- Right parasternal heave (present in this case)
- Findings on auscultation are:
  - i. An *ejection click (EC)* over pulmonary area which decreases on inspiration (Remember, this is a paradox, because right sided events increase during inspiration)
  - ii. P$_2$ is soft, and widely split.
  - iii. An *ejection systolic murmur (ESM)* over pulmonary area (2nd left space Fig. 30.1) and

left parasternal border, best heard during inspiration
  - iv. Sy may be audible
    - Do not forget to examine the other components of Fallot's tetralogy, if cyanosis and clubbing are present (Read Fallot's tetralogy as a case)

PROVISIONAL DIAGNOSIS

The physical signs suggest the diagnosis of pulmonary stenosis (lesion) probably congenital in origin (etiology) and patient is symptomatic with limited activity (functional status)

Q. What are the points in favor of your diagnosis?

Ans:
- Symptoms and signs of right heart failure (isolated)
- An ejection click in pulmonary area
- An ejection systolic murmur over pulmonary area
- P$_2$ is soft and widely split
- Raised JVP with prominent 'a' wave

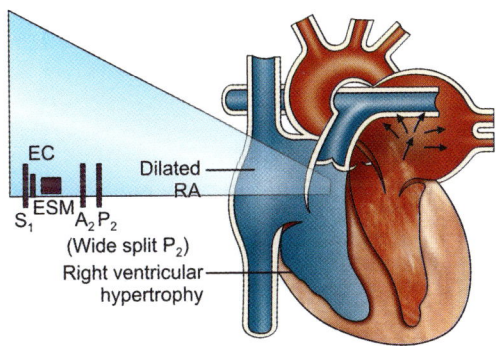

Fig. 30.1: Pulmonary stenosis; haemodynamic and auscultatory findings

QUESTIONS AND ANSWERS

Q. What are the causes of pulmonary stenosis?

Ans: 1. Congenital (commonest cause). It may be an isolated anomaly or may be a component of Fallot's tetralogy
2. Carcinoid syndrome

Q. What is normal diameter of pulmonary valve?

Ans: The normal pulmonary valve area in an adult is about 2 cm²/m² body surface area. There is no pressure gradient across the valve normally.

Q. What are types of pulmonary stenosis

Ans: • Valvular
• Subvalvular/infundibular
• Supravalvular

Q. What is Erb's point?

Ans: The third left space near to the sternum lies the Erb's point where the murmur of subvalvular (infundibular) stenosis is best audible.

Q. What are its complications?

Ans: • Right heart failure
• Infective endocarditis

Q. How would you assess the severity of pulmonary stenosis?

Ans: Read Table 30.1.

Q. Name the syndromes associated with pulmonary stenosis

Ans: 1. *Noonan syndrome:* It is characterized by short stature, downwards slanting eyeballs, hypertelorism, low-set ears, webbed neck, mental retardation, low hair line and pulmonary stenosis (present in about two-thirds cases)
2. *Watson's syndrome:* It is characterised by a triad of pulmonary stenosis, cafe-au-lait spots and mental retardation.
3. *William's syndrome:* (Read aortic stenosis). Supravalvular aortic stenosis is more common than subinfundibular pulmonary stenosis.

Q. What does foramen ovale become patent in pulmonary stenosis?

Ans: It is a small foramen which becomes closed during infancy but becomes patent under the effect of increased right atrial pressure resulting in shunting of blood from right to left atrium (R → L) resulting in cyanosis and clubbing of the fingers.

Q. How would you investigate this case?

Ans: *ECG:* The ECG will show P pulmonale (tall P waves) with right ventricular hypertrophy.

Echocardiogram: It will demonstrate the site of obstruction, its severity, enlarged right ventricle and paradoxical septal motion during systole

Color Doppler: It is used to assess the Severity by pressure gradient.

Chest X-ray: Pulmonary conus is prominent or enlarged due to post-stenotic dilatation

• Lungs are oligemic, pulmonary vascular markings are diminished

• Cardiac shadow normal or enlarged (due to presence of right ventricular failure or tricuspid regurgitation).

• Aortic knuckle is not prominent.

Q. How would you manage such a patient?

Ans: I. *Mild pulmonary stenosis* is usually asymptomatic, hence does not require treatment
II. *Moderate pulmonary stenosis:* Patient is treated medically for right heart failure and surgically, if indicated
  • Pulmonary balloon valvuloplasty is indicated in moderate disease with;
  i. Symptoms
  ii. Peak systolic gradient across the valve >50 mmHg
  iii. Right ventricular hypertrophy when the valve leaflets are not dysplastic or calcified.
  iv. Valve replacement is indicated when the valve leaflets are dysplastic or calcified.
III. *Severe stenosis* is managed surgically

Note: All the patients of pulmonary stenosis irrespective of severity should receive penicillin prophylaxis against infective endocarditis when undergoing elective dental or surgical procedure.

Table 30.1: Assessment of severity of pulmonary stenosis			
	Mild	*Moderate*	*Severe*
Orifice area	between/and 2cm²	0.5 – 1 cm²/m²	< 0.5 cm²/m²
Gradient	< 50 mmHg	50 – 80 mmHg	> 80 mmHg
Right ventricular systolic pressure	< 70 mmHg	75 – 100 mmHg	> 100 mmHg

31

Primary Pulmonary Hypertension (PPH)

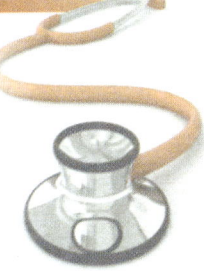

INSTRUCTION

Examine the cardiovascular system of the patient

SALIENT FEATURES

- Distended abdomen and edema feet

HISTORY

Ask for the following:
- Age and sex
- History of dyspnea, fatigue, syncope or dizziness
- History of palpitation, headache
- Puffiness of face and swelling of legs
- History of pain in abdomen (hepatomegaly), abdominal distension (ascites)
- History of drugs (antiobesity) or oral contraceptive
- History of consumption of plant products from, crotalaria species (particularly if patient is Caribbean)
- Family history of such a disease
- History of HIV (for HIV associated pulmonary hypertension)

EXAMINATION

General Physical Examination
- *Pulse and BP*: They may be normal.
- JVP is raised with prominent 'a' waves (in this case)
- Cyanosis and clubbing present if there is patent foramen ovale.
- Pitting edema over legs

Cardiovascular Examination
- Precordial and epigastric pulsations may be present due to RVH (present in this case).
- Apex beat is normally located.
- Right parasternal heave (present)
- P_2 may be palpable over 2nd left intercostal space.

On auscultation
- Loud P_2 over pulmonary area (present)

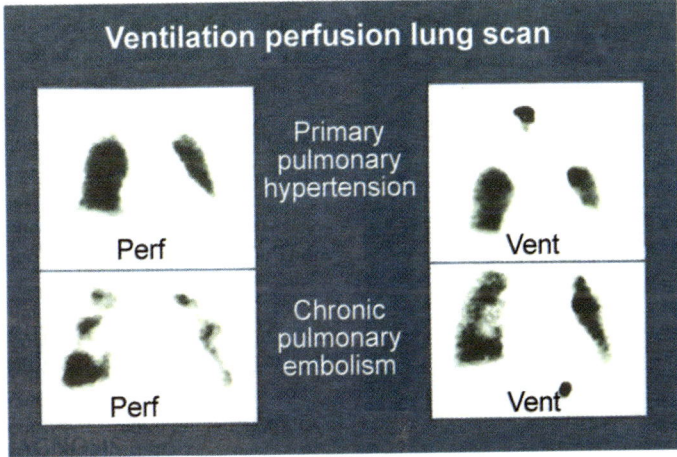

Fig. 31.1: Primary pulmonary hypertension. Perfusion (perf) and ventilation (vent) scan in a patient with thromboembolism who developed primary pulmonary hypertension shows perfusion defect in both the lungs with normal ventilation

- Early diastolic murmur of pulmonary regurgitation (present) best heard on inspiration (*Graham-Steell murmur*)
- Pansystolic murmur of tricuspid regurgitation, if it develops.

Examination of Other Systems
- *Respiratory system* for chronic respiratory disease (chronic cor pulmonale)
- *Abdomen* for hepatomegaly and ascites

PROVISIONAL DIAGNOSIS

The provisional diagnosis in this young female is primary pulmonary hypertension (lesion) the cause of which has to be found out. She is in congestive heart failure (functional status)

QUESTIONS AND ANSWERS

Q. **What are the points in favor of your diagnosis?**
Ans: 1. Raised JVP with prominent 'a' wave
2. Visible pulmonary arterial pulsations
3. Right parasternal heave
4. Right ventricular epigastric pulsations
5. Palpable P_2 in pulmonary area
6. On auscultation, loud P_2 and narrowly split second heart sound
7. Graham-Steell murmur
8. Ejection click

Q. **What are the causes of loud P2?**
Ans: • Primary pulmonary hypertension.
• Secondary pulmonary hypertension, irrespective of the cause
• Hyperkinetic circulation
• Eisenmenger's syndrome

Q. **What are the causes of pulmonary arterial hypertension?**
Ans: Read the question on classification of pulmonary hypertension
 I. *Diseases of the lungs*
  • COPD with or without chronic cor pulmonale
  • High-altitude
  • Sleep-apnea
 II. *Thromboembolism*
  Multiple pulmonary emboli (tumor, clot, foreign material)
 III. Disorders of pulmonary vasculature

Q. **What is normal pulmonary arterial pressure?**
Ans: Normal systolic pulmonary arterial pressure is 18–25 mmHg.

Q. **What is primary pulmonary hypertension?**
Ans: Primary pulmonary hypertension is defined as elevated pulmonary vascular resistance in the absence of other disease of the lungs or heart.

Q. **What are genetic abnormalities associated with primary pulmonary hypertension?**
Ans: 1. A mutation in BMPR2 gene (which encodes bone morphogenic receptor protein 2)
2. A cell surface receptor for transforming growth factor-β (TGF-β)
Two rare genes defects are:
• Activin-like kinase type (ALK–I)
• Endoglin (ENG)

Q. **What are pathological changes in pulmonary hypertension?**
Ans: Common changes are those of plexogenic pulmonary arteriopathy characterized by medial hypertrophy and concentric intimal fibrosis of the pulmonary arteries with complex plexiform lesions. Others may have occlusion of small pulmonary arteries caused by small thrombi or recurrent emboli

Q. **What are hypotheses for idiopathic pulmonary hypertension?**
Ans: 1. Excessive production of vasoconstrictor (thromboxane) than vasodilator (prostacyclin) substances by the endothelium.
2. Excessive endothelial 1 levels relative to nitric oxide.
3. Excessive *thrombosis in situ* caused by *increased platelets* activation plasminogen activator, inhibitor and decreased thrombomodulin
4. Increased serotonin levels
5. Down-regulation of K^+ channels in pulmonary artery smooth muscles
6. Monoclonal proliferation of endothelial cells

Q. **How would you grade pulmonary hypertension?**
Ans: It is graded on the basis of peak systolic pulmonary pressure and mean pulmonary artery wedge pressure.

Grade	Mean pulmonary artery wedge pressure
Normal	<20 mmHg
Mild	>20 mmHg
Moderate	>30 mmHg
Severe	>45 mmHg

Q. **How would you investigate such a case?**
Ans: 1. Measurement of protein C and S levels and presence of lupus anticoagulants, the factor V Leiden and D-dimer.

2. *Chest X-ray* for cardiomegaly, increased pulmonary artery size (prominent pulmonary conus), oligemic lungs, diseases of pulmonary vessels and lung

3. *Echocardiography* is a valuable tool to confirm the diagnosis and helps to find out the cause (congenital, and valvular heart disease), color Doppler helps to identify shunts, reveals tricuspid regurgitation

4. *High resolution CT scan of lungs* for parenchymal lung disease

5. *Ventilation and perfusion scan* for pulmonary thromboembolism. It is more sensitive than CT pulmonary angiography but does not help when there is underlying parenchymal lung disease

6. *Selective pulmonary angiography* is gold standard for diagnosis to delineate the pulmonary thromboembolism (hypoperfused areas), the location and the extent of the disease

7. *CT pulmonary angiography* for pulmonary artery enlargement, filling defects and visualization of pulmonary angiography

8. *Cardiac MRI* for imaging the RV and is also helpful to delineate congenital heart disease.

9. *Abdominal ultrasound* to screen the patient for portal hypertension, if suspected as the cause of pulmonary hypertension

Q. **How would you classify pulmonary arterial hypertension?**

Ans: The classification based on etiology is depicted in Table 31.1

Q. **How would you treat this condition?**

Ans: 1. *Diuretics* and salt restriction to decrease edema due to right ventricular preload.

2. *Vasodilators:* Calcium channel blockers (e.g. nifedipine or diltiazem) are the first drugs to be tried, if no response, then other vasodilators either phosphodiesterase inhibitors (sildenafil) or endothelial receptor blockers (bosentan or ambirsentan) are recommended.

3. Prostacyclin analogs (epoprostenol intravenously), or iloprost by inhalation or beraprost subcutaneously may be added to above regimen in case patient's symptoms are not relieved.

4. Anticoagulants (warfarin) to prevent *insitu* pulmonary thrombosis

5. Heart-lungs transplantation

Q. **What would you advise to such patients for future pregnancy?**

Ans: Women with significant pulmonary hypertension should not get pregnant, hence, permanent birth control measures should be adopted.

Q. **What are future advances being made in management of pulmonary hypertension.**

Ans: Advances in therapy are:
  i. Use of angiogenesis inhibitors
  ii. Growth factor inhibitors
  iii. Endothelial stem cell or progenitor stem cell therapy

Table 31.1: Classification of pulmonary arterial hypertension

I. *Idiopathic*, e.g. primary pulmonary hypertension

II. *Secondary pulmonary arterial hypertension*
  • *Passive or reactive* due to left sided heart lesions, e.g. mitral and aortic valve disease
  • *Hyperkinetic* due to high pulmonary flow in left to right shunts (ASD, VSD, PDA)
  • *Vasoconstrictive* (hypoxemia), e.g. chronic cor pulmonale, interstitial lung disease
  • *Obstructive* (reduction in pulmonary vascular bed) due to multiple thromboembolism
  • *Obliterative* (obliteration of pulmonary vasculature), e.g. pulmonary angiitis, sickle cell disease, collagen vascular diseases, etc.

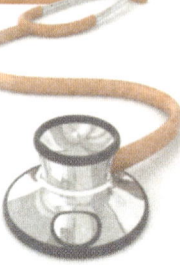

32

Chronic Cor Pulmonale

INSTRUCTION

Examine the chest of this patient

SALIENT FEATURES

- Breathlessness, pain abdomen and edema feet

HISTORY

Ask about the following:

- Cough, its frequency, seasonal relation, diurnal variation (nocturnal), etc.
- Sputum production, quantity, color, smell, consistency and history of hemoptysis
- Any recent change in the symptoms. History of recent fever, sore throat or loose motions
- History of swelling feet, abdomen (hepatomegaly)
- Ask for any aggravating or relieving factors

- Take full drug history, drug being taken and their effect

Past history

- Cough or expectoration in the past
- History of allergy or rhinitis or asthma in the past

Personal history

- History of smoking, alcoholism, exposure to dust or fumes

Occupational history

EXAMINATION

General Physical Examination (Figs 32.1A and B)

- Patient is orthopnoeic, sitting with hands on cardiac table and legs dangling/hanging from the bed to relieve breathlessness (Fig. 32.1A)

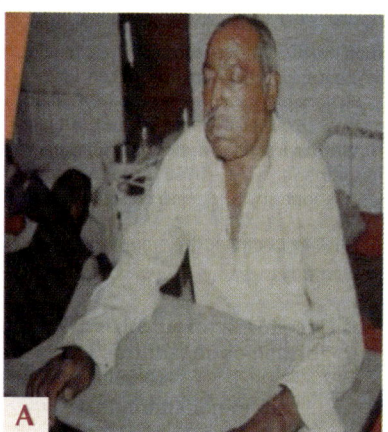

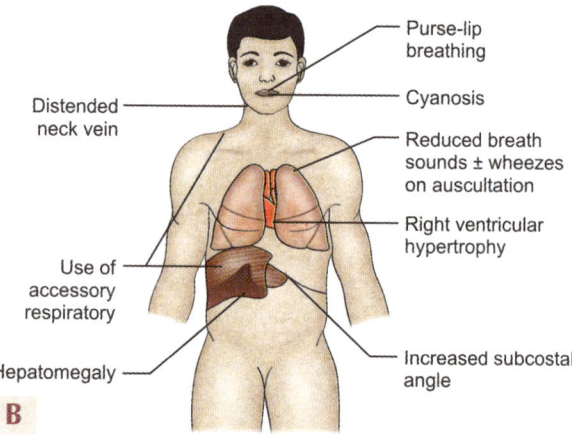

Fig. 32.1: (A) Chronic cor pulmonale. The patient has signs of COPD. Note the purse-lip breathing, cyanotic spells. The patient has facial edema and raised JVP. Note the common posture adopted by the patient with COPD and acute exacerbation with cor pulmonale to get relief from breathlessness; (B) Clinical signs of chronic cor pulmonale (diagram)

- Cyanosis is present in this case (Fig. 32.1A)
- Neck veins distended. JVP is raised. There may be v and y collapse due to TR (present in this case)
- Pulse and respiratory rate increased
- Warm extremities, clubbing of fingers and edema feet may be present (present in the case)
- Action of extra-respiratory muscles, i.e. there may be hyperactivity.

Systemic Examination (Fig. 31.1B)

1. Examination of Respiratory System

- Inspection, palpation and percussion will reveal evidences for COPD.
- Auscultation – reveals vesicular breathing with prolonged expiration. Crackles and rhonchi are scattered all over the chest (present in this case).

2. Examination of CVS

Inspection

- Apex beat may be normally placed or centrally placed or displaced outwards but not downwards or may not be visible
- No other visible pulsations

Palpation

- Apex beat may be palpable outside the mid-clavicular line (not palpable in this case)
- Parasternal heave present
- Right ventricular pulsations (palpable in epigastrium in this case).

Percussion

- Cardiac dullness may be masked or just limited to center (cardiac dullness was masked in this case)

Auscultation

- Heart sounds are normal
- Second heart sound is narrowly split (pulmonary hypertension present)
- There may be an ejection systolic murmur in P_2 area (present) and a pansystolic murmur in tricuspid area

3. Abdominal Examination

- Liver is enlarged, soft tender and may be pulsatile if TR present (liver was enlarged and tender in this case)
- There may be signs of ascites (fluid thrill and shifting dullness present).

PROVISIONAL DIAGNOSIS

The symptoms and signs suggest the diagnosis of cor pulmonale (lesion) caused by chronic obstructive pulmonary disease (etiology) and patient has congestive heart failure (functional status).

QUESTIONS AND ANSWERS

Q. What are points in favor of your diagnosis?

Ans: Sir, *first* of all history is suggestive of COPD, i.e. history of cough for most of the days in a week for 3 months in a year for 2 consecutive years.

Secondly symptoms such as breathlessness, cough, sputum production, hemoptysis and signs such as purse-lip breathing, cyanosis, action of extra-respiratory muscles, excavation of suprasternal and supraclavicular fossae, barrel-shaped chest or change in AP and transverse thoracic diameter ratio, decreased respiratory movements, diminished expansion and recession of intercostal spaces, reduced vocal fremitus, hyper-resonant note on percussion with pushing down of liver dullness to 7th intercostal space suggest COPD. On *auscultation*, harsh vesicular breathing with prolonged expiration, crackles and rhonchi favor obstruction to the respiratory passage.

Findings of distended neck veins with pulsations and raised JVP, enlarged liver, edema of legs and feet indicate right ventricular failure, therefore, after combining the two conditions the diagnosis become COPD with cor pulmonale with congestive heart failure.

Q. Define chronic cor pulmonale.

Ans: Chronic cor pulmonale is defined as right ventricular hypertrophy or dilatation secondary to the disease of the lung parenchyma, pulmonary vasculature, thoracic cage and ventilatory control.

Q. What are common causes of cor pulmonale.

Ans: Causes are:
  I. *Parenchymal lung disease*, e.g. COPD, interstitial lung diseases and pneumoconiosis, sleep apnea
  II. *Diseases* of pulmonary vasculature, e.g. pulmonary thromboembolism, primary pulmonary hypertension, pulmonary angiitis, vasculitis, collagen vascular disease
  III. *Diseases of thoracic cage*, e.g. kyphoscoliosis, obesity (picwickian syndrome), poliomyelitis.

Q. How would you investigate such a case?

Ans: Investigations required are as follows:
  1. *Chest X-ray*. It will show:
     - Cardiomegaly
     - Pulmonary conus is prominent
     - Hilar bronchovascular markings will be prominent with pruning of the peripheral pulmonary vessels

- Signs of COPD (emphysema) on X-ray will be evident
2. *ECG.* It will show
   - Low voltage graph
   - Right axis deviation, clockwise rotation
   - Right atrial hypertrophy (P-pulmonale)
   - Right ventricular hypertrophy (R > S or R:S > 1 in lead VI but both complexes will be small)
   - SI, SII, and SIII syndrome
   - Arrhythmias (MAT—multifocal atrial tachycardia is common)
3. *Echocardiography.* It will show increased right atrial and right ventricular wall thickness and enlargement of ventricular cavity. Interventricular septum is displaced leftward. Color Doppler may reveal functional TR.
4. *MRI* is useful to measure RV mass, wall thickness, and ejection fraction.
5. *Ventilation and perfusion scan* are helpful in confirming the diagnosis of chronic pulmonary vascular disease.
6. *Systemic venography and Doppler study* may reveal deep vein thrombosis.
7. *Cardiac catheterization* for measurement of pulmonary vascular pressures, calculation of pulmonary vascular resistance and response to vasodilator therapy.

Q.   What are complications of cor pulmonale?

Ans: Following are complications
- Right heart failure
- Secondary polycythemia
- Deep vein thrombosis
- Cardiac arrhythmias (multifocal atrial tachycardia, ventricular arrhythmias)

Q.   Is cor pulmonale high output failure? What are other causes of high output failure?

Ans: Initially, cor pulmonale is high output failure when hypoxia dominates leading to wide pulse pressure, later on due to involvement of myocardium, it becomes low output failure. Other causes of high output failure are:
   i.   Aortic regurgitation
   ii. Severe anemia (Hb < 4g%)
   iii. Severe thyrotoxicosis
   iv. Arteriovenous fistula
   v.   Paget's disease
   vi. Cirrhosis of liver
   vii. Beriberi heart disease

Q.   What is treatment of cor pulmonale?

Ans:
- *General measures,* i.e. back rest or prop up position, salt restriction and O_2 inhalation. Long term domiciliary O_2 therapy is helpful in patients with severe COPD as it reduces pulmonary artery hypertension.
- *Antibiotics* Acute respiratory infection is common precipitant of RV failure. Broad spectrum antibiotic may be used initially followed by antibiotic on the basis of sputum culture and sensitivity.
- *Bronchodilators* are used to relieve obstruction and to improve oxygenation.
- *Diuretics* are used to relieve obstruction and to improve oxygenation
- *Vasodilators* may be used to reduce preload.
- *Digitalis* should be used cautiously as it may induce arrhythmias in hypoxic myocardium

Q.   Does definition of cor pulmonale include right heart failure?

Ans: Right heart failure is not included in the definition of chronic cor pulmonale. It is a complication of cor pulmonale.

33

Tricuspid Regurgitation

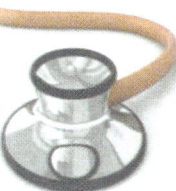

INSTRUCTION

Examine cardiovascular system

SALIENT FEATURES

- Ascites and edema feet

HISTORY

Ask the following points:

- History of IV drug abuse (right sided end-ocarditis)
- Trauma to the chest
- History of COPD (Chronic cough > 3 yrs with or without sputum)
- History of smoking
- History of recurrent attacks of asthma
- History of sore throat, skin infection or joint pains (acute rheumatic fever)

EXAMINATION

General Physical Signs

- Facial puffiness
- Neck veins are engorged. There is 'VY' collapse in jugular venous pulse (present). JVP is raised.
- Peripheral cyanosis (present)
- Pitting pedal edema (present)

Systemic Examination

Cardiovascular System

Inspection

- Left parasternal heave
- Epigastric right ventricular pulsations (present)

Palpation

- Palpable right ventricular heave
- Palpable P_2 in pulmonary area

Auscultation

- Apex beat is in normal position
- There is pansystolic murmur at the left sternal border (present), increases on inspiration (*Carvallo's signs* Fig. 33.1)

- P_2 is loud and narrowly split
- Right ventricular third heart sound (present)

Other Systems

- Respiratory system examination for signs of COPD or pulmonary hypertension
- Abdominal examination for enlarged pulsatile liver
- Presence of ascites (present)

N.B For demonstration of ascites and enlarged pulsatile liver read clinical methods by Prof S.N. Chugh.

PROVISIONAL DIAGNOSIS

This patient has tricuspid regurgitation (lesion) secondary to COPD and cor pulmonale (etiology) and has right heart failure (functional status)

QUESTIONS AND ANSWERS

Q. **What are points in favor of your diagnosis?**
Ans:
- All symptoms and signs of COPD and cor pulmonale are present
- Presence of epigastric pulsations and left parasternal heave indicate RVH

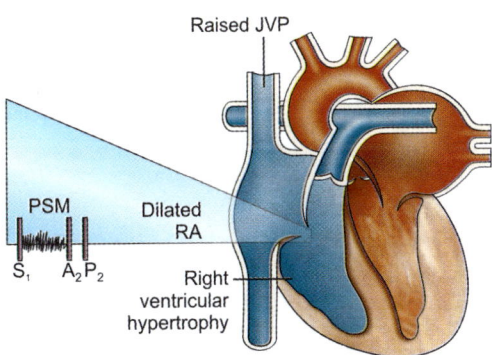

Fig. 33.1: Tricuspid regurgitation

- Pansystolic murmur increasing on inspiration, *VY* collapse on venous pulsations, pulsatile liver indicate tricuspid regurgitation
- Cyanosis, orthopnea, pitting ankle edema, enlarged liver, ascites indicate congestive heart failure/Right ventricular failure.

Q. What are causes of TR?

Ans: The causes of TR are;

1. Right ventricular dilatation secondary to pulmonary hypertension
2. Rheumatic heart disease (mitral/aortic or tricuspid valve disease)
3. Right sided endocarditis in drug abusers
4. Right ventricular infarction, right ventricular cardiomyopathy, endomyocardial fibrosis.
5. Carcinoid syndrome
6. Trauma to chest
7. Rare causes, i.e. right papillary muscle dysfunction, tricuspid valve prolapse.

Q. What are characteristics of TR?

Ans: The characteristic signs of TR are:

1. A pansystolic murmur in tricuspid area (right parasternal area/epigastrium) is heard which increases with inspiration.
2. *Signs of RVH:* There will be parasternal heave. Right ventricular pulsation may be felt in epigastrium.
3. Distended neck veins with typical '*V*' and '*Y*' collapse.
4. Pulsatile liver.
5. Hepatojugular reflux is positive.

Q. How would you differentiate MR from TR?

Ans: The differences are:

Feature	Mitral regurgitation	Tricuspid regurgitation
Pulse	Good volume jerky or normal volume	Normal pulse
JVP	Raised with 'V' prominent	Raised with 'VY' collapse
Palpation	Left ventricular heave	Right or Left parasternal heave
Auscultation	• Pansystolic murmur at apex	• Pansystolic murmur at left parasternal area
	• Murmur radiates to axilla	• Murmur may be heard in epigastrium and right sternal border
	• Intensity increases with expiration	• Intensity increases with inspiration

Other features	• 3rd heart sound	• 4th heart sound present
	• Liver may be enlarged without pulsations	• Liver is enlarged with pulsations (Pulsatile liver)
	• Lungs congested with crackles	• Lungs may or may not be congested, depending on its cause, i.e. Isolated or associated

Q. Which arrhythmia is common in TR?

Ans: Atrial fibrillation due to right atrial dilatation.

Q. What are the difference between functional and organic TR.

Ans: The differences are:

Functional TR	Organic TR
• Underlying cause is present	Organic TR is associated with mitral or aortic valve involvement
• Signs of pulmonary hypertension are present	Not present
• No association	Associated with tricuspid stenosis
• Pulmonary artery or RV pressure is usually >40 mmHg	PA or RV pressure is <40 mm Hg

Q. What do you understand by pulsatile liver? How will you demonstrate it?

Ans: Pulsatile liver means pulsations felt over the liver which could be;

1. *Intrinsic pulsations due to:*
   - Tricuspid regurgitation (systolic pulsations) either organic or functional
   - Hemangioma of the liver
2. *Transmitted pulsation from right ventricle due to*
   - Right ventricular hypertrophy

Method of demonstration of pulsations of liver: The presystolic or systolic pulsations of the heart can be transmitted to venous circulation in the liver in the presence of tricuspid incompetence, which can be detected as follows:

- Make the patient to sit in a chair, stand on the right side of the patient.
- Place your right palm over liver in right hypochondrium and left palm over the back in the same manner as used for bimanual palpation.

- Ask the patient to hold his breath after taking deep inspiration.
- The further separation of both hands over the abdomen indicates pulsatile liver.

Q. How would you quantify tricuspid regurgitation?

Ans: It is quantified on color Doppler imaging by determining the Jet area

I. Mild TR is indicated by flow disturbance in systole localised to Jet area < 5 cm^2

II. Moderate: Fills between 5 and 10 cm^2 of right atrium

III. Severe: Fills > 10 cm^2 of the enlarged right atrium.

Q. How would you investigate such a case?

Ans: 1. ECG will show P pulmonale and right ventricular hypertrophy

2. Chest X-ray will show dilated RA, dilated azygos vein and pleural effusion.

3. Echocardiogram assesses the right ventricular size, pressure and function. A paradoxically moving interventricular septum may be present due to volume overload

4. Catheterisation of right ventricle confirms the diagnosis. (Raised right ventricular and right atrial pressure).

Q. How would you treat such a case?

Ans: *Medical treatment* include salt restriction, diuretics and vasodilators. Find out the cause and treat it accordingly.

Surgical treatment is definite treatment; valve plication or annuloplasty and valve replacement performed depending on indication. Valve replacement is used when valve cannot be repaired.

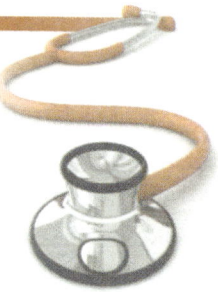

34

Congestive Heart Failure (CHF)

INSTRUCTION

Examine cardiovascular system

SALIENT FEATURES

- Ascites, edema, dyspnea and palpitation

HISTORY

Ask for the following:

1. Dyspnea on exertion, orthopnea and PND.
2. Nonproductive cough worst on recumbent position.
3. Fatigue, weakness, reduced exercise tolerance, syncope
4. History of swelling over the legs, puffiness of face, pain abdomen (congestive hepatomegaly), distension of abdomen (ascites)
5. Nocturia
6. History of irregular heart beats, fever, hemoptysis, chest pain, paralysis of limb (limbs)

EXAMINATION

General Physical Examination

- Pulse may be good, or low or normal volume. It is usually regular but becomes irregular in presence of atrial fibrillation or ventricular ectopics.
- Pulse pressure may be narrow or normal. Systolic BP is low.
- Cyanosis (peripheral or central or both) may be present
- Raised jugular venous pressure (Fig. 34.1)
- Pitting edema over the legs (Fig. 34.1)
- Cold and clammy extremities

Examination of CVS

Inspection

- Apex beat is normal or displaced down beyond 5th intercostal space outside the midclavicular line and is diffuse and less forceful.
- Pulmonary artery pulsations in 2nd left intercostal space may be seen.

Palpation

- Displaced down and out weak apex beat.
- A thrill at apex or aortic area may be palpable depending on the cause (e.g. mitral and aortic valve disease)

Percussion

- Left border of heart corresponds to apex beat, i.e. dullness does not extend beyond apex beat.

Auscultation

- First heart sound soft
- Systolic murmur at apex, soft, may be audible due to LV dilatation (functional murmur)
- End-inspiratory crackles at the bases of lungs (present).
- P_2 may normal or loud and narrowly split. Ejection systolic or an early diastolic murmur (Graham-Steell) at 2nd left space. These are signs of pulmonary arterial hypertension.
- Abdominal examination for tender hepatomegaly and ascites (Fig. 34.1)
  Now look for the signs of underlying disease such as:
  - Valvular heart disease, Eisenmenger's syndrome
  - Hypertension

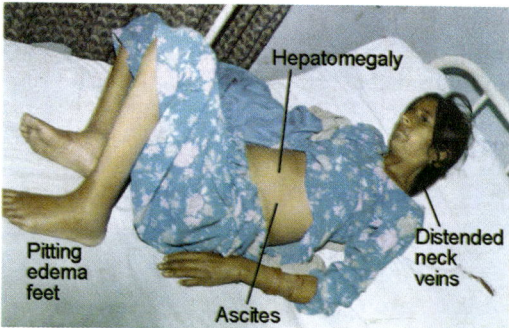

Fig. 34.1: Congestive heart failure (CHF)

– Thyrotoxicosis
– Severe anaemia, arrhythmias
– Constrictive pericarditis
– Cardiomyopathy

PROVISIONAL DIAGNOSIS

The history and physical signs suggest congestive heart failure (lesion) the cause of which has to be found out. Patient has limited activity due to dyspnea (functional status)

QUESTIONS AND ANSWERS

Q. What are points in favor of your diagnosis?
Ans: • Paroxysmal nocturnal dyspnea and distended neck veins (JVP raised)
  • Cardiomegaly with S3 gallop
  • Signs of congestion of lungs e.g. end inspiratory crackles at both the bases with rhonchi/wheezes
  • Ascites tender hepatomegaly and pitting pedal edema

Q. How do you define congestive heart failure (CHF)
Ans: When heart is not able to push sufficient amount of blood resulting in stagnation of blood in various viscera, it is called *congestive heart failure*. Congestive heart failure may left sided (lungs are congested) or right sided (all viscera except lungs are congested) or total (both right and left) heart failure (all organs are congested).

Q. What are diagnostic criteria for CHF?
Ans: **Framingham criteria** for diagnosis of CHF are:

Major criteria
  • Paroxysmal nocturnal dyspnea (PND)
  • Distended neck veins
  • Cardiomegaly
  • Rales
  • Acute pulmonary edema
  • S_3 gallop
  • Increased venous pressure (>16 cm H_2O)
  • Positive hepatojugular reflux

Minor criteria
  • Peripheral pitting edema
  • Night cough
  • Dyspnea on exertion
  • Hepatomegaly
  • Pleural effusion (hydrothorax)
  • Reduced vital capacity by 1/3 of normal

N.B To establish the diagnosis of CHF, at least one major and two minor criteria are required

Q. What are the causes of congestive heart failure?
Ans: The causes are
  I. *Ventricular outflow obstruction*, e.g. hypertension, aortic stenosis, pulmonary hypertension, pulmonary stenosis
  II. *Ventricular inflow obstruction*, e.g. mitral stenosis, tricuspid stenosis, endomyocardial fibrosis
  III. *Ventricular volume overload*
    • Mitral regurgitation, mitral valve prolapse
    • Aortic regurgitation and high output states
    • Left to right shunts (ASD, VSD, PDA)
  IV. *Depressed myocardial contractility*
    • Myocarditis, cardiomyopathy
    • Myocardial infarction/ischemia
    • Pericardial effusion, constrictive pericarditis
    • Tachyarrhythmias

Q. What are the causes of right and left heart failure?
Ans: Causes of right heart failure (RHF) are:
  1. *Pulmonary valve disease*
    • Pulmonary stenosis
    • Pulmonary hypertension due to any cause
    • Acute cor pulmonale (pulmonary thromboembolism)
    • Chronic cor pulmonale
  2. *Tricuspid diseases*
    • Tricuspid stenosis
    • Tricuspid regurgitation (dilated cardiomyopathy)
    • Ebstein anomaly
  3. *Depressed myocardial contractility*
    • Right ventricular infarction
    • Right ventricular dysplasia (right ventricular cardiomyopathy)
    • Myocarditis
  4. *Secondary to left heart failure*. The left ventricular failure ultimately may lead to right ventricular failure.

Causes of left heart failure
  • *Valvular diseases*, e.g. mitral stenosis, mitral regurgitation, MVP, aortic stenosis and aortic regurgitation
  • *Hypertension, coarctation of aorta*
  • *Cardiomyopathies*
  • *Myocarditis*
  • *Myocardial infarction/Ischemia*

Q. What are the causes of systolic heart failure?

Ans: Systolic heart failure means contractility is impaired
- Coronary artery disease
- Cardiomyopathies (restrictive), e.g. hypothyroidism, amyloidosis
- Myocarditis due to any cause
- Hypertension

Q. What are the causes of diastolic dysfunction?

Ans: Diastolic dysfunction means stiffness of heart resulting in impaired filling. The causes are;
- Elderly
- Restrictive cardiomyopathy
- Ventricular hypertrophies
- Hypertrophic cardiomyopathies

N.B These cause also can result in heart failure

Q. What do you mean by high output failure? What are its causes?

Ans: When high cardiac output does not meet the myocardial demands, it is called *high output failure.*

It is actually misnomer. It is called high output states now-a-days.

Causes: Read the causes in case discussion on chronic cor pulmonale

Q. What are the stages of heart failure?

Ans: It is classified into 4 stages depending on reversibility.
- I. *Stage A:* It includes patients at risk for developing heart failure (e.g. hypertension or CAD) without an evidence of structural abnormality. In majority of patients CHF can be prevented
- II. *Stage B:* Patients have structural heart disease but no current or past evidence of heart failure
- III. *Stage C and D:* Patient with an evidence of clinical heart failure

Q. How would you investigate?

Ans: The investigations done are:
1. *ECG* for ventricular hypertrophy, arrhythmias, myocardial ischemia/infarction
2. *Chest X-ray* (Fig. 34.2) for cardiomegaly, congested lung fields, presence of Kerley's lines, hydrothorax, pulmonary hypertension and calcification of valves
3. *Echocardiogram* is done to confirm the diagnosis (chamber enlarged) and to find out, the cause and to detect thrombus, vegetations, etc. (complications)
4. *BNP* (Brain Natriuretic peptide). The levels are elevated
5. *Radionuclide imaging* for accurate measurement of cardiac volumes, ejection fractions and regional wall abnormalities.

6. *Cardiac MRI*
7. *Cardiac catheterization,* if needed
8. *Cardiac biopsy* when cardiomyopathy or endomyocardial fibrosis is being suspected as its cause.

Q. What are the complications of CHF?

Ans:
1. Acute renal failure
2. Hypokalemia and hyponatremia (diuretic induced)
3. Pulmonary thromboembolism following deep vein thrombosis (DVT)
4. Arrhythmias
5. Systemic embolism following LV thrombus

Q. What are acute precipitants of CHF?

Ans:
- Acute respiratory infection
- Thyrotoxicosis (occult)
- Salt intake
- Mental stress
- Arrhythmias
- Noncompliance to treatment
- Pulmonary embolism
- Anemia
- Drugs, e.g. beta-blockers

Q. How would you treat CHF?

Ans:
- Salt restriction and diuretics
- ACE inhibitors or ARBs (angiotensin-receptor blockers)
- Betablockers
- Digitalis
- Vasodilators, nitrates
- Nesiritide. It is a recombinant form of human brain natriuretic peptide, a potent vasodilator that reduces preload.
- Positive inotropic agents

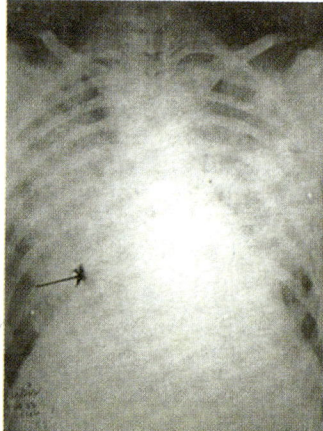

Fig. 34.2: Radiological findings in CHF

- Anticoagulants
- Antiarrhythmics, if arrhythmias are present

Q. **How will you treat digitalis toxicity?**

Ans: The steps of treatment are:
- Stop digoxin and diuretic
- Give potassium
- Give phenytoin for digitalis-induced arrhythmias
- Give digitalis Fab antibody

Q. **What is indication of beta blocker in heart failure?**

Ans: Usually beta blockers are contraindicated in heart failure but to slow the heart rate in AF or otherwise beta blockers are used in diastolic heart failure as they provide more time for ventricular filling.

The beta blockers used in heart failure include carvedilol, bisoprolol, nevibelol and metoprolol.

Q. **Which diuretic is preferred in CHF?**

Ans: You can use any diuretic but loop diuretics should be used with caution as it may cause metabolic alkalosis. Thiazides are better than loop diuretics.

Q. **What drugs should be avoided in CHF?**

Ans: Antiarrhythmics
- Betablockers and calcium channel blockers
- Tricyclic antidepressants
- NSAIDs and steroids
- Cyclo-oxygenase 2 inhibitors
- Daunorubicin
- Thiazolidinediones

Q. **What are devices used for heart failure?**

Ans: The devices are used as rescue therapy
1. Biventricular pacing device for intractable heart failure.
2. Implantable cardioverter defibrillator to prevent sudden cardiac death
3. Left ventricular transplantation
   - Before cardiac assist devices are used
   - As a bridge to recovery in patients with potentially reversible forms of CHF, e.g. myocarditis or peripartum cardiomyopathy
   - As a last resort, i.e. destination therapy

Q. **What is the indications of heart transplantation?**

Ans: Treatment failure or refractory to treatment and patients having NYHA class IV status.

35

Infective Endocarditis

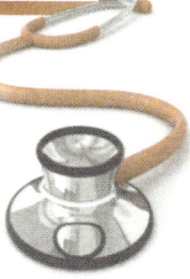

INSTRUCTION

Examine the patient cardiovascular system

SALIENT FEATURES

- Fever, palpitation and dyspnea in a patient with rheumatic heart disease

HISTORY

Ask for the following:

- Dyspnoea, palpitation, cough, chest discomfort due to basic heart disease, i.e. valvular (present) or congenital lesion
- Fever with chills, diaphoresis (present)
- Onset, duration of symptoms
- Symptoms of complications such as CHF or systemic embolization, e.g. cold extremity, hemiplegia, hematuria (present)
- Visual disturbance or visual loss
- History of procedure or dental extraction
- History of recent cardiac surgery
- History of IV drug misuse/abuse
- History of sepsis, skin infection
- Ask about past history of rheumatic (present) or congenital heart disease

EXAMINATION

General Physical Examination (Fig. 35.1)

- Toxic look. Patient is febrile and weak
- The *skin* may show purpuric spots, ecchymosis, Janeway lesion
- *Neck* for JVP and lymphadenopathy
- *Extremities* for
  - Clubbing of fingers
  - Janeway lesion (present)
  - Digital gangrene (present)
  - Splinter hemorrhages (Fig. 35.2) (present in this case).
  - Osler's nodes
  - Coldness of extremities (present)
  - Painful fingertips

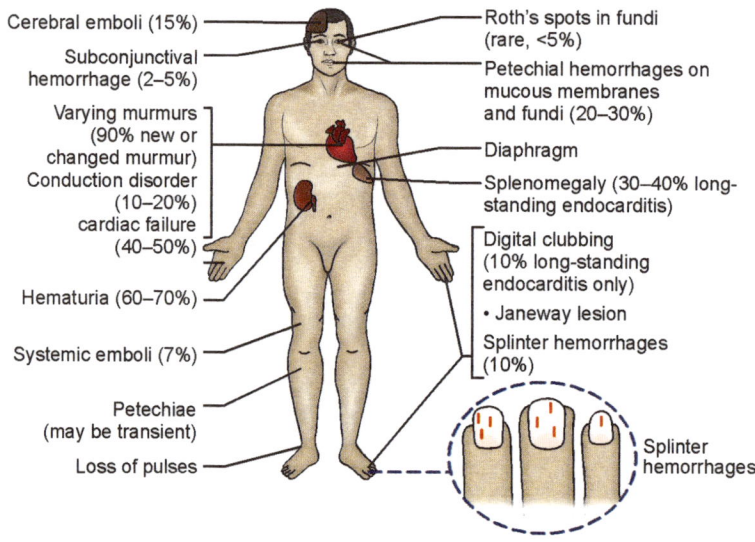

Fig. 35.1: Clinical features of endocarditis

- Eyes for subconjunctival hemorrhage, Roth's spots (present)
- Look for anemia, cyanosis, jaundice, edema
- Examine vitals, e.g. pulse, BP, respiration and temperature
- Palpate all the peripheral pulses.

Cardiovascular System
- *Inspection.* Look for signs of LHF (cardiomegaly)
- *Palpation.* Confirm the findings on inspection
- *Percussion* for cardiac dullness
- *Auscultation.* Auscultate for any murmur, change in previous murmur and appearance of new murmur in addition to findings of heart disease.

Other Systems
- *Nervous system* for motor or sensory deficit due to embolization (stroke). Examine ocular fundi
- *Respiratory system* for pulmonary embolism, infection, LVF
- *Kidneys* for pain and tenderness in renal area or hematuria (red urine)
- Abdomen for splenomegaly and hepatomegaly

PROVISIONAL DIAGNOSIS

The patient has infective endocarditis (lesion) with underlying rheumatic heart disease (etiology). Patient is in congestive heart failure (functional status)

QUESTIONS AND ANSWERS

Q. Enumerate physical signs of endocarditis in your case.

Ans: 1. Fever, tachypnea, tachycardia.
2. Coldness of extremities, digital clubbing, splinter hemorrhages, Janeway lesion, Roth's spots, Osler's nodes, gangrenous (embolic) fingertips, purpuric spots
3. Acute flank pain, hematuria (GN)
4. Splenomegaly (mild)
5. Anemia

Q. How do you define endocarditis? What are common causative organisms?

Ans: Infective endocarditis is due to microbial infection of a heart valve (native, prosthetic), the lining of a cardiac chamber, or blood vessels or a congenital septal defect or a congenital anomaly. The causative organism is either a bacterium (S. *viridans, Staph. aureus, Strep. fecalis HACEK*) or a fungus or a rickettsia (Q *fever endocarditis*).

Q. Name the conditions that produce clinical feature similar to endocarditis.

Ans: • Atrial myxoma
• Sickle cell disease
• SLE
• Nonbacterial endocarditis.

Q. What is basic difference between acute and subacute endocarditis

Ans: *Acute endocarditis* is usually bacterial in origin, has rapid onset, fulminant course causing destruction of cardiac structures, (perforation of valve cusps) and hematogenously seeds the extracardiac sites, and if untreated, progresses to death within weeks. *Subacute endocarditis* on the other hand follows an indolent course, causes structural cardiac damage slowly, rarely causes metastatic infection, and is gradually progressive unless complicated by a major embolic event or rupture of mycotic aneurysm.

Q. What are physical signs in the lungs in endocarditis?

Ans: • Read Table 35.1

Table 35.1: Systemic manifestations of infective endocarditis

Organ	Symptoms and signs
Heart	Dyspnea, palpitations, cough, pain chest • Tachycardia • Changing or appearance of new murmurs • Conduction defects • CHF, cardiomegaly • Muffling of heart sounds
Lung	• Hemoptysis, chest pain • Pleuritic rub due to embolic pulmonary infarct may be present • Crackers and whereas due to LVF
CNS	Headache, toxic encephalopathy, meningitis Monoplegia or hemiplegia due to embolization
Blood vessels	• Coldness of extremities • Loss of peripheral pulses due to embolization
Skin	• Petechial hemorrhages, purpuric spots Eyes, i.e. redness, visual disturbance • Subconjunctival hemorrhage, blindness, Roth's spots
Kidneys	• Hematuria, renal angle tender, acute flank pain,
Spleen	• Pain in splenic area, splenomegaly, • Splenic infarct (rub)
Blood	Pallor, lassitude, fatigue, anemia
Hands	• Digital gangrene, Clubbing of the fingers, splinter hemorrhages, Osler's nodes (painful tender swellings at fingertips) Janeway lesions (large nontender maculopapular eruption in palm and soles)

Q. What are signs in the heart?

Ans: • Read Table 35.1

Q. Enumerate major categories of endocarditis?

Ans: 1. Native valve infective endocarditis
2. Prosthetic valve infective endocarditis
3. Infective endocarditis in I.V. drug abusers
4. Nosocomial infective endocarditis

Q. What are systemic manifestations of endocarditis?

Ans: Systemic manifestations are given in Table 35.1.

Q. What are various pathogenic mechanisms?

Ans: • Infection and fluctuating toxemia due to adherence and growth of bacteria within cardiac lesion
• Formation of septic vegetation septic embolization
• Immune-complex mechanism
• Anemia

Q. What signs of endocarditis are seen in hands?

Ans: Read the above table

Q. What are clinical characteristics of acute bacterial endocarditis?

Ans: 1. It is commonly produced by *S. aureus* which can involve even normal valves
2. It is common in drug abusers in which right sided involvement occurs
3. Fever, toxemia, clubbing of the fingers
4. Perforation of valvular cusps (mitral and aortic) leading to valvular regurgitation.
5. Cardiac and renal failure develops rapidly.

Q. What is right sided endocarditis?

Ans: Main features are as follows:
• Commonly caused by *S. aureus*
• Tricuspid valve is commonly affected producing regurgitation. Pulmonary valve involvement is rare.
• Involvement of right ventricular wall is common in VSD.
• Common in drug addicts using I.V. line for drug delivery. It may occur in immuno-compromised patients and those with burns
• Prognosis is better
• Systemic embolization is rare. Lung infarction or infection (lung abscess, empyema, pneumonias) are common.

Q. What are the sites of endocarditis in valvular lesions?

Ans: The sites of endocarditis varies depending on the heart lesion (congenital/valvular) and are depicted in Fig. 35.2
A column of infected blood in the form of jet strikes at different sites in different cardiac disorders resulting in infective endocarditis.

Q. When do you suspect infective endocarditis in a patient with heart lesion?

Ans: Diagnosis of infective endocarditis is suspected in each and every patient of rheumatic valvular heart disease or a congenital heart disease developing fever, tachycardia, worsening dyspnea or congestive heart failure or an embolic episode, e.g. monoplegia/hemiplegia, etc.
In high risk patients, always look further for signs of endocarditis

Q. What are complications of endocarditis?

Ans: Common complications are:
1. *Heart failure:* Endocarditis may precipitate or aggravate the heart failure.
2. *Embolization* to any organ.
3. *Neurological complications.* Embolic stroke is the most common. Intracranial hemorrhage may occur due to ruptured mycotic aneurysm or rupture of an artery due to septic arteritis. Meningitis and brain abscess can occur.
4. Septicemia, metastatic abscesses
5. Valve destruction, e.g. acute regurgitation.

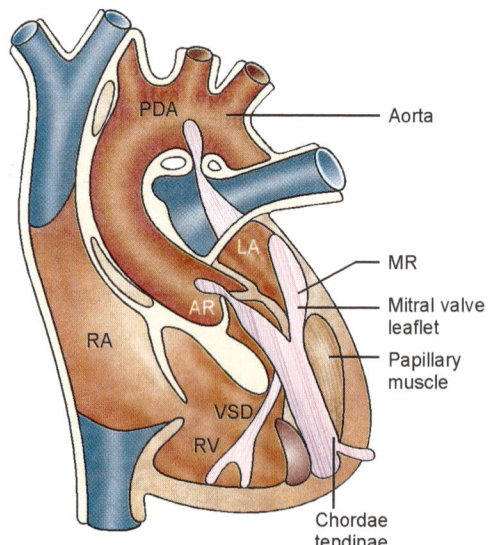

1. A lesion (vegetation) in the pulmonary artery in PDA
2. A lesion in the wall of right ventricle in VSD.
3. A lesion in the left atrium and LV in mitral regurgitation
4. A lesion in the left ventricle and on the mitral valve, chordae tendinae in aortic regurgitation

Fig. 35.2: Infective endocarditis in different cardiac lesions.

6. Local extension, e.g. myocarditis (abscess) and purulent pericarditis.

7. Glomerulonephritis

Q. **What are modified diagnostic Duke Criteria for infective endocarditis?**

Ans: This can easily be remembered by mnemonic—BE (for major) and FEVER (for minor criteria) as follows

1. *Major criteria*
   B. Blood cultures positive at least twice 12 hours apart
   E. Endocardial involvement (vegetations) on echocardiogram

2. *Minor criteria*
   F: Fever
   E: Evidence for microbiology
   V: Vascular findings
   E: Evidence on immunology
   R: Risk factors/Predisposing factors (drugs, valvular or congenital diseases)

Note: Read DUKE'S criteria in details for diagnosis in textbook of medicine by Prof SN Chugh

Q. **Name the risk/predisposing factors.**

Ans: 1. *Valvular heart diseases*, e.g. mitral, aortic, tricuspid. Mitral valve involvement is the commonest

2. *Congenital heart diseases*, e.g. VSD, PDA, bicuspid aortic valve. ASD does not predispose to it.

3. *Prosthetic valves*

4. *Immunocompromised state* (diabetes, steroids, immunosuppression, etc.).

5. *Intravenous habitual drug abusers* through infected needles/syringes

6. *Prior heart surgery*

Q. **How will you investigate a patient suspected of endocarditis?**

Ans: Investigation required are as follows:

1. *Blood examination.* There may be anemia (normocytic normochromic), leukocytosis raised ESR and high C-reactive protein.

2. Urine examination for albuminuria and microscopic hematuria.

3. Immune-complex and rheumatoid factor

4. *Blood culture*: Isolation of the microorganism from blood cultures is crucial not only for diagnosis but also for determination of antimicrobial sensitivity and planning the management. In the absence of prior antibiotic therapy; a total of 3 blood separate blood cultures ideally with the first separated from the last by at least 1 hour from different sites should be obtained from different venipuncture sites over 24 hour. If the cultures remain negative after 48 to 72 hours; two or three additional blood cultures, including a lysis-centrifugation culture, should be obtained, and the laboratory should be asked to pursue fastidious microorganisms by prolonging the incubation time and performing special subcultures. It is likely that 95–100% of all cultures obtained will be positive and that one of the first two cultures will be positive in at least 98% of patients. Blood culture obtained just prior to temperature peak will give a higher yield. Blood culture is likely to be sterile if patient has already received antibiotics.

5. *Echocardiogram.* Vegetations may be identified as small, sessile or polypoidal masses on heart valves or congenital defects. Transesophageal echocardiography offers the greatest sensitivity for detection of vegetations.

6. Serological tests, i.e. polymerase chain reaction can be used to identify some organisms that are difficult to recover on blood culture.

Q. **What are AHA (American Heart Association recommendations for endocarditis prophylaxis for dental procedures in cardiac conditions?**

Ans: Recommendations are:
1. Oral amoxycillin 2 g 1 hour before procedure.

In cases of allergy to penicillin, then
- Clindamycin 600 mg one hour before procedure or Cephalexin 2 g one hours before procedure or azithromycin/clarithromycin 500 mg one hour before procedure

In case of parenteral therapy
- Give amoxicillin 2 g I.M. 30 minutes before procedure or

In case of penicillin allergy, give
- Clindamycin 600 mg I.V. one hour before procedure or Cefazolin 1 g I.M. or I.V. 30 minutes before procedure.

Q. **How would you treat a patient suspected to have endocarditis?**

Ans: Until culture report become available, I.V. benzylpenicillin and gentamicin will be given on empirical basis. In severely ill patients, cloxacillin would be added to the regimen.

Q. What is marantic endocarditis?

Ans: *Marantic or Libman-Sacks endocarditis* is seen in SLE. It is a postmortem diagnosis. It is rarely detected clinically.

Q. What are indications of surgery?

Ans:

1. Valve replacement is indicated in patients who have relapsed after best antibiotic therapy (repeated blood cultures are positive)
2. Formation of valve abscess (drainage of abscess is indicated)
3. Heart blocks (2nd and third degree) in aortic valve endocarditis)
4. Replacement of prosthetic valve if there is valvular dysfunction/valve dehiscence
5. Development of sinus of Valsalva aneurysm
6. Fungal endocarditis

Q. What are recent recommendation for prophylaxis?

Ans: According to NICE guidelines (march 2008) prophylaxis should be recommended in those who are at increased risk of developing infective endocarditis including those with:

- Acquired valvular heart disease
- Valvular replacement done
- Structural congenital heart disease
- Previous infective endocarditis
- Hypertrophic cardiomyopathy

36

Absent Radial Pulse

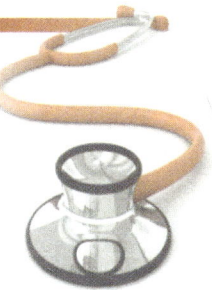

INSTRUCTION

Examine the patient's pulses

SALIENT FEATURES

- Gangrenous finger of left hand (Fig. 36.1)

HISTORY

Ask for the following points:

- History of any cardiac disease which predisposes to embolization, i.e. valvular disease, MI, cardiac aneurysm
- Systemic symptoms of vasculitis in the past, e.g. ask for past history of fever, tuberculosis, collagen vascular disease
- History of insertion of an arterial line for a procedure or sampling
- Past history of cardiac surgery (Blalock-Taussig shunt)

EXAMINATION

General Physical Examination

- Feel the hand. It is cold and clammy (in this case)
- Left radial pulse is weaker than right in this case
- There are few gangrenes finger tips (Fig. 36.1)
- Examine all other pulses, i.e. carotid, axillary, brachial, femoral, popliteal, posterior tibial and dorsalis pedis (For examination of various pulses read clinical methods in medicine by Prof SN Chugh)
- Now check the BP in both upper limbs. There is difference in BP more than 10 mm in both arms,

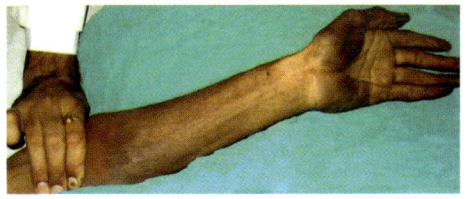

Fig. 36.1: Absent radial pulse (left hand)

i.e. systolic BP in right arm is more than left by 30 mmHg

PROVISIONAL DIAGNOSIS

The patient has cold clammy right hand, few gangrenous fingers, absent radial pulse (lesion) which is probably due to embolism (etiology). Patient is at risk of distant embolization (functional status)

QUESTIONS AND ANSWERS

Q. What are common causes of absent radial pulse?

Ans:
1. Aberrant (abnormally placed) radial pulse or a congenital anomaly.
2. Previous surgical cut-down and artery tied off at surgery
3. Brachial artery catheterization
4. Following procuring I.V. line for blood gas monitoring or arterial puncture.
5. Embolization into radial artery (endocarditis, L.V. thrombus, atrial fibrillation, L.V. aneurysm)
6. Subclavian artery stenosis
7. Cervical rib
8. Surgery (Blalock-Taussig shunt surgery)
9. Takayasu arteritis

Q. What are the causes of difference in pulse volume and BP between two arms or between the arms and legs?

Ans:
1. Aortic stenosis (supravalvular)
2. Coarctation of aorta
3. Occlusion of the artery supplying the limb
4. Dissecting aneurysm of aorta
5. PDA
6. Thoracic outlet syndrome
7. Cervical rib.

Q. What are the causes of radiofemoral delay?

Ans:
- Coarctation of aortic
- Aortoarteritis

Q. What are the causes of radio radial delay?

Ans:
- Valvular aortic stenosis
- Pre-ductal coarctation
- Dissecting aneurysm of aortic arch
- Occlusion of an artery of one upper limb.

Q. What is Adson's test? How would you perform it?

Ans: This test is used to test the compression of the axillary artery by scalene anterior muscle

Procedure
- Palpate the radial pulse and abduct the arm slightly
- Now ask the patient to hyperextend the neck and turn it to the affected side and inhale slowly
- Paresthesias or absent or weak pulse on palpation in this position indicates positive Adson's test
- Now ask the patient to turn head to opposite side (reverse Adson's test) to test the compression of axillary artery by middle scalene muscle

Q. What is aortoarteritis (Takayasu's syndrome)

Ans: It is nonspecific inflammatory arteritis involving the segments of the aorta and ostium of its main branches in young females. It is of four types based on the involvement of vessels.

It is associated commonly with rheumatic fever, infections (*streptococcal, tuberculosis*) and collagen vascular diseases. A positive mantoux test has been reported in 70–80% cases indicating tubercular antigen induced vascular injury by type IV reaction (delayed hypersensitivity)

It clinically presents with prodromal symptoms (fever, fatigue, arthralgia, GI upset) followed by vascular involvement, i.e. diminished or absent pulses in the upper limbs, higher BP and good pulses in the lower limbs and neurological manifestations

Q. What is Alien test? How would you perform it?

Ans: The Alien test is used to determine the patency of radial and ulnar artery (Fig. 36.2). This test is used before puncturing the radial artery for cannulation.

Procedure/method
- Occlude both the radial and ulnar arteries while patient raises the hand and makes fist (Fig. 36.2A)
- Now ask the patient extend the fingers, blanching of hand become visible due to occlusion of vessels (Fig. 36.2B)
- Now release the radial artery (Fig. 36.2C), colour of the hand returns to normal. If the colour does not return within 10 seconds, thrombotic occlusion of radial artery should be suspected.
- In thrombosis of ulnar artery, the hand remains blanched when this artery alone is released (Fig. 36.2D)

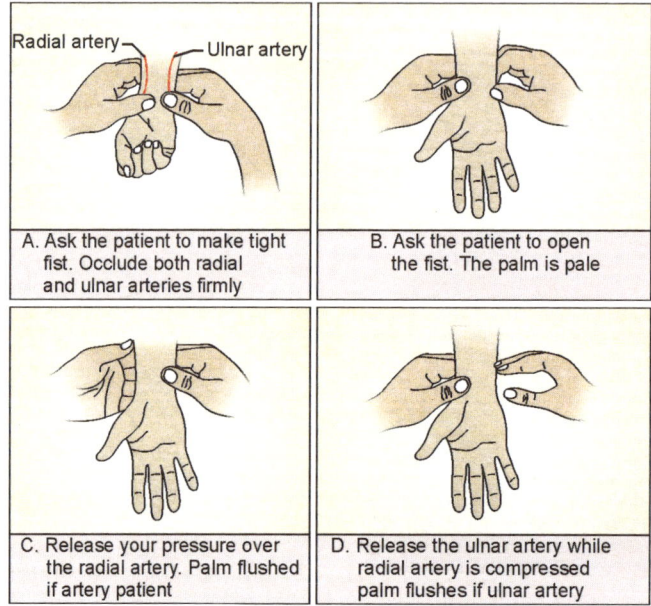

Radial artery — Ulnar artery

A. Ask the patient to make tight fist. Occlude both radial and ulnar arteries firmly

B. Ask the patient to open the fist. The palm is pale

C. Release your pressure over the radial artery. Palm flushed if artery patient

D. Release the ulnar artery while radial artery is compressed palm flushes if ulnar artery

Fig. 36.2: The Allen test for patency of the vessel

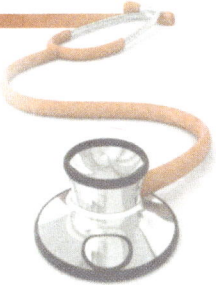

37

Dilated Cardiomyopathy

INSTRUCTION

Examine the cardiovascular system

SALIENT FEATURES

- Palpitation and dyspnea

HISTORY

Ask for the following:

- Cough, its frequency, nocturnal, etc.
- Sputum production, quantity, color, smell, consistency and history of hemoptysis
- Any recent change in the symptoms. History of recent fever, sore throat or loose motions
- History of swelling feet, abdomen (hepatomegaly)
- Ask for any aggravating or relieving factors
- Take full drug history, drug being taken and their effect

Past history

- History of delivery or abortion, diabetes

Personal and family history

- History of smoking, alcoholism
- No family history of such disease

EXAMINATION

General Physical Examination

- Patient is orthopneic, lying in prop up position.
- Cyanosis is present (in this case)
- Neck veins distended. JVP raised (Fig. 37.1). There may be v and y collapse due to TR (present in this case)
- Pulse and respiratory rate are increased
- Cold extremities and edema feet (Fig. 37.1) may be present (present in this case)

Examination of CVS

Inspection

- Apex beat may be normally placed or displaced outwards (to anterior axillary line in this case) but not downwards.
- No other visible pulsation all over the precordium

Palpation

- Apex beat may be palpable outside the midclavicular line (palpable in this case)
- Parasternal heave present
- Right ventricular pulsations may be palpable in epigastrium (present in this case)

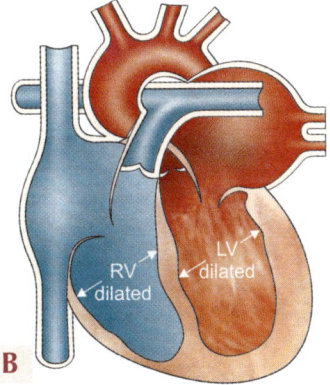

Fig. 37.1: (A) Patient of rheumatic heart disease with mitral stenosis and mitral regurgitation showing signs of congestive heart failure; (B) Diagram

Percussion

- Area of cardiac dullness is increased to anterior axillary line due to dilated heart. Dullness corresponds with apex beat.

Auscultation

- Heart sounds normal/feeble
- Second heart sound normally split
- There may be an ejection systolic murmur in P_2 area and a pansystolic murmur in tricuspid and mitral areas (present).

Abdominal Examination

- Liver is enlarged, soft, tender (Fig. 37.1) and may be pulsatile if TR present (liver was enlarged and pulsatile in this case)
- There may be signs of ascites (Fig. 37.1)

PROVISIONAL DIAGNOSIS

In view of clinical findings, patient has features of dilated cardiomyopathy, the cause of which has to be found out (idiopathic). Patient is markedly dyspneic (functional status)

QUESTIONS AND ANSWERS

Q. **Enumerate the points in favor of your diagnosis?**
Ans:
  - A middle aged female patient.
  - History of dyspnea, progressive in nature, orthopnea and PND
  - Signs of congestive heart failure without signs of pulmonary hypertension, e.g. raised JVP, tender hepatomegaly, ascites and pitting edema. There are end-inspiratory crackles in the lungs.
  - Signs of cardiomegaly, e.g. dilated heart with heaving apex beat which is down and out.
  - No evidence of any other cause of heart failure such as valvular, hypertensive, thyrotoxic and ischemic heart disease.
  - The features suggestive of mitral and tricuspid regurgitation (pansystolic murmur in both the areas) indicates dilated cardiomyopathy as simultaneous occurrence of both regurgitant lesions commonly occurs in dilated cardiomyopathy.

Q. **What is your differential diagnosis?**
Ans: Following myocardial diseases come into the differential diagnosis:
  - *Peripartum cardiomyopathy* (there will be history of delivery followed by signs and symptoms of CHF within 6 months)

- *Alcoholic cardiomyopathy* History of alcoholism, stigmatas of alcoholism and other associated diseases, e.g. cirrhosis or neuropathy)
- *Neuromuscular disease associated cardiomyopathy*, e.g. Friedrich's ataxia, Duchenne's muscular dystrophy, myotonic dystrophy, etc. (features of these neurological diseases will be present)
- **Myocarditis**—viral

Q. **Could it be rheumatic mitral regurgitation leading to tricuspid regurgitation?**
Ans: No. There are no signs of pulmonary hypertension (loud P_2, narrow splitting of 2nd heart sound, Graham-Steell murmur or an ejection systolic murmur).

Q. **What do you mean by cardiomyopathy?**
Ans: The cardiomyopathies are a heterogenous group of cardiac disorders primarily involving the myocardium and not associated with any other underlying cardiac cause such as ischemic heart disease, hypertension, thyrotoxicosis, valvular or congenital heart disease, pericardial disease, etc. Thus, cardiomyopathy is a diagnosis by exclusion of all other causes of heart disease.

Q. **How do you classify cardiomyopathies?**
Ans: WHO classified cardiomyopathy clinically into 3 main groups:
  i. **Dilated cardiomyopathy** characterized by ventricular enlargement, CHF, impaired systolic function, arrhythmias and embolization.
  ii. **Restrictive cardiomyopathy** characterized by restriction to left and/or right ventricular filling. It resembles constrictive pericarditis.
  iii. **Hypertrophic cardiomyopathy** characterized by left ventricular free wall hypertrophy along with septal hypertrophy without any dilatation of the ventricular cavity.

Q. **What are the causes of dilated cardiomyopathy?**
Ans: The common causes are:
  - Idiopathic
  - **Alcohol** induced cardiomyopathy
  - Peripartum cardiomyopathy
  - Ischemic cardiomyopathy
  - *Metabolic cardiomyopathy*, e.g. thyrotoxic, diabetic.
  - *Viral:* Chronic myocarditis, Chagas' disease

- *Drug induced*, e.g. doxorubicin, cocaine, cyclophosphamide
- *Neuromuscular diseases*, e.g. Friedrich's ataxia

Q. What is peripartum cardiomyopathy?

Ans: It develops during the last trimester or within 6 months after delivery, hence, the patient usually a multiparous woman over the age of 30 yrs develops symptoms and signs of CHF either 1 month before or immediately after delivery up to 6 months. The investigations revealed a dilated heart with depressed ejection fraction

Q. What would you advise to the patient with dilated cardiomyopathy about future pregnancies?

Ans: These patients if have dilated heart should avoid subsequent pregnancies which are likely to produce additional myocardial damage.

Q. What is alcoholic cardiomyopathy?

Ans:
- It occurs in chronic alcoholic who are heavy drinkers
- It presents with all symptoms and signs of congestive heart failure with dilated heart.
- The arrhythmias, e.g. atrial and ventricular commonly occur after a drinking binge.
- The progression of disease may stop following cessation of alcohol use.
- Other alcoholic stigmatas (parotid enlargement, gynecomastia, red tip of nose palmar erythema, spider nevi, etc.), cirrhosis or/and neuropathy may be present.

Q. How would you investigate such a case?

Ans:
  i. *ECG*. It will often show sinus tachycardia or atrial fibrillation, ventricular arrhythmias, left atrial enlargement, nonspecific ST-T changes and sometimes conduction defects and low voltage graph.
  ii. *Chest X-ray* will show cardiomegaly. There will be pulmonary venous congestion and interstitial/alveolar edema (Kerley's lines).
  iii. *Echocardiogram* (Fig. 37.2). It will show ventricular dilation with normal or thinned walls. The ejection fraction is markedly reduced.
  iv. *Radionuclide ventriculography*, usually, not required, may confirm ventricular dilatation and thinning/thickening of the walls.
  v. *Brain natriuretic peptide* levels are elevated.
  vi. *Cardiac catheterization* and *coronary angiography*. They are often performed to exclude ischemic heart disease (ischemic cardiomyopathy).
  vii. *Transvenous endomyocardial* biopsy. It is usually not necessary in idiopathic or familial cardiomyopathy. However, it is helpful in recognition of secondary cardiomyopathy due to amyloidosis and chronic myocarditis.

Q. How would you treat?

Ans: Treatment is symptomatic with:
- Salt restriction, diuretics, digitalis and ACE inhibitors
- Anticoagulation for systemic embolization
- Sophisticated therapy such as biventricular pacing (resynchronization therapy for intraventricular conduction delay, bundle branch blocks) and insertion of implantable cardioverter-defibrillator (ICD) for symptomatic ventricular arrhythmias
- Avoid alcohol and NSAIDs

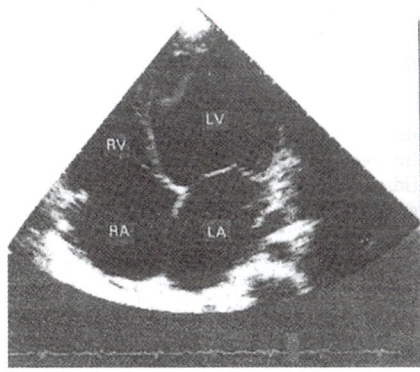

Fig. 37.2: Dilated cardiomyopathy. Echocardiogram (2D) shows the heart having a globular appearance with dilatation of all the 4 chambers.
LA = left atrium; LV = left ventricle; RA = right atrium; RV = right ventricle.

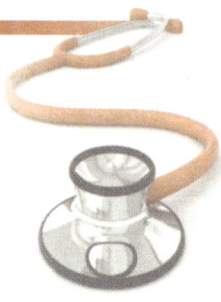

38

Hypertrophic Cardiomyopathy

INSTRUCTION

Examine the cardiovascular system.

SALIENT FEATURES

- Complaints of syncope, dizziness, palpitation

HISTORY

Ask for the following:

- History of dyspnea on exertion, progressive, PND and orthopnea
- Chest discomfort/pain usually exertional mimicking angina or may occur at rest

- Syncope in 25% cases
- Dizziness and palpitations
- Ask family history of similar illness and history of sudden death due to cardiac disease

Note: Premature death in young adults or athletes is common due to hypertrophic cardiomyopathy.

EXAMINATION

General Physical Examination

- Radial or carotid pulse is bifid or bisferiens or jerky type
- JVP shows prominent 'a' wave. JVP may be raised.

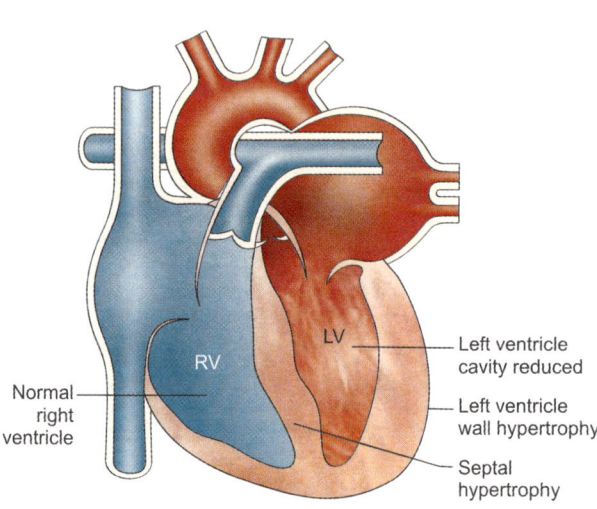

Normal right ventricle — RV

LV — Left ventricle cavity reduced

— Left ventricle wall hypertrophy

— Septal hypertrophy

A

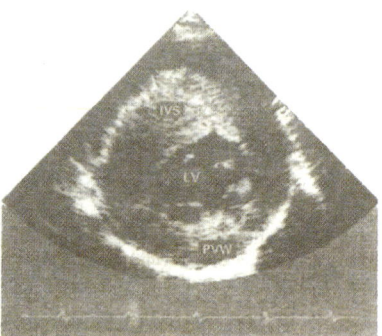

Short axis view

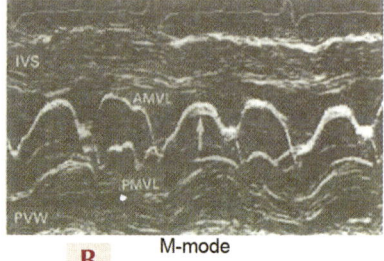

M-mode

B

Fig. 38.1: Hypertrophic cardiomyopathy. (A) Diagram; (B) Echocardiogram (short axis view) and M-mode showing mitral valve, thickened interventricular septum (IVS) and a small left ventricular (LV) cavity. The condition is associated with abnormal anterior motion of mitral valve leaflet (AMVL) indicated by an arrow.

- Blood pressure is normal or there may be wide pulse pressure
- Cyanosis and edema feet present if patient is in CHF

Cardiovascular System

- Double apical impulse (LV is divided into two portions producing double apex) may be visible and palpable.
- Left parasternal heave may be present
- Murmurs and sounds
  i. Pansystolic murmur at apex caused by mitral regurgitation radiating to axilla.
  ii. Soft first heart sound. Fourth heart sound may be present. Second heart sound is normal.
  iii. An ejection systolic murmur at left ventricular outflow tract along the left sternal border, accentuated by standing and Valsalva maneuver and softer on squatting (present in this case.)

  Remember: Aortic stenosis murmur decreases on Valsalva maneuver, but murmur of hypertrophic cardiomyopathy increases on Valsalva manoeuvre

Other Systems Examination

- *Respiratory system examination* will reveal end-inspiratory crackles and wheezes due to lung congestion.
- *Abdominal examination* may reveal hepatomegaly and ascites if patient is in CHF.

PROVISIONAL DIAGNOSIS

Patient has features suggestive of hypertrophic cardiomyopathy (lesion) probably familial in origin (etiology). Patient is in LVF (cardiac status).

QUESTIONS AND ANSWERS

Q. **What are the points in favor of your diagnosis?**
Ans: 1. Double apical impulse in a young adult.
2. Pansystolic murmur of mitral regurgitation
3. An ejection systolic murmur without click along the left sternal border which is heard better on standing

Q. **What is the cause of double apex beat?**
Ans: It is due to division of left ventricular cavity into two independent chambers by septal and ventricular wall hypertrophy which bulge during systole.

Q. **Why murmur of hypertrophic cardiomyopathy increases during standing and Valsalva maneuver?**
Ans: Hypovolemia (dehydration), standing and Valsalva decrease the LV cavity size, hence, accentuates obstruction (murmur) during systole.

Q. **Which maneuvers decrease the murmur of HOCM?**
Ans: Squatting, hand grip, passive leg elevation, Müller maneuver (deep inspiration against closed glottis) increase LV cavity size, thus reduce outflow obstruction, hence, reduce the murmur.

Q. **What do you understand by the term hypertrophic obstructive cardiomyopathy?**
Ans: It is a heredofamilial disorder seen in young characterized by reduction in the left ventricle cavity size due to septal and free ventricular wall hypertrophy.

Q. **What type of ventricular dysfunction is produced by HOCM?**
Ans: Diastolic dysfunction due to elevated LV pressure impairing LV filling.

Q. **What is genetics in HOCM?**
Ans: It is an autosomal dominant disorder with variable penetrance. It is caused by mutations of one of a large number of genes, most of which code for myosin heavy chain or proteins regulating calcium handling.

Q. **What is the type of HOCM in elderly?**
Ans: It is associated with hypertension in elderly.

Q. **What is the major difference between LV hypertrophy in athletes and LV hypertrophy of HOCM?**
Ans: LV hypertrophy in athletes is adaptive, does not produce diastolic dysfunction, hence differs from HOCM.

Q. **What is the cause of sudden death in HOCM?**
Ans: Arrhythmias which are malignant and do not respond to treatment.

Q. **Who are at higher risk of sudden death?**
Ans: 1. Patient with positive family history
2. Those with marked LV hypertrophy
3. Those who do not increase their systemic BP with exercise (poor response to exercise)
4. Patient with nonsustained VT
5. Patients with exertional syncope

Q. **What is recent recommendation about prophylaxis in HOCM?**
Ans: Now-a-days, it is recommended

Q. **How would you investigate such a case?**
Ans: 1. ECG (Fig. 38.2) may be normal or abnormal (large Q waves in inferolateral

leads mimicking myocardial infarction). Some patients may show LVH with strain pattern. Arrhythmias, conduction disturbance (RBBB) may be seen.

2. Echocardiogram (Fig. 38.1B) It is useful to determine the gradient, cavity size and function, valvular regurgitation, thickened interventricular septum and atrial diameters. The characteristic findings on M-mode echocardiogram is abnormal anterior mitral valve leaflet motion during systole.

3. *Chest X-ray PA view*: It may be normal or there may be mild cardiomegaly.

4. *Holter's monitoring.* 48 hour holter monitoring may detect arrhythmias, i.e. AF, PSVT, nonsustained VT and VT in asymptomatic patients.

5. *Endomyocardial biopsy.* It is indicated to exclude other cardiac muscle disorders, e.g. sarcoid heart disease and cardiac amyloidosis, otherwise it has no role

6. *Cardiac MRI.* It will show patchy areas of hyper enhancement, seen particularly at 10o' clock position in the short axis view at the confluence of anterior septum and anterior wall.

7. *Left heart catheterization* is rarely needed. In presence of LV outflow obstruction, aortic pressure tracing will show, rapid rise and fall followed by plateau (the spike and dome pattern).

Q. What are the conditions associated with HOCM?
Ans: • Duchenne muscular dystrophy
• Myotonias
• Friedreich's ataxia

Q. What are the complications of HOCM?
Ans: 1. Arrhythmias, e.g. atrial fibrillation, PSVT and malignant arrhythmias
2. Infective endocarditis
3. Systemic embolization following AF
4. Sudden death

Q. What do you know about epidemiology of this disease?
Ans: • It involves both sexes equally. It involves younger men and older women
• In children and adolescents, muscle hypertrophy often occurs during growth spurts, hence, frequent assessment at later age must be made before labelling them for HOCM.
• Myocardial hypertrophy does not progress after adolescent growth
• First degree relatives have 50% chance to inherit the disease gene. Therefore, genetic counselling is advised.

Q. How would you manage such a case?
Ans: 1. Treatment of symptoms by beta blockers, calcium channel blockers and diuretics.
2. Prophylaxis against infective endocarditis
3. Dual chamber pacing or DDD pacing for symptomatic patients resistent to treatment
4. Implantable cardioverter defibrillator to prevent sudden death
5. Cardioversion may be used for arrhythmias resistent to drugs
6. Surgery, i.e. septal ablation with alcohol or surgery (myomectomy) to relieve symptoms of intractable obstruction. Mitral valve replacement may be done for MR.
7. Counselling of the patients and relatives is essential.

N.B. Digoxin and vasodilators should be avoided in CHF due to this condition as they worsen outflow obstruction.

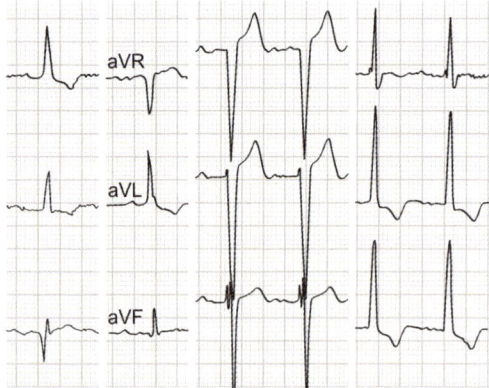

Fig. 38.2: Left ventricular hypertrophy in a patient with hypertrophic cardiomyopathy. The ECG shows
• Left axis deviation and intermediate heart position.
• R in aVL + S wave in V3 >28 mm (cornell criteria) $RV_5 + SV_1$ is >35mm (LVH)
• Associated ST – T changes
• First degree AV block present (P – R >2 sec)
• First degree AV block (PR interval is >20 sec)

Q. What is Brockenbrough-Braunwald-Morrow sign?
Ans: Diminished pulse pressure in post extrasystolic beat is called Brockenbrough-Braunwald sign. It is seen in aortic stenosis and HOCM.

39

Acute Coronary Syndrome

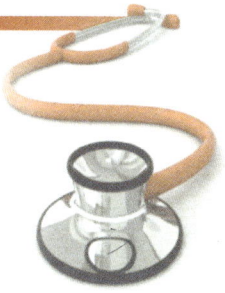

INSTRUCTION

Examine the cardiovascular system of this patient

SALIENT FEATURES

- Pain chest on exertion

HISTORY

Ask for the following:

- Have you ever had such type of pain or discomfort in the chest before?
- How would you describe the pain (burning, heaviness or tightness, stabbing, pressure?)
- Do you get this pain chest during walking at normal pace or does it come when you walk fast or in a hurry?
- Does the pain get relieved by rest or by nitroglycerine?
- Is this pain localized or radiate to some other sites?
- Can you pinpoint the pain with your finger?
- Does the food has any relation with pain?
- Are there any associated symptoms of retching, nausea, vomiting, sweating, syncope, palpitation, dyspnea?
- Is there any family history of ischemic heart disease? Did the patient had MI in the past?
- Is there any aggravating or relieving factor known?

EXAMINATION

General Physical Examination

- Facial appearance, e.g. depressed or normal
- Pulse (rate and rhythm) and BP (all the four limbs). Feel all other pulses (carotids, femoral)
- Eyes for xanthelasma, fundus examination for evidence of hypertension
- Neck for thyroid enlargement and JVP
- Skin for xanthoma
- Hands for nicotine staining (smoking)
- Look for signs of any cardiac or extracardiac disease
- Look for anemia

CVS Examination

Inspection

- No abnormality detected

Palpation

- Apex beat normal
- Chest expansion/movement normal
- Tenderness over chest (not present)

Percussion

- Percussion note/cardiac dullness (normal/abnormal)

Auscultation

- Auscultate for the presence of pansystolic murmur of papillary muscle dysfunction or a pericardial rub or a fourth heart sound.

Other Systems

Respiratory System: For any consolidation or evidence of pulmonary infarction or COPD.

Abdomen Examination: For any evidence of a mass or aortic pulsations

PROVISIONAL DIAGNOSIS

The middle aged male has central chest pain, constricting/squeezing in quality with no radiation, occurs on exertion and relieved by rest (Fig. 39.1). The provisional diagnosis is acute coronary syndrome, or angina pectoris (lesion) due to atherosclerotic coronary artery disease (etiology). She has Canadian Cardiovascular Society class II angina (functional status)

QUESTIONS AND ANSWERS

Q. **How would you grade angina?**
Ans: The Canadian Cardiovascular Society has graded angina into 4 functional classes:
Class I: Angina occurs on strenuous or prolonged exertion.

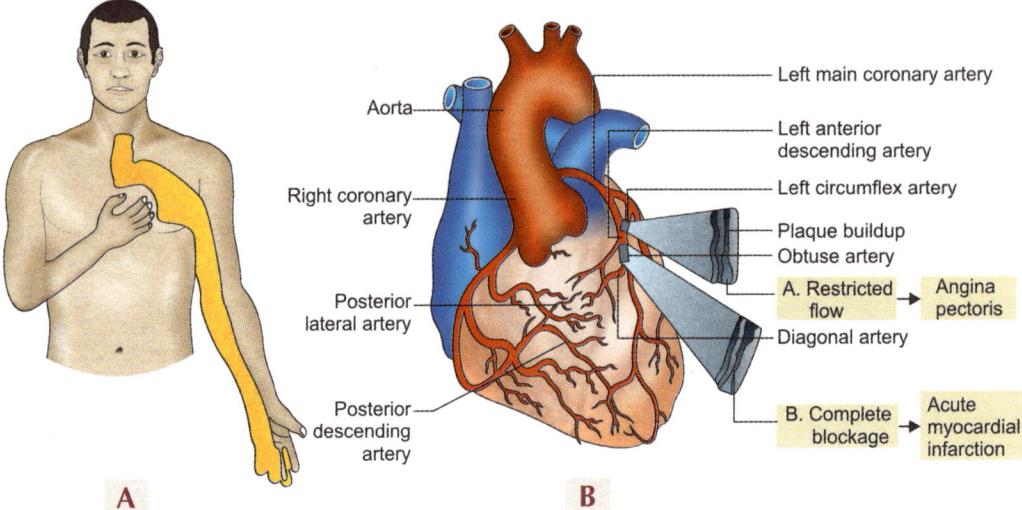

Fig. 39.1: Acute coronary syndrome. (A) Description of chest pain; (B) Evidence of coronary ischemia/thrombosis.
- Angina pectoris. Narrowing of branch left circumflex (left coronary artery) due to intermural plaque result in angina pectoris as a result of myocardial ischemia.
- Acute myocardial infarction. Complete blockage of left anterior descending due to superimposition of a thrombus over atheromatous plaque result in acute myocardial infarction.

Class II: Angina with slight limitation of ordinary normal activity (e.g. climbing more than one flight of ordinary stairs at normal pace).

Class III: Angina with marked limitation of ordinary activity, i.e. climbing more than one flight of stairs.

Class IV: Angina at rest with inability to perform any physical activity without discomfort.

Q.   What is the mechanism of angina pectoris?
Ans: • It is caused by increased myocardial oxygen demand triggered by physical activity.
- Coronary vasospasm is the other mechanism which causes transient decrease in O_2 supply.
- Nonocclusive intracoronary thrombi cause unstable angina pectoris.

Q.   What is Prinzmetal's angina?
Ans: It is a variant angina that occurs at rest, frequently at night induced by coronary vasospasm over and above atherosclerosis is the under-lying cause. It is characterized by transient elevation of ST segment (>4 mm) during pain which resolves with relief of pain.

Q.   What is differential diagnosis of central chest pain?
Ans: Read Table 39.1

Q.   What do you understand by the term acute coronary syndrome? What does it include?
Ans: Acute coronary syndrome refers to coronary events that occur due to narrowing of coronary arteries by atherosclerosis. It includes unstable angina/Non-ST elevation myocardial infarction and ST elevation myocardial infarction (STEMI).

Q.   What is microvascular angina (cardiac syndrome X)?
Ans: It refers to classic anginal symptoms with ST depression on stress ECG testing and a normal coronary angiogram in the absence of any demonstrable cardiac abnormality.

Q.   What is prevalence of angina?
Ans: The prevalence of angina is approximately 2% with an incidence of new cases each year approximately 1 per 1000.

Q.   What are the risk factors for acute coronary syndrome?
Ans: Risk factors are:
- Genetic [deletion polymorphism in the ACE gene (DD)]
- Advancing age and male sex

- Smoking
- Alcohol
- Diabetes
- Hypertension
- Hyperlipidemia

- Lack of exercise (sedentary lifestyle)
- Deficiency of antioxidant vitamins
- Homocysteinemia (Homocysteinuria)
- Oral contraceptive
- High levels of fibrinogen and factor VIII

Table 39.1: Differential diagnosis of central chest pain

Cause	Site	Quality/Severity/Timing	Aggravating/relieving factors
Angina pectoris	Retrosternal or across the chest, radiating to left arm, neck, shoulder, lower jaw, upper abdomen	Squeezing/pressing/ tightness in chest, moderate in intensity lasting for few minutes (1–3 min)	• Exertion, cold, heavy meal and psychological upset exacerbate it • Rest, nitroglycerine relieve it
Myocardial infarction	Same as above	Same as above. Pain is more severe and prolonged, associated with diaphoresis.	• Aggravating or relieving factors as described above • Underlying risk factor may be evident
Pericarditis	Central, limited to precordium, may radiate to shoulder or back	Sharp, cutting (knife like) pain, often severe and persistent	• Breathing, change is posture, coughing and lying may exacerbate it • Sitting and forward bending relieve it
Aortic dissecting aneurysm	Retrosternal, may radiate to back between scapulae	Tearing pain, severe and persistent	• Hypertension aggravates it, may be associated • No relieving factor • Associated features, e.g. syncope, an aortic diastolic murmur helps in the diagnosis
Gastrointestinal Causes			
Reflex esophagitis/ gastrointestinal reflux disease/ diffuse esophageal spasms	Retrosternal, may radiate to back	Burning/squeezing, mild to moderate in intensity	• Large meals, bending, lying emotional upset, spicy food aggravate it • Sitting up and antacid relieve it • Heart burn and acid taste in mouth are common accompaniments
Musuloskeletal Causes			
Myalgia	Often below the left breast	Stabbing or dull ache of fleeting nature, severity variable	• Movements of the chest aggravate it • There is local tenderness
Teitz' syndrome	Pain along the left costal margins	Sticking/stabbing, variable severity	• There may be tenderness and swelling of costochondral junctions (2nd to 4th ribs)
Psychogenic			
Cardiac neurosis	Precordial, below the left breast or whole of anterior chest	Stabbing, variable intensity, fleeting in nature	• Stress and effort precipitate it • Mental rest and anxiolytic relieve it • Anxious look, palpitations hyperventilation, frequent sighs are common associated symptoms

Q.   What are the common clinical patterns of angina?

Ans:
- *Classical* or *exertional angina pectoris.*
- *Decubitus angina* (angina on lying down) indicates angina with impaired LV function.
- *Nocturnal angina* (critical coronary artery disease or vasospasm are the causes)
- *Variant (Prinzmetal's) angina* (Rest angina without any provocation).
- *Unstable angina* (discussed below)

Q.   What are anginal equivalents?

Ans: These are symptoms of myocardial ischemia other than angina, carry same significance as angina. These include dyspnea, fatigue and faintness. They are more common in elderly and in diabetic patients.

Q.   What are angina precipitants?

Ans: Angina precipitants are:
- Physical exertion
- Heavy meals
- Recumbency (angina decubitus)
- Emotional disturbance
- Cold exposure
- Vivid dreams (nocturnal angina)
- Thyrotoxicosis
- Asymptomatic aortic valve disease
- Drugs, e.g. beta-adrenergic stimulants
- Tachycardia and tachyarrhythmias

Q.   What do you understand by the term unstable angina?

Ans: It refers to more severe and frequent angina superimposed on chronic stable angina, angina at rest or on minimal exertion or new onset angina < 1 month which is brought about by minimal exertion.

Q.   What is postprandial angina? What is its mechanism and significance?

Ans: Angina following meals is called *postprandial angina*. It results from the carbohydrate content of the meal. It indicates severe coronary artery disease and could occur as a result of intramyocardial stealing of blood from stenotic territories to normal territories following meal.

Q.   How would you investigate a case of angina?

Ans:
- **Hemoglobin** for anemia (anemia aggravates angina)
- **Resting ECG** (LV hypertrophy, ST–T changes, prior Q-wave MI).
- **Exercise ECG** for ST change (horizontal or downsloping ST segment depression > 1 mm staying for 60–80 ms or ST elevation) or an arrhythmia or production of symptoms.

- **Rest Echocardiogram** for any evidence of asymptomatic aortic stenosis or hypertrophic cardiomyopathy.
- **Exercise myocardial perfusion imaging/ exercise echocardiography** in patients having abnormal ECG at rest.
- **Coronary angiography** for coronary anatomy for any abnormality (atherosclerotic occlusion) or non-atherosclerotic causes (e.g. vasospasm, coronary anomaly/dissection/vasculopathy).

Q.   How would you treat a patient with chronic stable angina?

Ans: Treatment is denoted by mnemonic **ABCDE**
- **A**spirin, **A**ntianginal (nitrates, ranalozine, nicorandil) and ACE inhibitor therapy (Ramipril)
- **B**eta blocker and **b**lood pressure control
- **C**igarette smoking and **C**holesterol reduction.
- **D**iet and **D**iabetes control
- **E**ducation and **E**xercise

Q.   What is the prognostic significance of stress testing in evaluation of chest pain?

Ans: Stress testing determines high risk and low risk population of patients with chest pain suggestive of ischemic heart disease:

I. *Low risk group:* These are patients who can complete exercise testing using Bruce protocol without any change in ST segment and can achieve a maximum heart rate > 160/min without discomfort. These were found to have good prognosis (1 year survival in 99% and 4 years in 93%) and cardiac catheterization and CABG can be deferred.

II. *High risk group:* These are patients who were forced to stop exercise in Stage I and II (under 6 minutes). Survival rate was reduced to 85% at one year and 63% at 4 years.

Q.   What are glycoprotein II/IIIb inhibitors?

Ans: Glycoprotein II/IIIb inhibitors are antithrombotic agents useful for preventing thrombotic complications in patients with STEMI undergoing PCI.

Q.   Name the cardiac markers. What is their significance?

Ans: Cardiac markers are:
- CPK-MB. It peaks within 4–6 hours helps in early detection of MI
- Troponins I and T. They rise late, hence defect late infarction
- Myoglobin. It also rises in blood early during MI

Q. **What are other forms of treatment of acute coronary syndrome?**

Ans: 1. Percutaneous transluminal coronary angioplasty (PTCA) with stent placement
2. Coronary artery bypass surgery
3. Neurostimulation of spinal cord region that receives cardiac nerve fibers
4. External enhanced counterpulsation by wrapping 3 sets of pneumatic cuffs wrapped around lower extremities to achieve hemodynamic effect similar to intra-aortic balloon pump.

Q. **What resting ECG changes suggest ischemia or previous infarction?**

Ans: 1. Pathological Q waves
2. LBBB
3. ST segment depression and T wave flattening or inversion

Q. **What are the indications of CABG in acute coronary syndrome?**

Ans: ACC/AHA guidelines are:
1. Recommended in patients with:
   • Significant left main coronary artery stenosis

• Three vessels disease
• Left main coronary artery stenosis with ≥70% of stenosis of proximal left anterior descending and proximal left circumflex artery
• Two vessels disease with significant proximal left anterior descending stenosis and left ventricular EF < 30% or demonstrable ischemia on non-invasive testing.

II. Beneficial in patients with:
   • One or two vessels disease without significant proximal left anterior descending stenosis.

Q. **What is positive stress test?**

Ans: Criteria for positive stress test are:
1. Downsloping ST segment depression at least 1 mm for 80 ms after the J point.
2. ST elevation
3. Increase in QRS voltage
4. Failure of BP to rise during exercise
5. ventricular arrhythmia
6. Inability to increase heart rate
7. Typical ischemic symptoms during exercise

40

Acute Myocardial Infarction

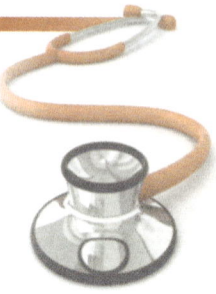

INSTRUCTION

This patient had history of acute severe chest pain, 2 days back, suspected to be having myocardial infarction. Examine the patient.

SALIENT FEATURES
- Acute pain chest

HISTORY

Ask about the following:
- Age, sex, occupation
- Shortness of breath, palpitation, dizziness or syncope
- Past history of heart attack (post-infarct angina)
- History of smoking, alcohol, oral contraceptive in females
- Past history of diabetes, hypertension, stroke, MI, hyperlipidemia, peripheral vascular disease (intermittent claudication)
- Past history of coronary artery disease or angina
- Family history of cardiovascular disease, hyperlipidemia, gout, etc.

EXAMINATION

General Physical Examination
- Record weight, height for BMI (obesity)
- Pulse for any abnormality, e.g. arrhythmia
- Blood pressure in both the arms during lying down and standing
- JVP for cardiac failure.
- Eyes for arcus senilis, xanthelasma
- Legs for edema, peripheral pulses and DVT

Systemic Examination
Cardiovacular System

- Look at the apex beat. Palpable double apex beat indicates ventricular aneurysm
- Auscultate the heart for pericardial rub, pan-systolic murmur (papillary muscle dysfunction or chordae tendinae dysfunction/rupture)

Other Systems
- **Respiratory system examination** for basal crackles and wheezes (left heart failure) or pleural effusion/hydrothorax
- **Abdominal examination** for tender hepatomegaly of CHF

PROVISIONAL DIAGNOSIS

This patient has features suggestive of myocardial infarction with papillary muscle dysfunction (lesion) caused by coronary thrombosis (etiology) and patient is not in cardiac failure (functional status).

QUESTIONS AND ANSWERS

Q. **What investigations would you like to see to confirm the diagnosis?**
Ans: I. ECG for ST segment changes of infarction
II. Serum cardiac markers whether elevated or not

Q. **What is Levine's sign?**
Ans: In acute MI, patient describes the pain by putting a clenched fist across the chest called Levine's sign.

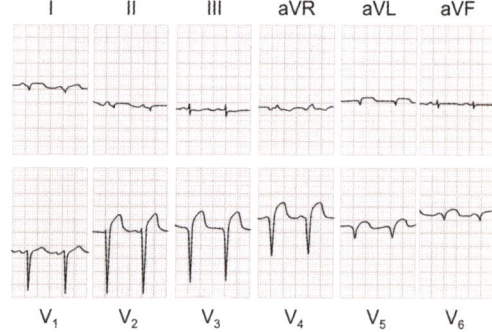

Fig. 40.1: ECG recorded from the patient shows acute anterial wall infarction

Q.   What are the risk factors for AMI?

Ans: These are same as discussed under acute coronary syndrome.

Q.   How would you diagnose AMI?

Ans: Out of the three, two criteria must be present.
I.   Symptoms of cardiac ischemia
II.   ECG change (Fig. 40.1)
III.   Elevated serum cardiac markers, e.g. troponin/CPK–MB

Q.   What are the other causes of raised troponins?

Ans: • Myocarditis
• Congestive heart failure
• Thromboembolism

Q.   What is Killip classification of heart failure?

Ans: This classification is used to characterize heart failure in AMI.

Killip I: Absence of 3rd heart sound and absence of crackles

Killip II: Presence of 3rd heart sound or crackles over < 50% of lung fields

Killip III: Crackles greater than 50% of lung fields

Killip IV: Cardiogenic shock

Q.   How would you localise myocardial infarction from ECG changes?

Ans: Localization based on ECG changes is given below

Site/Localization	ECG change
Anterior (Fig. 40.1)	ST elevation and/or Q wave in leads $V_1 - V_6$
Anterolateral	ST elevation and/or Q wave in leads I, aVL and $V_I - V_6$
Lateral (High)	ST elevation and/or Q wave in leads I, aVL, $V_5 - V_6$
Inferior	ST elevation and/or Q wave in leads II, III and aVF
Inferoseptal	ST elevation and/or Q waves in leads II, III, aVF and $V_1 - V_3$
Inferolateral	ST elevation and/or Q waves in leads II, III aVF and leads $V_5 - V_6$
True posterior	Tall R wave in $V_1 - V_2$ with ST depression (mirror image change of STEMI) with upright T waves in leads $V_1 - V_2$
Right ventricular Infarct	ST segment elevation in right precordial leads ($V_{3R} - V_{4R}$), usually occurs in conjunction with inferior infarction

Q.   What are the causes of ST elevation on ECG?

Ans: • Myocarditis
• Pericarditis
• Cardiac aneurysm
• Early repolarisation syndrome
• Intracranial bleed
• Pancreatitis

Q.   What is silent MI?

Ans: It is a painless infarct commonly seen in diabetics and elderly particularly women. It presents with complications.

Q.   What are the complications of MI?

Ans: I.   Immediate (within 24 hours)
1.   Heart failure/acute pulmonary edema
2.   Circulatory failure/cardiogenic shock
3.   Arrhythmias/conduction disturbance (common)
4.   Infarction of papillary muscle leading to acute mitral regurgitation
5.   Infarction of interventricular septum (acquired VSD)
6.   Murmal thrombosis and thromboembolism
7.   Pericarditis

II.   Late complications (after 24 – 48 hrs)
• Pericarditis
• Dressler's syndrome
• Ventricular aneurysm
• Deep vein thrombosis and pulmonary embolism
• Postmyocardial angina

Q.   Which myocardial infarction is associated with conduction disturbance?

Ans: Inferior myocardial infarction (Fig. 40.2).

Q.   What are the indications of thrombolysis?

Ans: 1.   Typical cardiac pain within 12 hours (preferably with in 6 hrs) and ST elevation in two contiguous ECG leads (>1 mm in limb leads or > 2 mm in chest leads)
2.   Cardiac pain with new/presumed new LBBB on ECG
3.   If ECG is equivocal on arrival, repeat ECG at 15–30 minutes reveals ST elevation.

Q.   What are the contraindications of thrombolysis?

Ans: I.   Absolute contraindications
1.   Active internal bleeding
2.   Suspected aortic dissection
3.   Recent head trauma and/or intracranial neoplasm
4.   Previous hemorrhagic stroke
5.   Previous ischemic stroke within past one year

6. History of allergic reaction to fibrinolytic agent
7. Trauma and/or surgery within past
2 weeks at risk of bleeding

II. Relative contraindications
1. Previous trauma more than 2 weeks
2. Uncontrolled severe hypertension
3. Non-hemorrhagic stroke over one yr
4. Known bleeding diathesis
5. Severe renal/liver dysfunction
6. Pregnancy or postpartum
7. Prior exposure to streptokinase
8. Menstrual bleeding or lactation

Q. Name the drugs available for thrombolysis?
Ans: 1. Streptokinase
2. Recombinant tissue-type plasminogen
activator (rt-PA, Alteplase)
3. Reteplase
4. Tenecteplase
5. APSAC (anistreplase)

Q. What are the complications of thrombolysis?
Ans: 1. Bleeding
2. Hypotension
3. Allergic reactions
4. Intracranial hemorrhage

5. Reperfusion arrhythmias
6. Systemic embolization

Q. What are the indications for primary coronary angioplasty?
Ans: 1. All patients with chest pain and ST
elevation or new LBBB. This is preferred
to thrombolysis.
2. ST elevation infarction (STEMI) where
thromsolysis is contraindicated.

Q. How would you diagnose right ventricular infarction?
Ans: RV infarction is diagnosed by:
1. Clinical signs of right heart failure
2. **ECG:** Changes of infarction (ST elevation
and/or Q waves) in right ventricular
leads $V_{3R}-V_{4R}$ in patients with inferior
wall infarction.
3. **ECHO:** Looking for RV dilatation and
wall motion abnormalities.

Q. What are TIMI Grades for coronary blood flow?
Ans: Grades 0 to 3 are used to determine the
coronary blood flow and luminal narrowing
following thrombolysis in myocardial infarction trial (TIMI).

Grade 0: No flow of contrast beyond the point
of occlusion

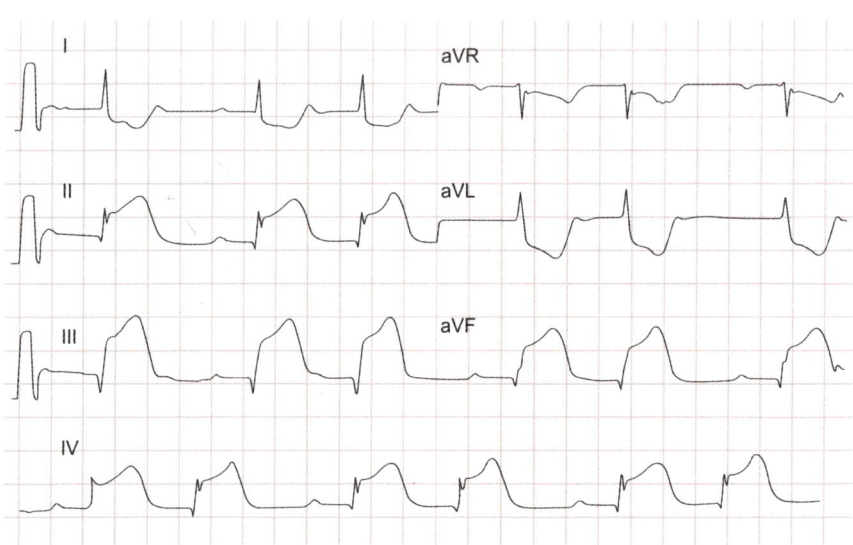

Fig. 40.2: Ventricular escape bigeminy in a patient with inferior wall infarction with bradycardia and AV block. The ECG shows
 i. Inferior wall infarction (ST elevation in leads II, III and aVF)
 ii. Bradycardia (HR <60/min)
iii. First degree AV block (PR interval 0.28 sec)
iv. Ventricular bigeminy. A normal sinus beat is conducted with prolonged P – R interval followed by an ventricular
   premature complex (escape beat) regularly.
N.B The ECG reversed to normal as patient recovered

Grade 1: Penetration with minimal perfusion (contrast fails to opacify the entire coronary bed distal to stenosis)

Grade 2: Partial perfusion (contrast opacifies the entire distal coronary artery but the rate of entry or clearance or both is slower in the perfused vessels).

Grade 3: Complete perfusion (contrast filling and clearance are as rapid in the previously blocked vessel as in normally perfused vessels)

Q. What is cooing or seagull murmur?

Ans: A soft blowing murmur produced by mitral regurgitation due to endocarditis or papillary muscle dysfunction/chordae tendinae dysfunction is called cooing murmur (Read endocarditis).

Q. What are the indications for drug eluting stents?

Ans: I. Taxus stent elutes paclitaxel to inhibit cell division

II. The cypher stent elutes sirolimus (previously known as rapamycin) an immunosuppressive agent that reduces inflammation

Q. What advice would you give to the patient at the time of discharge?

Ans: Advice will be given for secondary prevention as follows:

1. Cessation of smoking and alcohol.
2. Lifestyle modifications and cardiac rehabilitation program in which patients are advised to increase activity gradually over a period of 1–2 months.
3. Control of risk factors, e.g. obesity, diabetes, hypertension.
4. Aspirin and statins. Low dose aspirin is recommended along with statin to keep the lipid profile in check (LDL <70 mg/dl).
5. Betablockers. They reduce recurrence of MI, sudden death and all cause mortality.
6. ACE inhibitors, e.g. ramipril should be considered in all patients with uncomplicated MI. ACE inhibitors in full dose is recommended for an indefinite period in patients with CHF, an ejection fraction <40% or a large regional wall motion abnormality.
7. Regular and repeated follow up.

41

Acute Pericarditis (Pericardial Rub)

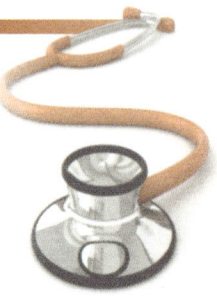

INSTRUCTION

Examine the patient's cardiovascular system

SALIENT FEATURES

- Acute chest pain

HISTORY

Ask for the following:

- History of fever, cough, sore throat
- Pain chest, central, worse in lying down and relieved by sitting and bending forward (postural relationship of pain). It does not radiate.
- History of angina/myocardial infarction
- History of chronic kidney disease/chronic renal failure (present)
- History of trauma
- History of tuberculosis, collagen vascular disorder, rheumatic fever
- History of drug intake

EXAMINATION

General Physical Examination

- Look for signs of chronic renal failure (facial edema, anemia, anorexia, uremic breath, pedal edema, etc.) which are present in this case
- Look for signs of hypothyroidism, collagen vascular disease, tuberculosis, RA

Examination of CVS

1. A pericardial rub may be palpable which is grating sound.
2. On auscultation, a scratching or grating sound is heard (Fig. 41.1) over the whole precordium. It has to be differentiated from coarse crackles. The rub does not have any relation to respiration or coughing, but is best heard with diaphragm with patient leaning forward and breath heard in expiration.

PROVISIONAL DIAGNOSIS

The patient has a pericardial rub (lesion) due to pericarditis secondary to chronic renal failure (etiology) and does not have pain (functional status).

QUESTIONS AND ANSWERS

Q. What are the common causes of pericarditis?

Ans:
    I. Infective pericarditis, e.g. bacterial (tuberculosis is the commonest cause, staphylococcal, pneumococcal, meningococcal), viral (Coxsackie, echo), fungal and parasitic

    II. Autoimmune pericarditis
- Collagen vascular diseases
- Rheumatic fever, rheumatoid arthritis

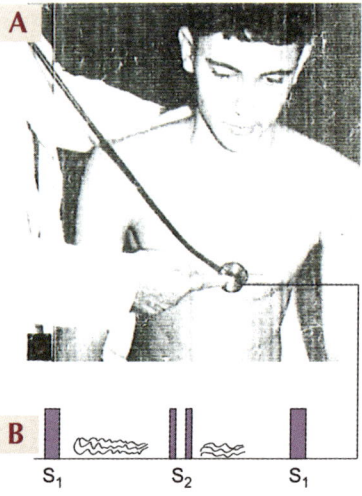

Fig. 41.1: Acute pericarditis. (A) Hearing for the pericardial rub in a patient with acute pericarditis; (B) A superficial scratching sound heard both in systole and diastole at left sternal edge with diaphragm and patient leaning forward

- Drugs, e.g. hydralazine, procain-amide, isoniazide
III. Postmyocardial infarction
IV. Traumatic
V. Bleeding into pericardium (anticoagulants, bleeding disorder)
VI. Metabolic, e.g. uremia, myxedema
VII. Miscellaneous, e.g radiation, sarcoidosis, amyloidosis, etc.

Q. What is pericardial rub? How does it differ from pleuropericardial rub or a continuous murmur?

Ans: It is an adventitious sound produced by rubbing of visceral and parietal pericardium, hence, has a rubbing or scratching quality. It may have presystolic, systolic or early diastolic components which means rub may be heard in a part of systolic or throughout systolic or in early diastole or both systole and diastole. It does not have any relation to respiration, hence, differs from pleuropericardial rub (Read the Clinical Methods in Medicine by Prof SN Chugh). Its differentiations from continuous murmur are given in Table 41.1.

Q. What are clinical characteristics of acute pericarditis?

Ans: Pain, a pericardial rub and characteristic ECG changes, ST segment elevation with concavity upwards in more than two or three standard leads and V_2–V_6 are clinical hallmarks (a triad) of acute pericarditis.

Q. What are the ECG changes in acute pericarditis?

Ans: Read Textbook of Electrocardiography by Prof SN Chugh
- There is sinus tachycardia, concave shaped ST segment elevation, PR segment depression in leads II, III and aVF.

Table 41.1: Differences between a continuous murmur and pericardial rub

Pericardial rub	Continuous murmur
• Rubbing or scratching high pitched sound	Soft musical or machinery sound
• Heard either in a part of systole or diastole	Heard both in systole and diastole
• Best heard in sitting position during expiration with patient sitting up and leaning forward	Heard in all positions
• Associated with pain	Not associated with pain
• Inconsistent and intermittent in character, i.e. may appear and then disappear for few hours	Consistent in character

Q. When does pericardial rub disappear in pericarditis?

Ans: As pericarditis indicates friction between two layers of the pericardium, the rub persists as long as friction persists in pericarditis, may disappear with appearance of massive pericardial effusion or development of chronic calcific pericarditis. It is possible to hear a pericardial rub in effusive pericarditis (pericarditis with minimal effusion).

Q. What are the causes of painless pericarditis?

Ans: Noninflammatory, nontraumatic pericarditis can be painless. The causes are:
1. Metabolic causes (diabetes, uremia)
2. Drug induced
3. Amyloidosis
4. Relief of pain by colchicine in pericarditis

Q. What do you understand by the term sub-acute effusive and constrictive pericarditis?

Ans: About 10% of patients with acute pericarditis pass on to transient subacute effusive-constrictive phase which may last for 2–3 months before it resolves either spontaneously or with treatment with NSAIDs. These patients have persistent pericardial rub, moderate pericardial effusion and as the effusion resolves, the pericardium becomes thickened, inflammed and non-compliant leading to symptoms and signs of constrictive pericarditis.

Q. What is Dressler's syndrome?

Ans: It is an autoimmune postmyocardial syndrome, occurs 2–3 weeks after infarction, is characterized by pyrexia, pericarditis and pleurisy. It responds to NSAIDs.

Q. What is post-pericardiotomy syndrome?

Ans: It is also an autoimmune syndrome like Dressler's syndrome, characterized symptoms of pericarditis from 1 to 6 months after surgery. It is presumed to be due to antibodies produced against pericardium and is related to cardiac trauma, surgery and irritation of pericardium by blood products. It also responds to NSAIDs and steroids (refractory cases). It does not produce constrictive pericarditis and pericardiectomy is rarely needed.

Q. What are the causes of recurrent pericarditis?

Ans: 1. Recurrent attacks of viral infection (Coxsackie)
2. Tuberculosis
3. Uremia
4. Neoplasia
5. Radiation
6. Collagen vascular disorder
7. Autoimmune

42

Constrictive Pericarditis

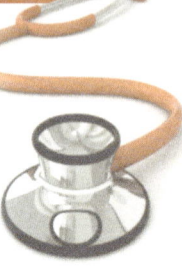

INSTRUCTION

Examine the cardiovascular system of this patient

SALIENT FEATURES

- Distended abdomen and edema feet

HISTORY

Ask for the following:

- History of chest pain
- Dyspnea, palpitation, fatigue
- Puffiness of face, edema feet
- Nausea, vomiting and pain in abdomen (hepatomegaly) and distension of abdomen (ascites)
- History of trauma
- Past history of tuberculosis, uremia, fever, radiation
- Past history of pericardiocentesis

EXAMINATION

General Physical Examination

- There may be puffiness of face (present)

- Pulse may be low volume, regular or irregular due to atrial fibrillation (common) 'Y' descents (Fig. 42.1A). Kussmaul's sign is positive in this case (level of JVP further rises on inspiration)
- Pedal edema over legs present (Fig. 42.1B)

Cardiovascular System

- Apex beat is neither visible nor palpable. There may be apical systolic contraction (Broadbent sign).
- Early pericardial diastolic knock (Fig. 42.1A) along the left sternal border may be heard which increases on inspiration.
- Cardiac sounds are feebly audible.

Examination of other Systems

I. *Respiratory system:* The lungs are clear but there are signs of right pleural effusion. There is a cavity in right lung (in this case)

II. *Abdominal examination:* There is tender hepatomegaly with signs of ascites (present, Fig. 42.1B)

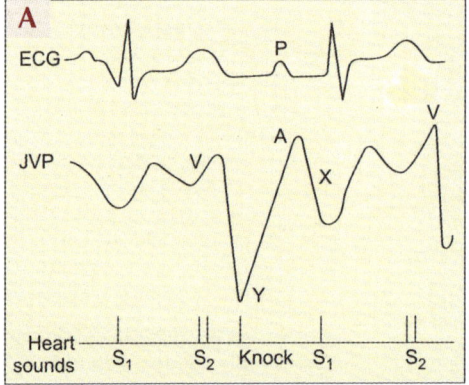

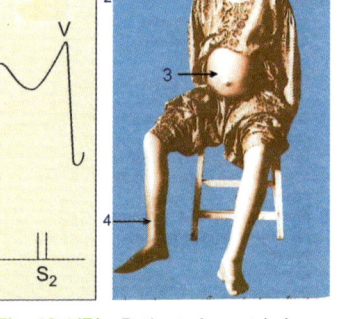

Fig. 42.1(A): Constrictive pericarditis: Analysis of jugular venous pulse. There is prominent 'Y' descent indicative of constrictive pericarditis. Note the timing of pericardial knock relative to S$_2$

Fig. 42.1(B): Patient of constrictive pericarditis with heart failure
1. Arrow at the level of neck indicates raised JVP (jugular venous pressure)
2. Prominent chest veins
3. Arrow at abdomen indicates ascites
4. Arrow at ankle indicates edema of feet and ankles

PROVISIONAL DIAGNOSIS

This patient has constrictive pericarditis (lesion) probably due to tuberculosis (signs of cavity and pleural effusion) of right lung (etiology). Patient has congestive heart failure (functional status).

Q. **What is differential diagnosis?**
Ans: The conditions that come into differential diagnosis are discussed in Table 42.1

QUESTIONS AND ANSWERS

Q. **What are the important common causes of constrictive pericarditis?**
Ans: 1. Tubercular pericarditis (most common)
2. Pyogenic infections of pericardium
3. Collagen vascular diseases
4. Neoplasm involving pericardium
5. Uremic pericarditis following hemodialysis
6. Radiation injury
7. Post-traumatic (hemopericardium)
8. Postsurgical

Q. **What is chronic constrictive pericarditis?**
Ans: The disorder results following healing of acute fibrinous or serofibrinous pericarditis or a chronic pericardial effusion leading to obliteration of the pericardial sac with granulation tissue and ultimately a firm scar encasing the heart is formed. Like pericardial effusion, it also interfers with filling of the ventricles (diastolic dysfunction)

Q. **What is restrictive cardiomyopathy? What are its causes?**
Ans: It is a rare disorder characterized by impaired diastolic function due to reduced ventricular compliance. The causes are:

I. *Myocardial causes*, e.g. infiltrative malignancies, amyloidosis, sarcoidosis, storage disease, hemochromatosis, and idiopathic

II. *Endomyocardial diseases*, e.g. endomyocardial fibrosis, carcinoid syndrome, hypereosinophillic syndrome, radiation, etc.

Q. **What is differential diagnosis of an early diastolic sound?**
Ans: • Early diastolic murmur
• S_3 gallop
• Opening snap
• Pericardial knock
• Tumor plop

Q. **How would you investigate this case?**
Ans: • *Chest X-ray (PA view)* for pericardial calcification and heart size.
• *ECG* for low voltage graph and an arrhythmia (AF)
• *Echocardiogram* may show thickened pericardium, normal ventricular dimensions, good systolic and poor diastolic ventricular function.
• *CT/MRI* shows normal myocardial thickness and pericardial thickening and calcification
• *Cardiac catheterization* shows 'square root' sign (equalization of pressure of all chambers, i.e. both atria and ventricles)

Q. **How would you treat this patient?**
Ans: 1. Medical treatment of congestive heart failure and pericardiectomy
2. Treatment of underlying cause, i.e. tuberculosis. Patient was put on ATT (anti tubercular therapy)

Table 42.1: Distinguishing features of constrictive pericarditis from other similar disorders

Feature A. Clinical	Constrictive pericarditis	Restrictive cardiomyopathy	Cardiac tamponade
• Pulsus paradoxus	Absent	Rare	Common
• Prominent 'Y' descent on JVP	Present	Rare	Absent
• Prominent 'X' descent on JVP	Present	Present	Present
• Kussmaul's sign	Present	Absent	Absent
• 3rd heart sound	Absent	Rare	Absent
• Pericardial knock	Often present	Absent	Absent
• ECG	Low voltage to normal graph	Low voltage graph to normal voltage	Low voltage graph with electrical alternans

43

Pericardial Effusion

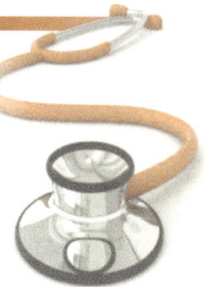

INSTRUCTION

Examine the cardiovascular system of the patient

SALIENT FEATURES

- Chest discomfort and dyspnea

HISTORY

Ask for the same points on the history discussed already for

Pericarditis and constrictive pericarditis. In addition ask for:

- Dry hacking cough, dyspnea
- Hoarseness and dysphagia (compressive symptoms)
- Chest discomfort and dyspnea

EXAMINATION

General Physical Examination

- Pulse is low volume (pulsus paradoxus)
- Pulse pressure is low
- Low systolic BP
- Cyanosis may or may not be present (not present in this case)
- JVP is raised with prominent 'X' descent (in this case)
- Kussmaul's sign absent
- Pitting pedal edema present

Cardiovascular System

Inspection

- Precordium may be bulging including xiphisternum
- Apex beat is not visible
- No other pulsations are visible

Palpation

- Apex beat is either feeble or not palpable (in this case)
- A pericardial rub may be palpable
- No other pulsations palpable

Percussion

- Increase in area of cardiac dullness (present). Shifting cardiac dullness may be present (area of cardiac dullness decreases on sitting)
- There is an area of dullness, on right side of sternum in 5th intercostal space (Rotch's sign present)
- An area of dullness in the left interscapular region with bronchial breathing and aegophony (Edward's sign). This is due to compression of base of the lung

Auscultation

- Heart sounds are muffled (in this case)
- A pericardial rub may be heard

Abdominal Examination

- Tender hepatomegaly (present)
- Ascites

PROVISIONAL DIAGNOSIS

The symptoms and signs in this patient suggest the diagnosis of pericardial effusion (lesion) probably caused by tubercular pericarditis (aetiology) and patient has limited activity due to congestive heart failure (functional status).

QUESTIONS AND ANSWERS

Q. Is patient in cardiac tamponade? What are the signs of cardiac tamponade?

Ans: Yes. It is defined as disturbance in early diastolic filling of ventricles due to sudden accumulation of large amount of pericardial fluid. Slow accumulation of large amount of fluid can also lead to cardiac tamponade.

All the signs of pericardial effusion are present with Beck's diagnostic triad consisting of:

1. Low arterial blood pressure
2. Raised JVP with 'X' descent
3. Silent heart

Q.   What are the points in favor of your diagnosis?

Ans: 1. Acute febrile onset
2. Symptoms and signs of CHF, e.g. dyspnea, raised JVP, hepatomegaly, ascites and edema
3. Absence of pericardial rub, prominent X descent
4. Negative Kussmaul's sign
5. Enlargement of area of cardiac dullness with feeble heart sounds

Q.   What is your alternative diagnosis?

Ans: • Dilated cardiomyopathy
• Myocarditis
• Myocardial infarction with pericardial effusion (pericarditis)

The differences between pericardial effusion and dilated cardiomyopathy are given in Table 43.1.

Table 43.1: Pericardial effusion vs dilated cardiomyopathy

Feature	Pericardial effusion	Dilated cardiomyopathy
Pulse	Pulsus paradoxus Narrow pulse pressure	Low volume pulse Narrow or normal pulse pressure
JVP	Raised with 'x' descent	Raised with 'VY' collapse
Early diastolic sound	Pericardial knock	Third heart sound
Heart sounds	Feeble	Audible
Apex beat	Neither visible nor palpable	Visible and palpable, heaving in character
Murmur	No murmur	Murmur of MR and TR may be present
Lungs	Normal	Lungs congested, basal rales and crackles present

Q.   How would you investigate such a case?

Ans: *Investigations*
1. *Chest X-ray:* The heart size is usually enlarged due to pericardial effusion (Fig. 43.1A). The shadow of superior vena cava is prominent. Lung fields are oligemic. Unilateral or bilateral pleural effusions may occur. Fluoroscopy may reveal diminished cardiac pulsations.

2. *The ECG:* There may be low voltage of QRS complex (low voltage graph), flattening or inversion of T waves and occasionally atrial fibrillation. There may be electrical alternans (Fig. 43.1C).
3. *Cardiac catheterization:* The pericardial pressure is elevated and is equal to right atrial pressure. This investigation is not required in cardiac tamponade.
4. *Echocardiography* (Fig. 43.2) shows echo free space.
5. *CT scan and MRI.*
6. *Diagnostic paracentesis.* Aspiration of pericardial fluid confirms the diagnosis (Fig. 43.1B) and helps to identify the cause. The aspirated fluid is sent for microscopic, biochemical and microbial examination.
7. *Pericardial biopsy.* It can be obtained during pericardiocentesis for histopathological diagnosis.

Q.   How would you treat pericardial effusion?

Ans: 1. To find out the underlying cause and treat it wherever possible.
2. *Pericardiocentesis (removal of fluid).* A small amount of fluid is removed for diagnostic purpose. For therapeutic purpose a large amount of fluid is removed to relieve cardiorespiratory embarrassment either through a rigid needle or by use of a plastic cannula. If the fluid withdrawn is purulent, then it should be drained with an indwelling tube connected to an underwater seal.
3. *Pericardiectomy* is the treatment of permanent nature in case of recurrent pericarditis or if chronic constrictive pericarditis develops

Q.   What are indications of pericardiocentesis (Fig. 41.1)?

Ans: I. **Diagnostic:** A small amount is removed for diagnostic purpose in small effusion, otherwise a portion of fluid during therapeutic paracentesis is sent for biochemical and culture analysis.
II. **Therapeutic:** When there is cardiac tamponade, fluid has to be removed. Pyogenic fluid is removed by catheter drainage.

Q.   What are the causes of recurrent pericardial effusion?

Ans: These are more or less same as for pleural effusion (read pleural effusion).

Q.   What are the causes of exudative and transudative pericardial effusion?

Ans: Again the causes are same as for exudative and transudative pleural effusion.

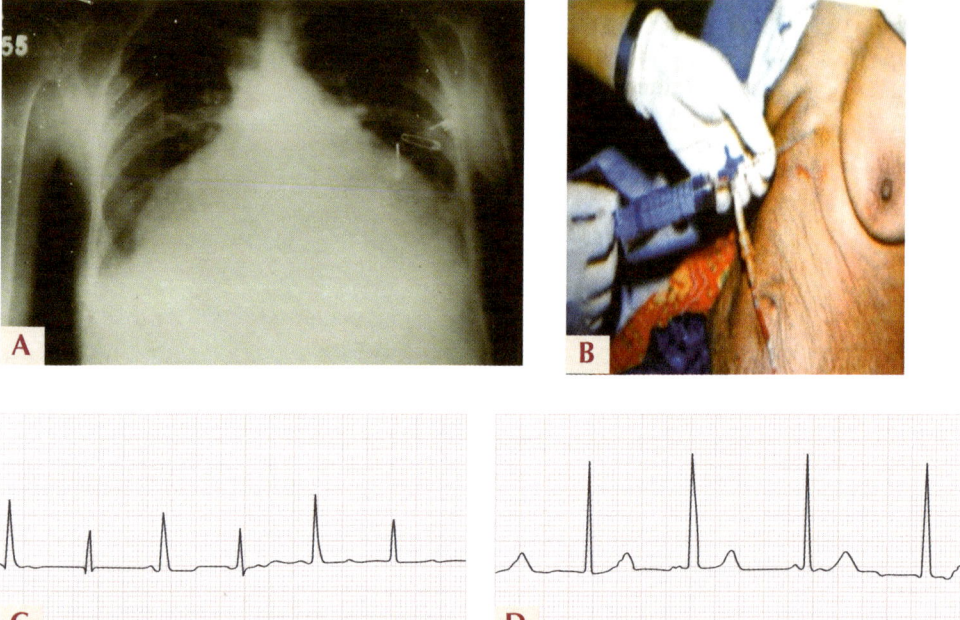

Fig. 43.1: Cardiac tamponade due to acute massive pericardial effusion.
(A) Chest X-ray (PA view) showing enlarged cardiac silhoutte (money-bag appearance);
(B) ECG strip showing the low voltage of QRS complexes with electrical alternans (a small QRS alternates with a large QRS complex);
(C) Pericardiocentesis;
(D) Restoration of QRS voltage after removal of pericardial fluid (pericardiocentesis) and disappearance of electrical alternans

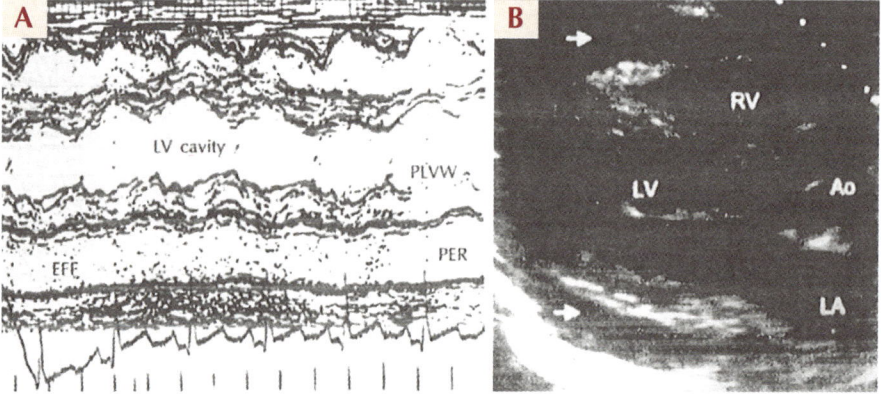

Fig. 43.2: (A) Echocardiogram from a patient with pericardial effusion. Fluid is seen as a relatively echo-free space (EFF) lying above the pericardium (PER). The effusion and pericardium both lie below the left ventricular (LV) cavity and the posterior left ventricular wall (PLVW); (B) Parasternal long-axis view showing effusion anterior to right ventricle and posterior to left ventricle (arrows)

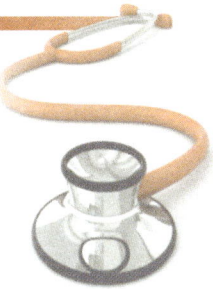

44

Myocarditis

INSTRUCTION

Examine the patient's cardiovascular system

SALIENT FEATURES

- Palpitation and dyspnea on exertion

HISTORY

Ask for the following:

- Patient may be asymptomatic
- Ask for history of myalgia, pleuro-pericardial chest pain, sore throat, arthralgia, palpitations and fever (present)
- Ask history of rheumatic fever, tuberculosis, sepsis, and typhoid fever
- Ask for history of syncope, dizziness (Lyme's disease)
- Ask for history of jaundice, hemorrhage and dark colored urine (Weil's disease)
- History of breathlessness, orthopnea, PND
- History of drugs, poison, chemical agents, radiation
- History of collagen vascular diseases

EXAMINATION

General Physical Examination

- Eyes for jaundice, subconjunctival hemorrhage
- Face for puffiness, edema
- Mouth for cyanosis, bleeding
- Neck for lymph nodes, thyroiditis, JVP—raised
- Skin for hemorrhages/petechiae
- Legs for pitting edema
- Record temperature, pulse, respiration and blood pressure for abnormality

Cardiovascular Examination

- *Inspection and palpation.* Apex beat is normal or feeble, may be deviated down and out due to presence of congestive heart failure
  Auscultation: There may be normal or feeble heart sounds, 3rd heart sound (gallop rhythm) and a midsystolic or a pansystolic murmur due to papillary muscle dysfunction. A pericardial rub may be heard if pericardium is also involved.

Other Systems Examination

- *Abdominal examination* for hepatomegaly and ascites (present)
- *Respiratory system examination* for crackles at both bases of lungs and wheezes (present)

PROVISIONAL DIAGNOSIS

In view of fever, arthralgia, upper respiratory infection; signs of congestive heart failure, the patient probably has acute myocarditis (lesion) due to viral infection (etiology) and is in state of congestive cardiac failure (functional cardiac status).

QUESTIONS AND ANSWERS

Q. Is it a case of myocarditis or myopericarditis?

Ans: As there is no pericardial rub, therefore, there are less chance of myopericarditis.

Q. Which investigations would you like to see and why?

Ans: 1. *ECG:* It is a gold standard for diagnosis of myocarditis (Fig. 44.1). Prolonged P–R interval, depressed ST segment, depressed P–R segment, QTc prolongation, T wave inversion are its characteristic features. An arrhythmia can also be seen.

2. *X-ray chest.* It may be normal or may show cardiomegaly and signs of CHF.

Q. What are the common causes of myocarditis?

Ans: 1. *Viral myocarditis,* e.g. Coxsackie B, CMV, EBV hepatitis, influenza, HIV

2. *Rickettsial myocarditis* (Q fever, spotted fever, typhus fever)

3. *Bacterial myocarditis,* e.g. diphtheria *Meningococcus, Mycoplasma, Salmonella,*

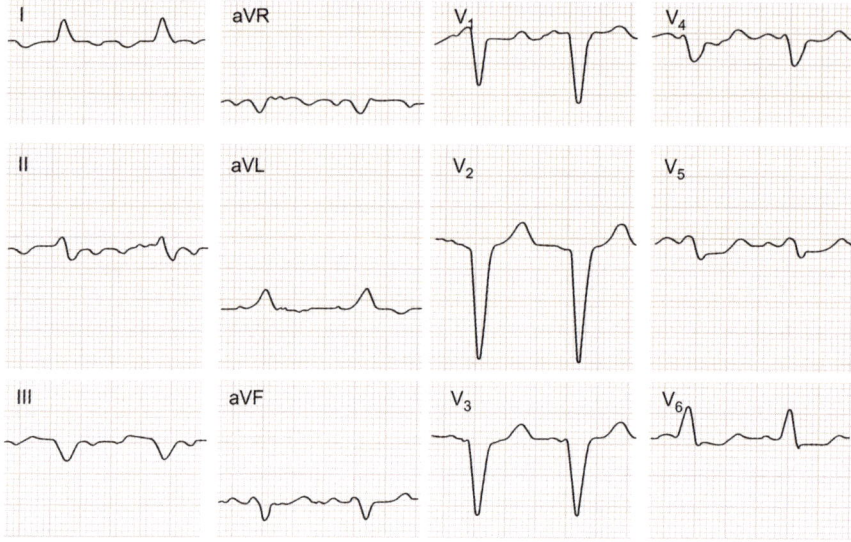

Fig. 44.1: Myocarditis. The ECG shows:
- Low voltage graph,
- Sinus tachycardia,
- Prolonged QTc (0.50 ms)

- LBBB pattern (wide slurred R in V_5 and S in V_1),
- Slurred wide QRS

acute rheumatic fever (streptococcal), tuberculosis

4. *Protozoal myocarditis*, e.g. trypanosmiasis (Chagas' disease), malaria, toxoplasma

5. *Fungal myocarditis*, e.g. *Aspergillus, Candida, Histoplasma*, etc.

6. *Toxic.* A variety of drugs can produce it, i.e. anthracyclines cocaine, catecholamine (*Tako-Tsubo cardiomyopathy*, etc.)

7. *Hypersensitivity myocarditis* due to drugs, e.g. antibiotics (penicillins, chloramphenicol, tetracyclines) antiepileptics, isoniazid, sulphonylurea, amphotericin, etc.

8. Physical injury, e.g. irradiation

9. Poisons, e.g. snake bite, scorpion bite, etc.

Q.   How would you investigate such a case?

Ans: 1. *Blood examination* for leucocytosis. ESR and CRP may be raised

2. *ECG* (already discussed)

3. *Chest X-ray (already, discussed)*

4. Echocardiogram, for ejection fraction, regional wall motion abnormality or global hypokinesia, and to exclude other diseases

5. Cardiac markers, e.g. CP–KMB and troponin may be raised

6. *Paired serum* viral *titres* and *serological tests* for other agents may indicate the cause

7. *Gallium scintigraphy* may reveal increased cardiac uptake

8. *MRI with gadolinium enhancement* reveals spotty areas of injury/uptake

9. *Endomyocardial biopsy.* It is usually not indicated

Q.   How would you treat it?

Ans: 1. Find out the cause and treat it specifically with appropriate antimicrobial therapy

2. Standard congestive heart failure treatment, e.g. salt restriction, diuretics, ACE inhibitors, vasodilators, digoxin, etc.

3. Corticosteroids and immunosuppressive drugs for autoimmune myocarditis

4. Intravenous immunoglobulins

5. Patients with acute cardiogenic shock may require short-term IABP (intra-aortic balloon counterpulsation) or left ventricular assist device

6. Extracorporeal membrane oxygenator may be temporarily required in fulminant cases

7. Chronic resistant cases are candidates for cardiac transplantation or long-term LV assist device

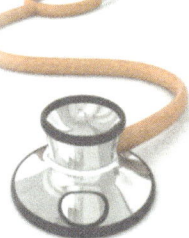

45

Systemic Hypertension

INSTRUCTION

Examine the patient's cardiovascular system

SALIENT FEATURES

- Complains of high BP

HISTORY

Ask for the following:

- Ask history of syncope, palpitations, dizziness
- Any history of chest pain or dyspnea on exertion
- History of intermittent claudication
- Any visual disturbance
- In female, ask history of hypertension during pregnancy
- Family history of hypertension
- Drug treatment if any
- History of renal or endocrinal disease

EXAMINATION

General Physical Examination

- *Facial appearance*, e.g. cushing face, myxedema, puffiness due to renal disease
- *Neck* for carotids pulsations, JVP, lymph node and thyroid enlargement
- *Pulse* (rate/volume and radiofemoral delay)
- *Blood pressure* in both upper arms, in standing and lying down. BP in the lower limbs. BP is high 180/120 mm Hg (Fig. 45.1) in this patient
- Fingers for staining (nicotine)
- Fundus examination for retinopathy (Grade II hypertensive changes present)

CVS Examination

Inspection

- Look at the apex beat, e.g. normally placed (in this case) or displaced
- Look for pulsations in suprasternal notch, precordium and epigastrium

Palpation

- Palpate the apex beat and note its location (normal or displaced), character and whether forceful or not and whether sustained or not?

Percussion

- Define cardiac dullness (normal or enlarged due to LVH)

Auscultation

- Hear heart sounds in all the areas especially 2nd right intercostal space (aortic area)
- Hear for any murmurs/rub
- Third heart sound (S_3)

Other Systems

1. *Abdominal Examination*

- For polycystic kidneys or for renal artery bruit
- Palpate liver for enlargement

2. *Respiratory system examination*

- For crackles and wheezes

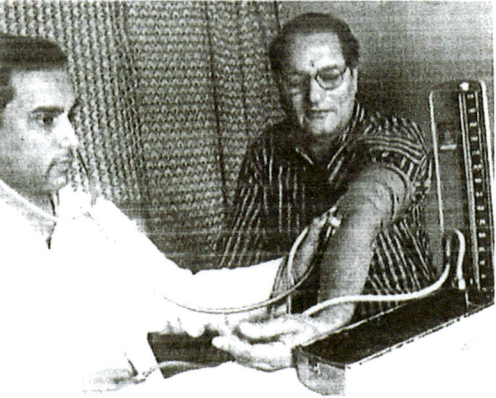

Fig. 45.1: A patient with hypertension

PROVISIONAL DIAGNOSIS

The patient has elevated BP (lesion), retinopathy and angina, hence diagnosis is hypertensive heart disease (etiology). There is no other target organ damage (functional status).

QUESTIONS AND ANSWERS

Q.   **How would you record the BP?**

Ans: • It is measured with sphygmomanometer (Fig. 45.1) which should be accurate and calibrated recently.

• Patient should rest for 10–15 minutes before measurement. Make the patient comfortably seated with the arms at the level of the heart. Take the blood pressure cuff of appropriate size of the arm. Cuff should be inflated higher than expected BP and then slowly deflated at 2 mm/sec and diastolic BP is measured to the nearest 2 mmHg. Diastolic BP is recorded as disappearance of the sound (*Krotokoff sound*) while systolic is measured as appearance of sound. At least 3 consecutive readings at an interval of 1 minutes are to be recorded before a patient is declared normal or hypertensive. If the patient is hypertensive, then two readings to be taken at each visit to determine BP threshold.

Q.   **What is normal and abnormal BP?**

Ans: JNC VIII classification (JNC VII criteria retained) of normal and abnormal BP is:

Category	SBP (mmHg)	DBP (mmHg)
Normal	<120	<80
Prehypertension	120–139	80–89
Stage I hypertension	140–159	90–99
Stage II hypertension	≥160	≥100

Q.   **What are recommendations of JNC VIII for initiation of therapy and goals of control?**

Ans: JNC VIII has not address prehypertension any hypertension. They have addressed only the therapeutic goals i.e initiation and control of hypertension.

Q.   **What are the common identifiable causes of hypertension?**

Ans: About 90% cases of hypertension do not have any identifiable cause hence labelled as idiopathic. The identifiable causes (10%) are:

Common identifiable causes of hypertension	
Renal	**Endocrinal**
• Chronic glomerulonephritis	• Cushing's syndrome
• Chronic pyelonephritis	• Excess of corticosteroid
• Renal artery stenosis	• Hypothyroidism
• Diabetic nephropathy	• Pheochromocytoma

Other

• Coarctation of aorta
• Toxemia of pregnancy
• Collagen vascular disease
• Drug induced, e.g. oral contraceptives and steroids

Q.   **What are the conditions that produce discrepancy of BP between the arms or between the arms and legs?**

Ans: • Coarctation of aorta
• PDA (patent ductus arteriosus)
• Supravalvular aortic stenosis
• Thoracic outlet syndrome
• Dissection of aortic aneurysm
• Arterial occlusion or stenosis of subclavian artery (discrepancy between arms)
• Aorto-arteritis
• Thrombotic occlusion or bifurcation of aorta (Lerisch's syndrome)

Q.   **What are the indications of ambulatory BP recording?**

Ans: • Unusual variability in BP recording
• Hypertension resistant to 3 or more drugs
• To exclude white coat hypertension
• When symptoms suggest that patient may have hypertension

Q.   **What is white coat hypertension?**

Ans: In some patients, the BP remaining otherwise normal increases to hypertensive range whenever they visit a doctor called *white coat hypertension*. They are usually labile hypertensive, need ambulatory BP recording before labelling them hypertensive patients.

Q.   **What is systolic hypertension?**

Ans: Isolated rise in systolic BP ≥ 160 mmHg with diastolic remaining <90 mmHg is called *systolic hypertension*. Old age, high output states and atherosclerosis are common causes of systolic hypertension.

Q.   **Define accelerated and malignant hypertension.**

Ans: *Accelerated hypertension* means a significant recent rise over previous hypertension levels associated with vascular damage on fundus examination (hemorrhage and exudate) without papilledema. The BP may range between 160 and 200 mmHg systolic and 100 and 120 mmHg diastolic. It is a hypertensive urgency. *Malignant hypertension* is defined as sustained high BP above 200/130 mmHg associated with vasculopathy and papilledema. It is a hypertensive emergency.

N.B Presence of papilledema in a patient with high BP indicates malignant rather than accelerated hypertension

Q. **What is hypertensive urgency and what is hypertensive emergency?**

Ans: • According to JNC VII report, the *hypertensive urgency* is a state of severely elevated BP (>200/120 mmHg) which is not associated with any organ dysfunction wherein BP can be controlled within hours with oral drug therapy given on an outpatient basis.

Hypertensive emergency means severely elevated BP (>200/130 mmHg) with symptoms and signs of organ dysfunction (encephalopathy, nephropathy, retinopathy) requiring parenteral drug therapy, close observation in ICU and immediate reduction of BP within hours.

Q. **Name few hypertensive emergency and hypertensive urgency conditions?**

Ans:

Hypertensive emergency	Hypertensive urgency
• Malignant hypertension or hypertensive encephalopathy	• Accelerated hypertension
• Acute aortic dissection	• Hypertension with coronary artery disease
• Pheochromocytoma-crisis	• Uncontrolled hypertension
• MAO inhibitors with tyramine interaction	• Hypertension in patients with kidney transplantation
• Intracranial bleed	• Pre-eclampsia

Q. **Name the organs involved in hypertension? What are the risks or complications of hypertension?**

Ans: Heart, kidney, brain and eyes are the common organs involved. The major risks of hypertension are its devastating complications such as myocardial infarction, aortic dissection, stroke, heart failure and renal failure.

Q. **How would you investigate a case with hypertension?**

Ans: The investigations done in hypertension are divided into two groups:

I. Basic (done in all the patients)
- Urine for protein, blood and glucose
- ECG for LVH and ischemia
- Hematocrit
- Blood glucose
- Blood urea, creatinine and electrolytes
- Chest X-ray for cardiomegaly or heart failure
- Lipidogram for any hyperlipidemia

II. Special investigations to screen for the cause
- *Renal ultrasound or IVP (intravenous pyelogram)* for kidney disease, e.g. polycystic kidneys, if suspected
- *Digital substraction angiography* for renal artery stenosis, if suspected
- *24 hour urine catecholamine* or *VMA* at least 3 samples for pheochromocytoma, if suspected
- *Urinary cortisol* and *dexamethasone suppression test* for Cushing syndrome, if suspected
- *Plasma renin activity* and *aldosterone levels* for Conn's syndrome if suspected
- *Angiography/MRI* for coarctation of aorta, if suspected

Q. **What should be optimal target BP?**

Ans: The optimal target BP to be achieved is <140/90 mmHg in all cases and <130/80 mmHg in patients with diabetes and kidney disease (UKPDS, HOT studies).

Q. **What do you understand by the term resistant hypertension? What are its causes?**

Ans: According to JNC VII, resistant hypertension is defined as failure to achieve BP control in patients who adhere to full doses of appropriate three drug regimen (including a diuretic). The causes are:
  i. Improper BP measurement
  ii. Excess sodium intake
  iii. Inadequate diuretic therapy (volume overload)
  iv. Excess alcohol intake
  v. Drug-induced, e.g. inadequate doses, non-compliance, over the counter use of drugs (self-medication with NSAIDs)
  vi. Unnecessary or concomitant use of other drugs, e.g. illicit drugs, sympathomimetics, oral contraceptives
  vii. Identifiable causes of hypertension (read the causes)

Q. **What lifestyle modifications would you advise to hypertensive?**

Ans: Lifestyle modifications are advised to all

prehypertensive and hypertensive patients. They include:

- **Diet:** Weight reduction in obese patients (BMI < 25 kg/m^2). Low fat diet for hyperlipidemics called DASH eating plan
- Regular physical exercise predominantly dynamic (brisk walking) rather than isometric (weight lifting)
- Limit alcohol consumption (< 14 units/week for women and < 21 units/week for men)
- Avoid smoking

Q. **What are British hypertensive society guidelines for initiating treatment for hypertension?**

Ans: The indications for starting drug treatment are:

- Sustained SBP over ≥160 mmHg or sustained diastolic BP ≥100 mmHg.
- Mild hypertension (SBP between 140 and 159 mmHg and diastolic BP between 90 and 99 mmHg) in presence of target organ damage, i.e. cardiovascular disease, stroke, diabetes.

Q. **What are first line agents for hypertension?**

Ans: A diuretic, thiazide or a calcium channel blocker or an angiotensin receptor blocker (ARBs), e.g. losarten, terlisartan, etc. are the drugs to start with.

Q. **What are the indications for specific class of antihypertensive?**

Ans: The class of drugs and their indications are given below:

Class of drug	Indication
1. Alpha blocker	1. Benign prostatic hypertrophy with HT
2. Angiotensin converting enzyme inhibitor, Angiotensin Receptor Blockers (ARBs)	2. Heart failure, LV dysfunction due to CAD, diabetic nephropathy and hypertension with LVF
3. Betablockers	3. MI, angina, heart failure in a patient with HT
4. Calcium channel blockers	4. Elderly hypertensive, heart failure, systolic hypertension
5. Central acting (methyldopa)	5. Pregnancy with HT

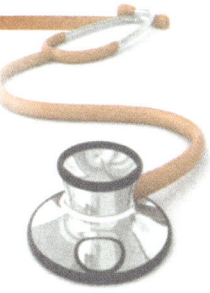

46

Irregular Pulse and Heart

INSTRUCTION

Examine the cardiovascular system

SALIENT FEATURES

- Irregular heart beats

HISTORY

Ask for the following:

- Palpitation, dizziness, syncope, sweating
- Dyspnea, fatigue
- History of pain chest (ischemic heart disease), headache, cough and expectoration
- Past history of sore throat, joint pain, arthralgia (acute rheumatic fever)
- History of consumption of drugs (digitalis, bronchodilators)
- History of excessive intake of tea, coffee
- History of weakness of limb/limbs
- History of thyroid disease

EXAMINATION

General Physical Examination

- *Patient* may be distressed
- *Pulse* is irregularly irregular. Pulse deficit is 14/min (in this patient)
- *Blood pressure* for hypertension
- *Face*, i.e. puffiness, malar flush
- *Eyes*, i.e. exophthalmos
- *Neck* for raised JVP, absent 'a' waves, thyroid enlargement (goitre)
- *Hands*, i.e. cold/warm and sweaty, acropachy, clubbing, tremors
- *Feet*, e.g. edema

CVS Examination

- Count the heart rate and pulse rate
- Now ask the patient to exercise, count the heart rate and calculate the pulse deficit
  There is no effect of exercise on HR, indicate irregularity due to atrial fibrillation not due to multiple VPCs
- Examine the heart on inspection, palpation, percussion and auscultation for any
  - i. Congenital heart disease
  - ii. Valvular lesion (mitral, aortic)
  - iii. Ischemic heart disease/cardiomyopathy
  - iv. Pericarditis/pericardial disease
  - v. Check all the signs of thyrotoxicosis
- Examine the patient for signs of thyrotoxicosis

PROVISIONAL DIAGNOSIS

The patient has atrial fibrillation (lesion) cause of which has to be found out. The patient is distressed due to irregularly irregular heart beats (functional status).

QUESTIONS AND ANSWERS

Q. How would you confirm your diagnosis?

Ans: ECG (Fig. 46.1) is the gold standard for diagnosis.

Q. How would you differentiate AF from multiple VPCs clinically?

Ans: If patient is not in heart failure, exercise the patient, VPCs after exercise tend to diminish in frequency while there is no effect on AF. The pulse deficit in AF is usually more than 10 but less in multiple VPCs.

Q. What are premalignant VPCs?

Ans: A premalignant VPC (VPCs) can provoke VT. These are:
1. VPC with R on T phenomenon
2. Ventricular couplet
3. Polymorphic VPCs or bidirectional VPCs

Q. What are the common causes of AF?

Ans: 1. Mitral valve disease (MS, MR) is the commonest cause in young and middle aged persons

2. Hypertension and ischemic heart disease (IHD) in elderly person
3. Hyperthyroidism (thyrotoxicosis) in old age
4. Congenital heart disease in young
5. Constrictive pericarditis
6. Cardiomyopathies, myocarditis
7. Pulmonary disease, e.g. COPD, pulmonary embolism
8. Cardiac tumor, cardiac surgery (uncommon)

Q. Name the congenital heart disease producing AF.
Ans: 1. Atrial septal defect
2. Ebstein anomaly

Q. Name few causes of irregular pulse.
Ans: 1. Atrial fibrillation
2. Multiple VPCs
3. Atrial flutter with changing blocks (2:1, 3:1)
4. Changing AV blocks

Q. Name a regularly irregular rhythm.
Ans: Bigeminus/Trigeminus/Quadrigeminus rhythm.

Q. How would you investigate this case?
Ans: I. The electrocardiogram is diagnostic (Fig. 46.1). The changes on ECG will be:
1. Irregular R–R intervals
2. Absent P waves. Instead of P waves, there are fibrillatory 'f' waves
3. There is undulation of baseline
4. Atrial rate is >300/min. Ventricular rate is variable
5. QRS complexes are narrow
II. *Echocardiogram* (transthoracic and transesophageal) is useful to determine the

atrial dimensions and left ventricular functions. It also helps to find out the underlying cause (valvular diseases, intracardiac thrombus, ischemic heart disease).
III. *Exercise test* to determine whether AF is precipitated by exercise.
IV. *Holter monitoring* to diagnose paroxysmal AF or any other atrial arrhythmia.
V. *Thyroid function tests* (T_3, T_4, TSH).

Q. Can heart rate be regular in AF?
Ans: Yes. Heart rate becomes regular in AF in presence of complete heart block. The undulation (wavy baseline) indicates presence of AF (Fig. 46.2)

Q. How would you broadly classify AF clinically?
Ans: 1. *Recent onset or first detected, first diagnosed AF*. It is an incidental finding on ECG.
2. *Recurrent AF* due to paroxysmal AF or persistent AF for few days (>7 days)
3. *Permanent AF* (cardioversion has failed and restoration of normal sinus rhythm is not possible)
4. *Secondary AF* due to other diseases, i.e. AMI, hyperthyroidism, cardiac surgery, pericarditis, myocarditis, pneumonia, pulmonary embolism, etc.
5. *Lone AF*. It occurs in the absence of any cardiac, pulmonary or thyroid disease before the age of 60 yrs

Q. How would you treat AF?
Ans: The aims of treatment are:
1. *The 4 C approach:*
   • **Control** of ventricular rate
   • **CHADS$_2$** score for anticoagulants
   • **Cause** to be found out
   • **Correct** the rhythm where possible (cardioversion or AF ablation)
II. *To slow the ventricular rate by:*
   a. *Drugs:* Beta-blockers or calcium channel blockers are used to slow the

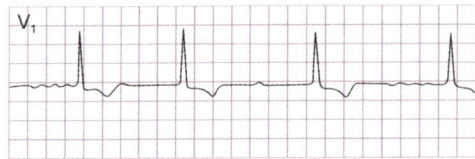

Fig. 46.1: Atrial fibrillation with slow ventricular response induced by digitalis. The electrocardiogram recorded after digitalis reveals:

Lead V_1 shows irregularly irregular heart rate of 62/min (digitalis effect). The digitalis increases the block to fibrillatory waves at AV node, but does not revert it. Therefore, the slower ventricular response in atrial fibrillation could be due to digitalis or high vagal tone (slow atrial fibrillation). At slow ventricular rate, the fibrillatory waves are nicely seen

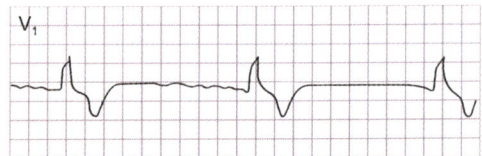

Fig. 46.2: Atrial fibrillation with complete AV block. There is undulation of baseline due to fibrillatory waves. The heart rate is 30/min. The R – R intervals instead of being variable have become constant due to block

ventricular rate in thyrotoxicosis, ischemic heart disease, hypertrophic cardiomyopathy, hypertension.

  b. *Radiofrequency ablation*: It is indicated when AF is either resistent to drug treatment or AF is paroxysmal and recurrent.

III. *Restoration of sinus rhythm*
  • By drugs, e.g. propafenone, flecainide, amiodarone, dofetilide and butilide, etc.
  • By cardioversion

IV. *Warfarin anticoagulation*: It is given if patient has mitral valve disease, or undergoing cardioversion, or is in LVF and old patients.

Q. **What is CHADS$_2$ score?**

Ans: Annual risk of stroke in patients with AF is stratified by a score called CHADS score. It has following components:

C	Congestive heart failure (recent onset)
H	Hypertension
A	Age ≥ 75 yrs
D	Dialysis
S	History of stroke or TIA

One mark is allotted to each first 4 components and two marks are given for previous stroke or TIA. Patents with mitral valve disease should be managed with adjusted dose of warfarin to achieve an international normalised ratio (INR) of 2 or 3.

For patients with CHADS score I, anticoagulation with either aspirin or warfarin is reasonable.

Q. **What is holiday heart syndrome?**

Ans: It is defined as recurrence of a supraventricular arrhythmia (AF and/or atrial flutter) following an alcoholic binge in chronic alcoholics. It is transient.

Q. **Name new antiarrhythmics for AF.**

Ans: 1. Vernakalant a new atrial selective agent effective for rapid cardioversion of recent onset AF
  2. Dronedarone—a derivative of amiodarone

Q. **What is the role of surgery in treatment of AF?**

Ans: Two procedures used for prevention of AF are:
  1. *The Maze procedure*. It involves multiple incisions in the atria to prevent re-entrant loops.
  2. The 'corridor' procedure effectively isolates both the left and right atrium leaving a strip of myocardium connecting the sinus node to AV node. This procedure does not prevent AF but isolates the atria.

Q. **What are the mechanisms of atrial fibrillation?**

Ans: 1. Ectopic atrial fibrillation produced by rapid discharge by an atrial ectopic focus
  2. Re-entry in the atrium (Fig. 46.3)

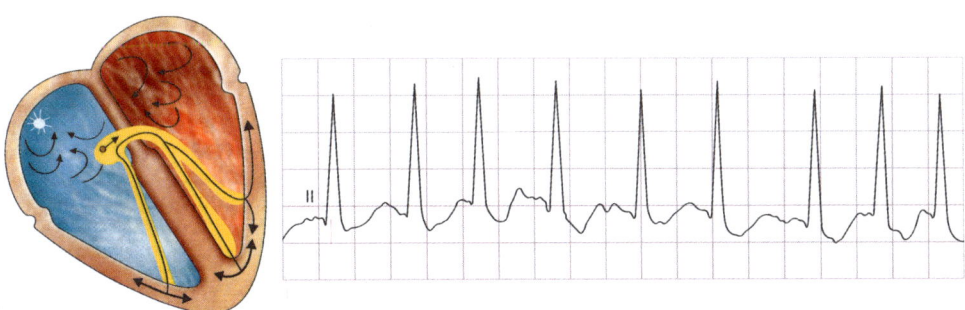

Fig. 46.3: Atrial fibrillation due to re-entry mechanism in atrium

47 Jugular Venous Pulse and Jugular Venous Pressure (JVP)

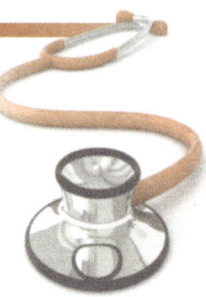

INSTRUCTION

- Perform general physical examination and relevant cardiovascular system examination

SALIENT FEATURES

- Distended neck veins

HISTORY

Ask for the following:

- Puffiness of face and edema feet
- Shortness of breath
- Pain abdomen (tender hepatomegaly) and distension of abdomen (ascites)

EXAMINATION

General Physical Examination

- Look at the neck veins at 45° inclination
  - I. *Measurement of JVP* (Read also the clinical methods in medicine by Prof SN Chugh)

    The steps for assessing the jugular venous pulse are as follows:
    1. Make the patient comfortable with the head resting on a pillow to relax the sternomastoid muscles.
    2. Raise the head of the patient to 45° in supine position (Fig. 47.1B) by putting the pillows behind the head or by raising the headend of the bed or examining table.
    3. Turn the patients's head slightly away from the side you are inspecting. Use good light for examination.
    4. Look at the neck veins from the side of the patient (Fig. 47.1 A).
    5. Identify the internal jugular pulsations especially on the right side. Focus on the pulsations and note the highest point of pulsations, if necessary, by means of abdominojugular reflux.
    6. Measure the JVP (Fig. 47.1C) by vertical distance in centimeter between the top of

venous pulsations and the sternal angle. This distance measured in centimeters above the sternal angle is the JVP.
7. Now readjust of the position of the patient, if necessary, to make the waveforms clearly visible.
8. Now identify the pattern of waveforms of venous pulsations and note any abnormality.

II. Comment on the various waveforms on jugular venous pulse (Fig. 47.2).

Waveforms. Identification of the jugular venous pulse waveforms requires experience. It has two positive waves; '*a*' wave and '*v*' wave, and two descents '*x*' and '*y*'. There is a third positive wave called '*c*' wave is not visible.

The '*a*' wave or first positive wave occurs due to right atrial contractions just before the first heart sound.

- The '*a*' wave becomes prominent in pulmonary hypertension, pulmonary stenosis, and tricuspid stenosis. Giant '*a*' wave (*cannon wave*) occurs due to forceful atrial contractions against closed tricuspid valve, is seen in complete heart block, supraventricular (junctional) tachycardia and ventricular tachycardia.
- The '*a*' wave is absent in atrial fibrillation.

The '*c*' wave, often not observed in the JVP is a positive wave produced by bulging of the tricuspid valve into the right atrium as right ventricular pressure rises.

The '*v*' wave is the third positive wave produced by the increasing volume of blood into the right atrium during ventricular systole when the tricuspid valve is closed. Tricuspid regurgitation causes the *v* wave to be more prominent (Fig. 47.2B) while tricuspid stenosis diminishes it.

The '*x*' descent is the first negative wave that follows '*a*' wave (*c* is not visible). This is

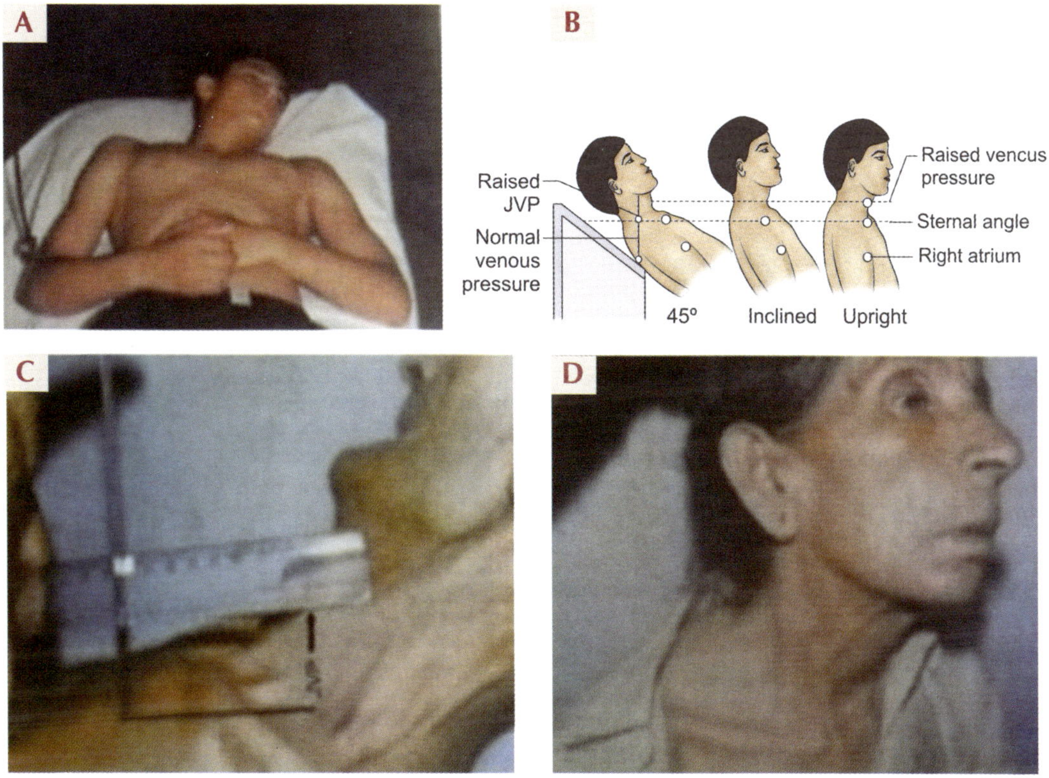

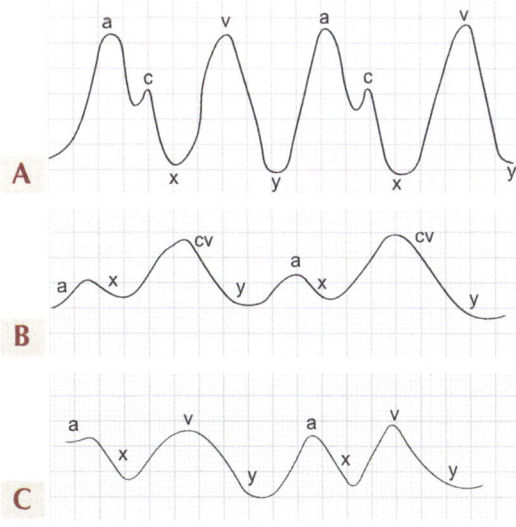

Fig. 47.1: JVP: (A) Inspection of distended neck veins; (B) Read JVP at inclination of 45° angle; (C) Measurement of raised JVP; (D) JVP beyond measurement, i.e. JVP raised beyond the angle of mandible

Fig. 47.2: Various waveforms on jugular venous pulse in different conditions. (A) Normal jugular venous pulse; (B) Jugular venous pulse in tricuspid regurgitation; (C) Jugular venous pulse (Y descent) in constrictive pericarditis

produced by atrial relaxation. It is accentuated in constrictive pericarditis, but is diminished in right ventricular dilatation and obliterated in tricuspid regurgitation.

The combination of a prominent 'v' wave and obliteration of 'x' descent results in a single large positive systolic wave, characteristically seen in tricuspid regurgitation.

The 'y' descent is the second negative wave (trough), produced by the opening of the tricuspid valve and the subsequent rapid inflow of the blood into the right ventricle.

- A sharp 'y' descent is seen in patients with constrictive pericarditis (Fig. 47.2C), or with right-sided heart failure.
- A slow 'y' descent indicates obstruction to the right ventricular filling, is seen in patients with tricuspid stenosis or right atrial myxoma.

The absent venous pulsations with prominent dilated neck veins and raised JVP are characteristically seen in *superior mediastinal compression or superior vena cava obstruction*.

III. Check the hepatojugular reflux.

Quick CVS Examination

- Cardiovascular system for the cause of congestive heart failure. Auscultate for heart sounds and murmurs.

Other System Examination

- *Respiratory system* for basal crackles and wheezes.
- *Abdominal examination* for tender hepatomegaly and ascites.

PROVISIONAL DIAGNOSIS

The patient has raised jugular venous pressure with prominent 'v' waves (lesion) caused by functional tricuspid regurgitation and patient is in congestive, heart failure (functional status).

QUESTIONS AND ANSWERS

Q. What are the causes of raised JVP?
Ans: The causes are:
- Right sided heart failure or congestive cardiac failure due to any cause
- Cor pulmonale
- Fluid overload (chronic renal failure)
- Constrictive pericarditis/pericardial effusion
- Tricuspid stenosis
- Superior vena cava obstruction (JVP is raised but pulsations may be absent)
- High output states, cirrhosis liver

Q. What is the effect of respiration on JVP? What is Kussmaul's sign?
Ans: Normally, the JVP decreases during inspiration, the paradoxical rise of JVP during inspiration (opposite to normal decrease) is called *Kussmaul's sign*, is most often caused by constrictive pericarditis, severe right-sided failure or right ventricular infarction.

Note. In patients with chronic obstructive lung disease (COPD), venous pressure may be elevated on expiration only. The veins collapse on inspiration (sucking effect). This finding does not indicate congestive heart failure.

Q. What is abdominojugular reflux test/maneuver?
Ans: In patients suspected of having right ventricular failure *(incipient failure)* who have a normal JVP at rest, the abdominojugular reflux test may be helpful. It is performed by applying firm pressure with the palm of the hand over the abdomen for 10 seconds or more. In normal persons, this maneuver does not alter JVP significantly but, when incipient or compensated right heart failure is present, the upper level of the pulsations usually increases, hence, positive test.

Q. How would you differentiate jugular venous pulsations from carotid artery pulsations?
Ans: Read clinical methods in medicine by Prof. SN Chugh. However, the difference are:

Jugular venous pulse	Carotid artery pulse
1. Better seen than felt	1. Better felt than seen
2. It has definite upper level which falls during inspiration	2. There is no definite upper level, no relation of pulse with inspiration
3. Jugular venous pulse has prominent 'x' descent which is an inward motion	3. Arterial pulse has just outward thrust/motion
4. It does not coincide with the apex beat	4. The pulse coincides with the apex beat which can be appreciated by simultaneously feeling the carotid pulse and apex beat

Palpitations (Supraventricular Tachycardia)

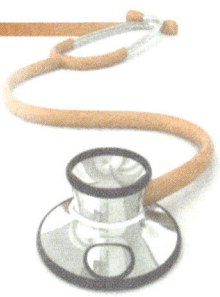

INSTRUCTION

- Examine the cardiovascular system

SALIENT FEATURES

- Palpitations, episodic

HISTORY

Ask about the following:

1. Ask about history of missed beats/sudden thumps
2. Age, onset and progression, supraventricular tachycardia is paroxysmal if due to bypass tract, occurs in young age while supraventricular tachycardias (AF, atrial tachycardia) occur in middle and old age. They are due to structural heart disease.
3. Ask about the frequency of episodes
4. Ask whether palpitations are regular or irregular
5. Does palpitation occur at rest or at work. Palpitations during work indicate structural heart disease.
6. Do the palpitations start on just going to sleep or on termination of exercise. These indicate AF
7. What is the duration of each episode?
8. Is there any accompanying pounding sensation in the neck. AVRT produces visibles neck pulsations
9. Is each episode is followed by polyuria? (SVT is followed by polyuria)
10. Is there any relation to exercise? (Polymorphic VT in long QT syndrome follows exercise)
11. What happens to palpitation on standing (AVNRT increases on standing)
12. Are there any provoking factors, i.e. tea, coffee, alcohol or drug (thyroid replacement, sympathomimetics, bronchodilators, etc.)
13. Are there any associated symptoms of chest pain, cough, expectoration, dyspnea, hemoptysis, sweating
14. Is there any associated syncope (syncope occurs during VT)
15. Are the palpitations provoked by anxiety or panic attacks (cardiac arrhythmias are provoked by panic attacks)
16. Is there any family history? Arrhythmias are common in familial cardiomyopathies

EXAMINATION

General Physical Examination

- Examine the pulse (radial and carotid) for rate and regularity. There is regular tachycardia at a rate of 183 bpm (in this patient)
- Look at JVP. Cannon waves are seen in junctional tachycardia and AV dissociation. Raised JVP indicates CHF. Absent '*a*' waves indicate AF.
- Look for signs of AF
- Look for signs of congestive heart failure (Left as well as right)
- Auscultate the heart for murmurs (MVP, valvular disease or MR/TR in dilated cardiomyopathy)

PROVISIONAL DIAGNOSIS

The patient has fast heart rate, i.e. tachycardia (lesion) accompanied by polyuria, indicating a supraventricular tachycardia (etiology). He/she is in distress due to palpitations (functional status).

QUESTIONS AND ANSWERS

Q. **Would you like to see an ECG?**

Ans: Yes. The ECG will confirm the diagnosis (Fig. 48.1). It will decide whether tachycardia is narrow complex or wide QRS complex tachycardia.

Q. **What would you see on ECG?**

Ans: • The presence of Q wave of old myocardial infarction will prompt the diagnosis of VT.

- An atrial ectopic may initiate the run of atrial tachycardia.
- The multiple origins of P waves (different shapes of P waves) and irregular R–R intervals indicates multifocal atrial tachycardia (MAT). Irregular R–R intervals with no visible P waves or presence of fibrillatory waves indicate AF. Large 'F' waves (flutter waves) with fixed AV block indicate atrial flutter.
- A short P–R interval, a delta wave on ECG before the episode (if previous ECG is available) suggest ventricular pre-excitation (WPW syndrome).
- Marked LVH with prominent Q waves in leads I, aVL and V_4–V_6 (septal hypertrophy) indicate hypertrophic cardiomyopathy (HOCM).
- Prolonged QT is harbinger of Torsade de pointes or polymorphic VT.
- Multiple VPCs indicate ventricular origin of tachycardia (VT).
- Brugada syndrome is precursor of tachycardia.
- Bradycardia and complete heart block.

Q. What is palpitation. What are its causes?

Ans: Consciousness of an apex beat is called *palpitation.* Usually it occurs due to tachyarrhythmias, but can occur with normal heart rate or slow heart rate.

Causes are:
- Extrasystoles (atrial, ventricular)
- Tachycardia/bradycardia
- Drugs (digoxin, bronchodilators, sympathomimetic, etc.)
- Sympathetic overactivity, e.g. anxiety, catecholamines—induced (pheochromocytomas), thyrotoxicosis/postural hypotension, exercise, hypoglycemia, fever, anemia
- Cardiac neurosis

Q. How would you investigate such a patient?

Ans: 1. *Blood test.* Hemoglobin, thyroid function, electrolytes (if patient on diuretic).
2. *12-lead ECG* for an evidence of abnormal rhythm. There is narrow QRS complex tachycardia (Fig. 48.1).
3. *Echocardiography* for any structure heart disease.
4. *Holter monitoring* to record the episodes of palpitations occurring during the day. Whether these episodes are associated with rhythm disturbance.
5. *Exercise ECG* in those patients whose palpitations are provoked by exercise. It will help to record arrhythmia induced by exercise.
6. *Loop (Event) monitors* have the highest yield for diagnosing arrhythmia.
7. *Electrophysiological studies* for anomalous tract when reciprocal tachycardia is suspected.

Q. What is drug of choice for AVNRT or supraventricular tachycardia?

Ans: Adenosine I.V. (6 mg stat) to be repeated if no response occurs).

Q. What are the causes of narrow QRS complex tachycardia?

Ans: 1. Atrial tachycardia
2. Nodal (AV nodal) tachycardia (AVNRT)
3. Multifocal atrial tachycardia
4. Atrial fibrillation
5. Atrial flutter

Q. What are the causes of wide QRS complex tachycardia?

Ans: 1. Ventricular tachycardia
2. Bundle branch tachycardia
3. Reciprocal tachycardia (WPW syndrome)
4. Supraventricular tachycardia with aberration
5. Idioventricular tachycardia
6. Ventricular flutter/fibrillation

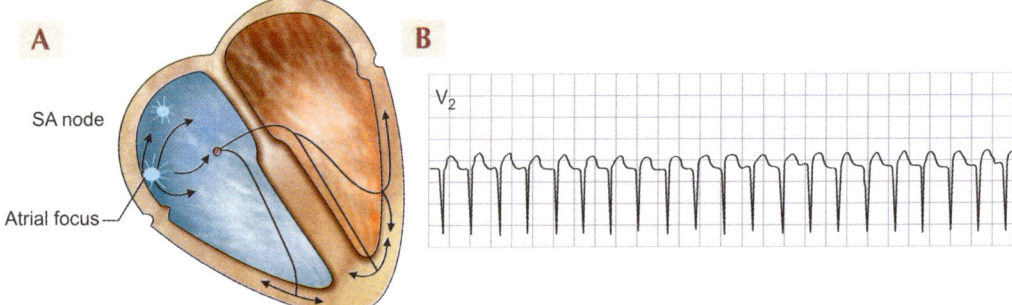

Fig. 48.1: Paroxysmal supraventricular tachycardia. (A) Diagram showing supraventricular focus of discharge; (B) Lead V_2 shows narrow QRS complex tachycardia

Q. What is the treatment of paroxysmal supra-ventricular tachycardia?

Ans: 1. The tachycardia is terminated by adeno-sine I.V or vagal maneuver [carotid mass-age (Fig. 48.2)].

2. For long-term management, β-blockers, verapamil or diltiazem can be used as maintenance therapy.

Alternatively, drugs used are flecainide, propafenone or sotalol.

3. DC cardioversion is indicated in patients with cardiovascular compromise.

Q. What is Brugada syndrome?

Ans: It is recognised entity as a cause of sudden cardiac death, characterized by a pattern of J-point ST elevation > 2 mm in leads $V_1 - V_2$. The heart is structurally and functionally normal. This is considered to be due to identifiable mutations in the sodium channel gene (30 – 40%). It classically presents in males (between 30 and 40 yrs of age) with symptoms of syncope and VF leading to cardiac arrest. No medical therapy is effective. ICD implant-ation provides the hope for survival.

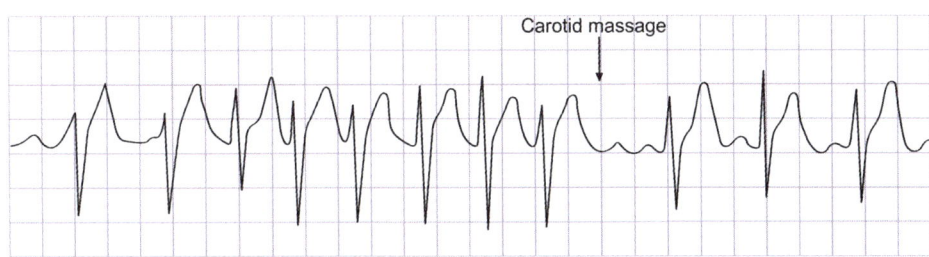

Fig. 48.2: Paroxysmal AV nodal extrasystolic tachycardia. The ECG lead shows first beat as sinus conducted beat followed by a run of paroxysmal AV nodal tachycardia (P waves are merged within QRS complexes). Carotid massage (↓) reverted the tachycardia

INSTRUCTION

- Examine the cardiovascular system of the patient

SALIENT FEATURES

- Pacemaker implanted

HISTORY

Ask for the following:

- History of slow heart beats.
- Past history of syncope (*Stokes-Adam attacks*) and heart block.
- Ask for the history of diseases which produce heart blocks, e.g. rheumatic valvular diseases, congenital heart blocks, ischemic heart disease, hypertensive heart disease.
- History of dropped beats and precordial thumps.
- Past history of conduction disturbance.

EXAMINATION

General Physical Examination

- Dropped beats or irregular heart beats (VPCs)
- Look for infraclavicular scar indicating pacemaker insertion (present)
- Palpate the infraclavicular area gently to confirm the presence of a pacemaker (present)

CVS Examination

- Record the heart beats which have pre-fixed rate around 60/min.
- Auscultate the heart for sounds which are louder. Heart rate is between 60 and 70/min regular.

PROVISIONAL DIAGNOSIS

The patient has pacemaker implantation (lesion) for complete heart block (etiology) which is functioning normally.

QUESTIONS AND ANSWERS

Q. What are the indications of permanent pacemakers?

Ans: The indications are:

Class I

- Sinus node disease/dysfunction characterized by sinus pauses, SA blocks producing syncope.
- Third degree or second degree AV blocks producing Stokes-Adam attacks.
- Persistent AF and asymptomatic pauses ≥5 second.
- VT with long QT syndrome.
- Recurrent syncope due to carotid sinus stimulation (hypersensitivity).

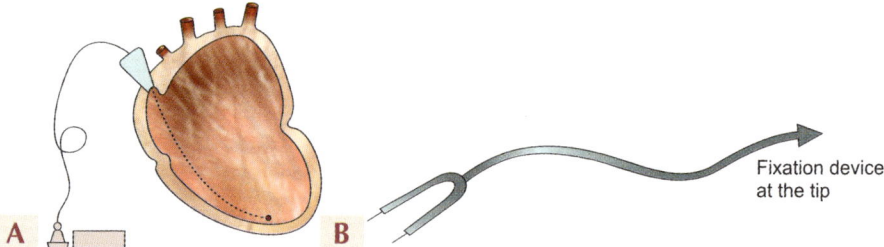

Fig. 49.1: Endocardial and epicardial pacing. (A) Endocardial permanent pacing: The generator set is implanted into subcutaneous space. The catheter is threaded into the right ventricle; (B) Permanent pacing catheter

Class II Indications
- Symptomatic sinus node disease or unexplained syncope
- Chronic bifascicular blocks
- Heart blocks producing pacemaker syndrome
- High risk patients with long QT syndrome
- Hypertrophic cardiomyopathy

Q.   What do you mean by permanent pacemaker?

Ans: Permanent pacemaker is connected to the heart by one or two electrodes and are powered by long-lasting (5–10 yrs) solid-state lithium batteries. Most of the pacemakers are designated to pace and sense the ventricles called VVI pacemakers which mean:

V : Ventricle paced

V : Ventricle sensed

I : Inhibited by ventricle signal

The pacemakers are inserted under local anesthesia and fluoroscopic guidance, subcutaneously under the pectoral muscles.

Q.   How would you decide pacing mode/modality?

Ans: The vast majority of patients should have an atrial-based pacing (i.e. either AAI or DDD). Ventricular-only pacing leads to greater incidence of AF and potential pacemakers syndrome (Fig. 49.2).

Q.   What are other uses of cardiac pacing?

Ans: 1. Dual chamber pacing has been used to optimize cardiac output and minimize outflow gradient in patients with cardiomyopathy.

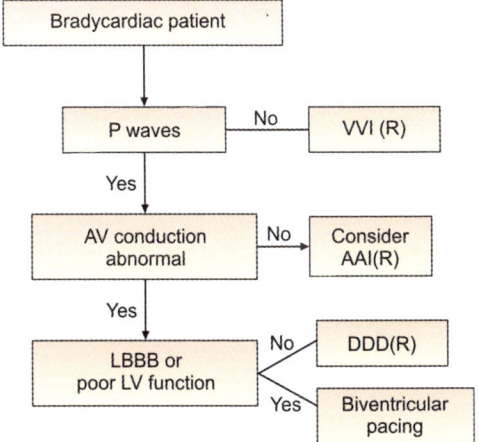

Fig. 49.2: Decision regarding pacing modality

2. Dual chamber pacing is being used in dilated cardiomyopathy with heart failure with intraventricular conduction delay to optimize atrioventricular delay and improve cardiac output-cardiac synchronization therapy.
3. Dual chamber atrial pacing can be used to prevent AF.

Q.   What are the complications of pacemaker?

Ans: I. *Complication at the time of implantation*
- Hematoma at the site
- Skin erosion and infection
- Pneumothorax or effusion
- Air embolism
- Axillary vein thrombosis

II. *Late complications*
- Lead displacement
- Lead erosion
- Lead damage/failure
- Device failure, electromagnetic interference
- Infection

III. *Others*
- Pacemaker syndrome
- Endless loop tachycardia

Q.   What are the potential sources of electromagnetic interference?

Ans: The potential sources of interference are:
1. Heavy electric motors and arc welding
2. Airport security devices and ham radios (The person should inform airport security staff that he/she has pacemaker)
3. Cellular phones and anti-theft devices or electronic article surveillance equipment. Patient is advised not to carry cellular phone in a pocket over the pacemaker.
4. MRI and lithotripsy. Patient with pacemakers should not be subjected to MRI and lithotripsy, radiotherapy, diathermy.

Q.   What is pacemaker syndrome?

Ans: It is a syndrome of low cardiac output, occurs with single chamber pacemakers (VVI) in whom sinus node function is normal. It results due to hemodynamic changes when ventricular pacing is not coupled with atrial contractions (atrial kick). This syndrome can also occur in any pacing mode where there is no ventriculo-atrial synchrony. Levels of natriuretic factor are high.

Symptoms include syncope/dizziness, light headedness, fatigue, exercise intolerance, malaise, lethargy and dyspnea.

The **treatment** is to restore atrioventricular synchrony by either reducing the pacing rate or inserting an atrial lead.

Q. What are the indications of lead removal?

Ans:
    I. *Life-threatening conditions*, e.g. septicemia, endocarditis, arrhythmias, lead migration, emboli.

    II. *Pocket infection, chronic draining sinus, lead erosion, venous thrombosis.*

    III. *Lead replacement.*

Q. Enumerate important indications of implantable cardiac defibrillator (ICD).

Ans:
1. Cardiac arrest as a result of irreversible ventricular tachyarrhythmias.
2. Spontaneous sustained VT.
3. Syncope of undetermined origin with inducible sustained VT on electrophysiological studies and when drug therapy is either not effective or not tolerated.
4. Nonsustained VT with coronary artery disease and inducible VT.

Q. What are sources of electromagnetic interference with ICDs?

Ans: MRI and lithotripsy.

Q. If a patient has an ICD device requires pacing, what would you do?

Ans: Placement of separate pacemaker in a patient with ICD is dangerous because of risk of pacemaker-defibrillator interactions. Nowadays ICDs have additional ability to terminate VT with anti-tachycardia pacing which is incorporated with ICD.

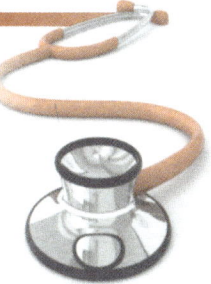

50

Gallop Rhythm

INSTRUCTION

Examine the cardiovascular system

SALIENT FEATURES

- Palpitation

HISTORY

Ask the following:

- Dyspnea, orthopnea, PND
- Palpitations, chest discomfort
- Swelling of legs

EXAMINATION

On auscultation there is tachycardia with an additional sound [third or fourth heart sound (Fig. 50.1). These sounds are audible with the bell of stethoscope as they are low pitched.

PROVISIONAL DIAGNOSIS

The patient has third heart sound with heart rate above 100/min, hence, has *gallop rhythm* (lesion) which indicates that patient has incipient cardiac failure (functional status).

QUESTIONS AND ANSWERS

Q. **What do you mean by gallop rhythm?**

Ans: When either S_3 or S_4 is associated with tachycardia, it is called gallop rhythm. Remember, just presence of S_3 or S_4 at normal heart rate does not constitute gallop rhythm.

Q. **What is summation gallop rhythm?**

Ans: When both S_3 and S_4 are present with sinus tachycardia, it is called *summation gallop rhythm*.

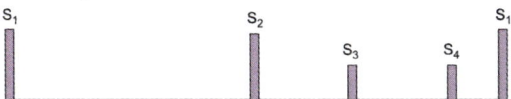

Fig. 50.1: Heart sounds

Q. **How a third heart sound is produced?**

Ans: It is produced by rapid ventricular filling during diastole.

Q. **How a fourth heart sound is produced?**

Ans: It is produced due to vigorous atrial contractions (atrial boost) during the end of diastole.

Q. **What are the causes of 3rd heart sound?**

Ans: 1. Left heart failure/left ventricular dysfunction

2. Physiological in children

3. Left ventricular dilatation without failure

4. Left to right shunts with rapid flow to left ventricle

5. Right ventricular 3rd heart sound indicates RV failure/dilatation

Q. **What are the causes of fourth heart sound?**

Ans: • Physiological in elderly

- Pathologically, it is due to:
  - AMI (acute myocardial infarction)
  - Aortic stenosis
  - Hypertension
  - Hypertrophic cardiomyopathy
  - Pulmonary stenosis

N.B The fourth heart sound indicates atrial stress only, does not denote heart failure unlike third heart sound.

Q. **How would you differentiate between a fourth heart sound and a split first heart sound and an ejection click?**

Ans: The fourth heart sound is not heard when pressure is applied on the chest piece of the stethoscope, but pressure does not obliterate the split first sound or the ejection click.

The click is better heard at the outlow tract and is high pitched sound. The fourth heart sound is low-pitched heard all over the precordium. Split first sound is high pitched heard at apex.

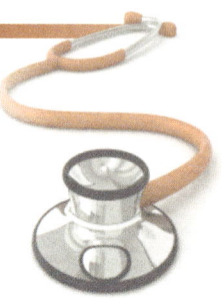

51

Slow Pulse Rate (Bradycardia)

INSTRUCTION

Examine the cardiovascular system

SALIENT FEATURES

- Slow heart beats

HISTORY

Ask the following:

- Is the patient athlete?
- Symptoms of slow pulse rate, i.e. dizziness, syncope, weakness, palpitations
- History of recent chest pain (MI)
- Is bradycardia episodic, if yes, ask its frequency, precipitating factors and other associated symptoms
- History of slowness of activity, edema of face and legs (myxedema)
- Ask history of drug intake specially beta-blockers, calcium channel blockers, digoxin, etc.
- Ask regarding nocturnal bradycardia—a feature of obstructive-sleep apnea
- Ask history of obstructive jaundice and raised intracranial tension

EXAMINATION

General Physical Examination

- Count pulse rate. It is <60/mm regular, good volume, normal in character (present).

- If rate is irregular, count the rate for full one minute and not the irregularity.
- Look at JVP for cannon '*a*' wave.
- Auscultate the heart. There is loud first heart sound called *cannon sound*.
- Look for the signs of hypothyroidism, liver disease, raised intracranial tension.

PROVISIONAL DIAGNOSIS

The patient has bradycardia (lesion) probably due to vagotonia (cause).

QUESTIONS AND ANSWERS

Q. What are the common causes of bradycardia?
Ans: I. **Physiological,** e.g. athlete, during sleep.
II. **Pathological**
- Acute inferior wall myocardial infarction
- Drugs, e.g. beta-blockers, digitalis, calcium channel blockers
- Hypothyroidism
- Obstructive jaundice
- Raised intracranial tension
- Hypothermia
- Hyperkalemia (uremia)
- Poisons—organophosphorus compound
- Hyperactive carotid sinus
- Idiopathic (ageing)

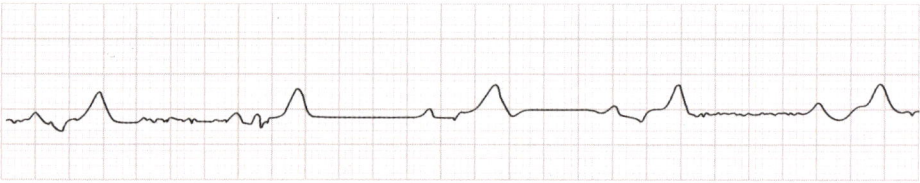

Fig. 51.1: Sinus bradycardia

Q. What is temporary cardiac pacing? What are its indications?

Ans: A temporary pacing catheter is connected to a temporary generator (Fig. 51.2) to pace the heart during following conditions:

1. Temporary pacing is done in reversible heart blocks in symptomatic patients, for example second and third degree heart blocks due to drugs, poisons and electrolyte disturbance

2. In patients with acute myocardial infarction developing second degree (mobitz 11) or complete heart block or bifascicular block

3. In symptomatic sinus bradycardia, atrial fibrillation with slow ventricular response

4. Transient sick sinus syndrome

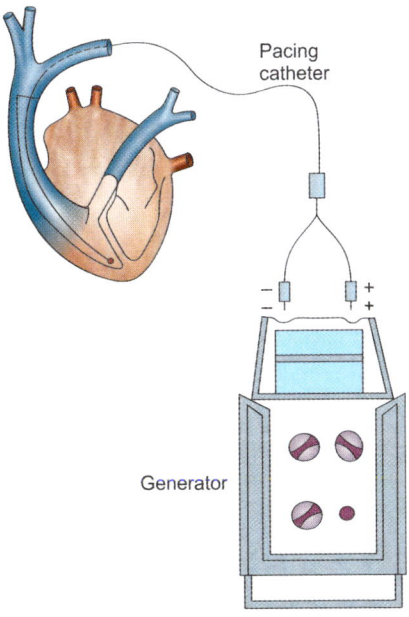

Pacing catheter

Generator

Fig. 51.2: Temporary pacing (diagram). A pacing catheter is connected to a temporary generator. A bridging cable of pacemaker extension cord (not shown) can be used between the generator and the catheter

Q. What are the indications of permanent pacing in bradyarrhythmias?

Ans:
1. Congenital heart blocks with symptoms (syncope)
2. Symptomatic sinus bradycardia
3. Symptomatic acquired second degree and complete heart block

Q. What do you understand by the term Stokes-Adams syndrome?

Ans: It is defined as attacks of syncope occurring in sitting position during complete heart blocks or during transition of change from second degree to complete heart block.

Q. What is chronotropic incompetence?

Ans: It is defined as failure to achieve a heart rate of 85% of the age-predicted maximum at peak exercise.

Q. What do you understand by the term complete heart block?

Ans: In complete AV block, there is bradycardia due to slow idioventricular rhythm. There is complete dissociation between atria and ventricles without any interference. No beat is transmitted from atria to ventricles. Atria and ventricles are driven by independent pacemakers.

Q. What are the causes of complete heart block?

Ans:
- Myocarditis, myocardial infarction (inferior wall) and cardiomyopathies
- Following cardiac surgery
- Drug-induced (digitalis, beta-blockers, amiodarone)
- Calcific aortic or mitral valve stenosis or both
- Cardiac tumors
- Idiopathic, e.g.
  - Lenegre's disease (fibrosis of conduction system)
  - Lev's disease (fibrosis of aortic or mitral valve ring)
- Connective tissue disease, e.g. SLE
- Miscellaneous conditions, e.g. amyloid heart disease, myxedema
- Following radiofrequency abalation of AV node

52

Dextrocardia

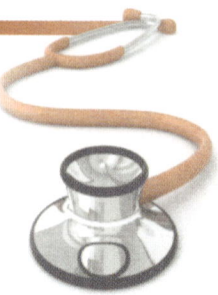

INSTRUCTION

Examine the patient's cardiovascular system

SALIENT FEATURES

- Asymptomatic

HISTORY

Ask for the following:

- Ask about the history of recurrent sinusitis (sneezing, cough) and bronchiectasis (cough with sputum production)
- History of recurrent fever
- History of infertility in married males (ciliary dysfunction of sperms)

EXAMINATION

General Physical Examination

- Elicit tenderness over the frontal sinuses and maxillary sinuses
- Look for clubbing of the fingers (bronchiectasis)
- Look at pulse and record BP

Cardiovascular System Examination

- Look at the apex beat on left side. It is absent (in this case). Now look at the apex beat on right side, it is present (in this case).
- Auscultate the heart from left side to right side. Heart sounds are better heard on the right side of the chest.
- Auscultate for murmurs and sounds for any associated cardiac abnormality.

Chest Examination

- Now ascertain the liver dullness by percussion of right fifth and sixth intercostal space. They are resonant due to presence of stomach (situs inversus) (in this case). Now percuss the same spaces on the left side, they are dull indicating liver on left side.

- Examine the lungs for crackles and wheezes (for bronchiectasis)

Other examination

- Examine the testes for size and consistency.

PROVISIONAL DIAGNOSIS

The patient has situs inversus (lesion) as a congenital anomaly (etiology). There is no other associated anomaly (functional status).

QUESTIONS AND ANSWERS

Q. What are the points in favor of situs inversus in your case?

Ans: Points in favor of situs inversus are:
1. Right-sided cardiac apex
2. Right-sided stomach
3. Right-sided descending aorta
4. The right atrium on the left (inverted P in lead I on ECG)

Q. What is situs solitus?

Ans: It is normal position of the heart.

Q. What will you want to see to confirm your diagnosis?

Ans: I. ECG (Fig. 52.1B). There will be negative P and QRS in lead I and AVL and positive in aVR. Negative QRS and T waves in all precordial leads (right ventricular complexes) will confirm the diagnosis after excluding pseudodextrocardia (misplacement of leads).

II. X-ray chest (PA view).
After checking the correct labelling of the side on X-ray, if left dome of the diaphragm is raised with gas bubble in the stomach and tip (apex) of the heart seen in right hemithorax will confirm the diagnosis.

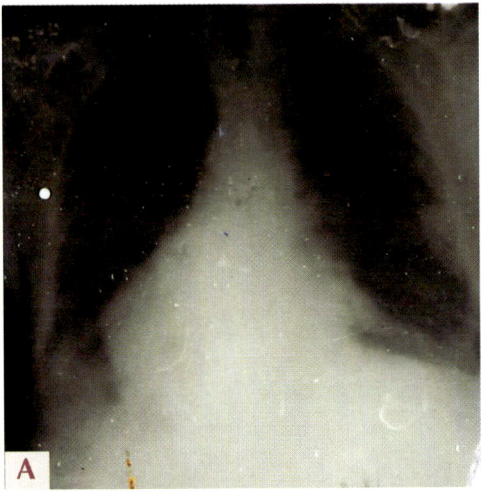
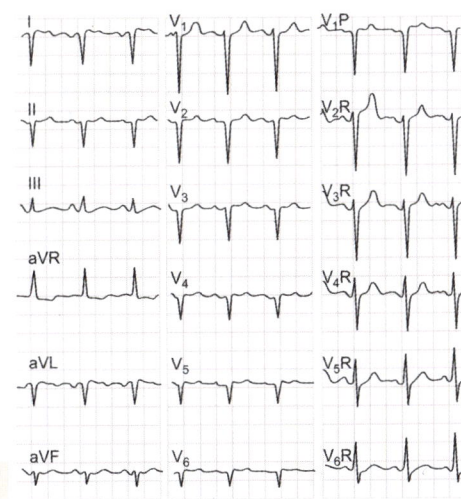

Fig. 52.1: Dextrocardia. (A) X-ray chest; (B) ECG

Q. What is technical dextrocardia (pseudo-dextrocardia)?

Ans: This occurs due to inadvertent interchange of right and left arm electrodes. This will produce dextrocardia in limb leads only (standard and unipolar leads).

The precordial leads will be normal. Therefore, in technical dextrocardia, there will be negative P waves and QRS complexes in leads I and aVL instead of aVR (AVR will record positive P–QRS–T complexes) like true dextrocardia. In technical dextrocardial, precordial leads will record normal P–QRS–T complexes which will be negative in true dextrocardia (a differentiating feature).

Q. What is Kartagener's syndrome?

Ans: The components are:
1. Dextrocardia/Situs inversus
2. Bronchiectasis
3. Sinusitis (sinus abnormality)
4. Immobile cilia syndrome (male infertility).

Q. What do you understand by the term dextroversion?

Ans: This is nothing but shift of the mediastinum to the right side, therefore, cardiac apex is on right side, otherwise there is no change in the position of heart chambers (left-sided aorta) and left side stomach.

Q. What are the causes of dextroversion?

Ans: • Removal of right lung or a part of lung
• Collapse of right lung or atelectasis of the lung

Q. What is levoversion?

Ans: It means:
1. Left sided apex
2. Right sided stomach
3. Right descending aorta

Q. What are extracardiac congenital anomalies associated with dextrocardia?

Ans: **Asplenia:** It is characterised by presence of Heinz bodies and Howell-Jolly bodies.

Polysplenia Syndrome:
It is common and consists of
• Abnormal bilobed lungs
• Abnormal gall bladder
• Bilateral symmetrical liver

Q. What are the other cardiac abnormalities associated with dextrocardia?

Ans: 1. Corrected transposition of great vessels
2. VSD
3. Pulmonary hypoplasia
4. Single ventricle
5. Single atrium
6. Endocardial cushion defect
7. Aortic abnormalities (right aortic arch/aortic atresia/obstruction)

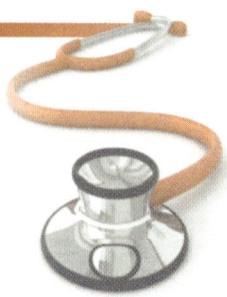

53

Patent Ductus Arteriosus (PDA)

INSTRUCTION

Examine patient's cardiovascular system

SALIENT FEATURES

- Palpitation since childhood

HISTORY

Ask about the following:

- History of dyspnea on exertion, palpitation, chest discomfort
- History of repeated chest infections, e.g. fever, cough and expectoration due to congestion of the lungs
- Maternal history of rubella
- Ask whether patient was born as premature baby or baby with low birth weight
- Ask whether patient was born at high altitude place
- History of prolonged childhood illness
- History of smoking/drug or alcohol intake by the mother

EXAMINATION

General Physical Examination

- Check the patient's height and weight
- *Pulse*: It is good volume collapsing pulse
- *BP*: Wide pulse pressure may be present
- *Neck*: Carotid pulsations are prominent. There is no thyroid enlargement
- Look for *anemia*, signs of *infective endocarditis*
- Look for *pedal edema*.
- Look for the features of Down's syndrome

Cardiovascular System Examination

- Apex beat may be normally placed or may be down and out of midclavicular line, heaving in character.
- A continuous or systolic thrill at left 2nd intercostal space (Fig. 53.1A present in this case).
- *On auscultation*, there is a continuous machinery murmur (starting from Ist heart sound and extending through the 2nd heart sound into diastole), waxing and waning in character, is heard along the left sternal edge below the clavicle (Fig. 53.1A present in this case).
- There may be reverse splitting of 2nd heart sound.

Respiratory System Examination

There may be signs of lung congestion (basal crackles)

PROVISIONAL DIAGNOSIS

The patient has symptoms and signs suggestive of PDA (lesion) which is a congenital heart disease (etiology) and patient does not have congestive heart failure (functional status).

QUESTIONS AND ANSWERS

Q. **What do you mean by a continuous murmur?**

Ans: A murmur which starts with the first heart sound, peaks at the end of systole, continues through second heart sound and also heard in diastole is called a *continuous murmur*. Therefore, it has both systolic and diastolic components.

Q. **What are the causes of a continuous murmur?**

Ans: 1. PDA (patent ductus arteriosus)
2. Rupture of the sinus of valsalva
3. Pulmonary arteriovenous fistula
4. Aortopulmonary window
5. Coronary arteriovenous fistula
6. Arteriovenous anastomosis of intercostal vessels

Note: All these conditions constitute the differential diagnosis of PDA

Q. **What murmurs can be confused with continuous murmur?**

Ans: Pansystolic murmur of MR or VSD when combined with early diastolic murmur of AR can be confused with a continuous murmur. These are two separate murmurs which are combined, therefore, there is no peaking of the murmur at the end of systole like continuous murmur. The continuous murmur has waxing and waning character which these murmurs do not have.

Q. What are the causes of a collapsing pulse?

Ans: Read clinical methods in Medicine by Prof. SN Chugh

Q. What happens to the continuous murmur when pulmonary hypertension develops?

Ans: Both systolic and diastolic components of the continuous murmur become softer and then diastolic component may disappear and only systolic murmur may be heard.

Q. What are the complications of PDA?

Ans: 1. Congestive heart failure
  2. Infective endocarditis. It occurs on the pulmonary side of ductus arteriosus
  3. Pulmonary hypertension and reversal of shunt called *Eisenmenger syndrome*
  4. Repeated lung infections due to congested lungs

5. Aneurysmal dilatation and calcification of the duct, which may lead to rupture.

Q. What other congenital heart diseases can be associated with PDA?

Ans: 1. VSD
  2. Pulmonary stenosis
  3. Coarctation of aorta

Q. How would you investigate your case?

Ans: 1. *ECG* for LVH (Fig. 53.1B) but can be normal.
  2. *Chest X-ray* will show characteristics of left to right shunt, i.e.
    • Cardiac shadow will be prominent due to left atrial and left ventricular enlargement
    • Pulmonary plethora
    • Proximal pulmonary arterial dilatation
    • Prominent ascending aorta
  3. *Echocardiography.* It will visualise the communicating duct between aorta and pulmonary artery.
  4. *Color Doppler Study* will reveal continuous flow in the pulmonary trunk.
  5. *Cardiac catheterization* is done to determine the presence and magnitude of the

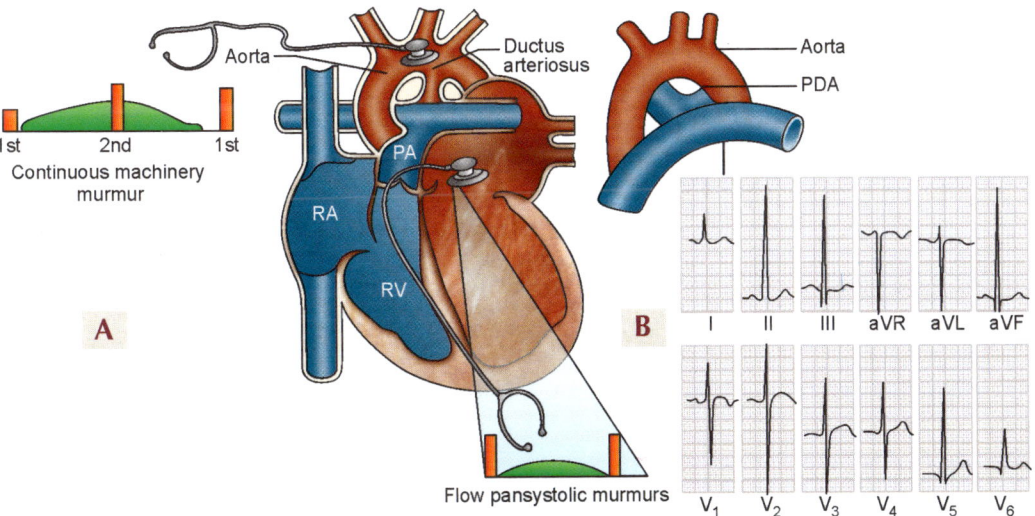

Fig. 53.1: Persistent (patent) ductus arteriosus. (A) Hemodynamic effects and auscultatory finding; (B) ECG shows:
  i. The QRS axis is normal downwards and to the left
  ii. There is horizontal heart position with deep q wave and tall R in leads II, III and aVF. The q waves in V_5–V_6 are accentuated
  iii. *Left ventricular volume overload:* It is evident from deep S wave in V_1 with tall R in V_5. RV_5 + SV_1 is > 35 mm. There are q waves in leads V_5–V_6 with upright T wave
  iv. *Evidence of biventricular hypertrophy:* There are large R and S waves in midprecordial leads (V_3–V_4) called *Katz-Watchel phenomenon* indicating biventricular hypertrophy

shunt and also to determine the pulmonary vascular resistance

6. *Cardiac MRI.*

Q. **How would you treat such patients?**

Ans: 1. Prophylaxis of infective endocarditis and treatment of congestive heart failure, if present.

2. For closure of the duct, indomethacin or ibuprofen—a prostaglandin E synthesis inhibitor may be administered within 1 – 3 weeks after birth.

3. Percutaneous closure of the duct by coils or occluders.

4. Surgical ligation or division of PDA is attempted in children or adults with large shunts.

Q. **What is the contraindication of surgery in PDA?**

Ans: The development of pulmonary arterial hypertension and reversal of shunt (Eisenmenger's syndrome) is contraindication for surgery.

Q. **In which congenital conditions, PDA presence is must?**

Ans: 1. Hypoplastic left heart syndrome

2. Critical aortic stenosis

3. Complex coarctation of aorta

54

Atrial Septal Defect (ASD)

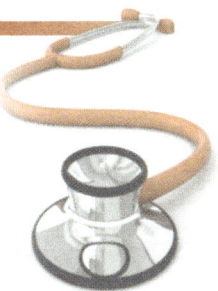

INSTRUCTION

Examine patient's cardiovascular system

SALIENT FEATURES

No symptom. Medical check up.

HISTORY

Ask about the following:

- Patient may not have symptoms
- Some patients may complain of fatigue, dyspnea
- Ask about palpitations for any arrhythmia
- Ask about fever, chest discomfort, cough and sputum especially in winters indicating recurrent lung infections
- Symptoms of pulmonary embolism (paradoxical embolisation)
- Symptoms right heart failure (tender hepatomegaly, edema feet) in large shunts
- Ask about syncope
- If the patient is child (there is possibility of ostium primum defect also), ask about symptoms of failure to thrive, delayed poor milestones development and symptoms of heart failure and infective endocarditis.

EXAMINATION

General Physical Examination

- Look for the symptoms and signs of Down's syndrome (Read Down's syndrome)
- Measure height, weight
- Record pulse, BP
- Look for any congenital deformity (congenital defects of the thumb in Holt-Oram syndrome)

Cardiovascular Examination

- Normal and diffuse apical impulse on inspection and palpation
- Left palasternal heave (present)
- Auscultatory findings are:

i. *Ejection systolic murmur* (Fig. 54.1A) in the second and third left intercostal space. This is flow murmur (present).
ii. *A mid-diastolic murmur*, soft, is heard in the tricuspid area. It is heard in large shunts due to high flow through tricuspid area (present).
iii. Wide and fixed second heart sound (present).
iv. Signs of right heart failure are usually not present.

PROVISIONAL DIAGNOSIS

The patient has atrial septal defect (ASD) (lesion) which is a congenital heart disease (etiology). She is not in congestive heart failure and there is no evidence of Eisenmenger's syndrome (functional status).

QUESTIONS AND ANSWERS

Q. What are the points in favor of your diagnosis?

Ans: 1. A young asymptomatic female
2. An ESM at pulmonary area
3. Wide and fixed S_2
4. A mid-diastolic murmur in tricuspid area

Q. What are the various types of ASD?

Ans: I. *Ostium primum defect.* It is characterised by defect in the interatrial septum with cleft mitral and tricuspid valves
II. *Ostium secundum defect* (commonest type)
III. *Sinus venosus defect*
IV. *Patent foramen ovale*

Q. What do you understand by the term patent foramen ovale?

Ans: In the fetus, an oblique valvular opening is present between right and left atria called *foramen ovale*. It persists throughout fetal

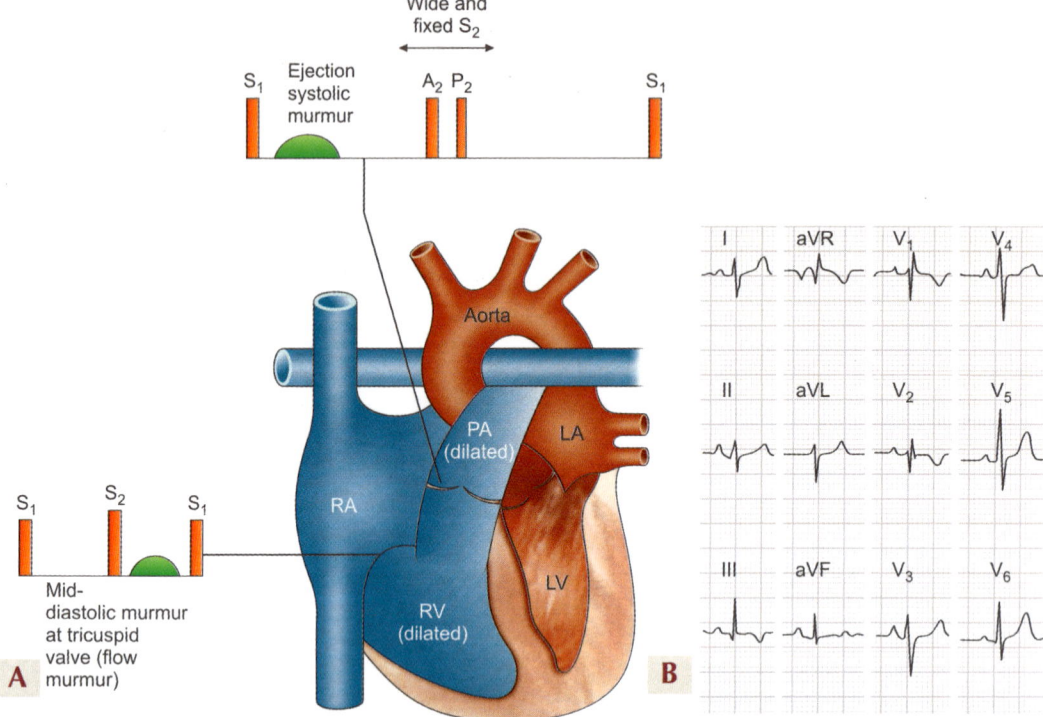

Fig. 54.1: Atrial septal defect (ostium secundum). (A) Diagram illustrating the defect and murmurs heard in ASD; (B) ECG: The electrocardiogram recorded from a 30 years old female shows P wave axis around +60°. The P wave is tall, wide and peaked in leads II and aVF and biphasic in V_1 with wide initial upright deflection. Indicating biatrial hypertrophy. There is rSR' pattern in V_1 which is not wide, indicates incomplete right bundle branch block. There is an associated ST depression and T wave inversion

life. After birth, the left atrium receives blood greater than in the right and this causes the closure of foramen ovale. If this does not close due to any reason, it is called *patent foramen ovale*.

Q. What is Holt-Oram syndrome?

Ans: It is an autosomal dominant syndrome characterised by ASD (ostium secundum defect) with a hypoplastic thumb and an accessory phalanx. This is due to mutation in chromosome $12q^2$.

Q. When does reversal of shunt occur in ASD?

Ans: It occurs either in 2nd or 3rd decade of life.

Q. What is the mechanism of fixed splitting of S_2 in ASD?

Ans: Fixed splitting means loss of effect of respiration. Normally splitting of second heart sound (S_2) widens during inspiration due to delay in closure of the pulmonary component.

In ASD, the volume of blood in right atrium is large which equalises the pressure of both atria, hence, respiration has no effect resulting in wide and fixed splitting.

Q. Enumerate the causes of widely split second heart sound?

Ans: The wide splitting of second heart sound (wide separation of aortic (A_2) and pulmonary component (P_2) of second heart sound occurs either due to delayed closure of pulmonary valve or early closure of aortic valve. The causes are:

I. *Delayed closure of pulmonary valve*
 • ASD
 • Pulmonary stenosis
 • RBBB

II. *Early closure of aortic valve (premature left ventricular emptying)*
 • Mitral regurgitation
 • VSD

Q.   What is Lutembacher syndrome?

Ans: ASD with acquired rheumatic mitral stenosis is called *Lutembacher syndrome*.

Q.   What investigations would you like to perform to confirm your diagnosis?

Ans: 1. *ECG* (Fig. 54.1B). The characteristic ECG findings in ostium secundum defect include right axis deviation with right incomplete bundle branch block.
   • In *ostium primum*, there is *left axis deviation* with *RBBB*.
   • In sinus venosus defect, there is a low atrial or junctional rhythm (Read Text book of Electrocardiography by Prof. SN Chugh)

2. *Chest X-ray* will show (i) large pulmonary conus, (ii) small aortic knuckle/knob, (iii) pulmonary plethora and (iv) enlarged RV and right atrium producing prominent cardiac shadow.

3. *Echocardiography*: Transthoracic (visualises the defect in ASD) and transesophageal and colour Doppler echocardiography help in localising the defect and also useful in identifying anomalous venous drainage and sinus venosus defect.

4. *MRI*

5. *Cardiac catheterisation*: It is usually not required for diagnosis. It can be done to measure the magnitude and direction of the shunt and to determine the severity and reversibility of pulmonary hypertension.

Q.   What do you mean by hilar dance?

Ans: It is a fluoroscopic finding seen in left to right shunt producing visible pulsations of pulmonary vessels.

Q.   Is prophylaxis for infective endocarditis recommended in ASD?

Ans: No. Infective endocarditis is unlikely in ASD (repaired/unrepaired).

Q.   Name the congenital heart disease in which pregnancy is contraindicated?

Ans: 1. Pulmonary hypertension (e.g. Eisenmenger's syndrome)

2. Heart failure

3. Congenital cyanotic heart disease with severe cyanosis (O_2 saturation < 80% at rest) and polycythemia (Hb > 18 g%)

4. Severe outflow tract obstruction, e.g. severe aortic stenosis

Q.   What do you know about endocardial cushion defects?

Ans: The endocardial cushion defects include the ostium primum defect in which there is ASD with cleft mitral or tricuspid valve resulting in mitral and tricuspid regurgitation. Commonly anterior leaflet of mitral valve is involved in ostium primum defect resulting in MR. The ECG shows left axis deviation with RBBB. The treatment is surgical closure of defect with repair of mitral valve.

Q.   What is treatment of ASD?

Ans: 1. In children with uncomplicated ASD, surgical closure is recommended between ages of 5 and 10 years to prevent right heart failure or arrhythmias.

2. Moderate ASD with left to right shunt of 1.5 : 1 or more require surgical closure to prevent RV dysfunction.

3. ASD with potentially reversible pulmonary vascular resistance demonstrated on vasodilator challenge or lung biopsy is another indication for surgical closure.

ASD is nowadays being closed by transcatheter button or clam-shell device.

Q.   What are complications of ASD?

Ans: 1. Atrial arrhythmias, e.g. atrial fibrillation (AF) and supraventricular tachycardia.

2. Pulmonary hypertension.

3. Eisemenger's syndrome with reversal of shunt.

4. Paradoxical embolisation.

5. Recurrent pneumonias especially in winters.

6. Infective endocarditis in ostium primum defect only.

55

Ventricular Septal Defect (VSD)

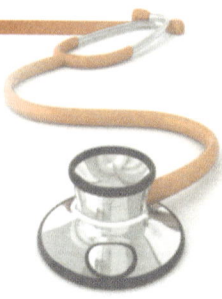

INSTRUCTION

Examine the cardiovascular system

SALIENT FEATURES

- Palpitation, winter cough

HISTORY

Ask for the following:

- History of dyspnea, fever, cough and reduced exercise tolerance
- History of cyanosis on exertion
- History of repeated chest infections especially in winters (present)
- Symptoms of infective endocarditis or past history of endocarditis
- Symptoms of Eisenmenger's syndrome, Down's syndrome

EXAMINATION

General Physical Examination

- Pulse may be normal
- BP may be normal or wide pulse pressure
- Neck for venous and arterial pulsations and JVP may show normal pulsations and normal pressure
- Look for anemia, cyanosis, edema, jaundice, etc.
- Look for clubbing fingers, edema feet

CVS Examination

Inspection
- Apex beat: dynamic or hyperkinetic (present) and laterally displaced
- Precordial pulsations may be present

Palpation
- Apex beat is hyperkinetic, ill sustained (present)
- Left ventricular thrust (present)
- Left parasternal heave (present) may be palpable
- A systolic thrill palpable across the sternum (present)

- P_2 may be palpable if pulmonary hypertension develops

Percussion
- Area of cardiac dullness may be widened due to LVH and apex beat corresponds with cardiac dullness
- Pulmonary area may be dull on percussion if pulmonary hypertension develops

Auscultation
- Both heart sounds are heard
- A pansystolic murmur heard (in this case) best in 3rd and 4th left intercostal spaces and radiates to the right across the sternum (Fig. 55.1). There is an associated thrill if defect is small (present)
- A mid diastolic flow murmur heard at the apex
- A Graham Steel's murmur heard if pulmonary regurgitation
- Second heart sound may be normal or loud due to pulmonary hypertension

Other System

Respiratory system
- For any evidence of consolidation or chest infection
- For signs of LVF, i.e. end-inspiratory crackles

Abdomen
- For hepatomegaly

PROVISIONAL DIAGNOSIS

The patient has ventricular septal defect (lesion) due to congenital heart disease (etiology) without pulmonary hypertension, CHF and bacterial endocarditis (functional status).

QUESTIONS AND ANSWERS

Q.   What are the points in favor of your diagnosis?
Ans: • Seasonal cough, fever and breathlessness

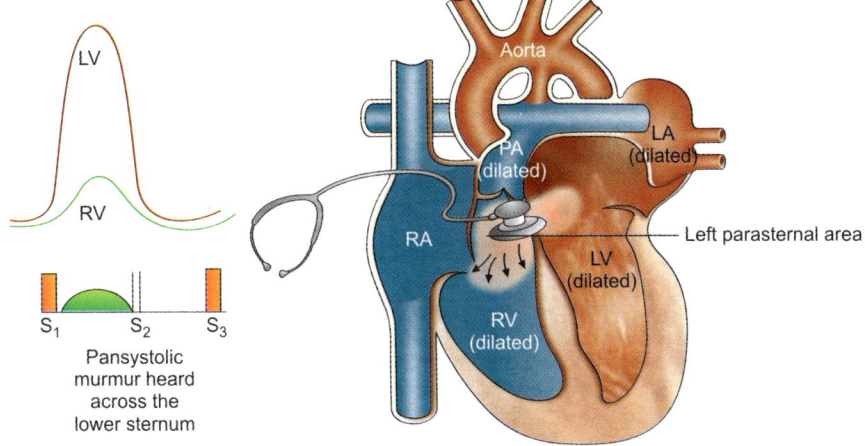

Fig. 55.1: Ventricular septal defect (VSD)

- A palpable systolic thrill across the sternum, palpable left parasternal heave
- A pansystolic murmur widely heard across the chest. P$_2$ is widely split
- No signs of CHF or LHF

Q.   What is differential diagnosis?

Ans: It has to be differentiated from:
- Mitral regurgitation
- Tricuspid regurgitation
- Papillary muscle dysfunction
- Cardiomyopathy (dilated)

Q.   Where is the defect in the septum?

Ans: • Commonly in the membranous portion of the septum
- Uncommonly in the muscular part of the interventricular septum

Q.   What are the causes of VSD?

Ans: • Congenital
- Acquired due to rupture of interventricular septum in a patient with myocardial infarction
- It may be a component of other congenital defect, e.g. septum primum, Fallot's tetralogy.

Q.   Does the defect close spontaneously?

Ans: Yes, it closes in early childhood in 50% cases if the defect is small.

Q.   What is the relation of murmur with size of the defect?

Ans: • Smaller the defect, longer is the murmur
- Larger the defect, shorter is the murmur

Q.   What is maladie de Roger?

Ans: A small membranous VSD with a loud pansystolic murmur with thrill across the sternum in a patient who is asymptomatic.

Q.   When does the duration of murmur decrease in VSD?

Ans: • The duration of murmur decreases if the defect lies in the muscular part of the septum
- The duration of murmur also decreases with development of pulmonary hypertension.

Q.   What are the causes of pansystolic murmur?

Ans: Read the causes in case discussion of MR.

Q.   What is Eisenmenger's complex?

Ans: Eisenmenger's complex is VSD with reversal of shunt ($R \rightarrow L$).

Q.   What will happen to the murmur in VSD if Eisenmenger's syndrome develop?

Ans: The murmur either disappears or becomes short systolic due to reduction in gradient across the defect.

Q.   Name common acyanotic congenital heart disease.

Ans: They are either with left to right shunt or with outflow tract obstruction.
- ASD, VSD, PDA
- Coarctation or aorta
- Congenital aortic stenosis
- Congenital pulmonary stenosis

Q.   What are the complications of VSD?

Ans: • Pulmonary hypertension with reversal of shunt (*Eisenmenger's complex*)

- Infective endocarditis
- CHF
- Repeated chest infections
- Aortic regurgitation in high VSD
- Right ventricular outflow tract obstruction (rare in only 5% cases).

Q.   How would you investigate such a case?

Ans: 1. *ECG:* It is normal in small VSD. In large defect, there may be LVH, left atrial hypertrophy and conduction defects (bundle branch block). For ECG, Read text book of Electrocardiograph by Prof S.N Chugh.

Note: Katz-Wachtel phenomenon (tall R and S in $V_3 - V_4$) is typically seen in VSD due to volume overloading of both the ventricles.

2. *Chest X-ray:* Cardiomegaly with pulmonary plethora (increased lung vascularity); if pulmonary hypertension develops then pulmonary conus is prominent with tapering of the peripheral pulmonary arteries and oligemic lung fields.

3. *Doppler echocardiography* (Fig. 55.2): Echocardiography will identify the presence and location of the defect while color flow study will identify the magnitude and the direction of shunting.

4. *MRI*

5. *Cardiac catheterisation.* It is not needed but indicated before surgical closure to know the severity of defect and to determine pulmonary vascular resistance.

Q.   What is indication of surgical closure of the defect?

Ans: Large defects should be corrected surgically as early as possible in early life when pulmonary vascular resistance is low, i.e.

pulmonary hypertension is still reversible or has not yet developed. The ratio of pulmonary to systemic resistance > 0.7 is contraindication for surgery.

Q.   Name the conditions where VSD is a part of them?

Ans: • Fallot's tetralogy
- Double-outlet right ventricle
- Truncus arteriosus
- Septum primum or endocardial cushion defects

Q.   Name the conditions frequently associated with it.

Ans: • PDA
- ASD
- Tricuspid atresia
- Pulmonary stenosis
- Coarctation of aorta
- Transposition of great vessels

Q.   What is the effect of pregnancy in women with VSD?

Ans: • Small defects do not cause any problem
- Patient with moderate or large defect and moderate pulmonary hypertension are at a risk of developing acute right ventricular failure and rapidly progressive worsening dyspnea in pregnancy. They should be managed for heart failure.
- Pregnancy should be avoided in patients of VSD with pulmonary hypertension.

Q.   Name the common congenital heart disease in order of prevalence.

Ans: 1. VSD
2. ASD (septum secundum)
3. Patent ductus arteriosus
4. Fallot's tetralogy

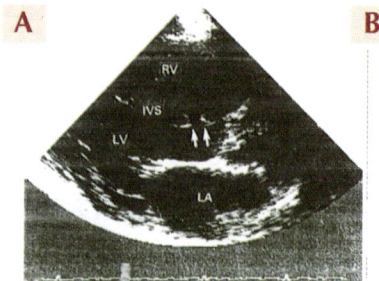 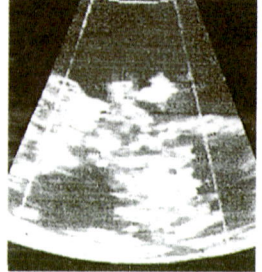

Fig. 55.2: (A) Two-dimensional echocardiogram (long-axis view) showing a ventricular septal defect (arrows); (B) Color Doppler would provide graphic demonstration of the left to right shunt. RV: right ventricle: IVS: interventricular septum, LV: left ventricle, LA: left atrium

56

Eisenmenger's Syndrome

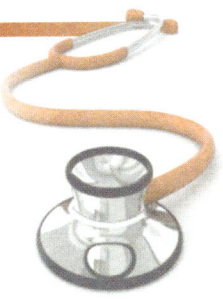

INSTRUCTION

Examine the cardiovascular system

SALIENT FEATURES

- Dyspnea and cyanosis (blue tongue)

HISTORY

Ask for the following:

- History of a congenital heart disease
- Note down the age at which symptoms appeared (symptoms usually do not appear until early childhood or early adulthood)
- Dyspnea on exertion and cyanosis (these occur once right to left shunt or bidirectional shunt develops)
- Impaired exercise tolerance
- Palpitations due to an arrhythmia (commonly due to AF)
- History of effort angina
- History of hemoptysis (due to pulmonary infarction as a result of paradoxical embolism)
- Syncope due to low cardiac output
- Symptoms of hyperviscosity and polycythemia, i.e. visual disturbance, headache, fatigue, paraesthesias, seizures, etc.
- Symptoms of right heart failure (i.e. raised JVP, pain abdomen, swelling of legs) if it develops

EXAMINATION

General Physical Examination

- Record pulse and BP
- There is clubbing of the fingers and central cyanosis (present)
- JVP is raised. Prominent 'a' waves are seen and 'v' wave may be prominent if TR is present

Cardiovascular Examination

- Left parasternal heave and palpable P₂ (present)
- Epigastric pulsations due to RVH
  Findings on auscultation of the heart are:

i. In pulmonary area, there is loud P_2, a pulmonary ejection click, Graham-Steell murmur [an early diastolic murmur) due to pulmonary regurgitation (Fig. 56.1)]
ii. Listen carefully to second heart sound to determine the splitting which points to the underlying cause of Eisenmenger's syndrome/complex as follows:
   a. VSD with reversal of shunt produces single second sound
   b. Fixed wide split second sound is heard in ASD
   c. Reversed splitting of second heart sound and differential cyanosis (cyanosis is seen only in lower limbs, not in upper limbs) indicate PDA with reversal of shunt

Abdominal Examination

- Look for hepatomegaly and pulsations of liver

PROVISIONAL DIAGNOSIS

The patient has Eisenmenger's syndrome with a shunt at ventricular level (lesion) which is congenital

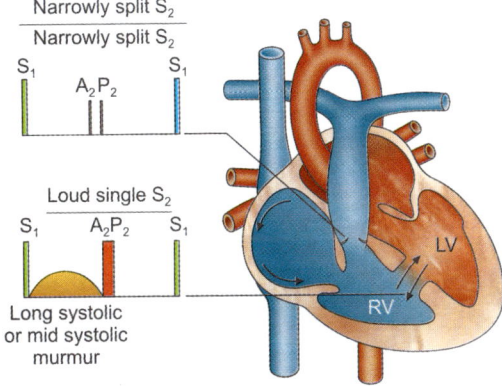

Fig. 56.1: Eisenmenger's syndrome (diag). There is VSD with reversal of shunt

in origin (cause). Patient has severe pulmonary hypertension and TR (functional status).

QUESTIONS AND ANSWERS

Q. What are the points in favor of your diagnosis?

Ans: 1. Cyanosis, clubbing of the fingers and polycythemia
2. Signs of pulmonary hypertension, i.e.
   - Palpable and Loud P_2
   - Single second heart sound
   - Graham-Steell murmur
   - Pansystolic murmur in tricuspid area with raised JVP, prominent 'v' waves

Q. What is Eisenmenger's syndrome?

Ans: Eisenmenger's syndrome is defined as pulmonary hypertension with a reversed or bidirectional shunt in patients with ASD, VSD, PDA, persistent truncus arteriosus, common atrioventricular canal.

Q. Enumerate some common cyanotic heart disease besides Eisenmenger's syndrome?

Ans: 1. Fallot tetralogy
2. Transposition of great vessels
3. Total anomalous pulmonary venous drainage
4. Common atrium
5. Persistent truncus arteriosus

Q. What is the age of onset of Eisenmenger's syndrome?

Ans: In VSD and PDA, the Eisenmenger's syndrome develops in infancy and childhood. In ASD, it develops in adulthood.

Q. What are the factors deleterious to pulmonary hypertension in these patients?

Ans: 1. Pregnancy
2. Dehydration as well as fluid overload
3. Renal/hepatic dysfunction
4. Hypoxia due to any cause, e.g. smoking, environment pollution
5. Systemic hypertension, Arrhythmias
6. Increased viscosity due to erythrocytosis or hypercoagulable states
7. Acute infections

Q. What are the complications of Eisenmenger's syndrome?

Ans: 1. Polycythemia, Hemoptysis (recurrent)
2. Right ventricular failure and TR

3. Thrombotic CVA due to increased viscosity
4. Infections, Infective endocarditis
5. Bleeding due to abnormal hemostasis
6. Paradoxical embolisation
7. Hyperuricemia

Q. How would you investigate such a case?

Ans: 1. *ECG:* There will be RVH with or without an atrial arrhythmia.
2. Chest X-ray will show dilated pulmonary artery, with narrow or 'pruned' peripheral vessels. There will be cardiomegaly (prominent RV).
3. *Echocardiogram:* It will reveal RV enlargement, pulmonary dilatation and underlying cardiac defect. Contrast echocardiography may be used to visualise the shunt.
4. *Cardiac catheterisation:* It is done to estimate the severity of intracardiac shunting, assessment of reversibility of shunting by vasodilators.

Q. What are bad prognostic factors?

Ans: 1. Recurrent syncopal attacks
2. RV systolic dysfunction
3. Low cardiac output
4. Hypoxaemia and polycythemia
Mortality rate is 80% after 10 years of diagnosis.

Q. Is pregnancy safe in these patients.

Ans: 1. It is not safe. It is associated with high rates of spontaneous abortions.
2. Mother mortality is also high.

N.B. Pregnancy is contraindicated and if occurs is best terminated at an early age. However, if pregnancy reaches full term, the vaginal delivery under careful supervision of the gynecologist and physician is necessary.

Q. What is the treatment of Eisenmenger's syndrome?

Ans: • Repeated phlebotomies in patients with secondary polycythemia (PCV >65%)
• Long-term I.V. epoprostenol
• Prostacyclin analogues and phosphodiesterase 5 inhibitors (e.g. sildenafil) may prove useful
• Bosentan has been found useful to improve exercise capacity on 6 minutes walk test
• Heart-lung (combined) transplantation

57

Fallot's Tetralogy

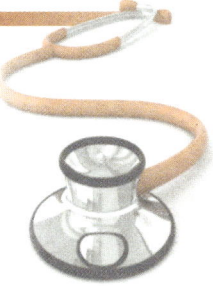

INSTRUCTION

Examine the cardiovascular system

SALIENT FEATURES

- Blue tongue and dyspnea on exertion

HISTORY

Ask for the following:

- Age of onset of symptoms
- History of syncopal attacks during exertion or while playing or during crying in children
- History of squatting (it gives relief to the patient)
- Shortness of breath (breathlessness) due to hypoxia (unoxygenated blood leading to decreased saturation)
- Reduced exercise capacity/tolerance
- Stunted growth and delayed milestones

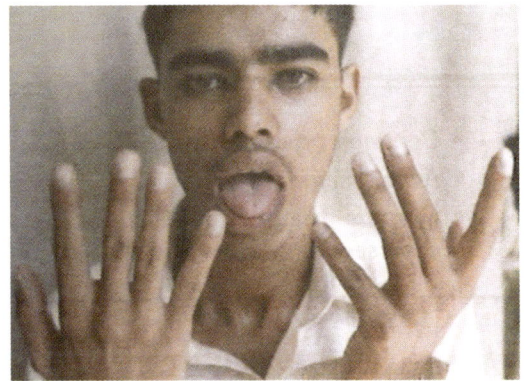

Fig. 57.1: Fallot's tetralogy. A young patient with cyanotic heart disease showing clubbing of the fingers. The bluish tinge of cyanosis is seen on tongue (central cyanosis). He was proved to be a case of tetralogy of Fallot on investigation

EXAMINATION

Cardiovascular System

- Central cyanosis and clubbing of the fingers (present in this case) (Fig. 57.1)
- Silent precordium on palpation due to balanced shunt and overriding of aorta (present)
- *On auscultation*, the findings in this case are:
    i. The second heart sound is single (pulmonary component absent)
    ii. An ejection systolic murmur heard at pulmonary area (present)
- Thoracotomy scar of Blalock-Taussig shunt
- If a scar is present look for the signs of Blalock-Taussig, shunt (a common operation done for Fallot's tetralogy)
    – As the surgery is done on the left side, hence the signs are confined to left side such as
        i. The left radial pulse is weak as compared to right

ii. The left arm is smaller than the right
iii. Pulse pressure is very low, hence, blood pressure is difficult to record.

PROVISIONAL DIAGNOSIS

The patient has Fallot's tetralogy (lesion), a congenital cyanotic heart disease (aetiology). Patient has frequent cyanotic spells and surgery has not been done (functional status).

QUESTIONS AND ANSWERS

Q. What are the components of Fallot's tetralogy?

Ans: It is a cyanotic heart disease having four following components such as: (i) *right ventricular hypertrophy* (ii) *VSD*, (iii) *overriding of aorta*, and (iv) *infundibular pulmonary stenosis:*

Q.   What is Fallot's trilogy and pentalogy?

Ans:

Fallot's trilogy includes:	Fallot's pentalogy includes:
• VSD	• ASD is added to Fallot's tetralogy to make it pentalogy
• ASD	
• Pulmonary stenosis	

Q.   Name few cyanotic heart diseases?

Ans: Read Eisenmenger's syndrome.

Q.   What is the cause of ejection systolic murmur in this case?

Ans: In Fallot's tetralogy, there is pulmonary stenosis which produces an ejection systolic murmur and single second heart sound. The pulmonary stenosis in Fallot's tetralogy may be infundibular (common) or valvular (uncommon).

Q.   Why cyanosis occurs in right to left shunt?

Ans: It is due to mixing of unoxygenated blood with oxygenated blood bringing down the O_2 saturation of the blood.

Q.   Why VSD in Fallot's does not produce murmur?

Ans: Murmur is produced due to presence of a flow gradient across a congenital defect or a valve. In Fallot's tetralogy, the shunt at VSD level is more or less balanced without much flow gradient across the defect, hence, murmur is not produced.

Q.   How does squatting position help in Fallot's tetralogy?

Ans: Squatting is the posture adopted by children with Fallot's tetralogy in which child sits with flexed hips and knees. It helps to reduce venous return of desaturated blood and increases the peripheral vascular resistance, thus, reduces right to left shunting and improves cerebral oxygenation. This posture reduces cyanotic spells.

Q.   What is the cause of cyanosis in Fallot's tetralogy?

Ans: This is due to mixing of the unoxygenated blood from right ventricle to left ventricle through VSD as the shunt between two ventricles is either bidirectional (blood flows from either ventricles depending on the pressure) or from right to left and the over-rided aorta gets mixed blood from both the ventricles leading to cyanosis.

Note: Right to left shunt produces cyanosis, left to right shunt does not.

Q.   What are the other anomalies associated with tetralogy of Fallot?

Ans: • Right sided aortic arch or double aortic arch
• ASD, so-called pentalogy of Fallot
• Coronary arterial anomalies
• Left sided superior vena cava
• Hypoplasia of the pulmonary arteries

Q.   What is Blalock-Taussig shunt?

Ans: It is surgery done for Fallot's tetralogy in which left subclavian artery is anastomosed to left pulmonary artery so as to increase the pulmonary flow.

Q.   What is the prognosis in Fallot's tetralogy?

Ans: The rate of survival in uncorrected defect decreases with age. At and beyond 20 yrs, the survival is just around 10%.

Q.   How would you investigate this case?

Ans: *ECG.* It will show RVH
Chest X-ray. It will show:
• Boot shaped heart with hypoplastic pulmonary conus with mild cardiomegaly
• Double aortic arch (30% cases)
• Decreased pulmonary vasculature

Q.   What is the treatment of Fallot's tetralogy?

Ans: 1. Total correction under the age of 1 yr. A second stage total correction can be performed when the child is of 2 yrs
2. *Blalock-Taussig shunt* (already discussed)
3. *Modified Blalock-Taussig shunt* is the interposition of a tubular graft between the subclavian and pulmonary arteries
4. The *Waterston shunt* (anastomosis of back of aorta with pulmonary artery)
5. The *Potts shunt* (anastomosis of descending aorta to the back of pulmonary artery)
6. The *Glenn operation* (anastomosis of superior vena cava to right pulmonary artery
7. *Pulmonary balloon valvuloplasty*

58

Coarctation of Aorta

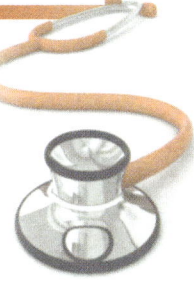

INSTRUCTION

Examine the cardiovascular system

SALIENT FEATURES

- Headache, dizziness and palpitation

HISTORY

Ask about the following:

- Patient may not complain of any symptom (asymptomatic)
- Ask about the symptoms of hypertension (headache, palpitations, nose bleeding, dizziness, dyspnea on exertion)
- Ask about intermittent claudication of legs
- Ask about symptoms of heart failure
- History of pregnancy (aortic dissection is common)

EXAMINATION

General Physical Examination

- Look at development of body proportion, i.e. upper part is well developed and muscular than lower part in coarctation of aorta
- JVP: It may be raised if patient has congestive heart failure
- *Pulse:* Radial pulse on left side is of low volume than the right. There may be radio-radial delay. The femoral pulses are also weak and delayed (radiofemoral delay)
- *Blood pressure:* It is higher in right upper limb than the left. The difference is > 10 mm (normal is < 10 mm). The systolic BP is higher in upper than lower limbs
- Look for edema feet
- Look for the features of Turner's syndrome (Read Turner's syndrome)
- Look for William's syndrome (elfin faces, peg-shaped incisors and mental retardation)

Cardiovascular System Examination

- Collaterals may be visible or there may be palpable pulsations in the upper part of back of chest especially in the scapular and interscapular region
- Pulsations may be visible in suprasternal notch. A systolic thrill may be palpable in this region
- Apex beat may be normal or displaced down and out, heaving in character due to hypertension
- Let parasternal heave may be palpable
- *On auscultation,* following findings may be present:
    i. A systolic ejection click in aortic area (due to bicuspid aortic valve a common association) is heard in 50% cases (present). An ejection systolic murmur may also be heard (present in this case)
    ii. Loud second heart sound (present)
    iii. A harsh systolic murmur heard along the left sternal border and in the back, particularly over the coarctation
    iv. A continuous murmur heard over the collaterals also in the back or over the left anterior chest (present)

Examination of Other System

1. *Abdominal examination* for hepatomegaly, ascites
2. *Respiratory system examination* for crackles and wheezes (LVF). They are present in this case
3. *Examine CNS* for cranial nerve palsy (3rd cranial nerve involvement) due to Berry aneurysm—an association of coarctation of aorta.

PROVISIONAL DIAGNOSIS

The symptoms and signs (hypertension, bicuspid aortic stenosis) suggest the provisional diagnosis of coarctation of aorta (lesion) due to congenital origin (etiology) with signs of left heart failure (functional status).

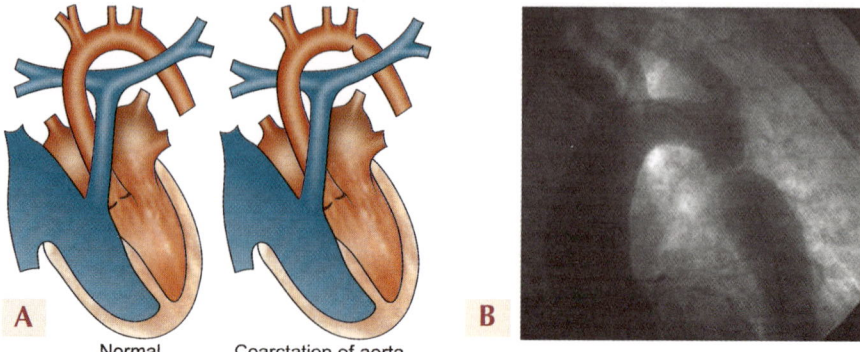

A Normal   Coarctation of aorta   **B**

Fig. 58.1: (A) Coarctation of aorta (diag.); (B) Aortogram showing coarctation

Q.   What are points in favor of your diagnosis?
Ans: • A young male presenting with hyper-
tension
  • Well built upper body part than lower
  • There is radio-radial and radio femoral
delay
  • BP in right upper limb more (>10 mm
than left
  • Presence of collaterals over the back
(scapular and interscapular region)
  • Asystolic ejection click and an ejection
systolic murmur in aortic area. A_2 is loud
  • A continuous murmur is also heard over
the collaterals

QUESTIONS AND ANSWERS

**Q.   What do you mean by coarctation of aorta?
What are its type?**
Ans: Coarctation of aorta just means narrowing of the
lumen of a part of aorta. It is of two types:
  I. *Preductal (infantile).* The constriction of
aorta is present between left subclavian
artery and patent ductus arteriosus.
  II. *Postductal (adult type).* The constriction of
aorta is after the origin of patent ductus
arteriosus, i.e. in the descending aorta.
  III. *Rare coarctation include:*
  • Coarctation of ascending aorta
  • Coarctation of distal descending tho-
racic aorta
  • Coarctation of abdominal aorta

**Q.   What do you understand by the term pseudo-
coarctation of aorta?**
Ans: It is just a kinked appearance of aorta in the
post-ductal region without stenosis and a
gradient. It is of no hemodynamic significance.

**Q.   What is sex distribution of coarctation of
aorta?**
Ans: Coarctation of aorta is two to five times
commoner in men and boys as in women and
girls.

**Q.   At which age does coarctation of aorta
manifest?**
Ans: 1. *Preductal coarctation* manifests in infancy with congestive heart failure.
  2. *Post ductal coarctation* manifests in adults
between 20 to 30 yrs with hypertension
and bicuspid aortic valve.

Q.   What is the cause of hypertension?
Ans: Hemodynamic effects and stimulation of
renin-angiotensin system.

**Q.   What are common associations of coarctation
of aorta?**
Ans: 1. Turner's syndrome (45 × 0)
  2. Bicuspid aortic valve
  3. VSD
  4. PDA
  5. Mitral stenosis or mitral regurgitation
  6. Berry aneurysms of *circle of Willis*

Q.   How would you investigate this patient?
Ans: 1. *ECG:* It will show LVH
  2. *Chest X-ray:* There will be symmetrical
notching of the ribs. The coarctation on
X-ray can be visualized by *characteristics
'3' sign* along the aortic shadow, i.e. the
upper bulge is due to dilatation of left
subclavian artery, the sharp indentation
in the middle is due to coarctation of
aorta and lower bulge of the sign is due to
post stenotic dilatation of aorta.
  3. *Echocardiography:* It may visualise the
coarctation. Doppler study will reveal a
pressure gradient across the coarctation
of aorta.

4. *CT and MRI scans* and *contrast aorto-graphy*. These investigations are useful to determine the precise anatomy of aorta, site of constriction, length of constriction, poststenotic dilatation and visualisation of the collaterals.

Q. **What is the cause of rib notching in coarctation?**

Ans: It occurs due to collateral flow through dilated, tortuous intercostal vessels passing on the under surface of the ribs, hence called posterior notching of the ribs. Anterior surface of the ribs is spared because anterior intercostal vessels do not run in the costal grooves.

Q. **Where would you see the notching of the ribs?**

Ans: The notching of the ribs is seen between 3rd and 9th intercostal ribs.

Q. **What are the other causes of rib notching?**

Ans: In addition to coarctation of aorta, other causes are;

1. Blalock-Taussig shunt/operation
2. Subclavian artery obstruction
3. Superior vena cava obstruction
4. Neurofibromatosis
5. Arteriovenous malformation of the lung and the chest wall

Q. **What are the complications of aortic coarctation?**

Ans: In coarctation, the complications result from hypertension such as:

1. Stroke
2. Premature ischemic heart disease
3. Left ventricular failure
4. Rupture of aorta
5. Infective endocarditis
6. Intracranial hemorrhage due to rupture of berry aneurysm
7. Death

Q. **What do you see on fundus examination in coarctation of aorta?**

Ans: It includes

1. Tortuous retinal vessels with frequent 'U' turns
2. Classical signs of hypertensive retinopathy, i.e. exudates, hemorrhages

Q. **What is the treatment of coarctation of aorta?**

Ans: 1. Treatment of hypertension
2. Treatment of LVF if present
3. *Balloon dilatation* with stent insertion is indicated in patients with native coarctation with suitable aortic anatomy with an echo peak gradient of >20 mmHg in the absence of extensive collaterals or < 20 mm Hg in their presence.
4. If aortic anatomy is unsuitable for dilatation and stenting, surgery is indicated (resection of a segment with end-to-end anastomosis). If narrow segment is too long, a tubular graft may be placed.

Q. **What happens to hypertension after surgery?**

Ans: Despite surgery, some patients continue to have persistent or recurrent hypertension and require monitoring and treatment. This is due to resetting of renin-angiotensin system.

Q. **What are the post operative complications?**

Ans: 1. Persistent/recurrent hypertension
2. Recurrent coarctation.

59

Ebstein's Anomaly

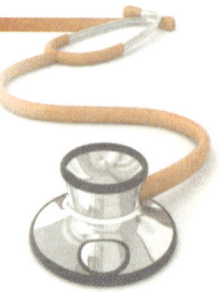

INSTRUCTION

Examine the cardiovascular system

SALIENT FEATURES

- Bluish tongue, distended abdomen and edema feet.

HISTORY

Ask about the following:

- Symptoms of right heart failure, i.e. swelling of abdomen, edema feet, pain abdomen, etc.
- History of palpitations (an arrhythmia)
- History of consumption of lithium ingestion by the mother
- History of exertional dyspnea or cyanosis

EXAMINATION

General Physical Examination

- Raised JVP with prominent pulsations but the large 'V' of tricuspid regurgitation is absent because the giant atrium absorbs most of the regurgitant volume from right ventricle
- Cyanosis is present (in this case)
- Edema feet is present.

Cardiovascular System Examination

- Left parasternal heave (not present)
- Loud first heart sound (present). Second sound is normal
- Pansystolic murmur of TR which increases on inspiration (present)
- Hepatomegaly which is tender. Hepatojugular reflux is present (in this case). Liver pulsations (pulsatile liver) may or may not be present (present)

PROVISIONAL DIAGNOSIS

The patient has symptoms and signs of tricuspid regurgitation without pulmonary hypertension, hence, the provisional diagnosis is Ebstein's anomaly (lesion) of congenital origin (etiology). Patient is in congestive heart failure (functional status).

QUESTIONS AND ANSWERS

Q. Why is this case not a Eisenmenger syndrome?

Ans: The absence of signs of pulmonary hypertension excludes this possibility

Q. What is Ebstein's anomaly?

Ans: It is characterised by downward displacement of the tricuspid valve into the right ventricle due to anomalous attachment of tricuspid leaflets.

Q. What is the hallmark of Ebstein's anomaly?

Ans: 1. The clinical hallmark is tricuspid regurgitation without pulmonary hypertension
2. Central cyanosis due to patent foramen ovale is present in cyanotic Ebstein's anomaly (present)
3. Inspite of TR, the right ventricle is hypoplastic

Q. What is the pathology of Ebstein's disease?

Ans: 1. The tricuspid leaflets are abnormal
2. The tricuspid ring is displaced downward, hence, there is atrialisation of a portion of right ventricle
3. The septal leaflet of tricuspid valve is deficient or absent. The posterior leaflet may also be deficient and there is large 'sail-like' anterior leaflet, which is pathological hallmark of this condition
4. 50% patients have either patent foramen ovale or a secundum type of ASD
5. 25% patients have one or more accessory pathways of conduction
6. The anomaly is said to be associated with maternal lithium ingestion

Q. **What is the mechanism of cyanosis in this patient?**

Ans: 50% patients have right-to-left shunt at atrial level either due to patent foramen ovale or ASD. These are cases of cyanotic Ebstein's anomaly.

Q. **What type of abnormal AV conduction occurs in Ebstein's anomaly?**

Ans: About 10% have WPW type (Kent bundle) of accelerated conduction (e.g. short P–R interval, delta wave and wide QRS). This can lead to reciprocal tachycardia.

Q. **How would you investigate such a case?**

Ans: 1. *ECG.* It shows RBBB, prolonged P–R interval, P pulmonale [right atrial hypertrophy (Fig. 59.1)], large P wave called Himalayan P waves, type B WPW (Wolff-Parkinson-White) syndrome

2. *Echocardiography* shows lower placement of tricuspid valve with abnormal posi-

tional relation between tricuspid and mitral valve with apical displacement of the septal tricuspid leaflet. There is TR on color Doppler.

Q. **What are the indications of surgery?**

Ans: 1. Severe functional limitation
2. Cardiomegaly with cardiothoracic ratio >60%
3. An atrial communication especially patent foramen ovale
4. Kent bundle conduction (Type 2 WPW syndrome)
5. Severe tricuspid regurgitation

Q. **What type of surgery is done in this condition?**

Ans: It includes either tricuspid valve replacement plus closure of patent foramen ovale or tricuspid annuloplasty with plication of atrialised portion of RV.

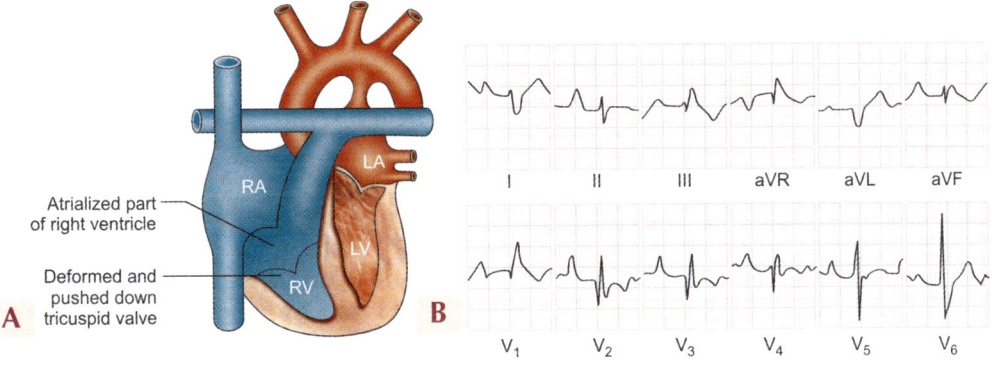

Fig. 59.1: Ebstein anomaly. (A) Diagram;
(B) The ECG recorded from 18-year-old boy shows:
  i. *First degree AV block:* The P-R interval is 0.28 sec
 ii. *Right bundle branch block (RBBB):* There is wide (>0.12 sec) rsR′ pattern in leads $V_1 - V_4$ with coving ST segment and inverted T waves. There is wide deep S wave in V_6
iii. *Right atrial hypertrophy:* There is tall peaked P waves in leads II, III, aVF, $V_2 - V_5$

NB: Tall P waves (Himalyan P waves in precordial leads) along with conduction defects are highly suggestive of Ebstein anomaly

60

Atrial Myxoma

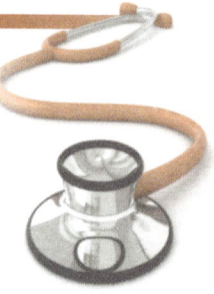

INSTRUCTION

Examine the cardiovascular system

SALIENT FEATURES

- Dyspnoea, cough and palpitation

HISTORY

Ask about the following:

- History of arthralgia, rash, Raynaud's pheno-menon
- History of chest discomfort, syncope (outflow obstruction)
- History of fever, palpitations, weakness, malaise, cachexia (tumor manifestations) (present in this case)
- History of cough, breathlessness, hemoptysis (left heart failure)
- Ask about symptoms of congestive heart failure (hepatomegaly, ascites, swelling of legs)
- Family history of such a disease
- Asked about increase or decrease in heart beats or missed beats (arrhythmias and conduction disturbance)
- Ask about nodule(s) in the breast (fibroadeno-mas)
- History of bleeding

EXAMINATION

General Physical Examination

- Look for lentigines and pigmented nevi
- Look for features of adrenal cortical hyperplasia, i.e. *Cushing's syndrome* (moon-facies, camel hump, striae, hirsutism, edema feet, etc.)
- Look for increase in height (*Gigantism*) or enlargement of acral parts (*acromegaly*)
- Especially look for manifestations of myxomas syndromes, i.e
  - *Carney complex* (e.g. spotty skin pig-mentation, myxoma, endocrine activity and neurofibromas)
  - *NAME syndrome* (nevi, atrial myxoma, neurofibroma and ephelides)

  - *LAMB syndrome* (lentigines, atrial myxoma and blue nevi)
- Look for clubbing of the fingers and other signs of endocarditis.

Systemic Examination

Cardiovascular System

- Examine the patients for signs of mitral stenosis (prolapse of atrial tumor into mitral ring) or regurgitation (due to atrial tumor-induced valvular trauma). There were features of MS in this case.
- Examine the patients with syncope or dizziness for subaortic or subpulmonic stenosis due to outflow obstruction by ventricular myxomas
- Examine for signs and symptoms of peripheral and pulmonary embolisation.
- The characteristic feature of atrial myxoma is tumor prop which is an early or mid-diastolic low pitched sound heard with the bell of stethoscope in upright position resulting from sudden striking of myxoma to ventricular wall across mitral ring (present in this case). This sound disappears with the change in position, i.e. upright to lying down position.

Respiratory System Examination

- Bilateral basal crackles and rales (present).

PROVISIONAL DIAGNOSIS

Symptoms and signs suggest atrial myxoma (lesion) congenital in origin (aetiology) with signs of left heart failure (functional status) without evidence of endocarditis.

QUESTIONS AND ANSWERS

Q. What are the points in favor of your diag-nosis?

Ans: 1. Constitutional symptoms, e.g. fever malaise, cachexia, etc.

2. Tumor plop (an early diastolic sound) appearing in sitting position and disappearing in lying down.
3. Sign of left heart failure, e.g. bilateral basal crackles.

Q. **What other characteristic features of atrial myxoma are absent in this case?**
Ans: 1. Signs of embolisation
2. Features suggestive of the cause, i.e. recognised atrial myxoma syndromes

Q. **What are the characteristic features of atrial myxomas?**
Ans: 1. Constitutional symptoms
2. Positional valvular obstruction (especially mitral valve) or regurgitation due to tumor-induced trauma
3. Embolisation due to endocarditis

Q. **What are associated conditions with myxomas?**
Ans: • Adrenocortical disease (Cushing's syndrome)
• Myxomatous mammary fibroadenoma
• Testicular tumors
• Pituitary adenomas
• Pigmented nevi/skin pigmentation
• Neurofibromas

Q. **What is pathology of myxoma?**
Ans: These are gelatinous structures constituting myxoma cells embedded in stroma rich in glycosaminoglycans. Most are pedunculated, solitary and located in atria in the vicinity of interatrial septum. Some myxomas occur in younger generation, usually multiple or have ventricular origin.

Q. **What is differential diagnosis of tumor plop?**
Ans: 1. Loud P_2
2. S_3 gallop
3. Opening snap
4. Pericardial knock

Q. **How would you investigate such a case?**
Ans: 1. *ECG* for atrial or ventricular hypertrophy, arrhythmias and conduction defects
2. *Echocardiogram* (Fig. 60.1): Both transthoracic or transesophageal are useful in the diagnosis of cardiac myxoma and allow the determination of the site of tumor and size of tumor
3. *Chest X-ray* for cardiac size and congestion of the lung (left heart failure)
4. *Cardiac MRI:* It will provide informations regarding size, shape, composition and surface
5. *Cardiac catheterisation and angiography:* It is not considered necessary because of risk of tumor embolisation

Q. **What is the genesis of cardiac myxoma?**
Ans: Most of the tumors are familial with autosomal dominant transmission, hence, echocardiographic screening of first-degree relative is appropriate particularly in young patients with multiple tumors or evidence of myxoma syndromes.

Q. **What are myxomas syndromes?**
Ans: These have already been described in examination.

Q. **What is the treatment of this condition?**
Ans: Surgical resection utilizing cardiopulmonary bypass is the curative treatment.

Q. **What is recurrence rate of myxomas?**
Ans: Myxomas recur in approximately 12 to 22% of familial cases and in about 1 to 2% of sporadic cases.

Tumor recurrence is attributed either to multicentric origin of the tumor or its inadequate resection.

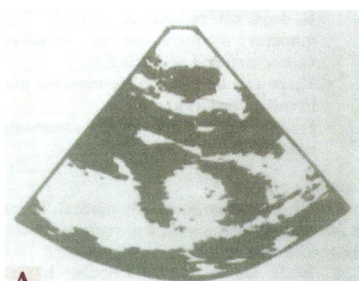 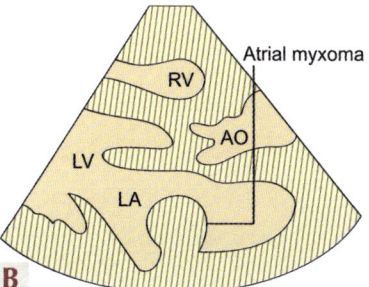

Fig. 60.1: Atrial myxoma. (A) The 2D-echocardiogram (four-chamber view); (B) Line diagram of left atrial myxoma
LA: Left atrium, LV: Left ventricle, RV: Right ventricle, AO: Aorta

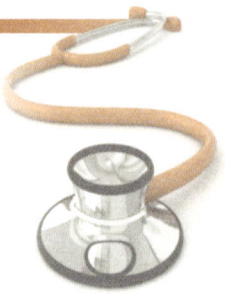

61

Aneurysm of Ascending Aorta

INSTRUCTION

Examine the cardiovascular system

SALIENT FEATURES

- Palpitation

HISTORY

Ask about the following:

- Substernal or neck pain
- History of dyspnea, stridor (tracheal compression), brassy cough (pressure on bronchus), edema of neck and arms, suffusion of face (superior vena cava obstruction), hoarseness (pressure over recurrent laryngeal nerve)
- History of palpitation and dyspnea (aortic regurgitation)
- History of trauma

EXAMINATION

General Physical Examination

- *Face:* Look for edema, suffusion, puffiness
- *Height* and *body proportions* for Marfan's syndrome
- *Elasticity of skin* and hypermobility of joints (*Ehlers-Danlos syndrome*)
- *Pulse* (good volume collapsing pulse), wide pulse pressure, dancing carotids and other signs of hyperdynamic circulation (aortic regurgitation)
- Look for signs of CHF

Cardiovascular System Examination

Inspection

- Pulsations may be visible in the suprasternal notch (present in this case)
- Apex beat may be visible, diffuse

Palpation

- Pulsations in suprasternal notch are palpable and are expansible (present in this case).
- Apex beat is sustained.

- Left parasternal heave is present due to aortic regurgitation and LVH dilatation.

Percussion

- There is widening of mediastinal dullness on percussion.

Auscultation

- There is an early diastolic murmur in aortic area. The A_2 is soft (Fig. 61.1).
- There is no Austin-Flint murmur
- No third heart sound

Respiratory System Examination

- No basal crackles and rales

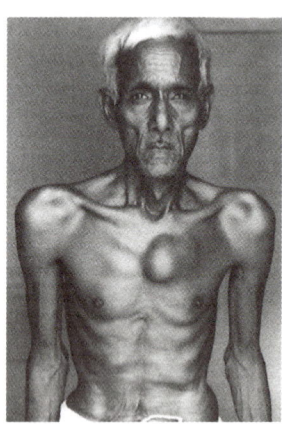

Fig. 61.1: A patient with visible swelling in left infraclavicular region, proved to be a case of aortic aneurysm involving ascending aorta and arch of aorta

PROVISIONAL DIAGNOSIS

The patient has visible pulsatile swelling in infraclavicular region with visible pulsations in suprasternal notch and mild aortic regurgitation (lesion) due to ascending aorta and aortic arch aneurysm (etiology). Patient is not in CHF (functional status).

QUESTIONS AND ANSWERS

Q. **What are the points in favor of your diagnosis?**

Ans: 1. Visible pulsatile swelling in left infraclavicular region.
2. Visible and palpable pulsations in suprasternal notch.
3. Symptoms and signs of aortic regurgitation.

Q. **Which simple investigation would confirm the diagnosis?**

Ans: Fluoroscopy for aortic dilatation and pulsations will confirm it.

Q. **What are the causes of aneurysm of aortic arch?**

Ans: • Atherosclerosis (old age)
• Connective tissue disorders, e.g.
  – Marfan's syndrome
  – Ehlers-Danlos syndrome
  – Cystic medial necrosis
• Syphilitic aneurysm (cardiovascular syphilis)
• Traumatic aneurysm
• Mycotic infections, e.g. *Staphylococcus*, *Salmonella*, SABE

Q. **What is the cause of aortic regurgitation in aortic aneurysm?**

Ans: Involvement of ascending aorta alone or along with the arch of aorta produces aortic regurgitation by dilatation of aortic root and annulus.

Q. **How would you investigate such a case?**

Ans: 1. *Plain X-ray chest* for calcification of the walls of aneurysm (Fig. 61.2) and dilatation of aortic knuckle.
2. *CT scan* to define anatomy and size of the aneurysm and to exclude other causes which can mimic aneurysm.

3. *MRI*
4. *Cardiac catheterisation* and *echocardiography* to describe the relationship of the coronary arteries to an aneurysm of ascending aorta.

Q. **What are the other conditions that can mimic ascending aorta/arch of aorta aneurysm?**

Ans: • Superior mediastinal neoplasm/lymph nodes
• Superior vena cava obstruction
• Mediastinal goitre

Q. **How would you treat?**

Ans: It is similar to abdominal aorta aneurysm (discussed as a separate case)

Q. **What are the complications of an aneurysm?**

Ans: • Rupture of aneurysm
• Thrombus and embolism leading to stroke
• Aortic regurgitation

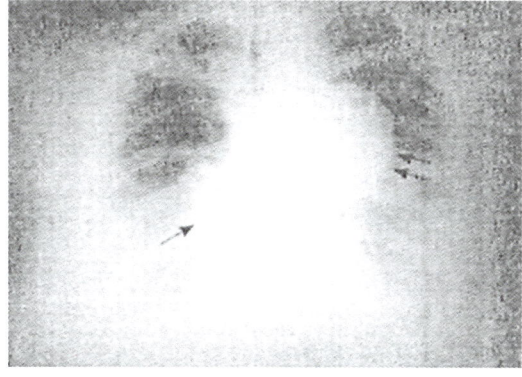

Fig. 61.2: Aortic aneurysm. Chest X-ray (PA view) shows aneurysm and dilatation of ascending aorta (↑) and arch of aorta (↑↑). There is ring like calcification of arch of the aorta.

62

Thromboangitis Obliterans (Buerger's Disease)

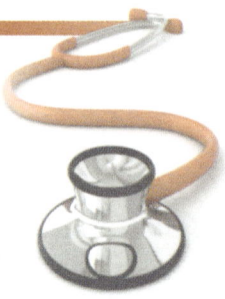

INSTRUCTION

Examine the patient's lower limbs and perform relevant cardiovascular system examination

SALIENT FEATURES

- Amputation of right great toe and left leg

HISTORY

Ask the patient (younger patients < 40 yrs) for:

- Intermittent claudication (not common)
- Rest leg and feet pain
- History of smoking (present in this case)
- History of gangrene of toes (present)
- History of amputations (present)
- History of diabetes, hypertension
- History of precipitating trauma
- History of non-healing foot/toe ulcers
- History of Raynaud's phenomenon (tricolor changes)

EXAMINATION

General Physical Examination

- Cold atrophic skin
- Loss of hair
- Amputated big toe and left leg (Fig. 62.1)
- Nails are thickened (trophic nail changes)
- Tender punched out ulcer on the fingers and big toe (present in this case)
- The painful ulcer is situated in the plantar surface over the head of big toe and first metatarsal (present)
- Amputation stump of left leg [amputation of lower leg and foot done (Fig. 62.1)]
- Pallor on elevation of the leg
- Peripheral pulses are feeble (present)
- Dorsalis pedis and posterior tibial arterial pulsations are not palpable on right side (in this case)
- Sluggish filling of toe capillaries

- Ischemic neuritis, e.g. numbness, paraesthesias, hyporeflexia, muscle atrophy

PROVISIONAL DIAGNOSIS

A 40 yrs male smoker has an amputated right big toe and left leg and ulcers on the toes as well as big toe (lesion) due to Buerger's disease (aetiology). He is afraid of repeated amputations (functional status).

QUESTIONS AND ANSWERS

Q.   **What are the points in favor of your diagnosis?**

Ans: 1. A male patient
      2. Chronic smoker
      3. Repeated amputations, on left side
      4. Non-healing arterial ulcer on right big toe after amputation and first toe
      5. Weak peripheral pulsations

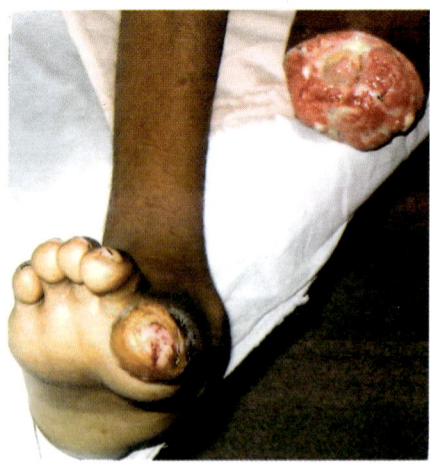

Fig. 62.1: Buerger's disease. It was the cause of repeated amputations in this patient

Q. What is Buerger's disease?

Ans: Buerger's disease is a segmental, inflammatory and thrombotic process of the distal most arteries and occasionally of the veins of extremities.

Q. What are the causes of gangrene of toes?

Ans:
- Peripheral vascular disease
- Raynaud's disease
- Bacterial endocarditis
- Vasculitis (small vessel)
- Repeated atheroembolisation
- Sickle cell anemia

Q. What is the diagnostic triad of Buerger's disease?

Ans: *Intermittent claudication* of affected extremity, *Raynaud's phenomenon* and *migratory superficial vein thrombophlebitis* constitute a diagnostic clinical triad.

Q. What are the causes of leg ulcer?

Ans:
1. Venous ulcer due to varicosity of veins
2. Neuropathic ulcers (diabetes, syringomyelia, leprosy, peripheral neuropathy)
3. Vasculitis (collagen vascular diseases)
4. Arterial occlusion, e.g. Buerger's disease
5. Sickle cell anemia
6. Neoplasm, e.g. Kaposi's sarcoma, basal cell carcinoma
7. Traumatic ulcer
8. Infections, e.g. cellulitis

Q. How would you demonstrate limb ischemia in this patient

Ans:
1. By elevation of the leg (right) for rubor
2. Demonstration of ankle-brachial pressure index

(For demonstration of clinical signs, read clinical methods by Prof SN Chugh)

Q. How would you investigate such a case?

Ans:
1. *Radiography* may show calcification of the arteries of legs.
2. *Doppler ultrasonography* to define the severity of arterial involvement.
3. *An ankle-brachial pressure index* measured by doppler device. An index <0.6 indicates arterial ischemia.
4. *Digital pulse volume recording* and *segmental plethysmography* to measure the changes in blood volume during systole and diastole in the segment of the limb being examined.
5. *MRI angiography*
6. *Aortography* shows narrowing and stenosis of the leg arteries.

Q. How would you manage Buerger's (arterial) ulcers?

Ans:
- Avoidance of smoking
- Control of diabetes, hypertension and obesity, if associated
- Avoid local heat to the limb. Keep the limb warm
- *Care of foot or feet*: Chiropody and foot care, proper foot wear
- Regular exercise to promote development of anastomotic collateral vessels
- Low dose aspirin
- Balloon dilatation when complicated by gangrene
- Grafting (prosthetic vascular grafts of autologous vein grafts)

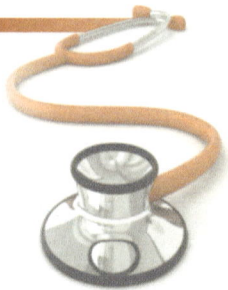

63 Chronic Obstructive Pulmonary Disease (COPD)

INSTRUCTION

Examine the chest for respiratory system

SALIENT FEATURES

- Cough, sputum and breathlessness

HISTORY

Ask for the following:

- Cough with expectoration, its onset, duration, the amount of sputum, postural relation.
- History of fever, chest pain, hemoptysis (Do not forget to look at the sputum cup).
- History recurrent chest infections.
- History of breathlessness, weight loss.
- *History of cigarette smoking.* Exposure to smoke from cigarette or biomass and solid fuel fires, atmospheric smoke is important factor in pathogenesis as well as in acute exacerbation of COPD. The smoke has adverse effect on surfactants and lung defence.
- Ask for *precipitating factors:* e.g. dusty atmosphere, air pollution and repeated upper respiratory tract infections. They cause acute exacerbations of the disease.
- *Family history:* There is increased susceptibility to develop COPD in a family of smokers than non-smokers.
- Alpha-1-antitrypsin deficiency can cause emphysema in non-smoker adult patients.

EXAMINATION

General Physical Examination

- Flexed posture (leaning forward) with pursed lip breathing (Fig. 63.1) and arms supported on their knees or table or bed.
- Central cyanosis, may be noticed in severe COPD (present in this case)
- Bounding pulses (wide pulse pressure) and flapping tremors on outstretched hand may be present is severe COPD with type 2 respiratory

failure. These signs suggest hypercapnia (carbon dioxide narcosis).

- Disturbed consciousness with apnoeic spells (CO_2 narcosis-type 2 respiratory failure).
- Raised JVP and pitting edema feet may be present if patient develops cor pulmonale with congestive heart failure.

Note: Edema feet without raised JVP indicate secondary renal amyloidosis due to pulmonary suppuration, e.g. bronchiectasis bronchitis, chest infections.

- Respiratory rate is increased (hyperpnea). There may be tachycardia (present)

Chest Examination

Inspection

Shape of the Chest: AP diameter is increased relative to transverse diameter (in this case)

- *Barrel-shaped chest (present).* The sternum becomes more arched, spines become unduly

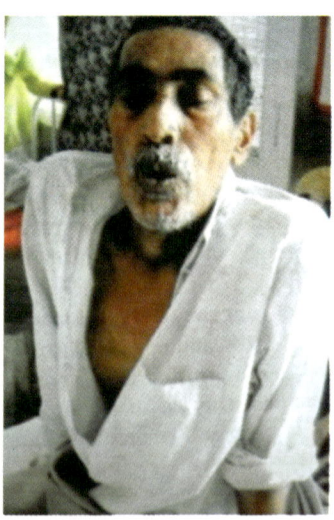

Fig. 63.1: Pursed-lip breathing in COPD

concave, the AP diameter is > transverse diameter, ribs are less oblique (more or less horizontal), subcostal angle is wide (may be obtuse), intercostal spaces are widened.

- *Movements of the chest wall* are bilaterally diminished.
- Pursed-lip breathing (present Fig. 63.1)
- Intercostal recession (in-drawing of the ribs)
- Excavation of suprasternal, supraclavicular and infraclavicular fossae during inspiration (present in this case)
- Widening of subcostal angle (present)
- Respiratory rate is increased. It is mainly abdominal. The alae nasi and extrarespiratory muscles are in action (present)

All these signs indicate hyperinflation of lung due to advanced airflow obstruction.

- Cardiac apex beat may or may not be visible.

Palpation

- Movements of the chest are diminished bilaterally and expansion of the chest is reduced (in this case).
- Trachea is central but there may be reduction in length of palpable trachea above the sternal notch and there may be trachea descent during inspiration (tracheal tug).
- Intercostal spaces may be widened bilaterally (present).
- Occasionally, there may be palpable wheeze (rhonchi) during acute exacerbation.
- Cardiac apex beat may not be palpable due to superimposition by the hyperinflated lungs.

Percussion

- A hyper-resonant note on both sides (present in this case).
- Cardiac dullness is either reduced or totally masked (masked in this case).
- Liver dullness is pushed down (below 5th intercostal space) in 6th intercostal space (in this case).
- There may be resonance over **Kronig's isthmus** and **Traube's area** (splenic dullness is masked).
- Diaphragmatic excursions are reduced on tidal percussion.
- Tactile vocal fremitus is reduced bilaterally (in this case). It can be normal in early cases.

Auscultation

- Breath sounds may be diminished in intensity due to diminished air entry (in this case).
- Vesicular breathing with prolonged expiration is a characteristic sign of COPD (present).
- Vocal resonance may be normal or slightly diminished on both sides equally.

- Rhonchi or wheeze are common (present in this case) especially during forced expiration (expiratory wheeze/rhonchi). Sometimes crackles may be heard during acute exacerbation of COPD.
- Check for forced expiratory time (FET). Ask the patient to exhale forcefully after full inspiration while your are listening over the trachea. If patient takes >6 sec., airway obstruction is indicated.

Examination of Abdomen

- Palpate the liver for hepatic enlargement or displacement.

PROVISIONAL DIAGNOSIS

The patient has features suggestive of COPD (lesion) caused by cigarette smoking (aetiology) and is cyanosed at rest (functional status).

QUESTIONS AND ANSWERS

Q. **What are the points in favor of your diagnosis?**

Ans:
- A 45 yrs male patient
- Smoker for the last 20 yrs
- History of chronic cough and expectoration for >8 yrs. with exacerbation on exposure to dust and smoke.
- No positive history of such disease in the family.
- **Examination reveals signs of both bronchitis and emphysema.**
  i. **Physical signs of bronchitis,** i.e. cyanosis, wheezing, rhonchi, vesicular breathing with prolonged expiration.
  ii. **Physical signs of emphysema** (e.g. barrel-shaped chest, pursed lip breathing, excavation of suprasternal and supraclavicular fossae, diminished vocal fremitus on both sides, hyper-resonant note, obliteration of liver dullness, central apex indicate hyperinflated lungs.

Q. **What is COPD?**

Ans: Chronic obstructive pulmonary disease is the internationally recognised term, includes chronic bronchitis and emphysema.

By definition, COPD is a chronic progressive disorder characterised by air-flow obstruction ($FEV_1 < 80\%$ predicted and FEV_1/FVC ratio < 70%) which does not change markedly over several months.

Q. **How do you define chronic bronchitis and chronic bronchitis with acute exacerbation?**

Ans: Chronic bronchitis is a condition characterised

by cough with or without expectoration on most of the days in a week for at least 3 months in a year for 2 consecutive year (WHO). Chronic bronchitis with acute exacerbation means, fever, persistent or recurrent mucopurulent sputum in the absence of localised suppurative lung disease, bronchiectasis.

Q. What is your differential diagnosis?

Ans: Based on the symptoms and signs, other two conditions that come into differential diagnosis are:

1. Bronchial asthma (Read Table 63.1).
2. Chronic asthmatic bronchitis. The features of bronchitis are more prominent than that of bronchial asthma.

Q. What is tidal percussion?

Ans: Read Clinical Methods in Medicine by Prof. SN Chugh.

Q. Which clinical signs indicate air flow obstruction?

Ans: *Measurement of forced expiratory time (FET).* This has been described under auscultation (Read examination)

Q. Name the accessory muscles of respiration.

Ans: *Alae nasi, sternomastoid, trapezius, serratus anterior, scaleni, latissimus dorsi, pectoralis* and *abdominal muscles* are accessory muscles of respiration seen working in a patient with severe COPD.

Q. How do you classify severity of COPD?

Ans: Severity of COPD is discussed in Table 63.2.

Q. How do you decide about which component of COPD is predominant, i.e. chronic bronchitis or emphysema?

Ans: Though COPD encompasses both chronic bronchitis and emphysema, but one may

Table 63.1: Differentiating features between bronchial asthma and COPD	
Bronchial asthma	*COPD (see Fig. 63.2)*
• Occurs in young age, seen in children and adults who are atopic.	Occurs in middle or old aged persons.
• Allergo-inflammatory disorder, characterised by reversible airflow obstruction, airway inflammation and bronchial hypersensitivity.	Inflammatory disorder characterised by progressive airway obstruction.
• Short duration of symptoms (weeks or months).	Long duration of symptoms, e.g. at least 2 years.
• Episodic disease with recurrent attacks.	Nonepisodic usually but acute exacerbations may occur which worsen the symptoms and disease further.
• Variable nature of symptoms is a characteristic feature.	Symptoms are fixed and persistent, may be progressive.
• Family history of asthma, hay fever or eczema may be positive.	No positive family history.
• A broad dynamic syndrome rather than static disease.	A chronic progressive disorder.
• Wheezing is more pronounced than cough.	Cough is more pronounced and wheezing may or may not be present.
• Shape of the chest remains normal because of dynamic airway obstruction but AP diameter may increase with severe asthma.	Barrel-shaped chest (AP diameter ≥ transverse) in patients with predominant emphysema.
• Pursed-lip breathing is uncommon.	Pursed-lip breathing common.
• Respiratory movements may be normal or decreased, tracheal tug absent. Accessory muscles of respiration may be active and intercostal recession may be present.	Respiratory movements are usually decreased with: • Reduced palpable length of trachea with tracheal tug. • Reduced expansion. • Excavation of suprasternal notch, supraclavicular and infraclavicular fossae. • Widening of subcostal angle. • Intercostal recession. • Accessory muscles of respiration hyperactive.

Table 63.2: Gold criteria for severity of COPD

Gold stage	Severity	Symptoms	Spirometry
0	At risk	Chronic cough, sputum	Normal
I	Mild	With or without chronic cough or sputum production	FEV_1/FVC <70% FEV_1 = 80% predicted
II	Moderate	With or without chronic cough or sputum production	FEV_1/FVC <70% FEV_1 = 50 to 79% predicted
III	Severe	—do—	FEV_1/FVC <70% FEV_1 = 30–49%
IV	Very severe	—do—	FEV_1/FVC <70% FEV_1 = <30%
			Or
			FEV_1 <50% predicted with respiratory failure or signs of right heart failure

GOLD: Global Initiative for Obstructive Lung Disease

predominate over the other. Clinically, patients with predominant bronchitis are referred as *"blue-bloaters"* (blue refers to cyanosis, bloater-edema) and with predominant emphysema as pink puffers (pink refers to absence of cyanosis, puffers-pursed lip breathing).

Q. What are the signs of advanced airflow obstruction?

Ans: Main signs are as follows:
- Dyspnea and even orthopnea with pursed lip breathing (a physiologic response to decreased air entry).
- Excavation of the suprasternal notch, supraclavicular fossae during inspiration, together with in-drawing (recession) of intercostal spaces.
- Barrel-shaped chest (AP diameter ≥ transverse diameter) with horizontality of the ribs.
- A reduction in the length of palpable trachea above the suprasternal notch.
- Contractions of extrarespiratory (accessory) muscles on inspiration.
- Central cyanosis.
- Expiratory filling of neck veins.
- Flapping tremors and bounding pulses.
- Wheeze (rhonchi) especially on forced expiration.

Q. What do you understand by the term emphysema? What are its bedside diagnostic signs?

Ans: Emphysema is defined as hyperinflation or overdistention of air spaces (e.g. alveoli)

distal to terminal bronchioles as well as destruction of the alveolar septae.

Bedside Diagnostic Signs are:
- Pursed lip breathing.
- Barrel-shaped chest.
- Apex beat is not visible.
- Diminished movement of chest with reduced expansion.
- Diminished vocal fremitus and vocal resonance.
- Hyper-resonant percussion note on both sides.
- Cardiac and liver dullness masked.
- Heart sounds may get muffled.
- Usually wheeze or crackles are absent.
- Liver may become palpable due to descent of diaphragm.

Q. Why does a patient of COPD has pursed lip breathing?

Ans: Pursed lip breathing can occur both in COPD and bronchial asthma. A patient purses, her/his lips to maintain high intrabronchial pressure over and above that exists within surrounding alveoli so as to prevent the collapse of bronchial wall by these surrounding distend alveoli.

Q. What are the complications of COPD?

Ans: Common complications are as follows:
- *Pneumothorax* due to rupture of bullae.
- *Recurrent pulmonary infections.*
- *Cor pulmonale.*

Table 63.3: Differences between chronic bronchitis and emphysema

Features	Predominant chronic bronchitis (blue bloaters)	Predominant emphysema (pink puffers)
Age at the time of diagnosis (years)	60 ±	50 ±
Major symptoms	Cough > dyspnea, cough starts before dyspnea	Dyspnea ≥ cough, cough starts after dyspnea
Sputum	Copious, purulent	Scanty and mucoid
Cyanosis	Common	Usually absent
Episodes of respiratory infection	Frequent	Infrequent
Episodes of respiratory insufficiency	Frequent	Occurs terminally
Hyperinflation of lungs	Absent	Present
Breath sounds	Vesicular beathing with prolonged expiration	Vesicular breathing with diminished intensity
Chest X-ray	Enlarged cardiac shadow with increased bronchovascular markings	Increased translucency of lungs (hyperinflation), central tubular heart, low flat diaphragm
Compliance of lung	Normal	Decreased
Airway resistance	High	Normal or slightly increased
Diffusing capacity	Normal to slight decrease	Decreased
Arterial blood gas	Abnormal in the beginning	Normal until late
Chronic cor pulmonale	Common	Rare except terminally
Cardiac failure	Common	Rare except terminally

- *Congestive cardiac failure* (raised JVP, hepatomegaly, cyanosis, ascites, peripheral edema with RVH).
- *Type 2 respiratory failure* (CO$_2$ narcosis) with flapping tremors, bounding pulses, worsening hypoxia and hypercapnia.
- *Secondary polycythemia* due to hypoxia.

Clinical Tips
1. A sudden worsening of dyspnea after prolonged coughing indicate pneumothorax due to rupture of bullae.
2. Edema of the legs in COPD indicates CHF or secondary renal amyloidosis
3. Flaps on outstretched hands indicate type 2 respiratory failure.

Q.   How will you investigate the patient?

Ans: The following investigations are usually performed:
1. *Hemoglobin*, TLC, DLC and PCV for anemia or polycythemia and infection.
2. *Sputum examination.* It is unnecessary in case of COPD but during acute exacerbation, the organisms (*Strep. pneumoniae* or *H. influenza*) may be cultured. Sensitivity to be done, if organisms cultured.
3. *Chest X-ray* (Fig. 63.2) will show:
   - Increased translucency with large voluminous lungs.

- Prominent bronchovascular markings at the hilum with sudden pruning/truncation in peripheral fields.
- Bullae formation.
- Low flat diaphragm. Sometimes, the diaphragm shows undulations due to irregular pressure of bullae.
- Heart is tubular and centrally located.

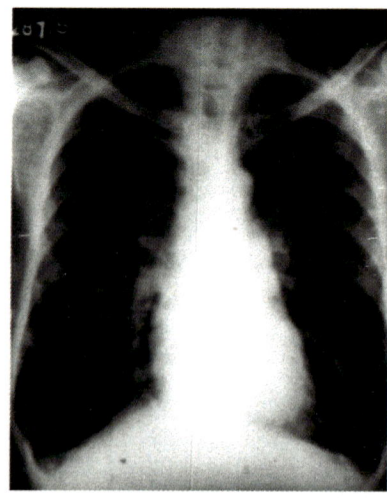

Fig. 63.2: Chest X-ray

Tip: An enlarged cardiac shadow with all of the above radiological findings suggests cor pulmonale.

4. *Electrocardiogram (ECG).* It may show:
   - Low voltage graph due to hyper-inflated lungs.
   - P-pulmonale may be present due to right atrial hypertrophy.
   - Clockwise rotation of heart.
   - Right ventricular hypertrophy (R>S in V1).

5. *Pulmonary function tests.* These show **obstructive ventilatory defect** (e.g. FEV_1, FEV_1 and FVC ratio and PEF all are reduced, **lung volumes**—total lung capacity and residual volume increased and transfer factor for CO is reduced).

6. *Arterial blood gas analysis may show reduced PaO_2 and increased $PaCO_2$* (hypercapnia).

7. *Alpha-1 antitrypsin levels:* Reduced level may occur in emphysema (normal range is 24 to 48 m mol/l).

Q. What is the role of high resolution CT scan in the diagnosis of emphysema?

Ans: It is most sensitive technique for diagnosis of emphysema. It is useful in evaluating symptomatic patients with normal pulmonary function except a low CO diffusing capacity.

Q. How would you differentiate COPD from restrictive lung disease on pulmonary from function tests?

Ans: Read Table 63.4.

Q. What do you understand by the term obstructive sleep-apnea syndrome?

Ans: Obstructive sleep-apnea syndrome is characterized by spells of apnea with snoring due to occlusion of upper airway at the level of oropharynx during sleep.

Apneas occur when airway at the back of throat is sucked closed during sleep. When awake, this tendency is overcome by the action of the muscles meant for opening the oropharynx which become hypotonic during sleep. Partial narrowing results in snoring, complete occlusion in apnea and critical narrowing in hyperventilation. The major features of this syndrome include, loud snoring, daytime somnolence, unfreshed or restless sleep, morning headache, noctural choking, reduced libido and poor performance at work, morning drunkenness and ankle edema. The patient's family report the pattern of sleep as "snore-silence-snore" cycle. The diagnosis is made if there are more than 15 apneas/hyperpneas in any one hour of sleep with fall in arterial O, saturation on ear or finger oximetry.

Q. What is the treatment of COPD?

Ans: Stable phase of COPD is treated by:
- **Cessation of smoking** and avoidance of precipitating factors.
- **Bronchodilator** — inhaled route of bronchodilatation is preferred than oral and parenteral route due to low side effects. Beta-agonists are commonly used. Tremors and trachycardia are common side effects.
- **Anticholinergics,** e.g. ipatropium bromide is not useful in chronic stable phase, is used in acute exacerbation for symptomatic relief.
- **Corticosteroids** —they are not useful in chronic phase, to be used for short-term in tapering doses in acute exacerbations.

Table 63.4: Pulmonary function tests in obstructive and restrictive lung defect		
Test	*Obstructive defect (COPD)*	*Restrictive defect (Interstitial lung disease)*
Forced expiratory volume during one second (FEV_1)	Markedly reduced	Slightly reduced
Vital capacity (VC)	Reduced or normal	Markedly reduced
FEV_1/VC ratio	Reduced	Increased or normal
Functional residual capacity (FRC)	Increased	Reduced
Peak expiratory flow (PEF)	Reduced	Normal
Residual volume (RV)	Increased	Reduced
Total lung capacity	Increased	Reduced
Transfer or diffusion factor for CO (T_{CO} and D_{CO})	Normal	Low
PaO_2	Decreased	Decreased
$PaCO_2$	Increased	Low or normal

- O_2 **therapy** — both the Medical Research Council Trial and Nocturnal O_2 therapy trial have documented the benefits of intermittent O_2 therapy for long hours in reducing the mortality in COPD.
- **Other agents:**
  i. N-Acetylecysteine is used as both mucolytic and antioxidant agent.
  ii. I.V alpha-antitrypsin therapy is available for severe deficiency of alpha 1-trypsin. Hepatitis vaccination is must prior to this therapy.
  iii. Lung transplantation is the last resort for end-stage lung disease.
  iv. *Surgical treatment*. Bullectomy can be done in severe bullous emphysema.

Q. What are the common precipitants of acute exacerbation?

Ans: Bacterial and viral respiratory infections.

Q. What are the organisms commonly associated with acute exacerbation?

Ans: *H. influenzae* and *S. pneumoniae* are the most common organisms
- *Moraxella catarrhalis, Chlamydia pneumoniae* and *Pseudomonas* are less common.

Q. What is the role of molecular genetics in COPD?

Ans: α_1-antitrypsin deficiency, increased production of tumor necrosis factor-alpha (TNF-α), increased generation of microsomal epoxide hydrolase during smoking are associated with increased risk of COPD.

Q. What is congenital lobar emphysema?

Ans: Infants rarely develop a check-valve mechanism in a lobar bronchus, which leads to rapid and life threatening unilateral overdistension of alveoli, called *congenital lobar emphysema*.

Q. What is unilateral emphysema? What are its causes?

Ans: Overdistension of one lung is called *unilateral emphysema*. It can be congenital or acquired (compensatory emphysema). Unilateral compensatory emphysema develops due to collapse or destruction of the whole lung or removal of one lung.

Macleod's or Swyer-James syndrome is characterised by unilateral emphysema

developing before the age of 8 years when the alveoli are increasing in number. This is an incidental radiological finding. In this condition, neither there is any obstruction nor there is destruction but there is overdistension of alveoli, hence, the term emphysema is not true to this condition. In this condition the number of alveoli are reduced which appear as larger airspaces with increased translucency on X-ray.

Q. What do you understand by the term bullous emphysema?

Ans: Confluent air spaces with dimension >1 cm are called *bullae*, may occasionally be congenital, but when occur in association with generalised emphysema or progressive fibrotic process, the condition is known as *bullous emphysema*. These bullae may rupture leading to pneumothorax.

Q. What is the treatment of COPD with acute exacerbation?

Ans: Read textbook of emergency medicine by Prof SN Chugh.

Q. What do you know about non-invasive ventilation?

Ans: Non-invasive ventilation is an alternative approach to endotracheal intubation to treat hypercapneic ventilatory failure which occurs in COPD. Non-invasive positive pressure ventilation (NIPPV) is delivered with a face mask to reduce the amount of internal dead space. Recently it has been shown that NIPPV reduces the hospital stay, need for endotracheal intubation and in hospital mortality in patients with acute exacerbation of COPD.

Q. What is the role of surgery in COPD?

Ans: 1. **Bullectomy:** It is indicated in selected patients with bullae larger than one third of the hemithorax and accompanying lung compression. It may improve oxygenation by improving gas exchange.
2. **Lung volume-reduction surgery:** It improves FEV_1, function of respiratory muscles, exercise capacity and quality of life.
3. **Single lung transplantation:** The criteria for lung transplantation have not been defined except end-stage lung disease.

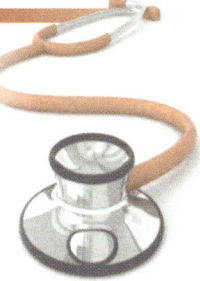

64 Lobar Consolidation

INSTRUCTION

Examine the chest of this patient

SALIENT FEATURES

- Sputum and hemoptysis, pain chest

HISTORY

Ask for the following:

- History of recent travel, local epidemics around point source suggest *Legionella* as the cause in middle to old age.
- History of large scale epidemics in the locality/region, associated sinusitis, pharyngitis, laryngitis suggest *Chlamydia* infection.
- History of underlying lung disease (bronchiectasis, fibrosis) with purulent sputum suggests secondary pneumonia (bronchopneumonia).
- History of past epilepsy, recent surgery on throat suggest aspiration pneumonia.

- History of co-existent debilitating illness, osteomyelitis or abscesses in other organs may lead to staphylococcal consolidation.
- History of contact with sick birds, farm animals suggest *Chlamydia psittaci* and *Coxiella burnetti* pneumonia.
- History of smoking suggests malignancy.
- History of recurrent episodes suggest secondary pneumonia.
- History of diabetes, intake of steroids or antimitotic drugs, AIDS suggest pneumonia in immunocompromised host.

EXAMINATION

General Physical Examination

- Red colored sputum (Fig. 64.1A)
- Toxic look, Fever (present)
- Tachypnea and Tachycardia (present)
- Cyanosis is absent
- Herpes labialis may be present
- Neck stiffness absent, if present, suggests meningitis as a complication

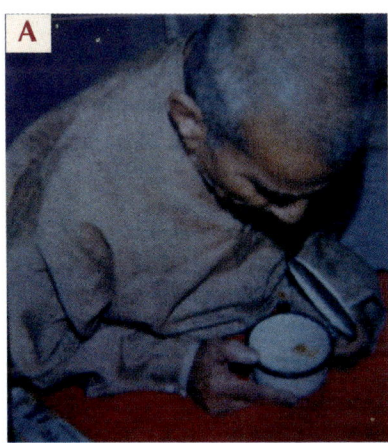
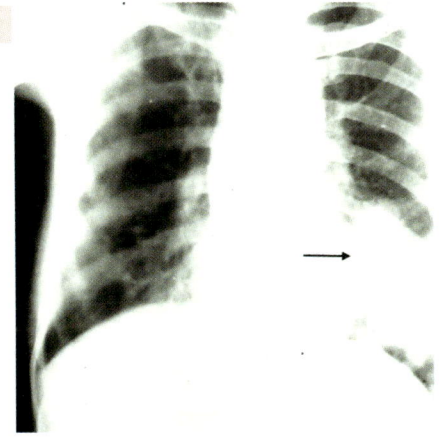

Fig. 64.1: Lobar consolidation. (A) Patient with sputum mixed with blood (hemoptysis); (B) Chest X-ray showing left lower lobe consolidation (→)

Systemic Examination

Inspection

- Shape of chest is normal
- In this case (Fig. 64.2), movements of left side of the chest are reduced
- Trachea central
- Apex beat normal
- No in-drawing of intercostal spaces; and accessory muscles of respiration are not working (active)

Palpation

- Restricted movement on the left side involved (present)
- Reduced expansion of the chest present on (left side in this case)
- Trachea and apex beat are normal in position
- Tactile vocal fremitus is *increased* on the left side over the part involved (in this case, in left lower chest)
- *Friction rub* may be palpable over the part of the chest involved (left lower chest)

Percussion

- Dull percussion note on the left side over the part of the chest involved (left lower anterior chest in this case).

Auscultation

The following findings will be present on the side and part involved (left lower anterior chest in this case).

- Bronchial breath sounds are present
- Increased vocal resonance with *bronchophony* and *whispering pectoriloquy*
- Aegophony (Not present)
- Pleural rub is present

PROVISIONAL DIAGNOSIS

The provisional clinical diagnosis in this case is left pneumonic consolidation (lesion) caused by pneumococcal infection (aetiology). Tuberculosis can also be the cause, hence, to be ruled out.

QUESTIONS AND ANSWERS

Q.　What is differential diagnosis?

Ans:　Read Table 64.1.

Q.　What is clinical triad of pneumonia?

Ans:　 i. *Cough and fever,*
　　　　 ii. *Chest pain* and
　　　　iii. *Hemoptysis* is a clinical triad of pneumonia.

Table. 64.1: Differential diagnosis of consolidation

I. Bronchogenic carcinoma
- Common in male, smokers, middle aged persons
- Hemoptysis is common.
- Cachexia/emaciation is present.
- Patient is not toxic.
- Clubbing may be present. There may be cervical lymphadenopathy.
- No shift of trachea or mediastinum unless there is associated pleural effusion.

II. Collapse of lung
- There is depression of the chest on the side involved. Movements are diminished on the involved side.
- Intercostal spaces are crowded. Trachea and mediastinum are shifted to same side.
- Impaired percussion note and decreased intensity of breath sounds.
- Patient is not toxic.
- History may be suggestive, e.g. aspiration, foreign body, trauma, postoperative condition.

III. Pleural effusion
- Gradual onset of cough and dyspnea.
- Chest may be prominent on the side involved.
- Trachea and mediastinum are shifted to opposite side.
- Stony dull percussion note with rising dullness in axilla.
- Vocal fremitus and vocal resonance are diminished over the area involved.
- There may a bronchial breathing (amphoric) or aegophony (increased vocal resonance) at the top of effusion posteriorly.

IV. Pulmonary infarct
- Sudden onset of chest pain, fever, hemoptysis.
- DVT may be present in leg(s).
- Patient is not toxic.
- Pleural rub may be present, P2 may become loud.
- ECG shows RVH or SI, QIII, TIII syndome.

Q.　What is the cause of chest pain in pneumonia?

Ans:　Chest pain in pneumonia is acute, occurs due to involvement of overlying pleura leading to friction between two layers of pleural.

Q.　What do you understand by the term consolidation? What are the stages of pneumonia and their clinical characteristics?

Ans:　Consolidation means solidification of the lung due to filling of the alveoli with inflammatory exudate. It represents second stage (red hepatisation) and third stage (gray hepatization) of pneumonia (Table 64.2).

Q.　Patient has consolidation on X-ray but is asymptomatic. How do you explain?

Ans:　Respiratory symptoms and signs in consolidation are often absent in elderly, alcoholics, immunocompromised and neutropenic patients.

Table. 64.2: Stages of pneumonia

I. *Stage of congestion*	Diminished vesicular breath sounds with fine inspiratory crackles due to alveolitis.
II. *Stage of red epatization*	All signs of consolidation present as mentioned.
III. *Stage of gray hepatization*	–do–
IV. *Stage of resolution*	• Bronchial breathing during consolidation is replaced either by bronchovesicular or vesicular breathing. • Mid inspiratory and expiratory crackles (coarse crepitations) appear. • All other signs of consolidation disappear.

Note: Children and young adults suffering from *Mycoplasma pneumonia* may have consolidation with few symptoms and signs in the chest, i.e. there is discrepancy between symptoms and signs with radiological appearance of consolidation or consolidation with non-patent bronchus may not produce physical signs on chest examination.

Q. What are the common sites of aspiration pneumonia?

Ans: The site of aspiration depends on the position of patient at the time of aspiration, i.e.

• Aspiration during supine position involves posterior segment of the upper lobe and superior segment of the lower lobe on the right side (right is more involved than left side).

• Aspiration in upright position involves basilar segments of both lower lobes.

Q. Enumerate the causes of consolidation.

Ans: Main causes of consolidation are as follows:
1. *Pneumonic* (lobar consolidation), may be bacterial, viral, fungal, allergic, chemical and radiation-induced.
2. Tuberculosis causes apical consolidation.
3. Malignancy (bronchogenic carcinoma).
4. Following massive pulmonary infarct (pulmonary embolism – may cause collapse consolidation).
5. Collagen vascular disorders.

Q. How pneumonia in young differs from pneumonia in old persons?

Ans: Pneumonias in young and old persons are compared in Table 64.3.

Table. 64.3: Differentiating features of pneumonia in younger and older persons

Pneumonia in young	*Pneumonia in old*
• Primary (occurs in previously healthy individuals)	Secondary (previous lung disease or immunocompromised state)
• Common organisms are; *Pneumococci, Mycoplasma, Chlamydia, Coxiella*	Common organisms are; *Pneumococci, H. influenzae, Legionella*
• Florid symptoms and signs	Few or no symptoms and signs
• Systemic manifestations are less pronounced	More pronounced systemic features
• Complications are less frequent	Complication are frequent
• Resolution is early	Resolution may be delayed
• Response to treatment is good and dramatic	Response to treatment is slow

Q. How do you classify pneumonias?

Ans: Pneumonias can be classified in various ways:

I. *Depending on the immunity and host resistance*
   • *Primary* (normal healthy individuals).
   • *Secondary* (host defence is lowered). It further includes:
      – Acute bronchopneumonia (lobar, lobular or hypostatic)
      – Aspiration pneumonia
      – Hospital-acquired pneumonia (nosocomial)
      – Pneumonias in immunocompromised host
      – Suppurative pneumonia including lung abscess

II. *Anatomical classification*
   • Lobar
   • Lobular (bronchopneumonia, bilateral)
   • Segmental (hypostatic pneumonia)

III. *Empiricist's classification (commonly used)*
   • *Community-acquired pneumonia (strep. pneumoniae, Mycoplasma, Chlamydia, Legionella, H. influenzae, virus, fungi, anaerobes, Mycobacterium).*
   • *Hospital-acquired pneumonia (Pseudomonas, B. proteus, Klebsiella, Staphylococcus, oral anaerobes).*
   • *Pneumonia in immunocompromised host (Pneumocystis carinii, Mycobacterium, S. pneumoniae, H. influenzae).*

Q. What are the characteristics of viral pneumonia?

Ans: Characteristics of viral pneumonia are:

- *Constitutional symptoms*, e.g. headache, malaise, myalgia, anorexia are predominant due to *influenza, para influenza measles* and *respiratory syncytial virus*).
- There may be no respiratory symptoms or signs and *consolidation* may just be discovered on *chest X-ray*.
- *Cough*, at times, with *mucoid expectoration*.
- *Hemoptysis, chest pain* (pleuritic) and pleural effusion are rare.
- Paucity of physical signs in the chest.
- *Chest X-ray* shows reticulonodular pattern instead of lobar consolidation.
- Spontaneous resolution
- WBC count is normal

Q. What do you understand about atypical pneumonia caused by *Mycoplasma pneumonia*?

Ans: *Mycoplasma pneumonia* is an important cause of community acquired pneumonia and epidemics of this pneumonia are common. The clinical features are

- Insidious onset, affects children and young adults. Incubation period is 1–3 weeks
- Commoner in winter season.
- Prodromal symptoms, e.g. headache, myalgia precede the pulmonary symptoms of pneumonia
- Clinically there are few signs in the chest
- Extrapulmonary manifestations are common, hence, called atypical
- Chest X-ray shows patchy consolidation. Hilar lymphadenopathy is common.
- Presence of cold agglutinins IgM type confirm the diagnosis

Q. What are the extrapulmonary manifestations of *Mycoplasma pneumonia*?

Ans: i. *Articular*, e.g. arthritis, arthralgia.
ii. *Cardiac*, e.g. pericarditis, myocarditis.
iii. *Blood*, e.g. autoimmune hemolytic anemia DIC.
iv. *Skin*, e.g. erythema nodosum, Stevens-Johnson's syndrome.
v. *Hepatitis and glomerulonephritis*.

Q. What are the characteristic of Staphylococcal pneumonia?

Ans: • Occurs at extremes of ages, coexisting debilitating illness, often complicates viral infection.
- Can arise from, or cause abscesses in other organs, e.g. osteomyelitis.
- Presents as bilateral pneumonia. Cavitation is frequent.

- X-ray chest shows lobar or segmental thin walled abscesses formation (pneumatoceles).

Q. What are the complications of bacterial pneumonia?

Ans: Common complications of pneumonia are:
- Pleural effusion and empyema thoracis
- Lung abscess, Meningitis, brain abscess
- Adult respiratory distress syndrome
- Circulatory failure (*Waterhouse Friedrichson's syndrome*)
- Septic arthritis, septicemia
- Pericarditis, congestive heart failure (myocarditis)
- Multiorgan failure, renal failure
- Peripheral thrombophlebitis
- Herpes labialis (secondary infection)

Q. What are the causes of recurrent pneumonia?

Ans: Recurrent pneumonias mean two or more attacks within a few weeks. It is due to either reduced/lowered resistance or there is a local predisposing factor, i.e.
- Chronic bronchitis
- Hypogammaglobulinemia
- Pharyngeal pouch
- Bronchial tumor
- GERD, achalasia cardia

Q. What is normal resolution? What is delayed resolution and non-resolution? What are the causes of delayed or non-resolution of pneumonia?

Ans: Normal resolution in a patient with pneumonia means disappearance of symptoms and signs within two weeks of onset and radiological clearance within four weeks. Delayed resolution means when physical signs persist for more than two weeks and radiological findings persist beyond four weeks after proper antibiotic therapy. *Non-resolution* means radiological findings persisting beyond eight weeks after proper antibiotic therapy. Causes are:
- Inappropriate antibiotic therapy.
- Presence of a complication (pleural effusion, empyema), underlying disease
- Depressed immunity, e.g. diabetes, alcoholism, steroids therapy, neutropenia, AIDS, hypogammaglobulinemia, old age.
- Partial obstruction of a bronchus by a foreign body like denture or a malignant tumor.
- Fungal or atypical pneumonia.
- Pneumonia due to SLE and pulmonary infarction or due to recurrent aspirations in GERD or cardia achalasia.

Q. How will you investigate a patient with community acquired pneumonia (CAP)?

Ans: 1. **Radiology:** Chest X-ray detects consolidation in most of the cases (Fig. 64.1). Air bronchogram may be diagnostic (Fig. 64.2). If pneumonia is suspected on clinical grounds and no opacity is seen on initial chest X-ray, it is useful to repeat either X-ray after 24-48 hours or perform CT scan. High resolution CT scan detects opacities in patients suspected of pneumonia but chest X-ray is normal.

2. **Blood culture:** The most common isolates, in ascending order before antibiotic therapy are; *S. pneumonia, S. aureus* and *E. coli.*

3. **Sputum stains and culture:** Gram's staining of sputum is used for presumptive etiologic diagnosis. Other types of sputum stainings are also useful for determining the cause of CAP. A variety of stains for acid-fast bacilli are used to diagnose tuberculosis. *Pneumocystis pneumonia* common in HIV patients can be diagnosed with monoclonal antibody staining. Special strains are also available for fungi, etc.

   Sputum should be sent for culture and sensitivity. Bronchoscopy and bronchoalveolar lavage may be attempted in case there is no sputum.

4. **Detection of antigens in urine:** Urine antigen test by ELISA is used to diagnose *Legionnaires disease.* Similarly, *S. pneumonia* urinary antigen detection by ELISA is also useful.

5. **Serology:** The detection of IgM antibody or demonstration of 4-fold rise in titre of antibody in blood to a particular agent between acute and convalescent phase is considered a good evidence that this agent is the cause of pneumonia. The various serological tests used include complement fixation, indirect immunofluorescence and ELISA. The following etiological agents are often diagnosed serologically, i.e. *Mycoplasma, C. pneumoniae, Chlamydia, Legionella* spp, *C. burnetti,* viruses (adeno, influenza, parainfluenza).

6. **Polymerase chain reaction (PCR):** A multiplex PCR allows detection of DNA of *Legionella* spp, *M. pneumoniae* and *C. pneumoniae.*

7. **Blood counts:** Leukocytosis with polymorphonuclear response indicates bacterial infection.

Q. What do you know about bronchopulmonary sequestration?

Ans: It is a congenital condition in which a portion of non-functioning lung tissue is detached from the normal lung and is supplied by an anomalous systemic artery which arises from the aorta or one of its branches, the segment/tissue has no bronchopulmonary connection/communication. The sequestration may be extralobar (sequestrated segment has separate pleural lining which separates it from the lung) or intralobar (portion or segment shares its pleura with the adjacent normal lung). The patients with lung sequestration present with cough, recurrent pneumonia and occasional hemoptysis.

Q. How do you diagnose pleural effusion in a patient with consolidation?

Ans: The clues to the diagnosis are:
- History suggestive of pneumonia (fever, chest pain, hemoptysis, cough) and persistence of these symptoms beyond 2–4 weeks.
- Signs of pleural effusion, e.g. stony dull percussion note, shifting of trachea and mediastinum to opposite side.
- The obliteration of costophrenic angle in presence of consolidation on chest x-ray (a pathognomonic sign).

Q. What is the mechanism of trachea being shifted to same side in consolidation?

Ans: Usually, trachea remains central in a case of consolidation, but may be shifted to the same side if;
- Consolidation is associated with collapse on the same side (Collapse consolidation due to malignancy).
- Consolidation is associated with underlying old fibrosis on the same side.

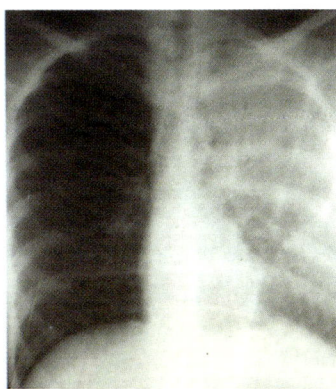

Fig. 64.2: Pneumonia chest X-ray shows left lung with air bronchogram

65

Bronchogenic Carcinoma

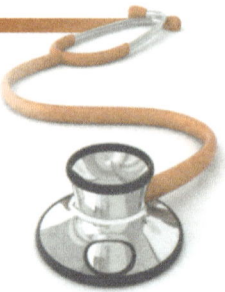

INSTRUCTION

Examine the patient's chest

SALIENT FEATURES

• Cough, pain chest and hemoptysis

HISTORY

Ask the following:

1. Cough, dyspnea, hemoptysis and chest pain (symptoms of primary tumor present).
2. History of fever, weakness, cachexia, weight loss, anorexia (malignancy).
3. History of hoarseness (present), suffusion of face, puffiness of face, chemosis and dysphagia (symptoms and signs of mediastinal obstruction).
4. History of hiccough (phrenic nerve involvement).
5. Ask about symptoms and signs of metastatic and non-metastatic manifestations of malignancy (common with adenocarcinoma).
6. History of smoking.

EXAMINATION

General Physical Examination

• Look at the face for puffiness, chemosis, suffusion, cyanosis, etc.
• Look at JVP. It is raised if malignancy produces superior vena cava obstruction. The waves on the jugular venous pulse will become absent if there is SVC obstruction (Read SVC obstruction).
• Neck for lymph nodes enlargement (present)
• Fingers for tar staining and clubbing.
• Edema feet and muscle wasting due to cachexia, (present).

Chest Examination

1. The chest examination in bronchogenic carcinoma may produce physical signs of con-

solidation, collapse and pleural effusion commonly. They have been discussed as separate cases. This patient has signs of collapse consolidation

PROVISIONAL DIAGNOSIS

The patient has consolidation of left upper lobe (lesion) probably due to bronchogenic carcinoma (aetiology) and has dyspnea at rest (functional status).

QUESTIONS AND ANSWERS

Q. What are the points in favor of the diagnosis?

Ans: 1. *Short duration of symptoms*, e.g. cough, expectoration, pain chest and hemoptysis.
2. Fever, weakness, anorexia, weight loss, night sweets.
3. Signs of left lobe collapse consolation (read next question) with hoarseness of voice and lymphadenopathy.
4. Edema and cachexia.

Q. What will be the features in malignant consolidation?

Ans: Common features in malignant consolidation are:
• Patient will be old and usually a smoker.
• History of dry persistent hacking cough, dyspnea, hemoptysis, pleuritic chest pain.
• There will be weight loss, emaciation due to malignant cachexia.
• Cervical lymphadenopathy may be present.
• Trachea will be central, but is shifted to same side if there is associated collapse or to the opposite if associated with pleural effusion.
• All signs of consolidation, i.e. diminished movements, reduced expansion, dull

percussion note, bronchial breathing may be present if bronchus is occluded. The bronchial breathing can occur from the adjoining patent bronchi. The bronchial breathing will, however, be absent if there is partial bronchial obstruction.

• Signs and symptoms of local spread, i.e. to pleura (pleural effusion), to hilar lymph nodes (dysphagia due to esoph-ageal compression, dysphonia due to recurrent laryngeal nerve involvement, diaphragmatic paralysis due to phrenic nerve involvement, superior vena cava compression), brachial plexus involve-ment (i.e. pancoast tumor producing monoplegia), cervical lymphadenopathy (Horner's syndrome — cervical sym-pathetic compression) may be evident.

• Sometimes, signs of distant metastases, e.g. hepatomegaly, spinal deformities, fracture of rib(s) are present.

• Nonmetastatic manifestations may occur.

Q.   What are the pulmonary manifestations of bronchogenic carcinoma?

Ans: It may present as;

• Localised *collapse* of the lung due to par-tial bronchial obstruction.

• *Consolidation*—a solid mass lesion.

• *Cavitation*—Secondary degeneration and necrosis in a malignant tumor leads to a cavity formation.

• *Mediastinal syndrome*—It will present with features of compression of struc-tures present in various compartments of mediastinum (superior, anterior, middle and posterior). These include:

• *Superior vena cava obstruction* with ed-ema of face, suffused eyes with chemosis, distended non-pulsatile neck veins, and prominent veins over the upper part of the chest as well as forehead (read case discussion on Superior Mediastinal Com-pression).

• Dysphonia and bovine cough due to compression of recurrent laryngeal nerve, stridor due to tracheal obstruction.

• Dysphagia due to esophageal compres-sion.

• Diaphragmatic paralysis—phrenic nerve compression.

• Intercostal neuralgia due to infiltration of intercostal nerves.

• Pericardial effusion due to infiltration of pericardium, myocarditis (arrhythmias, heart failure).

• Thoracic duct compression leading to chylous pleural effusion.

• Brachial plexus compression (pancoast tumor) producing monoplegia.

Q.   What are the extrapulmonary non-metastatic manifestations of carcinoma lung?

Ans: The paraneoplastic/non-metastatic extra-pulmonary manifestations occur in patients with *oat cell carcinoma* and are not due to local or distant metastatic spread. These are:

a. **Endocrinal** (hormones produced by the tumor)

   ACTH—Cushing's syndrome

   PTH—Hypercalcemia

   ADH—Hyponatremia

   Insulin-like peptide—Hypoglycemia

   Serotonin—Carcinoid syndrome

   Erythropoietin—Polycythemia

   Sex hormone—Gynecomastia

b. **Skeletal:** Digital clubbing

c. **Skin,** e.g. Acanthosis nigricans, pruritus

d. **Neurological:**

   • Encephalopathy

   • Myelopathy

   • Myopathy

   • Amyotrophy

   • Neuropathy

e. **Muscular:**

   • Polymyositis, dermatomyositis

   • Myasthenia — myopathic syndrome (*Lambert-Eaton syndrome*)

f. **Vascular:**

   • Migratory thrombophlebitis

g. **Hematological:**

   • Hemolytic anemia

   • Thrombocytopenia

Q.   Where do the distant metastases occur and what are the modes of spread in bronchogenic carcinoma?

Ans: It spreads to distant organs in three ways:

• *Lymphatic spread* involves mediastinal, cervical and axillary lymph nodes.

• *Hematogenous spread* involves liver, brain, skin, bone and subcutaneous tissue.

• *Transbronchial spread* leads to involve-ment of other side.

Q.   How would you investigate a patient with suspected malignant consolidation?

Ans: • *Sputum cytology:* It provides high yield for endobronchial tumors such as squamous cell and small cell carcinoma.

- *Chest X-ray* (Fig. 65.1). May reveal collapse of a part or whole lung
- *Pleural fluid* for biochemistry and cytology (malignant cells).
- *Bronchoscopy* gives a higher yield when tumor is accessible endobronchially.
- *CT scan* of the chest and upper abdomen for hilar lymphadenopathy, extent of growth, involvement of other structures and liver metastases.
- *Bone scan* for bone metastases.

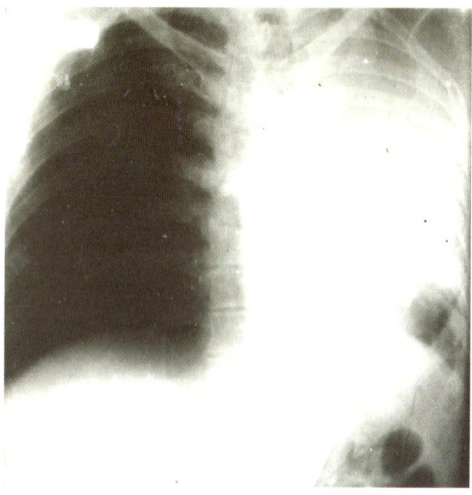

Fig. 65.1: Bronchogenic carcinoma. X-ray chest (PA view) showing malignant collapse of the left lung with hypertrophic emphysema (Rt lung)

- *PET scanning* is highly sensitive and specific for mediastinal staging.
- *Pulmonary function tests* so as to evaluate the patient for treatment.

Q. **What is the aim of staging bronchogenic carcinoma?**

Ans: The main aim of staging is to identify candidates for surgery, since this approach offers higher potential cure for lung cancer. The staging assessment covers 3 major issues; distant metastases, state of the chest and mediastinum and the condition of the patient.

Q. **What is the role of surgery in lung cancer?**

Ans: Surgery is beneficial in peripheral non small cell carcinoma. Its role is limited in small cell carcinoma.

Q. **Which tumors respond to chemotherapy?**

Ans: Small cell carcinoma. The drugs used include cyclophosphamide, doxorubicin, cisplatin, etoposide and vincristine. The combination of etoposide and cisplatin appears to have the best therapeutic index of any regimen.

Q. **What are the indications of radiotherapy in bronchogenic carcinoma?**

Ans: • Pain either local or metastatic
- Breathlessness due to bronchial obstruction
- Dysphagia
- Hemoptysis
- Pancoast tumor
- Mediastinal compression/superior vena cava obstruction
- Before and after surgery

66

Pleural Effusion

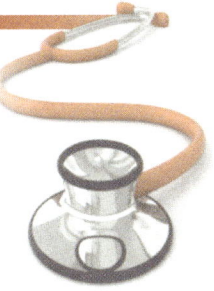

INSTRUCTION

Examine the patient's chest

SALIENT FEATURES

- Complains of dyspnea and chest discomfort

HISTORY

Ask for the following:

- History of fever, cough, rigors, removal of fluid in the past. History of hemoptysis
- History of trauma
- Past/present history of tuberculosis, malignancy
- Occupational history (exposure to asbestos)
- Any skin rash, swelling of joints, lymphadenopathy
- Any history of dysentery in the past
- Is there history of edema, pain abdomen, distension of abdomen (ascites), edema legs?
- Any menstrual irregularity in female
- History of drug taken or being taken.

EXAMINATION

General Physical Examination (GPE)

- Any puffiness of face or malar flush.
- Fever, tachypnea, tachycardia (pyogenic infection)
- Patient prefers to lie in lateral position of uninvolved side (left side in this case)
- *Emaciation, clubbing* of fingers and tar stain.
- Cervical lymph nodes may be palpable if effusion is tubercular.
- Neck veins may be full due to kinking of superior vena cava or raised JVP.
- Signs of underlying cause, e.g. rheumatoid hands or butterfly rash (SLE).
- Edema may be present if pleural effusion is due to a systemic disorder.

- Look for any rash, arthritis/arthralgia.
- Note the vitals, pulse, BP, temperature and respiration.
- Comment on aspiration mark, mastectomy scar or radiation mark, if present.

Chest Examination (Fig. 66.1B)

Inspection
- Respiratory rate (increased).
- Restricted respiratory movements on affected side (right side in this case).
- Intercostal spaces are full and appear widened on the affected side (right side in this case).

Palpation
- Diminished movements on the side involved (right side in this case).
- Chest expansion on measurement is reduced.
- Trachea and apex beat (mediastinum) shifted to opposite side (left side in this case).
- Vocal fremitus reduced or absent on affected side (right side in this case).
- No tenderness.
- Occasionally, in early effusion, pleural rub may be palpable (not present).

Percussion
- Stony dull note over the area of effusion on the affected side (right side in this case).
- Rising dullness in axilla (S shaped Ellis' curve) due to capillary action.
- Skodiac band of resonance at the upper level of effusion because of compensatory emphysema.
- No shifting dullness.
- No tenderness of ribs.

Auscultation
- Breath sounds are absent over the fluid (right side in this case).
- Vocal resonance is reduced over the area of effusion (right side in this case).
- Sometimes, *bronchial breathing* (tubular — high pitched), *bronchophony, whispering pectoriloquy*

and *egophony* present at the upper border (apex) of pleural effusion (present over right interscapular region in this case).
- Pleural rub can be heard in some cases (not present).

PROVISIONAL DIAGNOSIS

The diagnosis is pleural effusion right side (lesion) probably due to tuberculosis (etiology). Patients complains of breathlessness on exertion (functional status).

QUESTIONS AND ANSWERS

Q.   **What are the points in favor of your diagnosis?**

Ans: The features in support of diagnosis are:
   i. Diminished movements on the involved side.
   ii. Trachea and mediastinum shifted to opposite side.
   iii. Stony dull percussion note with rising dullness in right axilla.
   iv. Vocal fremitus reduced on the side involved.
   v. Breath sounds absent over the effusion but there is a patch of bronchial breath sound with egophony at the top of effusion on the back on right side.

Q.   **What are the causes of dullness at lung base?**
Ans: • Pleural effusion
     • Thickened pleura
     • Collapse of lung
     • Raised hemidiaphragm due to amebic liver abscess or ascites

Q.   **What do you understand by pleural effusion?**
Ans: Normal pleural space on each side contains 50 to 150 ml of fluid but excessive collection of fluid above the normal value is called *pleural effusion* which may or may not be detected clinically. Fluid between 150 and 300 ml can be detected radiologically by chest X-ray (obliteration of costophrenic angle). More than 500 ml fluid can be detected clinically.
     Note: USG of the chest is the earliest means of detecting the small amount of fluid.

Q.   **What is transudative or exudative pleural effusion?**
Ans: Biochemically, the fluid may be transudate or exudate; the differences between the two are summarised in Table 66.1.

Q.   **What are the causes of transudative and exudative pleural effusion?**
Ans: The causes are given in Table 66.2

Table 66.1: Characteristics of pleural fluid

Fluid	Transudate (SFAG > 1.1)	Exudate (SFAG < 1.1)
1. Appearance	Clear, light yellow	Straw-colored, turbid or purulent, milky or hemorrhagic
2. Protein	<3 g% or <50% of serum proteins	>3 g% or >50% of serum proteins
3. Serum fluid albumin gradient	>1.1	<1.1
4. Glucose	Normal	Low
5. pH	>7.3	<7.3
6. Cells (WBCs)	<1000/mm^3	Usually >1000/mm^3
7. Fluid LDH	<2/3rd of serum LDH	>2/3rd of serum LDH
8. Fluid/serum LDH ratio	<0.6	>0.6
9. Fluid adenosine deaminase	Low	High
10. Fluid cholesterol	Low (<60 mg/dl)	High (>60 mg/dl)
11. Culture	Sterile	May yield organism

SFAG: Serum fluid albumin gradient.

Table 66.2: Causes of pleural effusion depending on the fluid characteristic

Common	Uncommon
I. Transudate (SFAG > 1.1)	
• Congestive heart failure • Cirrhosis of liver • Nephrotic syndrome • Hypoproteinemia due to any cause • Pericardial effusion	• Superior vena cava obstruction • Myxedema • Peritoneal dialysis • Meig's syndrome
II. Exudate (SFAG < 1.1)	
• Infections, e.g. tubercular, bacterial (pneumonia), viral	• Chylothorax • Pancreatitis • Esophageal perforation
• Malignancy, e.g. bronchogenic (common), mesothelioma (rare), lymphoma rare	• Subphrenic abscess • Post-cardiac injury syndrome
• Collagen vascular disorders e.g. SLE, rheumatoid arthritis, Wegener's granulomatosis • Pulmonary emboli • Sarcoidosis, Asbestosis	• Uremia • Radiation injury • *Drug-induced effusion,*
• Ruptured liver abscess into pleural space	*e.g.* nitrofurantoin, gold, bromocriptine, procarbazine, amiodarone

Q. **What does raised fluid ADA level indicate?**

Ans: Tubercular effusion or effusion due to rheumatoid arthritis.

Q. **Name the drugs causing pleural effusion?**

Ans: Read Table 66.2.

Q. **What do you understand by the term chylous, pseudochylous and chyliform pleural fluid?**

Ans: The milky or white-looking fluid may be chylous, pseudochylous, chyliform or cholesterol fluid, the difference among them are listed in Box I.

Q. **What are the causes of hemorrhagic effusion?**

Ans: *Hemorrhagic effusion (Hemothorax, e.g. blood stained fluid or fluid containing RBCs)* is caused by:

BOX I: Differences between various types of milky fluid

Chylos (milky) effusion (Triglyceride > 1000 mg% with many large fat globules)
- Nephrotic syndrome
- Filariasis
- Tubercular
- Myxedema
- Malignancy
- Trauma to chest wall
- Lymphoma

N.B Ether extraction dissolves fat and leads to clearing; confirms true chylous nature of fluid.

Chyliform (fat present is not derived from thoracic duct but from degnerated leukocytes and tumor cells). The *causes are*:
- Tubercular
- Carcinoma of lung and pleura

Pseudochylous. Milky appearance is not due to fat but due to albumin, calcium, phosphate and lecithin. *Causes are*:
- Tuberculosis
- Nephrosis
- Heart disease
- Malignancy

N.B Alkalinisation dissolves cellular protein and clears the fluid thus differentiates it from true chylous.

Cholesterol effusion (Glistening opalescent fluid due to cholesterol crystals). *Causes are*:
- Long standing effusion, e.g. tuberculosis, carcinoma, nephrotic syndrome, myxedem and post myocardial infarction.

- Neoplasm, e.g. primary mesothelioma or secondaries in the lung with pleural involvement
- Chest trauma (during paracentesis)
- Tubercular effusion
- Leukemias and lymphoma
- Pulmonary infarction
- Bleeding diathesis:
  - Anticoagulant therapy
  - Acute hemorrhagic pancreatitis

Q. **What are the causes of unilateral (right) and bilateral pleural effusion?**

Ans: I. **Bilateral pleural effusion.** The causes are:
- Congestive heart failure

- Collagen vascular disease, e.g. SLE, rheumatoid arthritis
- Lymphoma and leukemias
- Bilateral tubercular effusion (rare)
- Pulmonary infarction

II. **Unilateral right side pleural effusion.** The causes are:
- Rupture of acute amebic liver abscess into pleura
- Cirrhosis of the liver
- Congestive cardiac failure
- Meig's syndrome — fibroma of ovary with pleural effusion and ascites

Q. **What are the causes of recurrent pleural effusion?**

Ans:
- Malignancy lung (e.g. bronchogenic, mesothelioma)
- Pulmonary tuberculosis
- Congestive heart failure
- Collagen vascular disorder

Q. **What is Meig's syndrome?**

Ans: It comprises right sided transudative pleural effusion associated with an ovarian tumor usually benign (e.g. fibroma).

Q. **What is phantom tumor (pseudotumor)?**

Ans: This is an interlobar effusion (effusion in interlobar fissure) producing a homogenous opacity on chest X-ray. This mimics a tumor due to its dense opacity, but disappears with resolution of effusion, hence, called *phantom tumor.* This is occasionally seen in congestive heart failure and disappears with diuretic therapy.

Q. **What is subpulmonic effusion? When would you suspect it?**

Ans: A collection of fluid below the lung and above the diaphragm is called *subpulmonic effusion.* This is suspected when diaphragm is unduly elevated on one side on chest X-ray. Chest X-ray taken in lateral decubitus position shows pleural effusion (layering out of the opacity along the lateral chest wall) which confirms the diagnosis.

Q. **How do you explain the position of trachea either as central or to the same side in a case with pleural effusion?**

Ans: Remember that negative intrapleural pressure on both sides keeps the trachea central, but it is shifted to opposite side when a positive pressure develops in one of the pleural space, therefore, midline trachea despite pleural effusion on one side could be due to:
- *Mild pleural effusion* (insignificant positive pressure develops).

- *Loculated or encysted pleural effusion* (positive pressure develops but not transmitted to opposite side — no pushing effect).
- *Bilateral pleural effusion* (both pleural cavities have positive pressure that neutralise each other's effect).
- *Pleural effusion associated with apical fibrosis* (fibrosis pulls the trachea to same side and neutralises the pushing effect of pleural effusion on the same side).
- *Malignant pleural effusion with absorption collapse* due to endobronchial obstruction. Due to collapse, trachea tries to shift towards the same side, but pushing effect of effusion keeps it central in position.
- *Collapse consolidation* due to any cause (Isolated collapse and isolated consolidation has opposing effects).

Q.   What are the signs at the apex (upper level) of pleural effusion?

Ans: The following signs develop only and occasionally in moderate (500–1000 ml) pleural effusion.
- *Rising dullness*; S-shaped Ellis curve in axilla.
- *Skodiac resonance* — a band of hyperresonance due to compensatory emphysema.
- *Bronchial breathing* — high pitched tubular with bronchophony, whispering pectoriloquy and aegophony.
- *Pleural rub* — rarely.

Q.   What are the causes of recurrent filling of pleural effusion after paracentesis?

Ans: Recurrent filling of the pleural effusion means appearance of the fluid to same level or above it on X-ray chest within few days (rapid filling) to weeks (slow filling) after removal of the fluid. That is the reason, a chest X-ray is taken before and after removal of the fluid to know the result of the procedure, its complications and later on its refilling. The causes are:
1. *Rapid refilling of pleural effusion*
   - Malignancy and acute tuberculosis
2. *Slow refilling*
   - Tubercular effusion on treatment.
   - Congestive cardiac failure — slow response or no response to conventional diuretics
   - Collagen vascular disorders
   - Meig's syndrome

Q.   What are the pathogenic mechanism of pleural effusion?

Ans. 1. Involvement of pleura by malignants infiltration, involvement by primary tumor or inflammatory process resulting in increased permeability.
2. Disruption of fluid containing structures in pleural cavity such as thoracic duct, esophagus, blood vessels with leakage of contents into pleural space.
3. Rupture of subpleural lung abscess or amoebic liver abscess into pleura.
4. Abnormal hydrostatic or lower osmotic pressure on an otherwise healthy pleura leading to transudation into pleural cavity.

Q.   What are the complications of pleural effusion?

Ans: Common complications are:
- *Thickened pleura* (healed effusion).
- *Empyema thoracis* — spontaneous or iatrogenic (introduction of infection with improperly sterilized needle).
- *Non-expansion of the lung* — Usually, after removal of pleural fluid, there is reexpansion of the compressed lung immediately, but sometimes in long standing cases, it may not occur.
- *Acute pulmonary edema* develops with sudden withdrawal of a large amount of fluid. It is uncommon.
- *Hydropneumothorax* is again iatrogenic (procedural complication) due to lung injury and leakage of air into pleural space during pleural aspiration.
- *Cachexia* may develop in longstanding and malignant pleural effusion.

Q.   What are clinical differences between thickened pleura and pleural effusion?

Ans. The differences are:

Thickened pleura	Pleural effusion
• Chest is normal or retracted on the side involved	• Chest is normal or prominent on side involved
• Movements are diminished.	• Movement of chest are markedly diminished.
• No shift of trachea or mediastinum	• Trachea and mediastinum is shifted to opposite side
• Percussion note is impaired with no rising dullness	• Percussion note is stony dull and there is rising dullness
• Breath sounds are just diminished over the side involved	• Breath sounds are absent over the area of effusion

Q. What are causes of lymphadenopathy with pleural effusion?

Ans. Common causes are:
- *Tubercular lymphadenitis* with pleural effusion (lymph node in cervical, axillary, mediastinal regions may be enlarged).
- *Lymphomas* (effusion with generalised lymphadenopathy and splenomegaly).
- *Acute lymphoblastic leukemia* (cervical and axillary lymph nodes enlargement).
- *Malignancy lung* (scalene node, Virchow's gland, mediastinal lymph node).
- *Collagen vascular disorder* (generalised lymphadenopathy).
- *Sarcoidosis* (cervical, bilateral hilar lymphadenopathy).

Q. What are differences between tubercular and malignant pleural effusion?

Ans. Tubercular and malignant pleural effusions are differentiated in Table 66.3.

Table 66.3: Differentiating features between tubercular and malignant pleural effusion

Tubercular	Malignant
A. Clinical characteristics:	
• Commonest cause of effusion in all age groups	Common cause in old age
• Slow, insidious onset, can be acute or sudden	• Acute sudden onset
• Slow filling	• Rapid filling
• Cough, fever (evening rise), hemoptysis, night sweats are common complaints	• Cough, hemoptysis, dyspnea, tightness of chest are presenting symptoms
• Cervical, axillary lymph nodes may be enlarged	• Scalene nodes or Virchow's gland enlarged
• Weakness, loss of weight present	• Marked cachexia and prostration.
• Clubbing uncommon	• Clubbing common
• No signs of local compression	• Signs of local compression, e.g. superior vena cava trachea esophagus, and phrenic nerve may be accompanying symptoms
• Localized crackles or rhonchi may be present depending on the site and type of lung involvement	• Localized wheeze or rhonchi common than crackles
B. Fluid characteristics	
• Straw-coloured exudate	• Hemorrhagic, exudate.
• Lymphocytes present	• Malignant cells may be present along with RBCs
• Cob-web coagulum on standing	• RBCs may settle down on standing if hemorrhagic

Q. How will you investigate a case of pleural effusion?

Ans. A pleural effusion being of varied etiology, needs investigations for confirmation of the diagnosis as well as to find out the cause.

1. *Routine blood tests* (TLC, DLC and ESR). High ESR and lymphocytosis go in favor of tubercular effusion.
2. *Blood biochemistry:*
   - Serum amylase for pancreatitis.
   - Autoantibodies for collagen vascular disorders.
   - Rheumatoid factor for rheumatoid arthritis.
3. *Chest X-ray* (PA view, Fig. 66.1A) shows:
   - A lower homogenous opacity with a curved upper border which is concave medially but rising laterally towards the axilla.
   - Obliteration of costophrenic angle. It is the earliest sign hence, present in all cases of pleural effusion irrespective of its cause except loculated or encysted effusion.
   - Shift of trachea and mediastinum to opposite side.
   - Lateral view is done to differentiate it from lobar consolidation.
   - Lateral decubitus view is taken in case of subpulmonic effusion.
   - Repeat X-ray chest after therapeutic aspiration of fluid.
4. *Sputum examination:*
   - For AFB and malignant cells.
5. *Mantoux test:* It is not much of diagnostic value, may be positive in tuberculosis, negative in sarcoidosis, lymphoma and disseminated (miliary) tuberculosis or tubercular effusion in patients with AIDS.
6. *FNAC of lymph node,* if found enlarged.
7. *Ultrasonography*
8. *CT scan and MRI* are usually not required for diagnosis, but can be carried out to find out the cause wherever appropriate, and to differentiate localised effusion from pleural tumor.
9. *Aspiration of pleural find for* confirmation of diagnosis (Fig. 66.1B).

   At least 50 ml of fluid is to be removed and subjected to:
   - biochemistry (transudate/exudate), LDH, ADA, cholesterol and pH of fluid if empyema is suspected.

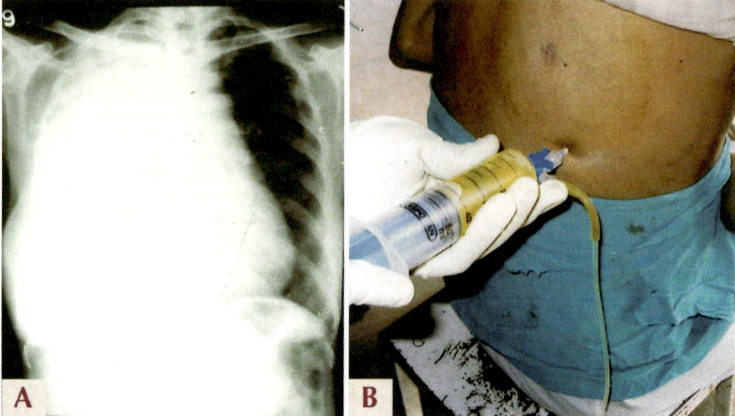

Fig. 66.1: Pleural effusion. (A) X-ray chest showing pleural effusion right side; (B) Removal of pleural fluid from a patient with right-sided pleural effusion

- cytology (for malignant cells, RBCs, WBCs and pus cells).
- smear examination (e.g. Gram stain, Ziehl-Neelsen stain, special stains for malignant cells).
- culture for AFB. Recently introduced BACTEC system gives result within 7 days. Amylase level when malignancy or pancreatitis is suspected.

10. *Bronchoscopy* in a suspected case of bronchogenic carcinoma.
11. *Pleural biopsy* for histopathological examination (confirms the aetiology) and mycobacterial culture
12. *Thoracoscopy* to inspect the pleura so as to find out the cause. It is done rarely.

Q. **What are the uses of ultrasonography in pleural effusion?**

Ans. Uses other than hilar lymphadenopathy are:
1. For diagnosis of loculated effusions.
2. For guided thoracocentesis, closed pleural biopsy or insertion of a chest drain.
3. To differentiate pleural fluid from pleural thickening.

Q. **Name the conditions in which fluid pH and glucose concentration are low.**

Ans.
- Empyema thoracis
- Malignancy lungs
- Tuberculosis of lung
- Rheumatoid pleural effusion
- SLE with effusion

67

Empyema Thoracis

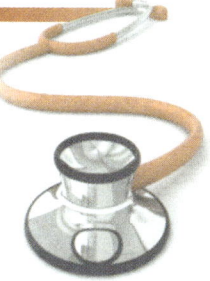

INSTRUCTION

Examine the patient's chest

SALIENT FEATURES

- Fever, chest pain, breathlessness

HISTORY

Ask about the following:

- Fever (swinging temperature), sweats, weakness
- Pleuritic chest pain and breathlessness, tachypnea
- History of palpitation, tachycardia (present)
- History of cough with purulent (fetid) sputum (lung abscess, bronchiectasis)
- History of chest injury (hemithorax)
- History of tapping the pleural effusion or presence of a scar
- History of recurrent pneumonia or aspirations (aspiration pheumonia)

EXAMINATION

General Physical Examination

- Patient is febrile, having a toxic look, sunken cheeks
- Pulse shows tachycardia: BP is normal
- Respiratory rate (increased in this case)
- Look at the sputum cup which shows fetid purulent sputum
- Clubbing of the fingers (present)
- Oedema feet due to hypoproteinemia
- Muscle wasting due to toxemia (present)

Chest Examination (Fig. 67.1)

Inspection and Palpation

- Trachea is central or deviated to same side or opposite side (left side in this case)
- Respiratory rate (high in this case)

- Decreased movement on the affected side (right side in this case)
- In-drawing of ribs/intercostal recession on the affected side (right side in this case)

Percussion

- Stony dull note on percussion on the affected side. There is no rising dullness (Dullness is flat, does not rise in axilla in this case).
- Intercostal spaces are normal or narrow (thickened pleura).
- Vocal fremitus is decreased on the affected side (right side in this case).

Auscultation

- Decreased or absent breath sounds on the affected side (right side).
- Decreased vocal resonance (right side).

PROVISIONAL DIAGNOSIS

In view of signs of pleural effusion with features of toxemia, the patient probably has empyema thoracis right side (lesion) due to pyogenic infection (aetiology), and has intercostal tube inside for drainage (functional status).

QUESTIONS AND ANSWERS

Q. What are the points in favor of your diagnosis?

Ans:
- Patient has a toxic look and prostration
- Signs of toxemia (fever, tachypnea and tachycardia). There is hectic rise of temperature with chills and rigors
- Digital clubbing
- Intercostal spaces are full and tender (right side)
- All signs of pleural effusion are present on right side with flat dullness in axilla. This is due to collection of thick pus rather than

clear fluid which does not obey the law of capillary action

- The skin is red, edematous and glossy overlying empyema (recent onset)
- There may be a scar mark of an intercostal drainage (tube aspiration is being done in this case)
- Rarely, a subcutaneous swelling on the chest wall may be seen called *empyema necessitans*. The swelling increases with coughing (not present in this case)

Q. What is empyema thoracis?

Ans: Collection of pus or purulent material or infected pleural fluid in the pleural cavity is called *empyema thoracis*.

Q. What are its causes?

Ans: The causes are:
1. *Diseases of the lung* (infection travels from the lung to the pleura either by contiguity or by rupture)
   - Lung abscess
   - Pneumonia
   - Tuberculosis
   - Infection
   - Bronchiectasis
   - Bronchopleural fistula
2. *Diseases of the abdominal viscera* (spread of infection from abdominal viscera to pleura)
   - Liver abscess (ruptured or unruptured)
   - Subphrenic abscess
   - Perforated peptic ulcer
3. *Diseases of the mediastinum.* There may be infective focus in the mediastinum from which it spreads to the pleura.
   - Cold abscess
   - Esophageal perforation
   - Osteomyelitis
4. *Trauma with superadded infection*
   - Chest wall injuries (gun-shot wound, stab wound)
   - Postoperative
5. *Iatrogenic infection introduced* during procedure
   - Chest aspiration
   - Liver biopsy
6. *Blood-borne infection,* e.g. septicemia

Q. How would you differentiate between empyema and thickened pleura?

Ans: Thickened pleura develops during the resolution or healing of empyema thoracis.

The difference are:

Thickened Pleura	Empyema Thoracis
1. Signs of toxemia absent	Signs of toxemia, e.g. fever present
2. Chest is retracted on the affected side	Chest is normal in shape
3. Trachea is shifted to same side	Trachea is central
4. Intercostal spaces are narrowed	Intercostal spaces are normal.
5. Impaired note or dullness	Stony dull note
6. Breath sound are diminished	Breath sound are absent

Q. How would you investigate such a case?

Ans: 1. *Complete hemogram.* The hemoglobin may be low.
2. *Total leucocyte count.* There is neutrophilic leucocytosis.
3. **Chest X-ray.** This will show the radiological signs of pleural effusion (read pleural effusion) but the presence of a catheter/drainage tube mark on radiology confirms the diagnosis.
4. *Sputum examination* for pus cells.
5. **Pleural fluid aspirate** and its analysis. Fluid removed is thick, white in color, may be looking exudative or pus like. Biochemistry of the fluid shows raised pleural protein, low sugar and neutrophila in the fluid. It should be sent for culture and sensitivity. A Gram staining should be done on the bed side.
6. **CT scan.** It will visualise the underlying cause as well as confirm thick fluid and the presence of thickening of the pleura or fibrotic bands crossing the pleural cavity.

Q. What is the role of pleural fluid cytology in diagnosis of pleural effusion?

Ans: • **Pleural fluid cell count:** Counts >50,000 with neutrophilia are seen in para-pneumonic effusion or empyema, whereas low count <1000 cells/HPF indicates transudate (noninfective aetiology).
- *Pleural fluid lymphocytosis* indicates tuberculosis, malignancy, collagen vascular disease, lymphoma and sarcoidosis.
- *Computerized interactive morphometry* (analyses the size and nuclei of cells in a centrifuged specimen of fluid) differentiates between malignant cells and reactive lymphocytosis.

Q.   What is the treatment of empyema thoracis?

Ans: 1. *Antibiotics* according to pus culture and sensitivity.

2. *Drainage of the fluid.* A large bore needle should be used to drain the fluid during diagnostic aspiration. If fluid is thick and pus like, tube thoracostomy drainage (Fig. 67.1) of the empyema is indicated.

3. *Intrapleural instillation of fibrinolytic agent* (streptokinase or urokinase) to liquefy the pus and improve the drainage.

4. *Decortication* is indicated if above measure fails or when empyema is recurrent.

Q.   What is the clinical hallmark that differentiates between pleural effusion and empyema?

Ans: The basic clinical difference between pleural effusion and empyema is:

1. The presence of signs of toxemia, flat stony dull percussion note, absence of rising dullness, clubbing of fingers, no shift of trachea or mediastinum indicate empyema rather than pleural effusion.

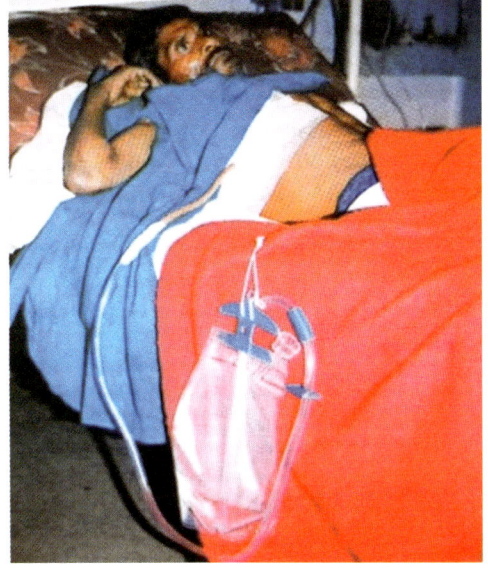

Fig. 67.1: Intercostal tube drainage in empyema thoracis

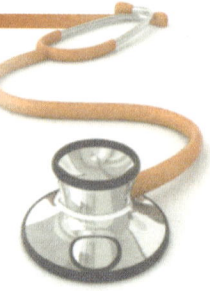

68

Pleural Rub

INSTRUCTION

Examine the patient's chest.

SALIENT FEATURES

- Pain chest on left side which increases on coughing and during deep breathing

HISTORY

Ask about the following:

- Patient is disturbed, winces frequently due to pain and puts the left hand over the left chest to reduce pain.
- Is pain sharp and localised?
- Ask whether pain increases on coughing, sneezing or respiration (yes, in this case)
- Ask the factors which relieve the pain.
- Does the pain radiate to shoulder, neck, etc.?
- Ask about cough and expectoration, fever and sore throat or URC.
- History of hemoptysis.
- History of use of oral contraceptives.

EXAMINATION

General Physical Examination

- Patient is distressed due to pain, wants to mobilise the chest on left side with left hand to reduce pain.
- There is tachypnea and sweating.
- *Pulse shows* rapid rate, good volume no, abnormal character.
- BP is normal.

Chest Examination

- A pleural rub (scratching sound) is palpable in the left upper part of the chest.
- *On auscultation*, heart sounds and breath sounds are normal. There is superficial scratchy, grating sound heard on deep inspiration and expiration (Fig. 68.1).
- Ask the patient to cough and listen to the abnormal sound and note any change in the character. If there is no change then it is pleural rub (no change in this patient).
- Listen for gallop rhythm, if present.

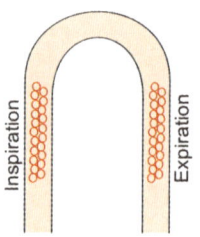

A. Crackles
   (Discontinuous
   rusting or
   bubling sounds)

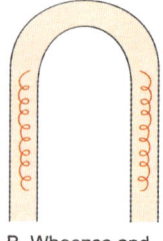

B. Wheezes and
   rhonchi (musical
   continuous sounds)

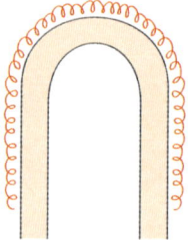

C. Pleural rub
   (extrapulmonary
   rubbing or
   cracking continuous
   sound)

Fig. 68.1: Characteristics of common pulmonary and extrapulmonary sound (diagram)

PROVISIONAL DIAGNOSIS

The patient has pleurisy (pleural rub) the cause of which has to be found out. Patient is in distress due to pain (functional status).

QUESTIONS AND ANSWERS

Q. **What are the causes of pleural rub?**

Ans. The causes are:
1. Pleurodynia
2. Heard over a patch of consolidation
3. Pulmonary embolism (infarction)
4. Following pleural biopsy
5. Mesothelioma or malignant infiltration into pleura

Q. **Could it be pericardial rub?**

Ans: No. Points against are:
1. *Location.* It is peripherally located
2. *Relation to respiration.* It increases both during inspiration and expiration.
3. *No relation of heart sounds.*
4. *No evidence of heart disease,* e.g. myocarditis or percarditis

Q. **What are the differences between pleural rub and crackles?**

Ans. Read the Clinical Methods in Medicine by Prof. SN Chugh.

The differences are summarised in Box I

Box I: Differences between pleural rub and coarse crackles

Pleural rub	Coarse crackles
• Rubbing or scratching or grating sound	Bubbling or clicking sound
• Audible in both phases of respiration	May be inspiratory, or inspiratory and expiratory
• Equal intensity during inspiration and expiration or louder during expiration	Usually louder during inspiration
• Heard over a small area over the chest	Heard over a large area over the chest
• No change in character after coughing	May change its character or intensity on coughing
• Gets accentuated by firmly pressing the chest piece of stethoscope over the chest wall	No accentuation
• Associated with pain and tenderness	Usually not associated
• Caused by rubbing of the roughened pleural surfaces	Coarse crackles are due to air bubbles flowing through the secretions

Q. **What is triad of dry pleurisy?**

Ans: *Pain, fever* and *pleural* rub is a clinical triad of dry pleurisy.

Q. **What is pleurodynia (Bornholm disease)?**

Ans: It is fibrinous pelurisy caused by infection with *coxsackie B virus.* It is mostly a dry pleurisy characterised by clinical triad (*fever, pain* and *pleural rub*). Some patients may have small effusion not detected clinically. The condition is self-limiting and resolves within 2 weeks.

Q. **How would you investigate such a case?**

Ans: Investigations will be done to confirm the diagnosis and to find out its cause:
1. *Complete hemogram* and total leukocyte count.
2. *Sputum examination,* e.g. Gram stain, culture and sensitivity and staining for AFB.
3. *Chest X-ray* for pleural effusion. Wedged-shaped shadows of an infarction may be present in peripheral lung fields (pulmonary embolism).
4. *ECG.* It may be normal or may show signs of pulmonary embolism i.e. RV strain, bundle branch block, P-pulmonale, S_I, Q_{III}, T_{III} syndrome, etc.
5. *Investigations for pulmonary embolism* if suspected, i.e.

   i. Detection of D-dimers

   ii. Blood gas analysis

   iii. Ventilation perfusion scan

   iv. MRI angiography

Q. **How would you treat this patient?**

Ans: 1. Pain relief with analgesics.
2. Treat the underlying cause. For pulmonary infarct, anticoagulation (low molecular heparin) is the initial and immediate treatment followed by oral anticoagulation. Oral anticoagulant therapy is monitored by INR which is kept 2–3 times than normal.
3. Streptokinase or urokinase to dissolve the thombus.
4. Interruption of inferior vena cava by filter in recurrent pulmonary embolism.
5. Embolectomy—surgical procedure for large embolus.

For pleural effusion:

Remove the fluid. Appropriate antibiotic therapy for infection. Malignancy is treated medically, surgically or by radiotherapy.

69

Bronchial Asthma

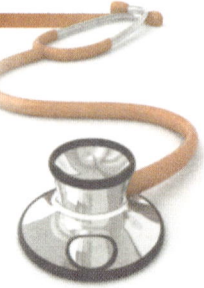

INSTRUCTION

Examine the patient's chest

SALIENT FEATURES

- Acute attack of breathlessness

HISTORY

Ask for the following:

- Present history should cover the present symptoms in details. Note seasonal or noctural attacks of asthma. Is there worsening of symptoms in the morning (morning dipping)?
- Ask whether breathlessness and wheezing reversible.
- Ask about heaviness or tightness of chest.
- Ask about exacerbation of cough and sneezing at night or on exercise.
- History of rhinitis, hay fever, nasal obstruction (polyps).
- Improvement in wheezing and breathlessness with bronchodilators.
- Ask about any precipitant, e.g. emotion, dust, smoke, drugs, pollution, viral infections, pets, pollens, etc.
- *Past history* of cough and cold in the childhood, chronic exposure to dust and smoke. Any history of recurrent attacks of nasal discharge, sneezing and angioneurotic edema.
- *Personal history,* e.g. smoking, alcohol, occupation, habits, diet (food allergy).
- *Family history* of bronchial asthma, hay fever and eczema.

EXAMINATION

General Physical Examination

- *Resting position:* Patient is dyspneic and tachypneic during acute attack, sits in prop up position and uses extrarespiratory muscles for respiration.

- *Pulse:* Tachycardia is usually present in acute attack. Marked tachycardia and bounding pulses indicate CO_2 narcosis (retention). Presence of *pulsus paradoxus* indicates severe acute asthma.
- *BP* and *temperature* normal.
- *Cyanosis* is present in severe acute asthma (present in this case).
- *Level of consciousness:* Patients with mild attacks are fully conscious, but anxious looking. Marked anxiety, drowsiness and restlessness indicate increasing severity of airway obstruction (present).
- *Respiration:* Rate is more, respiration is rapid and shallow.
- *Speech:* If the patient can speak easily and in full sentences, the dyspnea is mild. Monosyllabic speech suggests moderate dyspnea (present in this case). Inability to speak sentences without stopping to take a breath indicate severe asthma.
- *Flapping tremors (asterixis)* on outstretched hands, papilledema, and bounding pulses indicate CO_2 narcosis (absent in this case).
- *Nasal examination* for polyp or allergic rhinitis. Throat examination for septic focus.
- *Skin examination* for allergy.

Chest Examination

Inspection

- Patient is dyspneic at rest.
- Accessory muscles of respiration and alae nasi are working (present)
- Respiratory rate is increased.
- Audible wheezing.
- Excavation of suprasternal notch and supraclavicular fossae may be present with recession of intercostal spaces during inspiration.
- Shape of the chest normal (in this case), but there may be pigeon shape chest in long standing childhood asthma.
- Tracheal tug absent.
- Inspect the sputum cup (mucoid sputum present).

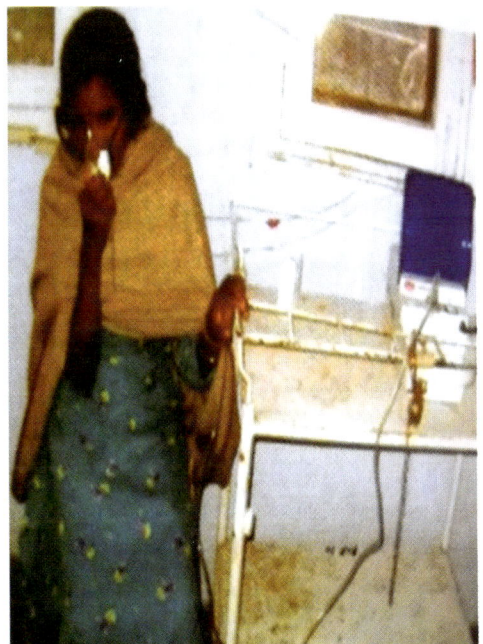

Fig. 69.1: A patient of acute severe asthma being nebulized

Palpation

- Trachea is central.
- Apex beat may not be palpable due to over in-flated lungs.
- Movements of the chest are bilaterally and symmetrically decreased (in this case).
- Expansion of the chest on the *measurement* is reduced (in this case).
- Vocal fremitus is reduced uniformly on both the sides.
- Wheeze/rhonchi may be palpable (not palpable as patient is being nebulised).

Percussion

- Resonant note all over the chest (present).
- Liver dullness intact at normal 5th intercostal space in right mid-clavicular line.
- Normal cardiac dullness (in this case).

Auscultation

- Vesicular breathing with prolonged expiration present all over the chest (in this case).
- Vocal resonance reduced uniformly all over the chest.
- Polyphonic expiratory and inspiratory wheezes (rhonchi) are heard over the chest (present).
- Coarse crackles are heard at both the bases (in this case).
- No pleural rub.

PROVISIONAL DIAGNOSIS

Patient has history of nasal allergy and has bilateral snorous wheezes (lesion) due to nasobronchial allergy, i.e. asthma (aetiology) and is breathless at rest i.e. acute attack of bronchial asthma (functional status).

QUESTIONS AND ANSWERS

Q. **What are the points in favor of your diagnosis?**

Ans: The points in the favor of diagnosis are:
  i. *Episodic nature* of cough, wheeze, breath-lessness and tightness in chest.
  ii. *Exacerbation* of cough or wheeze at night or after exercise.
  iii. *Precipitation of attacks* during summer, dusty and rainy seasons (*seasonal attacks*).
  iv. History of atopy (eczema, hay fever) or rhinitis (seasonal) present.
  v. *Examination of chest* shows tachypnea, excavation of suprasternal and supra-clavicular, fossa; reduced movements and expansion of chest, indrawing of intercostal spaces. Resonant percussion note on both sides, and bilateral scattered wheezes and rhonchi. There is vesicular breathing with prolonged expiration.

Q. **What are the conditions which can produce similar clinical findings?**

Ans: The differentiation of asthma from other diseases associated with dyspnea and wheezing is not difficult, following conditions come to one's mind during an attack of asthma.
  1. **Chronic bronchitis/COPD:** The differences between asthma and chronic bronchitis have been discussed. (read the differences in case no 63).
  2. **Upper airway obstruction by a tumor or laryngeal edema:** In this condition, there is usually *stridor* and there are harsh respiratory sounds limited to the area of trachea not all over the chest as heard in bronchial asthma. Diffuse wheezing is absent. Indirect laryngoscopy and bronchoscopy confirm the diagnosis.
  3. **Endobronchial disease** due to a tumor, tuberculosis, foreign body or broncho-stenosis produce paroxysms of coughing with persistent wheezing limited to one area of the chest.
  4. **Left ventricular failure** (cardiac asthma) produces cough, dyspnea, PND with

moist basal rales, gallop rhythm, blood stained sputum and other signs of heart failure (cardiomegaly, murmurs).

5. **Carcinoid syndrome.** Episodic flushing, diarrhea, pruritus, salivation along with diffuse wheezing in the chest are its characteristics. Cardiac lesions may also occur. The diagnosis is confirmed by measurement of urinary or plasma serotonin or its metabolites in urine.

6. **Recurrent pulmonary thromboembolism:** Recurrent episodes of dyspnea, particularly on exertion with or without hemoptysis can occur in pulmonary embolism. Sometimes, wide spread wheezing simulating asthma may occur causing confusion with it. Lung scans and pulmonary angiography may be necessary to confirm the diagnosis.

7. **Eosinophilic pneumonia:** Acute eosinophilic pneumonia is characterized by episodes of cough, fever, chills, dyspnea and wheezing following an exposure to an antigen. Neutrophila, eosinophilia and lymphopenia can occur. Chest X-ray shows nodular infiltrates or reticulonodular opacities. Pulmonary function tests reveal restrictive defect. High resolution CT scan is diagnostic.

Q. **What do you understand by the term bronchial asthma?**

Ans: *Bronchial asthma* is defined as a transient obstructive pulmonary disorder characterized by chronic airway inflammation and increased responsiveness of tracheobronchial tree to a variety of stimuli resulting in temporary narrowing of the air passages leading to symptoms of cough, wheeze, tightness of chest and dyspnea. Airflow obstruction is reversible with treatment.

Q. **What do you understand by extrinsic and intrinsic asthma?**

Ans: Bronchial asthma comprises two common distinct patterns; (i) episodic asthma in which acute attacks are precipitated by allergens or infection by respiratory virus. These attacks are short-lived and patient in between attacks is symptom free. These attacks are common in children who are atopic hence, called *extrinsic asthma.* (ii) The other pattern is persistent asthma in which there is chronic wheeze and breathlessness, these cases resemble patients of chronic bronchitis. These individuals are nonatopic, and asthma develops in old age — called *intrinsic asthma.*

Q. **Name some triggering factors for asthma.**

Ans: 1. *Allergen,* e.g. pollen, house dust, animal dander, feathers in pillows or quilts.
2. *Drugs,* e.g. beta-blockers.
3. *Insect web, food / food items, chemicals / pollutants.*
4. *Occupational factors:*
   • Metal salts, e.g. platinum, chromium, nickle.
   • Wood and vegetable dusts, e.g. grain flour, cast or bean, coffee beans, gum acacia, etc.
   • Industrial chemicals and plastics e.g. dyes.
   • Biological enzymes, e.g. laundry detergents and pancreatic enzymes.
5. *Infections,* e.g. viral, bacterial.
6. *Exercise* (exercise-induced asthma).
7. *Emotional stress.*

Q. **What is wheeze? What are its types?**

Ans: Read Clinical methods by Prof. SN Chugh.

Q. **What are the causes of recurrent bronchospasm?**

Ans: • Bronchial asthma
• Carcinoid tumor
• Recurrent pulmonary emboli
• Chronic bronchitis with acute exacerbation
• Recurrent LVF (cardiac asthma)

Q. **What are the causes of wheezes?**

Ans: 1. Bronchial asthma
2. COPD, predominantly chronic bronchitis
3. Left ventricular failure (cardiac asthma)
4. Bronchial tumor
5. Eosinophilic lung disease (pulmonary eosinophilia)
6. Carcinoid syndrome
7. Recurrent thromboembolism
8. Anaphylaxis
9. Systemic vasculitis with pulmonary involvement
10. Mastocytosis

Q. **What is persistent rhonchus/wheeze? What are its causes?**

Ans: A localized wheeze persisting in a localized area could be due to
• Bronchostenosis
• Foreign body obstruction
• Bronchial adenoma

Q. **What are the differences between extrinsic and intrinsic asthma?**

Ans: Table 69.1 differentiates atopic (extrinsic) and non-atopic intrinsic asthma.

Table 69.1: Differentiating features of extrinsic and intrinsic asthma

Extrinsic asthma (atopic)	Intrinsic asthma (non-atopic)
• Episodic, sudden onset	Non-episodic, chronic or persistent
• Early onset or childhood asthma	Late onset or adult asthma
• More wheeze, less cough	More cough, less wheeze
• Mostly seasonal	Mostly non-seasonal
• Attacks may occur at any time of the day or night.	Mostly attacks occur at night (nocturnal)
• Diurnal pattern, e.g symptoms and peak expiratory flow show morning dipping with subsequent recovery	Non-diurnal pattern
• Non-exercise induced attacks	Exercise-induced attacks
• Positive family history of an allergic disorder	No family history
• Skin hypersensitivity tests positive	Skin tests negative
• Sodium cromoglycate is most effective	Not effective

Q.   What is an acute severe asthma?

Ans: This term has replaced the previous horrifying term *status asthmaticus.* It is defined as either an acute attack of prolonged asthma or paroxysmal attacks of acute asthma where there is no remission of attacks in between and they are not controlled with conventional bronchodilators. It is a life-threatening emergency, needs proper diagnosis and urgent treatment. The **diagnosis** is suggested by:

- Acute dyspnea, orthopnea with wheeze, tachycardia, tachypnea and perspiration.
- Central cyanosis.
- Dry (unproductive) cough with mucoid expectoration.
- Respiratory distress with hyperactivity of extrarespiratory muscles (accessory muscles of respiration).
- Pulsus paradoxus.
- Diminished breath sounds due to reduced air entry and minimal or absence of high-pitched polyphonic rhonchi (wheezes).
- PEFR (peak expiratory flow rate) is <50% of predicted or patient's best.

Q.   How would you decide the severity of asthma clinically?

Ans: It is decided by:

I. *Bed side clinical parameters:*

- Pulse rate and respiratory rate.
- Pulsus paradoxus (present/absent).
- Tachypnea (rapid shallow respiration) present or absent.
- Able or unable to speak in sentences (i.e. one sentence in one breath).
- PEFR more than or less than 50% of predicted or <100 L/min.
- Central cyanosis (present/absent).
- Exhaustion, confusion, obtunded consciousness (present/absent).
- Bradycardia, hypotension (present or absent).
- *"Silent chest", feeble respiratory effort.* Indicate life-threatening asthma.

Q.   What are the complications of asthma?

Ans: • *Severe acute asthma* (*status asthmaticus*).
- *Recurrent pulmonary infections.*
- *Sputum retention syndrome* leading to atelectasis of lung.
- *Pneumothorax.*
- *Emphysema,* can occur in long-standing asthma.
- *Respiratory failure (type II common).*
- *Chronic cor pulmonale.*
- *Precipitation* of syncope, hernias, prolapse, subconjunctival hemorrhage due to repeated coughing.

Q.   How does bronchial asthma differ from chronic bronchitis?

Ans: Read Table 69.2.

Q.   What are the indications of steroids in asthma?

Ans: 1. *Nocturnal asthma* (sleep is disturbed by wheeze).
2. Persistence of morning tightness until mid-day.
3. Symptoms and peak expiratory flow deteriorates progressively each day.
4. Maximum treatment with bronchodilators.
5. When there is need of emergency nebulisers.

Q.   Name the inhalational steroids.

Ans: Beclomethasone, Budesonide, Ciclesonide, Fluticasone, Triamcinolone

Q.   What are the indications for mechanical ventilation with intermittent positive pressure ventilation?

Ans: • Worsening hypoxia ($PaO_2 < 8$ kPa) despite 60% inspired O_2
- Hypercapnia ($PaCO_2 > 6$ kPa)
- Drowsiness
- Coma

Table 69.2: Differences between bronchial asthma and chronical bronchitis

Feature	Asthma	Chronic bronchitis
Onset	Acute	Slow, insidious
Age	Childhood, adolescents and middle age	Usually middle age or old patients
Pathogenesis	Allergic	Allergic-inflammatory
H/o Smoking	Absent	Present
Family history	May be positive	Negative
H/o Allergy e.g. rhinitis, hay fever, eczema	Present	Absent
Duration of symptoms	No fixed duration	At least of 2 years duration
Nature of symptoms and signs	Intermittent, episodic	Persistent, acute exacerbation can occur
Seasonal variations	Present	Absent
Symptoms	Dyspnea > cough	Cough > dyspnea
Signs	Wheezes/rhonchi are more pronounced than crackles	Both wheezes and crackles are present
Sputum and blood eosinophilia	Common	Uncommon
Pulmonary function tests	Usually normal	Usually abnormal

Q.   What preventive measure would you advise to the patient of bronchial asthma?

Ans: Preventive measures are:

- Try to avoid exposure to flowering vegetation.
- Keep bed room windows closed.
- Vacuum cleaning of the matress daily.
- Shake out the blankets and bedsheets daily.
- Dust bed room thoroughly.
- Avoid contact with animal pets, e.g. dogs, cats, horses, etc.
- Substitute foam pillows and terylene quilts.
- Avoid all preparations of relevant drugs.
- Do not allow the insect web to collect.
- Identify dietary precipitants and eliminate them from diet.
- Avoid exposure to chemicals/pollutants. Change of an occupation, if necessary

Q.   What is step-care regimen for management of chronic asthma in adults?

Ans. British thoracic society regimen is depicted in Fig. 69.2.

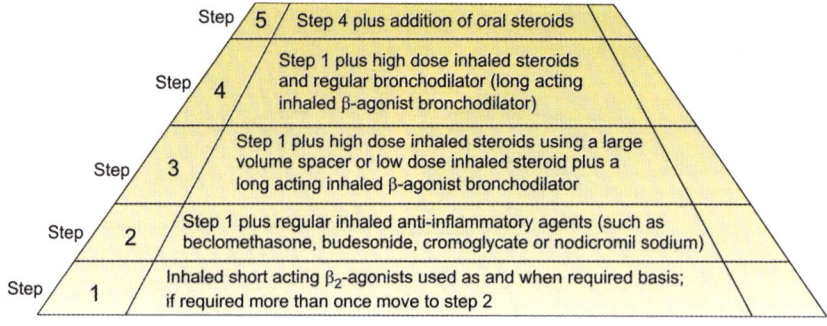

Step 5   Step 4 plus addition of oral steroids

Step 4   Step 1 plus high dose inhaled steroids and regular bronchodilator (long acting inhaled β-agonist bronchodilator)

Step 3   Step 1 plus high dose inhaled steroids using a large volume spacer or low dose inhaled steroid plus a long acting inhaled β-agonist bronchodilator

Step 2   Step 1 plus regular inhaled anti-inflammatory agents (such as beclomethasone, budesonide, cromoglycate or nodicromil sodium)

Step 1   Inhaled short acting β_2-agonists used as and when required basis; if required more than once move to step 2

Fig. 69.2: Pyramid of step-care treatment of chronic bronchial asthma

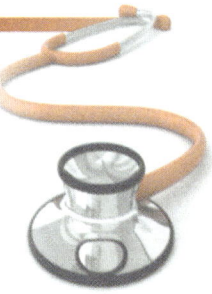

70

Bronchiectasis

INSTRUCTION

Examine the patient's chest.

SALIENT FEATURES

- Massive fetid sputum, fever and cough

HISTORY

Ask for the following:

- Write the complaints in chronological order and detail them.
- Ask specifically about the amount of sputum, color, consistency, smell, etc.
- Ask the history of recurrent hemoptysis.
- History of fever, night sweats.
- Is there any relationship between posture and cough?
- Past history of tuberculosis or childhood measles, mumps or whooping cough.
- Past history of recurrent fever or chest infection or asthma.
- Any history of edema feet, swelling of the abdomen, etc.
- Any history of fever, headache, vomiting, or neurological deficit.
- History of weight loss.

EXAMINATION

General Physical Examination

- Patient may be dyspneic and has lots of coughing (coughing-couging-coughing). Examine the sputum cup for expectoration (Fig. 70.1). Sputum contains large amount of expectoration (in this case).
- Bony cage is normal.
- Toxic look and fever if present indicate severe infection.
- Pulse rate may be increased.
- Respiratory rate may be high.
- Nutrition may be poor due to hypoproteinemia as a result of massive expectoration.

- Cyanosis may be present, if disease is bilateral and severe or patient develops respiratory failure or cor pulmonale.
- Clubbing of fingers and toes common (present in this case); may be grade I to IV.
- Edema feet if there is cor pulmonale or hypo-proteinemia (present in this case).

Chest Examination (Fig. 70.1)

Inspection

- The affected side of the chest (right lower part in this case) may be retracted
- There may be diminished movement on the side involved (right side)
- There is wasting of muscles of thorax.
- Look for the apex beat for dextrocardia (apex beat is at normal place).

Palpation

- Chest may be retracted with diminished movements and crowding of the ribs in the lower parts (s). There may be palpable wheeze or

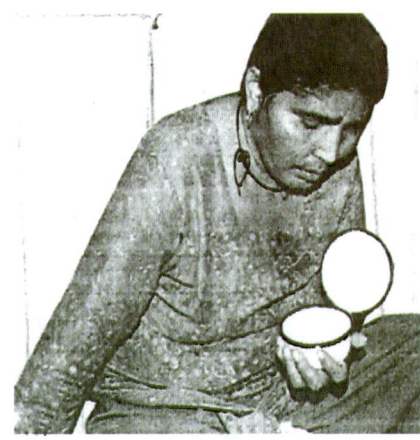

Fig. 70.1: A patient of bronchiectasis with massive fetid expectoration and foul-smelling breath (Halitosis)

rhonchi and coarse mid-inspiratory and expiratory crackles (present in this case).

Percussion

The percussion note is impaired over the area involved (right lower chest).

Auscultation

- Breath sounds may be bronchial, with coarse, bubbling leathery mid inspiratory and expiratory crackles (right lower zone in this case).
- Vocal resonance may be increased.

N.B All the signs will be seen on both sides in bilateral disease.

Abdominal Examination

- For hepatomegaly and/or splenomegaly (for secondary amyloidosis).

PROVISIONAL DIAGNOSIS

The symptoms and signs suggest the diagnosis of bronchiectasis (aetiology) and patient has bilateral pedal edema due to hypoproteinemia (functional status).

QUESTIONS AND ANSWERS

Q. **What are the positive points in favor of your diagnosis?**

Ans: 1. Long history of cough with massive purulent expectoration, more in the morning and in lying down position;
2. Cyanosis and clubbing of fingers.
3. Retraction of lower part of the right chest.
4. Diminished chest movements of right side of chest (lower part).
5. Presence of coarse, bubbling crackles and wheezes over right lower part.

Q. **What are your other possibilities?**

Ans: 1. *Lung abscess* — read case discussion on lung abscess.
2. *Tubercular cavity filled with exudate* (Read case discussion).
3. *Resolving pneumonia/necrotising pneumonia*
4. *Empyema thoracis* with bronchopleural fistula.
5. Cystic fibrosis
6. Chronic bronchitis

N.B All these conditions lead to massive sputum.

Q. **What do you understand by the term bronchiectasis?**

Ans: *Bronchiectasis* is a localized irreversible dilatation and distortion of bronchi. Although the definition is based on histopathological

changes, yet clinical diagnosis is applied when chronic and recurrent infections occur in the dilated airways resulting in collection of secretions within them leading to massive expectoration, more so in the morning. It may be focal and unilateral or diffuse and bilateral.

Q. **What are its pathological types (Reid's classification)?**

Ans: Pathological types of bronchiectasis seen on bronchoscopy and CT scan are:
1. *Cylindrical bronchiectasis.* The bronchi are uniformly dilated.
2. *Varicose bronchiectasis.* The affected bronchi have irregular or beeded pattern of dilatation.
3. *Saccular (cystic) bronchiectasis.* The bronchi have ballooned or cystic appearance.

Q. **What are the causes of bronchiectasis?**

Ans: The causes of bronchiectasis are:
1. *Postinfective,* e.g. postpneumonic, following measles, whooping cough and post-tubercular (tubercular bronchiectasis common in upper lobe).
2. *Mechanical bronchial obstruction (obstructive bronchiectasis)* as in endobronchial tuberculosis, carcinoma, extrinsic lymph node compression.
3. *Allergic bronchopulmonary aspergillosis.*
4. *γ-globulin deficiency*, e.g. congenital or acquired.
5. Immobile cilia syndrome (*Kartagener's syndrome*).
6. Cystic fibrosis.
7. *Neuropathic disorders* namely Riley-day syndrome, (Chagas' disease).
8. Idiopathic.

Q. **What are the major pathogens in bronchiectasis?**

Ans: Major pathogens are:
- *S. aureus, H. influenzae, Pseudomonas aeruginosa*

Q. **What is the common site for localized disease?**

Ans: Left lower lobe and lingula.

Q. **What is Kartagener's syndrome?**

Ans: It consists of the following:
- Sinusitis
- Dextrocardia
- Bronchiectasis
- *Primary ciliary dyskinesia.* The abnormal sperm motility due to improper ciliary function, males are generally infertile.

Q. **Where does bronchiectasis occur in allergic bronchopulmonary aspergillosis?**

Ans: The bronchial dilatation occurs in more proximal bronchi (proximal bronchiectasis) due to type III immune complex reactions.

Q. **What other abnormalities may be associated with bronchiectasis?**

Ans: 1. Congenital absence of bronchial cartilage (*Campbell syndrome*).
2. Tracheobronchomegaly.
3. Azoospermia.
4. Chronic sinopulmonary infection.
5. Congenital kyphoscoliosis.
6. Situs inversus and paranasal sinusitis (Kartagener's syndrome).

Q. **What is dry or wet bronchiectasis?**

Ans: Chronic cough with massive purulent sputum, more in the morning and in one of the lateral or lying down position and dilated airways on CT scan indicate *wet bronchiectasis*. The term *dry bronchiectasis* refers to either asymptomatic disease or a disease with recurrent non-productive cough associated with hemoptysis and bronchiectasis in an upper lobe.

Q. **How will you investigate bronchiectasis?**

Ans: Following investigations are done:
- **Hemoglobin, TLC, DLC, ESR:** There may be normocytic normochromic anemia with leukocytosis.
- **Sputum for culture and sensitivity:** The sputum culture is useful guide for active infection. Sputum for eosinophilia provides a clue to asthma and/or bronchopulmonary aspergillosis.
- **Urine examination** for proteinuria if amyloidosis is being suspected.
- **Blood culture and sensitivity** if there is an evidence of bacteremia or septicemia.
- **Chest X-ray (PA view):** The chest X-ray (Fig. 70.2) may be normal with mild disease or may show prominent (dilated) cystic spaces (saccular bronchiectasis) either with or without air fluid levels, corresponding to the dilated airways. These dilated airways are often crowded together in parallel, when seen longitudinally, appear as "*tram-tracks*", and when seen in cross section appear as, "*ring shadows*". These may be difficult to distinguish from regions of honeycombing in patients with severe interstitial lung disease.
- **Bronchography (a gold standard for diagnosis)** shows an excellent visualization of bronchiectatic airways, but, nowadays it is not done because of availability of high resolution CT scan.

- **High resolution CT scan** will show dilated airways in one or both of the lower lobes or in an upper lobe. When seen in cross-section, the dilated airways have a ring-like appearance.
- **Fiberoptic bronchoscopy:** It is done to find out the cause. When the bronchiectasis is focal, fibreoptic bronchoscopy may show an under-lying endobronchial obstruction. Bronchiectasis of an upper lobe is common in tuberculosis and bronchopulmonary aspergillosis.
- **Pulmonary function tests**. Pulmonary function tests are useful to define the extent, severity of the disease, need for bronchodilators and to plan surgery.
- **Specific tests for aspergillosis,** i.e. precipitin test and serum IgE.

Q. **What are the complications of bronchiectasis?**

Ans: Common complications are as follows:
- Recurrent pneumonias
- Bacteremia and septicemia.
- Massive hemoptysis leading to pulmonary apoplexy.
- Cor pulmonale.
- Secondary amyloidosis.
- Meningitis or brain abscess.
- Aspergilloma (fungal ball) in a bronchiectatic cavity.

Q. **What do you know about spiral CT?**

Ans: This is a rapidly evolving technique to image the chest and has the advantage of imaging truly contiguous sections; with the result completely seamless reconstructions are possible. This may allow virtual-reality bronchoscopic imaging.

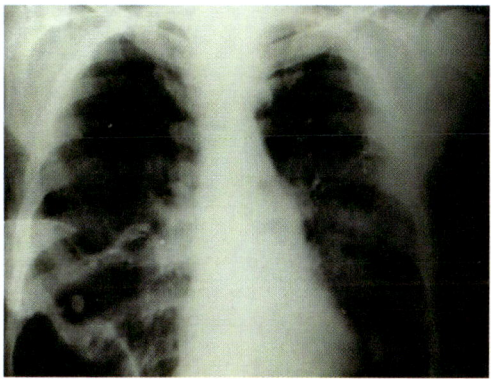

Fig. 70.2: X-ray chest showing dilated air space as ring shadows in lower parts of both lungs (more marked on right side)

71

Cystic Fibrosis

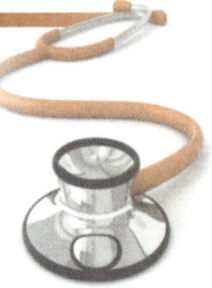

INSTRUCTION

Examine the chest of this patient

SALIENT FEATURES

- Foul breath and large amount of sputum

HISTORY

Ask about the following:

- Age and sex
- History of cough and expectoration with duration, nature of the sputum and hemoptysis (long duration).
- Ask about GI symptoms in details, i.e. abdominal pain, nausea, appetite, frequency of stool, color, consistency, greasy, smell (offensive in this case), etc.
- Ask history of rectal prolapse, smell of stool (offensive in this case), symptoms of intestinal obstruction.
- History of heat stroke, sweating, salt depletion.
- History of sterility in male and decreased fertility in female.

EXAMINATION

General Physical Examination

- General condition is usually poor (malnourished).
- Foul breath (halitosis) due to fetid sputum (present).
- Central cyanosis (present).
- Elicit sinus tenderness or look for nasal polyp.
- Finger clubbing and edema feet (present)
- Anemia and asthenia (present).

Chest Examination

- Chest is bilaterally symmetrical with diminished movements on both sides.
- AP diameter of chest is more than transverse diameter.
- On auscultation, there are bilateral coarse crackles (present).

PROVISIONAL DIAGNOSIS

The symptoms and signs suggest the diagnosis of cystic fibrosis (aetiology). Patient has cyanosis and tachypnea indicating respiratory insufficiency (functional status).

QUESTIONS AND ANSWERS

Q.   **What are the points in favor of your diagnosis?**

Ans: 1. Male patient.
2. Presence of purulent massive sputum, fever and cyanosis.
3. Steatorrhea (offensive fatty stool).
4. Sterility present.
5. Anaemia and asthenia

Q.   **What would you like to check to substantiate the diagnosis?**

Ans: 1. Urine for sugar (diabetes mellitus)
2. Fecal fat content
3. Sweat sodium

Q.   **What are the clinical manifestations of cystic fibrosis?**

Ans: In children and adults, the clinical manifestations are:

I. **Respiratory manifestations,** e.g. recurrent respiratory infections, sinusitis, nasal polyps, bronchiectasis, pneumothorax, recurrent hemoptysis, allergic bronchopulmonary aspergillosis.

II. **Cardiovascular manifestations,** e.g. cor pulmonale.

III. **GI manifestations,** e.g. steatorrhoea, ileal obstruction, biliary cirrhosis, gallstones, intussusception, rectal prolapse.

IV. **Miscellaneous,** e.g. sterlity in males and infertility in females, diabetes mellitus, hypertrophic pulmonary osteoarthropathy.

Q. What is the cause of male sterility in cystic fibrosis?

Ans: Congenital bilateral absence of vas deferens with azoospermia.

Q. What is the cause of steatorrhea in cystic fibrosis?

Ans: Pancreatic insufficiency due to blockage of pancreatic duct by an abnormal mucus results in steatorrhea. Biliary tract obstruction and obstruction of cystic duct also contribute to it.

Q. How would you treat steatorrhea?

Ans: • Low fat diet
- Pancreatic supplements
- H_2-receptors antagonist

Q. What pathogens are responsible for purulent sputum in cystic fibrosis?

Ans: The pathogens are:
1. *H. influenzae*
2. *Staph. aureus*
3. *Burkolderia cepacia*
4. *Pseudomonas aeruginosa*

Q. What is the mode of inheritance in cystic fibrosis?

Ans: It is transmitted by autosomal recessive manner.

Cystic fibrosis is caused by abnormalities in a membrane chloride channel by a defect in the gene encoding CFTR (cystic fibrosis transmembrane conductance regular protein) which resides on long arm of chromosome 7. The mutation of this gene on chromosome 7 leads to failure of the chloride channel to open in response to cyclic AMP.

Q. What is the basic defect in airways of these patients?

Ans: In cystic fibrosis, there is alteration in chloride transport as these channel do not open resulting in 3-fold increase in the reabsorption of Na^+ from the airway into the cytoplasm of the cells. Water also moves with sodium from the lumen into the cells resulting in thick, tenacious mucus which impairs mucociliary function resulting in retention of secretion and repeated infections.

Q. What is the significance of sweat testing?

Ans: A sweat sodium concentration >60 mmol/L is indicative of cystic fibrosis.

Q. What is the risk of cancer in these patients?

Ans: Patients with cystic fibrosis have an increased risk of malignancies of GI tract, hence persistence of GI symptoms in these cases should be investigated carefully.

Q. What are the causes of death in this condition?

Ans: Repeated pulmonary complications, e.g. pneumonia, pneumothorax, bronchiectasis result in chronic respiratory failure and death.

Q. How would you investigate this case?

Ans: 1. *Chest X-ray.* It may reveal apical bronchiectasis, pneumonia, pneumothorax or prominent bronchovascular markings, rounded peripheral opacities and focal atelectasis.
2. *CT scan* will confirm the presence of bronchiectasis (Fig. 71.1).
3. *Arterial blood gas analysis* may show hypoxia and compensated respiratory acidosis.
4. *Pulmonary function tests* may reveal a mixed obstructive and restrictive pattern.
5. *Sputum for culture and sensitivity* may result in isolation of the organism if sputum is purulent.
6. *Pilocarpine iontophoresis sweat test* reveals elevated sodium and chloride levels (>60 mEg/L) in the sweat of the patients with cystic fibrosis. Two tests on different days are required to confirm the diagnosis.
7. *Others tests* include:
   - Nasal membrane potential difference.
   - Semen analysis for oligo or azoospermia.
   - Pancreatic function test for exocrine pancreatic insufficiency.
   - Genotyping for gene mutations.

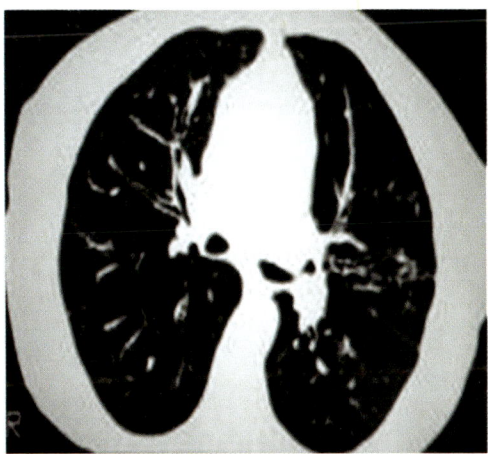

Fig. 71.1: Cystic fibrosis. High-resolution CT image shows bronchial wall thickening (tram lines), predominantly in the upper lobes

Q. How would you treat chest complications in such a case?

Ans: Treatment is a multidisciplinary approach as follows:

1. Treatment of chest problems is done by antibiotics, postural drainage, bronchodilators and physiotherapy (chest percussion or vibration techniques, positive expiratory pressure (PEP) or flutter valve breathing devices, etc.). Inhaled recombinant human deoxyribonuclease (rhDNase, dornase alpha) improves FEV_1, and reduces the exacerbations in cystic fibrosis. The ultimate and final treatment is lung transplantation.

Q. What recent advances have been made in the treatment of cystic fibrosis?

Ans: 1. High dose ibuprofen in patients with mild disease taken consistently for 4 yrs significantly slows the progression of the disease.

2. Inhalation of human recombinant DNAase (dornase-alpha 2.5 mg) which degrades DNA in the bronchial secretion, improves FEV_1, reduces the exacerbation of the disease and curtails the need for antibiotics.

3. Inhalation of hypertonic saline accelerates mucus clearance and improves lung functions and reduces pulmonary exacerbations.

4. Improved hydration of bronchial secretion by (i) blocking the reabsorption of sodium from the bronchial lumen by amiloride and (ii) stimulating the secretion of chloride with triphosphate nucleotides (of adenosine or uridine) improves mucociliary function.

5. Immunisation against various organisms, i.e. *pseudomonas, pneumococci* and *influenza*.

6. *Gene therapy.* The gene transferred in a carrier known as ribosome, or in an adenovirus to the nasal epithelium has shown promising results.

7. Lung transplantation.

Q. What would you advise to a patient with cystic fibrosis who wishes to conceive?

Ans. i. The couple will be offered genetic counselling. The genetic status of the man will be determined, whether he is a carrier. Chorionic villous sampling will be considered as there is risk 1 in 2 to the infant born to this couple to have cystic fibrosis and they may wish to consider selective termination in the first trimester. There are hazards of general anaesthesia for termination of pregnancy, which should be told to them. Termination of pregnancy will be possible either with spinal anesthesia or with medications.

ii. Women with severe disease if wants to conceive, cannot complete the pregnancy. This is made clear.

iii. In women with FEV_1 <60%, there are increased chances of premature delivery, respiratory complications and even death of mother.

iv. Pregnancy after heart-lung transplantation offer better health and increased longevity of the mother but keeping in mind the risk of organ rejection and exposure of fetus to immunosuppressive drugs, the pregnancy should not be attempted by women with transplants.

72

Fibrosing Alveolitis

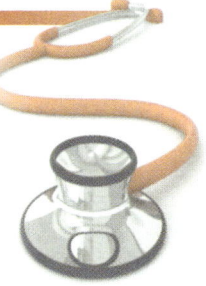

INSTRUCTION

Examine the patient's chest

SALIENT FEATURES

• Exertional dyspnea, cough and sputum

HISTORY

Ask about the following:

• Progressive exertional dyspnea (present).
• Persistent dry cough (present in this case).
• Fever, weight loss, fatigue (present).
• Symptoms of cor pulmonale (abdominal pain due to hepatomegaly, ascites, swelling legs).
• Past history of tuberculosis or lung suppuration.
• Any history of radiation exposure.
• Any history of joint pain, arthralgia, rash.
• Drug history.
• Occupational history, e.g. coal miner, stone cutter, farmer or industrial worker.
• Past history of rheumatic heart disease or any other cardiac disorders.

EXAMINATION

General Physical Examination

• Dyspnea, orthopnea (present).
• Tachypnea.
• Central cyanosis (present).
• Clubbing of the fingers (present).
• Signs of occupation.
• Raised JVP and ankle edema if severe disease.
• Examine *hands* for rheumatoid arthritis, systemic sclerosis.
• *Face:* Look for butterfly rash for dermatomyositis, typical rash of SLE, pinched faces of systemic sclerosis and lupus pernio of sarcoidosis.
• *Mouth:* Look for aphthous ulcers of Crohn's disease, dry mouth of Sjögren's syndrome.

Chest Examination

Inspection
• Bilateral symmetrical reduction in chest movements (present in this case).
• Accessory muscles of respiration may be hyperactive.

Palpation
• Reduced bilateral chest movements (present).
• Reduced expansion of the chest (present).
• Bilateral reduction of vocal fremitus (present).

Percussion
• Dullness on percussion at lung bases on both sides (present).

Auscultation
• Bilateral crackles (end-inspiratory) at both the bases (lower zones) of the lungs which may disappear or become quieter on leaning forward, but do not disappear on coughing unlike those of pulmonary edema (present).
• Vesicular breathing diminished in intensity (present).
• Vocal resonance bilaterally diminished (present).

Other System Examination

• On CVS examination signs of right heart failure (raised JVP, loud P2, hepatomegaly, central cyanosis and pitting edema) may or may not be present, if present, indicates chronic cor pulmonale.

PROVISIONAL DIAGNOSIS

The patient complains of progressive dyspnea, has bilateral basal fine end-inspiratory crackles (lesion) caused by fibrosing alveolitis (aetiology) and has orthopnea (functional status).

Q. **Summarize your findings in favor of your diagnosis?**

Ans: A middle aged coal miner presented with progressive dyspnea, cough, fever, malaise and weight loss. There is tachypnea, tachycardia, central cyanosis and clubbing of fingers. Chest examination shows reduced bilateral chest movements, expansion and vocal fremitus. The lung bases are dull on percussion. On auscultation, there is vesicular breathing with fine, basal end-inspiratory crackles.

QUESTIONS AND ANSWERS

Q. **What is your differential diagnosis?**

Ans: Differential diagnosis lies between the causes of bilateral interstitial fibrosis (read the cause of fibrosis). The common conditions to be differentiated are:
- Collagen vascular diseases, e.g. SLE, RA, dermatomyositis, systemic sclerosis
- Idiopathic interstitial fibrosis
- Farmer's lung, extrinsic allergic alveolitis
- Respiratory bronchiolitis
- Pneumoconiosis
- Silicosis
- Asbestosis
- Chronic pulmonary oedema
- Lymphangitis carcinomatosa

Q. **What are the causes of crackles at the lung bases with clubbing?**

Ans: 1. Bronchogenic carcinoma
2. Bronchiectasis
3. Asbestosis
4. Pulmonary edema

Q. **What are the causes of interstitial fibrosis?**

Ans: Interstitial fibrosis is bilateral fibrosis of alveolar walls and septa. Causes are:
- A. *Pulmonary origin:*
  - *Hypersensitivity*
    - Diffuse fibrosing alveolitis (Fig. 72.1)
    - Farmer's lung
  - *Collagen vascular disorders*
    - SLE
    - Systemic sclerosis
    - Rheumatoid arthritis (rheumatoid lungs)
  - Lymphangitis carcinomatosis
  - Drug-induced, e.g. busulfan, bleomycin, nitrofurantoin, methysergide, hydralazine, hexamethonium, amiodarone.
- B. Idiopathic
- C. *Miscellaneous*
  - Sarcoidosis
  - Aspiration pneumonitis
  - Histiocytosis
  - Tuberous sclerosis
  - Xanthomatosis

Q. **What is Hamman-Rich syndrome? What are its clinical features?**

Ans: Diffuse interstitial fibrosis or fibrosing alveolitis of acute onset, progressive course of unknown etiology is called *Hamman-Rich syndrome*. It is characterised by progressive dyspnea, dry cough, fever, weight loss and signs of bilateral fibrosis of the lung.

Q. **What are the causes of end-inspiratory crackles?**

Ans: Read respiratory system in clinical methods in medicine by Prof. SN Chugh.

Q. **How will you investigate a patient with cryptogenic fibrosing alveolitis?**

Ans: The common investigations are:
1. *Routine blood tests.* ESR is high.
2. *Blood* for *rheumatoid factor* and *anti-nuclear antibodies.* Immunoglobulins are raised.
3. *Chest X-ray (PA view) shows:*
   - Diffuse pulmonary opacities in the lower zones peripherally.
   - The hemidiaphragms are high and the lungs appear small.
   - In advanced disease, there may be "honey-comb" appearance of the lungs in which diffuse pulmonary shadowing is inerspersed.
4. *High resolution CT* scan may show honey-combing (Fig. 72.1) and scarring, most marked peripherally in both the lungs or there may be ground glass appearance. CT scan is useful in early diagnosis when chest X-ray may not show the radiological changes. MRI is useful to determine disease activity.
5. *Pulmonary function test.* There is restrictive ventilatory defect. The carbon monoxide transfer factor is low and lung volumes are reduced.

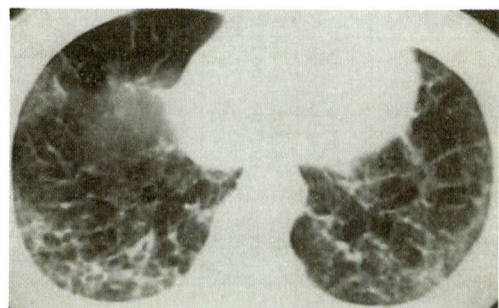

Fig. 72.1: Extrinsic allergic alveolitis. CT scan shows ground glass appearance and honeycombing of the lungs (traction bronchiectasis)

6. *Bronchoalveolar lavage* may show a large number of lymphocytes and *transbronchial biopsy* may sometimes be helpful.
7. *Open lung biopsy* for histological patterns of idiopathic cases of interstitial lung disease. In early stages, there is mononuclear cell infiltration in alveolar wall with interstitial fibrosis; in late stages, honey combing, bronchial dilatation and cysts are seen.

Q.   What is respiratory bronchiolitis?

Ans: Respiratory bronchiolitis is an interstitial lung disease of smokers in which there is accumulation of pigment-laden macrophages in the respiratory bronchioles and adjacent alveoli leading to mononuclear cell infiltration and fibrosis. It may reverse on cessation of smoking. Clinical picture is similar to cryptogenic fibrosing alveolitis.

Q.   What is farmer's lung?

Ans: It is an occupational lung disease caused by an inhalation of organic dust (mouldy hay, straw, grain), characterised by features of extrinsic allergic alveolitis (e.g. headache, muscle pains, malaise, pyrexia, dry cough and breathlessness without wheeze) which may progress to irreversible pulmonary fibrosis.

The pathogenic mechanism is local immune response to fungal antigen, e.g. *micropolyspora faenaei or Aspergillus fumigatus*. The **diagnosis** is confirmed on serology and high resolution CT scan.

Q.   What is coal-worker's pneumoconiosis?

Ans: The disease follows prolonged inhalation of coal dust, hence, is an occupational lung disease seen in coal-workers. The condition is subdivided into *simple pneumoconiosis* and *progressive massive fibrosis*.

The **simple coal miner's pneumoconiosis** is reversible (if miner leaves the industry), non-progressive and radiologically characterised by nodulation without cavitation. On the other hand, **progressive massive fibrosis** — is irreversible, progressive and radiologically characterised by large dense masses, single or multiple, occur mainly in upper lobes associated with cavitation.

Q.   What is Caplan's syndrome?

Ans: It consists of association of *rheumatoid arthritis* with *coal worker's pneumoconiosis* and rounded *fibrotic nodules (nodular shadowing)* 0.5 to 5 cm in diameter distributed mainly in the periphery of the lung fields.

Q.   What is silicosis?

Ans: This disease is caused by inhalation of silica dust or quartz particles, characterised by progressive development of hard nodules which coalesce as the disease progresses followed by fibrosis. The clinical and radiological features are similar to coal worker's pneumoconiosis though changes tend to be more marked in the upper lobe. The *egg-shell calcification* of enlarged hilar lymph nodes is a distinct feature. Tuberculosis may be a complication ensuring caseation and calcification. The disease progresses even when the exposure to dust ceases (relentless progression).

Q.   What is asbestosis? What are its possible effects on respiratory tract?

Ans: *Asbestosis* is an occupational lung disorder, occurs due to exposure to fibrous mineral asbestos in certain occupations such as in the mining and milling of the mineral. The main types of asbestosis are:
- *Chrysolite* (white asbestos — a common factor)
- *Crocidolite* (blue asbestos — uncommon factor)
- *Amosite (brown) asbestos* — a rare factor

The possible effects of asbestosis are depicted in Fig. 72.2.

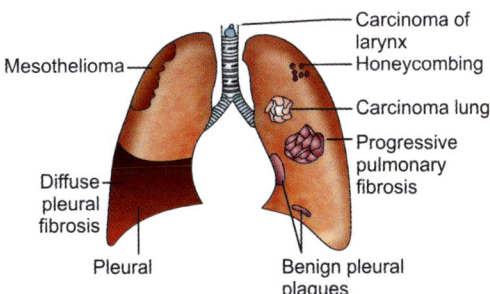

Fig. 72.2: The effects of asbestosis on respiratory tract (diag)

73

Cavity with Fibrosis

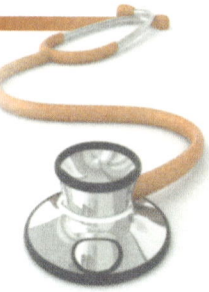

INSTRUCTION

Examine the patient's chest

SALIENT FEATURES

- Complains of fever, hemoptysis. Had tuberculosis in the past.

HISTORY

Ask about the following:

- Age and sex
- Cough, fever and night sweats, weakness, etc. for manifestations of *tubercular cavity.*
- Cough, massive expectoration, fever, purulent sputum with postural and diurnal variation (for lung *abscess* or *bronchiectasis).*
- Cough, hemoptysis, breathlessness, fever, weight loss, anorexia (for *malignancy* as the cause of cavity).
- Onset and progression of the symptoms.
- Past history of tuberculosis or lung malignancy, ankylosing spondylitis.
- Past history of pneumonia (e.g. fever, cough, hemoptysis and pain chest) or lung suppuration (cough with mucopurulent or purulent sputum).
- Any history of headache, vomiting, visual disturbance or neurological deficit.
- Any history of radiation.

EXAMINATION

General Physical Examination

- Patient may be ill-looking, emaciated.
- Repeated coughing and bringing out a large amount of sputum.
- Tachypnea and tachycardia.
- Fever.
- Clubbing of fingers and toes.
- Weight loss.
- Edema feet if secondary amyloidosis develops and involves the kidneys.

Chest Examination

Inspection
- Diminished movement on the side involved (right side in this case).

Palpation
- Movements of the chest reduced on the side involved (right side in this case).
- Expansion of the chest is reduced if cavity is large.
- Shift of trachea and mediastinum to the same side if there is a large cavity with fibrosis (shifted to right side in this case).

Percussion
- Dull percussion note over the cavity. Rest of the lung is normally resonant.

Auscultation
- Amphoric or cavernous bronchial breathing over the cavity (cavernous breathing in this case).
- Increased vocal resonance over the area of cavity with bronchophony (present).
- Mid-inspiratory and expiratory crackles (present).
- Post-tussive crackles (present in this case).
- Crackpot sounds.

Note: All the above mentioned signs will be present only if the cavity is large, superficial and communicates with bronchus. Deep seated cavity may not produce any physical sign.

PROVISIONAL DIAGNOSIS

The symptoms of cough, fever, hemoptysis of 6 months duration and signs of cavitation (lesion) in this patient suggest a tubercular cavity in the right lung (aetiology). Patient has intermittent hemoptysis and dyspnea (functional status).

QUESTIONS AND ANSWERS

Q. **What are the points in favor of cavity?**

Ans: 1. Dull percussion note
2. Cavernous bronchial breathing
3. Increased vocal resonance, bronchophony and whispering pectorlique
4. Inspiratory and expiratory crackles
5. Post-tussive crackles

Q. **What are the a signs of fibrosis in your case?**

Ans: • Shift of trachea to same side
• Retraction of right infraclavicular region with crowding of ribs
• Reduced movement on right side (apical region)
• Dull percussion note
• Crackles

Q. **What is your differential diagnosis?**

Ans: 1. **Bronchiectasis** (could be tubercular). Read clinical case discussion on bronchiectasis.
2. **Resolving consolidation** will produce massive expectoration and bronchial breath sounds.
3. **Lung abscess.** Read symptoms and signs of lung abscess in separate case discussion.
4. **Malignancy lung.** Cough, hemoptysis, weakness, weight loss, cachexia along with signs of a cavity and hilar lymphadenopathy are pointers to its diagnosis.

Q. **What do you understand by the term "cavity" and pseudocavity?**

Ans: Pulmonary cavity is an area of liquefaction necrosis within the lung parenchyma in communication with a patent bronchus. The cavity may be empty or may be filled with secretions and infected material.

Pseudocavity means appearance of a cavity on chest X-ray which may be obtained with summation of shadows of vessels, ribs and calcification.

Q. **Name five common causes of cavity in the lung.**

Ans: 1. Tubercular cavity
2. Lung abscess, bronchiectasis
3. Malignancy lung
4. Pulmonary infarction
5. Wegener's granulomatosis

Q. **What are the various types of cavity seen in the lung?**

Ans: Types of cavities are as follows:
1. **Thin-walled:** A cavity is surrounded by a thin margin of lung tissue. The margin may be irregular, shaggy in lung abscess (*staphylococcal*) and bronchogenic carcinoma while it is smooth and regular in tuberculosis, lung cyst, hydatid cyst and fungal infection.
2. **Thicked walled** (Fig. 73.1): A thick wall is formed by thick exudative material or heaps of cells such as in *lung abscess, tuberculosis* and *bronchogenic carcinoma.*

Q. **What are the physical signs of a cavity?**

Ans: Typically, a superficial large cavity communicating with the bronchus produces signs which depend on whether the cavity is empty or filled with fluid at the time of examination. The signs of cavity are given in Table 73.1.

Table 73.1: Physical signs over a cavity		
Sign	*Empty*	*Filled*
• Movement of chest on the side and area involved	Diminished	Diminished
• Retraction/flattening of chest	Present	Present
• Tactile vocal fremitus and vocal resonance	Increased	Decreased
• Percussion note	Crackpot sounds	Diminished
• Breath sounds	Amphoric/ cavernous	Diminished
• Whispering pectoriloquy	Present	Absent
• Post-tussive crackles/rales	Absent	Present

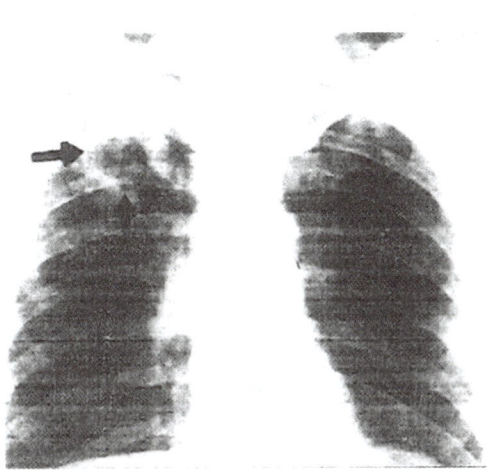

Fig. 73.1: Chest X-ray (PA view) showing a thick walled cavity with fibrosis (right side)

Q. **What is post-tussive crackles?**

Ans: These are crackles which are heard after coughing due to dislodgment of secretions in a cavity. They are characteristic of a tubercular cavity.

Q. **What is amphoric breath sounds? What are its causes?**

Ans: Read Clinical Methods by Prof. SN Chugh.

Q. **Which type of breathing occurs over a cavity?**

Ans. • Thin walled large cavity with narrow bronchus produces **amphoric bronchial breathing.**

• Thick walled cavity with patent (narrow or wide) bronchus produces **cavernous breathing.**

Q. **What are the complications of a tubercular cavity?**

Ans: • A source of intercurrent infections.
• Meningitis (tubercular) or miliary tuberculosis.
• Secondary amyloidosis in case of long-standing cavity.
• Hydropneumothorax.
• Chronic cavity may lead to malnutrition or hypoproteinemia.

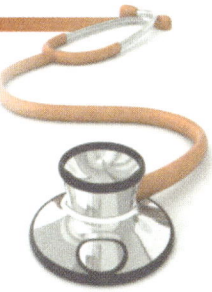

INSTRUCTION

Examine the patient's chest

SALIENT FEATURES

- Massive fetid sputum

HISTORY

Ask about the following:

- Fever, sweating, palpitations, tachypnea.
- Copious purulent or mucopurulent sputum with diurnal (more in the morning) and posturnal (more in lying down than sitting position) relation (a characteristic feature of pulmonary suppuration)
- Hemoptysis.
- Pain chest due to pleuritis if pleura involved.
- Ask about symptoms of underlying disease, e.g. tuberculosis, amebic liver abscess, malignancy lung.
- Ask about symptoms of meningitis (neck stiffness, vomiting, visual disturbance) and empyema thoracis.
- Ask about history of unconsciousness epilepsy, throat surgery or any other surgery under general anaesthesia (predisposing factors)

EXAMINATION

General Physical examination

- Toxic look
- Fever, sweating, tachycardia, tachypnea (present)
- Poor nutrition
- Cyanosis
- Clubbing of the fingers (present)
- Edema of legs if secondary renal amyloidosis or hypoproteinemia due to massive expectoration develops
- Foul smelling (fetid) sputum and breath (halitosis)

- Source of infection in upper respiratory tract, e.g. tonsillar or parapharyngeal abscess or throat sepsis may be evident
- Cervical lymphadenopathy may be present

Chest Examination

- All the signs present in a cavity filled with secretion/necrotic material will be present as discussed above in Case No. 73.
- In case of ruptured lung abscess, either the signs of empyema thoracis, or pyopneumothorax will be present. (Read empyema thoracis)
- In case of ruptured amebic liver abscess, there will be history of expectoration of anchovy sauce sputum with tender hepatomegaly.
- In case of malignancy, there will be marked weight loss, cachexia, hemoptysis with signs of collapse or consolidation. In addition, there may be features of metastatic spread to the mediastinal lymph nodes or evidence of compression of neighbouring structures.

PROVISIONAL DIAGNOSIS

The presence of fever, chest pain, copious sputum with signs of cavitation suggest lung abscess (lesion) following aspiration pneumonia (aetiology). Patient has toxemia with tachypnea, tachycardia (functional status).

QUESTIONS AND ANSWERS

Q. What are the points in favor of your diagnosis?

Ans:
- History of fever, chest pain, hemoptysis one month back.
- Persistence of fever, chest pain followed by massive expectoration.
- Foul breath.
- Sputum cup shows fetid, large amount of sputum.

- All signs of cavity are present, i.e. localised coarse crackles on the right lower lung with a patch of bronchial breathing.

Q. **What do you understand by the term lung abscess?**

Ans: **Definition:** It is defined as collection of purulent material in a localized necrotic area of the lung parenchyma. It is a suppurative lung disease.

Q. **What are the causes of lung abscess?**

Ans: I. **Primary lung abscess:** It is usually caused by necrotising pneumonia due to following organisms.
  a. *Pyogenic,* e.g. *Staph. aureus, Klebsiella. streptococci.*
  b. *Tubercular bacilli*—a tubercular cavity with collection of purulent material.
  c. *Fungi,* e.g. *Aspergillus, Histoplasma.*
  d. *Amebic lung abscess* secondary to liver abscess.

  II. **Secondary cavitation followed by infection:**
  - Thromboembolism with lung cavitation.
  - Metastatic lung abscesses.
  - Bronchogenic carcinoma with lung abscess.
  - Infected congenital cyst.

Q. **What are the sites of lung abscess?**

Ans: The site of an abscess depending on the position of patient at the time of abscess formation are tabulated (Table 74.1).

Table 74.1: Localization of lung abscess

1. Patient in lying down position
  - Right lung (commonest site)
    e.g. posterior segment of upper and superior segment of lower lobe
2. Patient in upright position
  - Basal segments of both the lobes

Note: The lung abscess is more common on right side due to less obliquity of right bronchus.

Q. **How will you investigate a case with lung abscess?**

Ans: The tests done are:
  - *Blood examination* for anemia and leukocytosis. Raised ESR suggests infection especially tuberculosis (markedly elevated).
  - *Sputum examination* for isolation of the organisms (Gram staining, Ziehl-Neelsen stain), for cytology including malignant cell; and culture and sensitivity.
  - *Blood culture* to isolate the organism. It is mostly sterile.

- *Urine examination* for proteinuria, pus cells and casts. Albuminuria indicates secondary renal amyloidosis.
- *Chest X-ray* (PA view) will show:
  - An area of consolidation with breakdown and translucency. The walls of the abscess may be outlined (Fig. 74.1).
  - The presence of a fluid level inside the translucent area confirms the diagnosis (Fig. 74.1).
  - Empyema, if develops, will be detected by radiological appearance of a pleural effusion (read radiological appearance of pleural effusion).
- *Bronchoscopic aspiration* for diagnosis. The aspirate is subjected to cytology, microbiology and culture.
- *Aspiration of empyema* — if develops.
- *MRI* of upper lobe.

Q. **How would you differentiate lung abscess from loculated empyema on CT scan?**

Ans: Read Fig. 74.2

Q. **What does edema indicate in a patient with lung abscess?**

Ans: 1. *Hypoproteinemia* due to loss of protein through massive expectoration.
  2. *Malnutrition/malabsorption.*
  3. *Renal amyloidosis* leading to albuminuria and nephrotic syndrome.

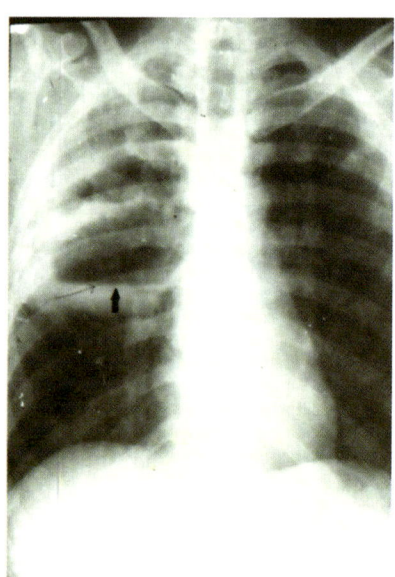

Fig. 74.1: Chest X-ray PA showing lung abscess on right side (↑)

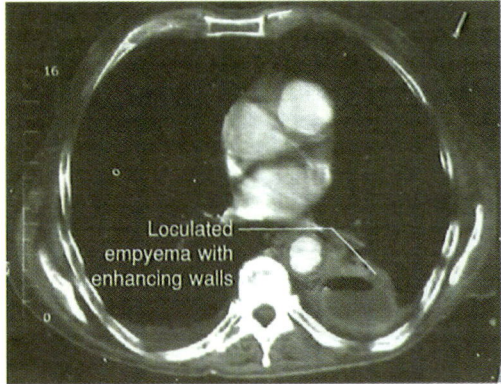

Loculated empyema with enhancing walls

CT features differentiating empyema from lung abscess

Loculated empyema	Lung abscess
• Lenticular shape	• Round shape.
• Uniform enhancing wall	• Non-uniform thick wall
• Compression of adjacent lung	• No compression of surrounding lung
• Obtuse angle with chest wall	• Acute angle with chst wall
• Separation of pleural layers	• May contain locules of gas in the wall

Fig. 74.2: CT scan shows loculated empyema. Read its features differentiating if from lung abscess discussed above

4. *Cor pulmonale* and *congestive cardiac failure*, through rare, may develop in some cases when the disease is extensive or bilateral.

Q. How does a lung abscess lead to brain abscess? What is the commonest site?

Ans: Lung abscess leads to meningitis and brain abscess by hematogenous spread. These abscesses are common in the posterior frontal region or parietal lobes.

Q. Which is the imaging procedure for upper lobe lesions?

Ans: MRI is better for upper lobe lesions than CT scan of the chest, otherwise MRI is less useful than CT scan because of poorer imaging of lung parenchyma and inferior spatial resolution.

Q. How would you treat such a case?

Ans: 1. *Postural drainage of the cavity*, sitting position is best for upper lobe cavity

2. Antibiotics for infection, first broad spectrum with anaerobic cover, then according to culture and sensitivity

3. Expectorants and mucolytic agents

4. Bronchoscopic aspiration, if accessible

5. Surgical resection, if localised and no complication

75

Old Pulmonary Tuberculosis

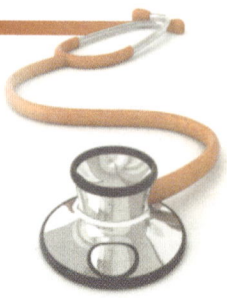

INSTRUCTION

Examine the patient's chest

SALIENT FEATURES

- Cough, fever, hemoptysis, night sweats and weakness.

HISTORY

Ask for the following:

- Write chief complaints in chronological order.
- Note the onset and progression of the symptoms.
- History of fever, cough, hemoptysis, breathlessness, pain chest/discomfort, any neurological deficit.
- Any history of weight loss, decreased appetite, night sweats or evening rise in temperature (present).
- Ask complaints pertaining to other systems.

EXAMINATION

General Physical Examination

- Ill-look, emaciated
- Look for phlyctenular conjunctivitis.
- Look for cervical or axillary lymphadenopathy.
- Look for anemia, jaundice, cyanosis and edema feet.
- Look for JVP, trachea, etc.
- Note any clubbing of the fingers.
- Any joint involvement.

Chest Examination

Inspection

- Shape and symmetry of chest, note any bulging or retraction (bilateral infraclavicular retraction present).
- Look at the movements of chest at every quadrant of chest. Compare both sides with each other (movements of upper parts of both sides reduced).

- Look at the apex beat e.g. location.
- Look for any distended veins or scar mark or mark for aspiration over the chest.
- Count the respiratory rate and note the type of breathing.
- Look for pulsations in supraclavicular fossa, epigastrium or other sites.

Palpation

- Palpate the apex beat to confirm its position.
- Palpate the trachea for any deviation.
- Note the expansion of the chest and measure it.
- Compare the vocal fremitus on both the sides.
- Palpate the intercostal space for any widening or narrowing.
- Palpate the crepitus, or crackles or rub if any.

Percussion

- Percuss the lungs for resonance. Note is dull in infraclavicular regions.
- Define cardiac and liver dullness.
- Percuss 2nd left and right intercostal spaces for dullness or resonance.
- Percuss directly the clavicles and supraclavicular areas for resonance.

Auscultation

- Hear the breath sounds and note the character and intensity and compare them on both the sides.
- Hear for any added sounds, e.g. crackles (present), wheezes and rub, etc.
- Vocal resonance to be compared on both sides for increase or decrease
- Elicit other specific signs depending on the underlying disease, e.g. succussion splash, coin test, etc.

Other Systems

- Examine the spine for deformity and tenderness.
- Examine abdomen for fluid or any organ enlargement.

- Examine eyes for phlyctenular conjunctivitis or choroid tubercles.
- Elicit the signs of meningitis if suspected.

PROVISIONAL DIAGNOSIS

The patient has fever, cough, hemoptysis and crackles at both apices (lesion) due to post primary apical tuberculosis (aetiology). Patient has weakness and anemia (functional status).

QUESTIONS AND ANSWERS

Q. What are the points in favor of your diagnosis of bilateral apical fibro-exudative tuberculosis?

Ans: The points in favour are:
- Depressed chest in both the infraclavicular regions.
- Trachea is not shifted due to bilateral lesions.
- No mediastinal shift.
- Percussion note over the areas involved is impaired.
- Fine crackles are heard at both the apices
- No bronchial breath sounds.

Q. What do you understand by the term post primary tuberculosis? How does, it differ from progressive primary complex?

Ans: About 85–90% of patients develop latent infection (i.e positive tuberculin test or radiographic evidence of self-healed tuberculosis (primary focus) and within this group 5–10% reactivate during their life-time resulting in post-primary disease predominantly pulmonary (50% smear positive). Reactivation of these smear positive pulmonary tuberculosis cases may result in post primary disease/tuberculosis. The difference between progressive primary complex and post-primary tuberculosis are enlisted in Table 75.1.

Table 75.1: Difference between progressive primary and postprimary tuberculosis

Progressive primary complex	Postprimary tuberculosis
• Common in children	• Common in adults
1. Hilar lymphadenopathy present	Absence of lymph node enlargement
2. Subpleural focus or focus in any part of the lung	Usually apical fibrosis
3. Cavitation rare	Cavitation common
4. Fibrosis uncommon	Fibrosis common
5. Miliary tuberculosis common	Miliary tuberculosis uncommon
6. Direct extension of primary focus	Reactivation of smear positive pulmonary disease

Q. What are the clinical presentations of post-primary pulmonary tuberculosis?

Ans: Clinical presentations are as follows:
- Asymptomatic (diagnosed on chest X-ray).

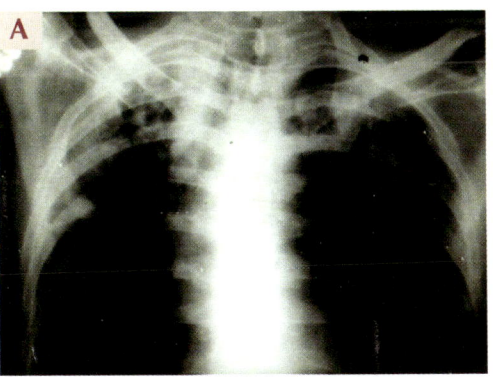
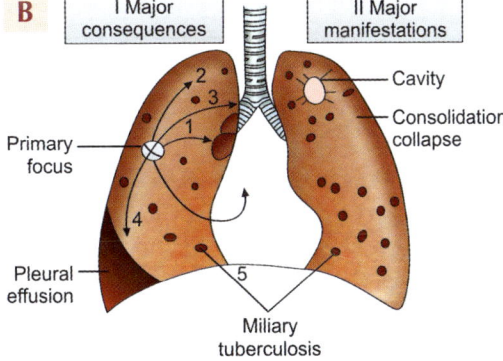

Fig. 75.1: (A) Old pulmonary tubercular lesions: There is bilateral fibrocalcified lesion;
(B) Primary pulmonary tuberculosis. Consequences if left untreated are (diagram)
1. The primary focus may spread to hilar or mediastinal lymph node to form primary or Ghon's focus
2. Direct extension of primary focus into other part of the lung
3. Extension of primary focus to bronchus
4. Extension of primary focus to pleura
5. Dissemination into blood stream leading to miliary tuberculosis

- Chronic cough, hemoptysis with signs and symptoms of exudation/infiltration or a cavity or collapse/fibrosis.
- Pyrexia of unknown origin (PUO).
- Unresolved pneumonia (consolidation).
- Pleural effusion, pleural calcification.
- Weight loss, night sweats, evening rise of temperature, general debility (cryptic tuberculosis).
- Spontaneous pneumothorax.

Q. What is the time table of tuberculosis?

Ans: As already described, in 85–90% cases the primary complex heals spontaneously with or without calcification. In 10–15% cases, multiplication of tubercular bacilli is not contained, further spread leads to lymph nodes enlargement resulting in local pressure effects or lymphatic spread occurs to the pleura or pericardium or rupture into adjacent bronchus or pulmonary blood vessel. The time table of tuberculosis is given in Table 75.2.

Table 75.2: Time table of tuberculosis

Time from infection	Manifestation
3–8 weeks	• Primary complex, positive tuberculin skin test, erythema nodosum
3–6 months	• Collapse and bronchiectasis, adult pulmonary tuberculosis, miliary tuberculosis
Within 1 year	• Pneumonia, pleural effusion
Within 3 years	• Tuberculosis affecting bones, lymph node, joints, GI tract and genitourinary
From 3 years onwards	• Post-primary disease due to reactivation or reinfection
Around 8 years	• Urinary tract disease

Q. Who are at high risk of tuberculosis?

Ans:
- Asian immigrants
- Older persons
- Alcoholics, debilitated persons and destitutes
- Immunocompromised individuals, i.e. AIDS and diabetic patients
- Professional, e.g. doctors, nurses, physiotherapist.
- Close contacts (e.g. family members of a open case)

Q. What is cryptic tuberculosis? What is its presentation?

Ans: The term 'cryptic' means 'hidden'. A patient of tuberculosis with normal chest radiograph is called *cryptic tuberculosis*. Its presentation is as follows:
- Age over 60 years.

- Intermittent low grade fever (PUO) with night sweats and evening rise.
- Unexplained weight loss, general debility.
- Hepatosplenomegaly (seen in 25% cases only).
- Normal chest X-ray.
- Negative tuberculin skin test.
- Leukemoid reaction or pancytopenia.
- Confirmation is done by biopsy (liver or bone marrow).

Q. What are the stigmata of tuberculosis (evidence of present or past infection or disease)?

Ans: Stigmata associated with the tuberculosis are as follows:
- Phlyctenular conjunctivitis.
- Erythema nodosum.
- Tubercular lymphadenopathy with or without scars and sinuses.
- Thickened, beaded spermatic cord.
- Scrofuloderma.
- Positive Mantoux test.
- Localized gibbus, spinal deformity, paravertebral soft tissue swelling.

Q. What are the chronic complications of pulmonary tuberculosis?

Ans: Common chronic complications of pulmonary TB are:

1. **Pulmonary complications:**
   - Massive hemoptysis resulting in anaemia
   - Cor pulmonale
   - Fibrosis/emphysema (compensatory)
   - Recurrent infections
   - Tubercular empyema
   - Lung/pleural calcification
   - Obstructive airway disease (endobronchial)
   - Bronchiectasis
   - Bronchopleural fistula

2. **Non-pulmonary complications:**
   - Empyema necessitans
   - Laryngitis
   - Enteritis following ingestion of infected sputum
   - Anorectal disease following ingestion of infected sputum
   - Amyloidosis (secondary)
   - Poncet's polyarthritis

Q. How will you investigate a case of pulmonary tuberculosis?

Ans: Investigations are as follows:

1. *Routine blood examination,* i.e. TLC, DLC and ESR. Raised ESR and C-reactive protein suggest tuberculosis.

2. *Mantoux* test is non-specific (low sensitivity and specificity).

3. *Sputum* (induced by nebulized hypertonic saline if not expectorated), or *gastric lavage* (mainly used for children) or *bronchoalveolar lavage* for acid fast bacilli isolation (Ziehl-Neelsen stain and culture).

4. *Chest X-ray* (AP, PA, lateral and lordotic views) for radiological manifestations of tuberculosis in the lungs. The varied manifestations are:
   • Soft fluffy shadow (confluent)
   • Apical infiltration
   • Dense nodular opacities
   • Miliary mottling shadows (military tuberculosis)
   • A cavity or multiple cavities (irregular, thick walled)
   • Fibrocaseous lesion
   • Tuberculoma
   • Calcification—lung and/or pleura
   • Bronchiectasis especially in the upper zones
   • Mediastinal (unilateral) lymphadenopathy (enlarged hilar lymphnodes)
   • Primary complex in children

5. *CT scan* for diagnosis and differential diagnosis

6. *PCR (polymerase chain reaction)* with blood or any other fluid

7. *ADA (adenosine deaminase)* levels increase in tuberculosis

8. *Transbronchial biopsy*

Q. **Which test gives an early diagnosis of tuberculosis?**

Ans: Polymerase chain reaction (PCR) gives rapid diagnosis.

Q. **How would you investigate close contacts of a patient with tuberculosis?**

Ans: Close contacts are investigated as follows:
   • First confirm the history of close contacts with the patient having open tuberculosis.
   • Enquire about BCG vaccination.
   • Perform Mantoux or Heaf testing.
   • Advise chest X-ray examination.

Q. **How would you treat newly diagnosed sputum positive tuberculosis?**

Ans: 1. Isolation of the patient in a single room for 2 weeks if smear positive.
   2. Barrier nursing care.

3. For new smear-positive or new cases of pulmonary tuberculosis are put on WHO—DOTS regimen category I which comprises of
   • HRZE daily/thrice a week for 2 months (double dose of the drug).
   • Assess sputum for AFB. If negative use two drugs (HR) for 4 months.
   • If sputum remain positive, extend four drugs regimen for one month more, then use 2 drugs (HR) for 2 months and if sputum is negative continue it for 2 months more or if positive, shift to category II.

Q. **What are the indications of BCG vaccination?**

Ans: • Previous unvaccinated contacts.
   • Persistently Mantoux test negative contacts below 35 years of age.

Q. **What are the indications of chemoprophylaxis?**

Ans: 1. Mantoux test positive persons with no clinical or radiological evidence of tuberculosis.
   2. Children under 5 years of age who are close contacts of smear positive adult patient.
   3. Immunocompromised contacts irrespective of immune status.

Q. **Which drug is used for chemoprophylaxis?**

Ans: Isoniazid is used in usual dosage for one year.

Q. **What is miliary tuberculosis? What is the status of immunity in this disease?**

Ans: It is defined as dissemination of tuberculosis through the blood stream producing miliary tubercles in various organs. Immunity is lowered in it, hence, dissemination occurs. Mantoux test is negative which confirms lowered immunity.

Q. **What is the treatment of multidrug resistant tuberculosis?**

Ans: Drug resistant tuberculosis may be primary or acquired during treatment with inappropriate regimen or due to irregular treatment. MDR (multidrug resistant) tuberculosis is a big problem in Asia. Although 6 months regimen of RZE (excluding H) is effective for patients with initial isoniazid resistance, all the 3 drugs to be continued for 6 months.

For patients resistant to isoniazid (H) and rifampicin (R), combinations of a fluoroquinolones, ethambutol (E), pyrazinamide (Z) and streptomycin (S) is given for 18–24 months and for at least a months after sputum culture conversion. For those resistant to streptomycin, injectable amikacin can be used in its place.

For patients resistant to all first line drugs, cure may be obtained with combination of 4 second line drugs (ethionamide, cycloserine, quinoline and PAS) including one injectable agent for full 24 months.

Q.   Name new antitubercular drugs.

Ans: Following drugs are being evaluated:
  • Rifapentine—a rifamycin antibiotic is bacteriostatic similar to rifampicin. Other drugs include gatifloxacin, moxifloxacin clarithromycin, linezolid and oxazolidi-nones.

76

Pneumothorax

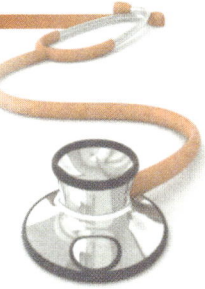

INSTRUCTION

Examine the patient's chest.

SALIENT FEATURES

- Acute dyspnoea at rest

HISTORY

Ask about the following:

- History of acute onset of dyspnea at rest and non-progressive.
- History of pain chest or tightness of chest.
- History of palpitation and tachypnea.
- History of asthma, COPD, ARDS, pneumonia and trauma to chest.
- Ipsilateral acute pleuritic pain.
- History of recent pleural aspiration or insertion of subclavian line or recent surgery on head and neck.
- History of Marfan's syndrome (tall stature).
- History of HIV (sexual contact).
- History of positive pressure ventilation.
- Any history of IHD (chest pain in the present or past).
- Any history of prolonged immobilisation or calf pain (pulmonary thromboembolism).
- Past/history of COPD, asthma, tuberculosis, hemoptysis or trauma.
- History of similar episodes in the past.

EXAMINATION

General Physical Examination

- *Posture:* Patients prefer to lie on the uninvolved side in lateral decubitus position or propped up position.
- Restlessness.
- Tachypnea (respiratory rate is increased), dyspnea at rest (present in this case).
- Tachycardia.
- Central cyanosis indicates tension pneumothorax.

- Lymph nodes may or may not be palpable.
- Trachea may be shifted to opposite side (sternomastoid sign or Trail's sign positive in this case).
- Accessory muscles of respiration may be actively working.
- Ear, nose, throat should be examined.
- Note the vitals, i.e. pulse, BP, temperature and respiration. Presence of hypotension or shock indicates tension pneumothorax, creates an emergency situation and warrants removal of the air.
- Look for clues regarding etiology, e.g.
  - Pleural aspiration site
  - Infraclavicular region for a bruise from the central line
  - Marfanoid features
  - Inhaler or peak flowmeter by bedside to ascertain asthma or COPD.

Chest Examination

Inspection

- Diminished movements on the side involved (right side in this case).
- Intercostal spaces widened and full on the side involved (right side in this case).
- Apex beat displaced to opposite side (left side).
- Accessory muscles of respiration are hyperactive and stand out prominently in tension pneumothorax.

Palpation

- Shift of trachea and apex beat (mediastinum) to the opposite side (e.g. left side in this case).
- Diminished movements on the side involved (e.g. right side).
- Expansion of chest decreased (on manual or tape measurement).
- Tactile vocal fremitus is reduced on the side involved (right side).

Percussion

- Hyperresonant percussion note on the side involved (right side).

- Obliteration of liver dullness if right side is involved (obliterated in this case), splenic dullness if left side is involved (not applicable in this case).

Auscultation

- Markedly diminished vesicular breathing or absent breath sounds on the side involved (right side in this case). Bronchial breathing indicates bronchopleural fistula (open pneumothorax).
- Vocal resonance diminished over the area involved (right side).
- No adventitious sound.
- Coin test may be positive.

PROVISIONAL DIAGNOSIS

The patient has pneumothorax (lesion) secondary to COPD (aetiology) and is dyspnoeic at rest but does not have chronic cor pulmonale (functional status).

QUESTIONS AND ANSWERS

Q.   What are points in favour of your diagnosis?
Ans: The points in favor of diagnosis are:
  i. Prominent chest on the right side involved with diminished movements.
  ii. Shifting of trachea and mediastinum to opposite side (left side in this case).
  iii. Reduced vocal fremitus and vocal resonance on the side involved (right side).
  iv. Hyperresonant percussion note with diminished/absent breath sounds on the side involved (right side in this case).

Q.   What is pneumothorax?
Ans: Presence of air in the pleural cavity is called *pneumothorax.*

Q.   Could it be a large bulla instead of pneumothorax right side?
Ans: No. The differentiating features are tabulated (Table 76.1)

Table 76.1: Differentiating features of bulla from pneumothorax

Large air cyst or bulla	Pneumothorax
May be congenital or acquired	Acquired usually
Mediastinum not shifted (trachea is central)	Mediastinum shifted to opposite side (trachea shifted to opposite side)
No underlying collapse of the lung on chest X-ray	Collapse of the lung occurs in pneumothorax. It will be evident by a thin line on chest X-ray

Q.   What are various types of pneumothorax? What are their causes?
Ans: Read Table 76.2.

Q.   What are the causes of recurrent pneumothorax?
Ans: This refers to occurrence of second episode of pneumothorax within few weeks following the first episode. The causes are;
- Rupture of apical subpleural blebs or emphysematous bullae.
- Cystic fibrosis.
- Rupture of lung cysts.
- Rupture of bronchogenic carcinoma or esophageal carcinoma.
- Catamenial pneumothorax.
- AIDS.
- Interstitial lung disease.

Q.   What do you understand by the term subcutaneous emphysema? What are its causes?
Ans: Subcutaneous emphysema (or surgical emphysema) refers to presence of air in the subcutaneous space either formed by necrotizing inflammation of the tissue by gas-forming organisms (gas gangrene) or by leakage of air from the lungs or neighboring hollow structures. The causes are:
- Pneumothorax.
- Rib fracture or flail chest with leakage of air.
- Fractures of paranasal sinuses.
- Perforation of a hollow viscus, e.g. esophagus or larynx (spontaneous or procedural).
- Gas gangrene.

Always look for subcutaneous emphysema in a case of pneumothorax by palpation with pressure of fingers for palpable crepitus over the side involved.

Q.   What are the complications of pneumothorax?
Ans: Common complications of pneumothorax are:
- Hydropneumothorax.
- Empyema thoracis, pyopneumothorax.
- Hemopneumothorax.
- Thickened pleura.
- Acute circulatory failure—cardiac tamponade in tension pneumothorax.
- Atelectasis of the lung.
- Surgical emphysema and pneumomediastinum.

Q.   How would you grade the degree of collapse in pneumothorax?
Ans: British thoracic society grading is:

Table 76.2: Types of pneumothorax and their clinical features

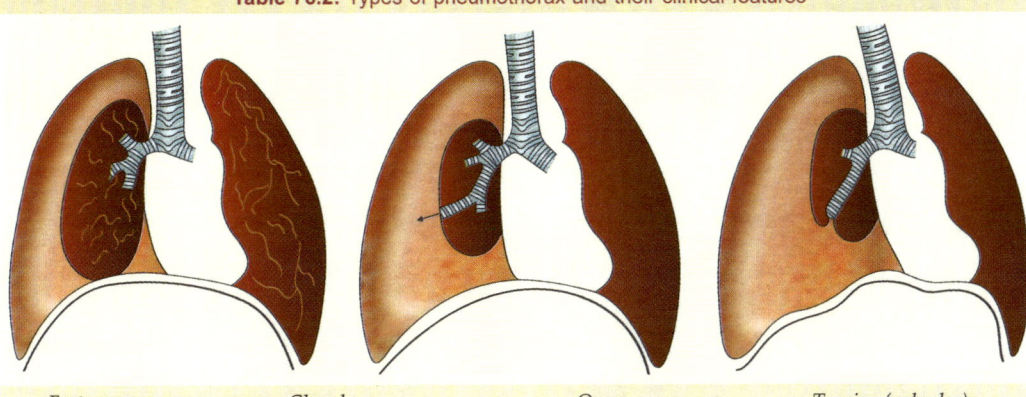

Features	Closed	Open	Tension (valvular)
Pathogenesis	The rupture site (opening) gets closed and underlying lung is collapsed (deflated). There is no communication between bronchus and the pleural space	The opening between the bronchus and pleural space does not close, remains patent, hence, called *bronchopleural fistula*	The communication between bronchus and pleural space persists and acts as a check valve (air can get in but cannot get out)
Mean pleural pressure	Negative (less than atmospheric pressure) hence, air can get absorbed and lung re-expands	Mean pleural pressure is atmospheric, hence, lung cannot reexpand. Secondly, due to patent communication, pneumothorax is likely to be infected leading to *pyopneumothorax*—a common complication	Mean pleural pressure is positive, goes on building due to constant air entry during inspiration resulting in compression collapse with mediastinal shift and imparid venous return leading to cardiac tamponade
Causes	• Rupture of subpleural blebs or emphysematous bullae COPD • Spontaneous due to congenital bleb rupture • Rupture of pulmonary end of pleural adhesion • Secondary to lung disease • Chest injury (blunt/penetrating)	• Tubercular cavity • Lung abscess • Necrotizing pneumonia • Chest trauma • Barotrauma • Empyema thoracic • Lung resection	• It can occur due to any cause • Catamenial pneumothorax (endometriosis in female)

- *Small;* where there is small rim of air (translucent area) around the lung.
- *Moderate;* when the lung is compressed towards the hilum (Fig. 76.1) by a large translucent area containing air.
- *Complete;* Airless lung, separate from diaphragm (aspiration is necessary).
- *Tension;* Any pneumothorax with signs of cardiorespiratory distress.

Q. When would you suspect tension penumothorax?

Ans: Tension pneumothorax should be suspected with any of the following signs:

- Severe progressive dyspnea.

- Tachypnea (RR > 30 min), tachycardia (HR > 130/min), cyanosis.
- Hypotension, pulsus paradoxus.
- Marked mediastinal shift.

Q. How will you investigate a patient with pneumothorax?

Ans: Investigations are done for sake of diagnosis and to find out the cause.

1. *Chest X-ray (PA view*, Fig. 76.1) should be done first of all before any other investigation in case of suspected pneumothorax. It is done in erect position, sometimes expiratory film is taken especially in small pneumothorax. The radiological features are:

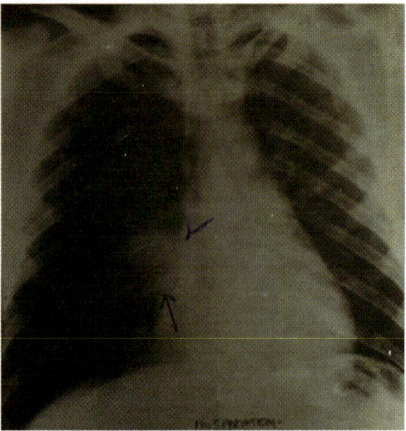

Fig. 76.1: Pneumothorax — Chest X-ray showing right sided pneumothorax. The collapsed lung is indicated by arrows

- Increased translucency of the lung on the side involved with absence of peripheral lung markings.
- The underlying lung is collapsed which is separated from airless peripheral translucent shadow (pneumothorax) by a pencil — sharp border.
- Mediastinum is shifted to opposite side.
- Costophrenic angle is clear.
- Underlying lung disease may be apparent such as a tubercular cavity.

2. *Routine blood tests,* e.g. TLC, DLC, ESR, (raised ESR with relative mononuclear leukocytosis suggest tubercular etiology).
3. *Mantoux test* may be positive in tuberculosis.
4. *Sputum for AFB* (3 consecutive specimens).
5. *Pulmonary function tests* (FEV$_1$, FEV$_1$/VC ratio, PFR, etc. for COPD).

Q. How would you perform a pleurodhesis?

Ans: By injecting talc into pleural cavity via intercostal tube.

Q. In which patient, pleurodhesis is not performed?

Ans: In patients with fibrosis, pleurodhesis is not attempted as they need lung transplantation in future and pleurodhesis would make it technically not feasible.

Q. What are indications of open thoracotomy?

Ans: It is considered when one of the following is present.
- A third episode of spontaneous pneumothorax.
- An occurrence of bilateral pneumothorax.
- Failure of the lung to expand after tube thoracotomy.

Q. How would you manage this patient?

Ans: As this patient has a large pneumothorax, hence aspiration is needed. Large pneumothorax with normal lungs are managed by simple aspiration rather than an intercostal tube drainage, aspiration is less painful than intercostal drainage, leads to shorter admission and reduces the need for pleurectomy with no increase in recurrence rate.

Following simple aspiration, an intercostal tube with underwater seal drainage is used. The tube should be left for 24 hr. When the lung has re-expanded, clamp the tube for 24 hr. If repeat chest X-ray shows that lung remains expanded, the tube can be removed if not, suction should be applied to the tube.

If pneumothorax fails to resolve within one week, surgical pleurodhesis should be considered.

Note: Small pneumothorax (< 20% in size) spontaneously resolve within weeks.

77

Bronchopleural Fistula (Hydro/ Pyopneumothorax)

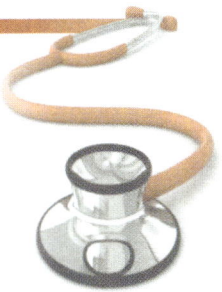

INSTRUCTION

Examine the patient's chest

SALIENT FEATURES

- Cough, breathlessness and sputum. Complains of abnormal sound in the left hemithorax while walking

HISTORY

Ask for the following:

- Dyspnea at rest, cough
- Pain chest or heaviness in chest
- Splashing sound during jumping (present)
- Fever, high grade with chills and rigors if pyopneumothorax
- History of fever or injury in the past
- History of tuberculosis in the past
- Any history of pain chest, hemoptysis or a cardiac disorder
- Any history of drainage of fluid in the past

EXAMINATION

General Physical Examination

- Patient is orthopneic
- Fever (afebrile)
- Tachypnea, tachycardia
- Cyanosis
- Clubbing of fingers present in pyopneumothorax
- Accessory muscles of respiration may be active
- Shift of trachea and mediastinum to opposite side—*Sternomastoid sign or Trail sign* may be positive (present)

Chest Examination

Inspection

- Signs similar to closed penumothorax

Palpation

- Signs similar to open pneumothorax (Read previous case discussion)

Percussion

- A horizontal fluid level, above which percussion note in hyperresonant and below which it is stony dull—hence, there is a clear cut transition between a hyperresonant to stony dull note (present on left side in this case)
- Shifting dullness (present) because fluid has space (occupied by air) to shift
- Coin test positive

Auscultation

- Succession splash (present in this case)
- Amphoric bronchial breathing is present in bronchopleural fistula—a common cause of hydropneumothorax (present in this case)
- Tingling sounds heard

PROVISIONAL DIAGNOSIS

The patient has hydropneumothorax (lesion) caused by bronchopleural fistula (aetiology). Patient is dyspneic at rest (functional status).

QUESTIONS AND ANSWERS

Q. **What are the points in favor of your diagnosis?**

Ans: • History of fluid movement in the chest while walking.
  - Presence of a clear cut level defined on percussion above which there is hyper-resonant note and below it stony dull note on left side.
  - Shifting dullness
  - Succussion splash is present. Coin test is positive in this case.
  - Amphoric bronchial breathing (diagnostic)
  - Tingling sound on ausculation

Q. **What is hydropneumothorax?**

Ans: The presence of both air (above) and fluid (below) in a pleural cavity is called *hydropneumothorax*. If instead of fluid, pus collects along with air, then it is called *pyopneumothorax*. Similarly collection of air and blood is called *hemopneumothorax*.

Q. **What is your differential diagnosis?**

Ans: Following conditions may mimic hydropneumothorax:

1. **Pyopneumothorax** (there will be fever, signs of toxemia in addition to hydropneumothorax).

2. **Pleural effusion** (Read Table 77.1).

3. **Eventration of diaphragm** with herniation of stomach into chest (this will produce succussion splash with resonant percussion note. Borborgymi sounds may be heard over the chest).

4. A **large lung abscess** partially filled with exudate will produce signs of cavity

and coarse crackles are characteristics. (Read Table 77.2).

Q. **What are causes of succession splash?**

Ans: Read clinical methods in medicine by Prof. SN Chugh.

Q. **What is bronchopleural fistula?**

Ans: Actually it is communication between atmosphere via nose and pleura via the bronchus. It is an open type of pneumothorax in which repeated infections are common and results in *hydro* or *pyopneumothorax*. All signs of hydropneumothorax are present. Amphoric bronchial sounds indicate a patent communication and confirm the diagnosis.

Q. **What are the differences between hydropneumothorax and pleural effusion?**

Ans: Read Table 77.1.

Q. **What are the causes of hydropneumothorax?**

Ans: Common causes of hydropneumothorax are:
  - Rupture of subpleural tubercular cavity (the most common cause).

Table 77.1: Differentiating feature of hydropneumothorax and pleural effusion

Hydropneumothorax (Fig. 77.1)	Pleural effusion
• Shifting dullness present	Shifting dullness absent
• Horizontal fluid level, i.e. there is transition between hyperresonant note (above and stony dull note (below)	No such level
• Succussion splash present	No succussion splash
• Tingling sounds especially after cough may be audible	No such sound
• Coin-test sound in upper part of hydropneumothorax may occasionally be positive	Coin—test negative
• Diminished breath sounds and vocal resonance except in bronchopleural fistula where amphoric breath sounds may be heard	Sometimes, a tubular bronchial breathing with increased vocal resonance (bronchophony, whispering pectoriloquy and egophony) present over the top of effusion

Table 77.2: Differentiating features between pyopneumothorax and lung abscess

Pyopneumothorax	Lung abscess
• Cough and expectoration minimal	Copious purulent expectoration is a predominant feature
• Shift of the mediastinum and trachea to opposite side	No shift of trachea or mediastinum
• Added sounds are absent	Added sounds such as crackles will be present
• Chest X-ray will show horizontal level starting from the periphery	A horizontal fluid level does not touch the periphery of the lung
• Vocal fremitus, breath sounds and vocal resonance diminished or absent	Vocal fremitus and vocal resonance may be decreased (cavity full of pus) or increased if lung abscess is empty and superficially placed. There can be a bronchial breathing as heard over a cavity. communicating with bronchus

- Rupture of lung abscess—actually, it causes pyopneumothorax.
- Penetrating chest injury with infection—again a cause of hemo-pneumothorax.
- Acute pulmonary infarction (embolism).
- Following cardiac surgery.
- *Iatrogenic,* i.e. introduction of the air during aspiration of pleural effusion.
- *Pneumothorax.* Actually broncho-pleural fistula (open pneumothorax) of tubercular etiology is the most common cause, but sympathetic collection of fluid in closed and tension pneumothorax may also lead to hydropneumothorax.

Q. **What are the causes of bronchopleural fistula?**

Ans: Hydropneumothorax is not synonymous with bronchopleural fistula. Common causes include:

- Rupture of tubercular cavity into pleural space (communicating bronchus patent)
- Rupture of lung abscess into pleura with patent bronchus
- Trauma to chest or barotrauma
- Necrotizing pneumonia leading to empyema thoracis
- Following lung resection

Q. **How would you explain absent shifting dullness in a case of hydropneumothorax?**

Ans: Hydropneumothorax contains air above (occupying a large space) and fluid below (occupying smaller space), both in moderate amount and are separated by a horizontal level (Fig. 77.1). Shifting dullness is present because fluid has space to shift by displacing air. Therefore, shifting dullness in hydropneumothorax will be absent if above mentioned conditions are not fulfilled thick pus or blood in the pleural space or adhesions in the space.

Q. **What are the characteristic features of pyopneumothorax?**

Ans: The patient will have all the clinical features of hydropneumothorax *plus:*

- Presence of toxic look and prostration.
- Hectic fever with chills and rigors.
- Tachycardia, tachypnea and clubbing of fingers.
- Intercostal tenderness and tenderness during percussion (patient winces during percussion).

Q. **Are empyema thoracis and pyopneumothorax synonymous?**

Ans: Yes, clinical features of both empyema thoracis and pyopneumothorax are similar.

Q. **How will you differentiate between a lung abscess and pyopneumothorax?**

Ans: Read Table 77.2

Q. **How will you investigate a patient with pyopneumothorax?**

Ans: Investigations are as follows:

1. *Routine blood tests* such as TLC, DLC and ESR for leukocytosis.
2. *Sputum examination* for culture and sensitivity.
3. *Chest X-ray (PA view)* will show:
   - A horizontal fluid level.
   - Increased radiolucency above the horizontal level without lung markings with a homogeneous opacity below the horizontal level (Fig. 77.1).
   - Shifting of trachea and media-stinum to the opposite side.

   N.B. X-ray should be taken in upright position to show a fluid level:
   - The collapsed lung due to compression from outside is usually hidden within homogeneous opacity of fluid and may not be visible on X-ray.
4. *Aspiration of fluid* or the thick exudate (pus) will be done which is sent for culture and sensitivity.

Q. **What is coin test and how would you elicit it?**

Ans: Read Clinical Methods in Medicine by Prof. SN Chugh.

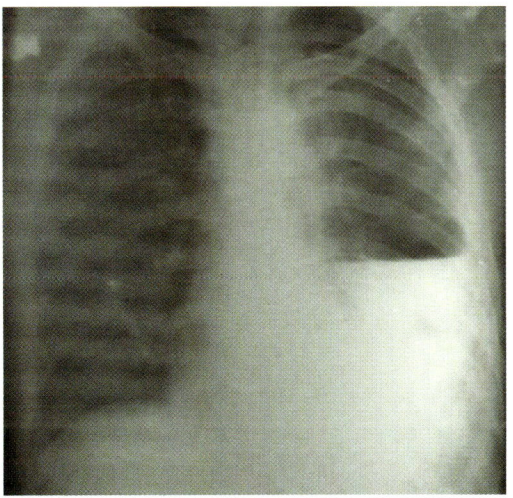

Fig. 77.1: Hydropneumothorax; chest X-ray (PA view) shows hydropneumothorax (left side)

Q. How will you treat a patient with hydro-pneumothorax/bronchopleural fistula?

Ans: 1. *Water-seal intercostal tube drainage* by putting a Foley's catheter into pleural space and connecting it with water-seal. The fluid will be drained and the air is also expelled with it while remaining air will get absorbed automatically.

2. *Antibiotics depending* on the cause. If cause is tubercular, institute ATT.

3. *Surgery* is done in resistant cases especially with pyo or hemopneumothorax.

78

Collapse of the Lung

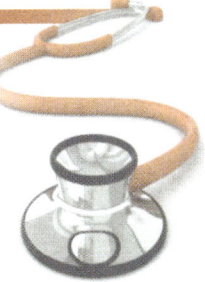

INSTRUCTION

Examine the patient's chest

SALIENT FEATURES

- Dyspnoea on exertion with cough

HISTORY

Ask about the following:

- Onset of symptoms with duration
- Pain chest or deformity of chest
- Breathlessness (at rest or on exertion)
- Dry cough and fever
- Malaise, night sweats, evening rise in temperature and weight loss
- Past history of tuberculosis or malignancy or asthma
- Any history of swelling in the neck, axilla or groin (lymphadenopathy)
- Past history of mumps, measles and whooping cough during childhood
- Past history of rheumatic heart disease or pericardial disease (fever, chest pain)

EXAMINATION

General Physical Examination

Look for the followings:
- Patient may be dyspneic, orthopneic if major bronchus is involved
- Central cyanosis
- Tachypnea, tachycardia
- Fever (develops in fibrosing alveolitis or in bronchogenic carcinoma)

Chest Examination

Inspection

- Flattening or depression of the chest on affected side (right upper part, i.e. infraclavicular region)

- Crowding of the ribs and narrowing of intercostal spaces over upper part of chest (present in this case)
- Diminished movements on the side involved (present)
- Shifting of trachea (Trail sign), apex beat towards the side involved (present in this case
- Kyphoscoliosis may result in long-standing collapsed lung with fibrosis
- Drooping of shoulder if apex of the lung is collapsed (present in this case)

Palpation

- Shifting of trachea and mediastinum to the same side (present)
- Reduced movements of the chest on involved side (right side)
- Reduced expansion of the chest on side involved (right side)
- Vocal fremitus on the affected side may be;
    - Diminished or absent if bronchus is totally occluded
    - Increased if bronchus is patent

Percussion

- Impaired or dull note on the side affected (right side in this case)

Auscultation

Collapse with obstructed bronchus (central collapse)
- Diminished or absent breath sounds
- Diminished/absent vocal resonance
- No added sounds

Collapse with patent bronchus (peripheral collapse)
- Tubular bronchial breath sounds
- Increased vocal resonance with bronchophony and whispering pectoriloquy
- Coarse crackles may be heard occasionally

PROVISIONAL DIAGNOSIS

The patient has a collapsed upper part of right lung (lesion) the cause of which has to be found out. The patient is breathless at rest (functional status).

QUESTIONS AND ANSWERS

Q. What are the points in favor of your diagnosis?

Ans: Points in favour of diagnosis are:
- Depressed chest and decreased movements on the right side involved.
- Shift of trachea and mediastinum to the right side.
- Dull percussion note on the site involved. (infraclavicular region)
- Breath sounds are diminished on the affected part of lung. (upper lobe)

Q. What is the probable cause in this case?

Ans: It could be tubercular due to following reasons:
- Gradual onset of weight loss, anorexia, fever with evening rise and night sweats.
- Physical signs are localized to apical region of upper lobe.
- No signs of toxaemia or cachexia.

Q. What is Brock syndrome?

Ans: Collapse of lung due to compression of right middle lobe bronchus by an enlarged lymph node is called *Brock syndrome*.

Q. What is your alternate diagnosis?

Ans: The only condition from which collapse is to be differentiated is pulmonary fibrosis (Table 78.1).

Table 78.1: Differentiating features of lung collapse and fibrosis

Feature	Collapse	Fibrosis
Onset	Acute	Chronic
Chest wall	Flattened	Retracted
Breath sounds	Absent	Feeble but never absent
Crackles	Absent	Present

Q. What do you understand by the term collapse of the lung?

Ans: Pulmonary collapse or atelectasis is defined as *"airlessness with shrinkage"* of a part or the whole lung. Atelectasis may be present since birth (*atelectasis neonatorum*) due to failure of the lung to expand, or may occur anytime during life (acquired atelectasis) due to absorption of air secondary to obstruction, compression, contraction or surfactant loss.

Q. What are various types of collapse?

Ans: Localised/hemithoracic loss of lung volume (collapse of the lung) can occur with patent bronchus or with occluded bronchus (obstructive collapse) or there is compression of the lung from outside (intrapleural positive pressure), hence, collapse is of two main types:

1. *Obstructive collapse (absorption or resorption collapse).* It occurs due to absorption of air distal to obstruction in the alveoli. The site of obstruction can be central or peripheral.
   - i. *Central obstructive collapse* is with obstructed major bronchus
   - ii. *Peripheral obstructive* (absorption) *collapse* is always with patent surrounding bronchus.
2. *Compression collapse (Relaxation collapse).* It occurs from relaxation of the lung due to pleural disease (e.g. pleural effusion, pneumothorax and hydropneumothorax).

Q. What are the causes of collapse of the lung?

Ans: 1. *Obstructive (absorption collapse)*
   - **A. Central (major bronchus):** The causes are:
     - Bronchial adenoma or carcinoma
     - Enlarged tracheobronchial lymp nodes (malignant, tubercular)
     - Inhaled foreign body, misplaced endotracheal tube
     - Mucus plugging (asthma, aspergillosis)
     - Aortic aneurysm
     - Giant left atrium
     - Congenital bronchial atresia
     - Stricture/stenosis
     - Pericardial effusion
   - **B. Peripheral (divisions of bronchus/ bronchi):**
     - Pneumonias

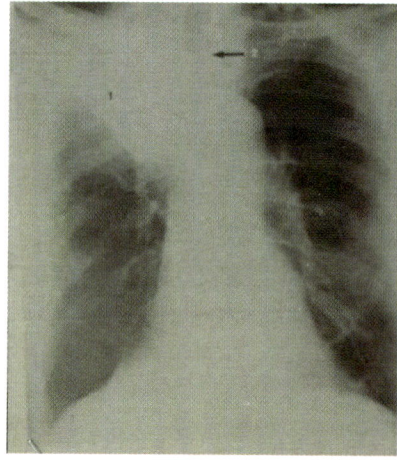

Fig. 78.1: Chest X-ray showing collapse of right upper lobe. There is compensatory emphysema of left lung and right lower lung

- Mucus plugging (sputum retention)
- Asthma
- Pulmonary eosinophilia.

2. *Compression collapse (relaxation collapse)*
  - Pleural effusion
  - Pneumothorax
  - Hydropneumothorax, pyopneumo-thoax haemopneumothorax.

Q. **What are the clinical differences between central obstructive and peripheral obstructive collapse?**

Ans: Remember that peripheral collapse does not involve the major bronchus, involves divisions of a bronchus or bronchi with the result the collapse occurs with patent bronchus (i.e. surrounding bronchi are patent) while, central obstruction of a major bronchus leads to collapse of all its division, hence, the whole lobe is airless with no patent bronchus. The differentiating features are summarised in Table 78.2.

Q. **What are the clinical pulmonary presentations of bronchogenic carcinoma?**

Ans: Clinical pulmonary presentations of bronchogenic carcinoma are:
- Collapse of a lobe or lung
- Collapse consolidation
- Cavitation
- Mediastinal compression/syndrome, superior vena cava syndrome
- Pancoast's tumor—apical carcinoma may involve brachial plexus producing monoplegia
- Consolidation—a solid tumor
- Pleural effusion—rapid filling, hemorrhagic

Q. **How will you investigate a patient with lobar collapse?**

Ans: Investigations of lobar collapse are:
- *Routine blood examination.*
- *Sputum examination*—cytology, microbiology and culture.
- *Chest X-ray (PA and lateral view).* It will show:
  - Homogeneous opacity of the collapsed lung.
  - Displacement of trachea and cardiac shadow (mediastinum) to the diseased (involved) side.
  - Crowding of the ribs with reduc-tion of intercostal spaces due to loss of volume of the lung on the side involved.
  - Elevation of hemidiaphragm o the side involved.
  - Pleural effusion on the side involved if collapse is due to malignancy of lung.
  - Sometimes, the radiological features of underlying cause (hilar lymphadeno-pathy), foreign body may be evident.
- *CT scan* to find out the cause.
- *Bronchoscopy* to find out the cause and to take biopsy.
- *Scalene node biopsy,* if lymph node enlarged or malignancy lung suspected.
- *Pleural fluid examination* if pleural effusion present.

Q. **What are the complications of collapse?**

Ans: Common complications of collapse are:
- Secondary infection.
- Spontaneous pneumothorax from ruptured bullae of compensatory emphysema on the uninvolved side of the lung.

Table 78.2: Differentiating features of central obstructive and peripheral obstruction collapse of lung

Feature	Central obstructive collapse (occluded bronchus)	Peripheral obstructive collapse (patent bronchus)
• Shift of trachea and mediastinum	To the same side	To the same side
• Elevated dome of the diaphragm	On the same side	On the same side
• Breath sounds	Absent on the side involved	Tubular (bronchial) breath sounds
• Vocal resonance	Decreased/absent on the side involved	Increased vocal resonance with whispering pectoriloquy
• Common cause	• Tumor or lymph node or a foreign body	• Mucus plugging, ipsilateral bronchial cast or clot
• CT scan or chest X-ray	Collapse with loss of open bronchus sign—Golden's "S" sign	Collapse with open bronchus
• Signs on the other side	Signs of compensatory emphysema i.e. hyperresonant note, vesicular breathing with prolonged expiration	No signs of compensatory emphysema on the other side

79

Pickwickian Syndrome

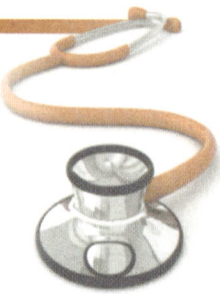

INSTRUCTION

Examine the patient's chest

SALIENT FEATURES

- Over weight and difficulty in breathing

HISTORY

Ask about the following:

- Daytime somnolence
- Non-refreshing sleep
- History of weakness, tiredness, fatigue
- Snoring at night
- History of breathlessness, distension of abdomen and swelling of feet (right heart failure)
- History of headache, visual disturbances (hypertension)
- Poor concentration and loss of libido
- History of nocturnal angina
- Retrosternal burning, chest discomfort (gastroesophageal reflux)
- Ask about *past history* of stroke
- *Family history* of obesity

EXAMINATION

General Physical Examination

- Measure the height and weight. Calculate the BMI
- BP may be elevated (170/100 mm Hg in this case)
- Short mandible (mandibular hypoplasia)
- Cyanosis (present): Patient is plethoric
- JVP raised
- Measure the neck circumference
- Measure skin fold thickness (increased)
- Edema feet (present)

Chest Examination

- Chest is bilaterally symmetrical and movement are reduced. Expansion of chest is reduced.

Vesicular breathing but intensity of breath sounds is decreased.

CVS Examination

- Apex beat is neither visible nor palpable
- P_2 is loud
- Second heart sound is normally split

Abdominal Examination

- Abdominal wall is thick. Liver is enlarged. No ascites

PROVISIONAL DIAGNOSIS

The patient has marked obesity (BMI 36 kg/m^2) and daytime hypersomnolence with signs of pulmonary and systemic hypertension (lesion), the provisional diagnosis is Pickwickian syndrome. He has signs of right ventricular failure (functional status).

QUESTIONS AND ANSWERS

Q. **What is Pickwickian syndrome?**

Ans: It is an idiopathic obesity—hypoventilation syndrome.

Q. **What is the cause of alveolar hypoventilation in Pickwickian syndrome?**

Ans: Alveolar hypoventilation results from a combination of blunted respiratory drive and increased mechanical load imposed on chest by obesity.

Q. **What is the cause of cyanosis in such a patient?**

Ans: Cyanosis results as a result of obstructive apnea which is present in most of the cases within bracker (sleep-induced hypoventilation).

Q. **What is the abnormality in blood gas analysis in such patients?**

Ans: 1. Hypoxaemia
2. Hypercapnia (CO_2 retention)

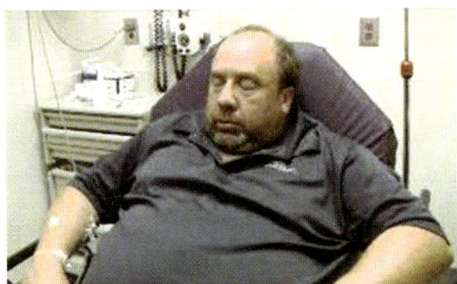
Fig. 79.1: Pickwickian syndrome

Q. **What happens to serum leptin levels in Pickwickian syndrome?**

Ans: They are elevated.

Q **What is the frequency of obstructive sleep apnea in this syndrome?**

Ans: About 50% patients of Pickwickian have obstructive sleep apnea with snoring at night.

Q. **Where is the obstruction in obstructive sleep apnoea?**

Ans: It is caused by narrowing of the upper airway by apposition of the tongue and the palate with posterior pharyngeal wall.

Q. **What is significance of neck circumference?**

Ans: Neck circumference is used as predictor of probability of having a positive sleep test result in obese (polysomnography) patient. Neck circumference is adjusted if patient has hypertension, i.e. 4 cm is added (in this case); 3 cm is added to a habitual snorer and in patients with gasps at night.
Adjusted neck circumference indicate as follows:
  i. <43 cm indicate low clinical probability.
  ii. Between 43–48 cm indicate intermediate probability (4–8 times probability).
  iii. >48 cm indicates more than 20 time probability (high probability).

Q. **What is obstructive sleep apnoea syndrome?**

Ans: Obstructive-sleep apnoea syndrome is defined as intermittent cessation of air-flow at upper airway due to obstruction resulting from opposition of tongue palate and pharyngeal wall. This obstruction during sleep results in snoring.

Q. **What is central sleep apnoea syndrome?**

Ans: It is a transient abolition of central respiratory drive to the ventilatory muscles.

Q. **What is the cause of pulmonary hypertension in this syndrome?**

Ans: Hypoxemia is pulmonary vasoconstrictor, results in pulmonary hypertension and subsequently cor pulmonale.

Q. **What does systemic hypertension indicate in this case?**

Ans: Metabolic syndrome.

Q. **What is metabolic syndrome?**

Ans: Read it as a separate case in Endocrinology.

Q. **What is the treatment of this syndrome?**

Ans: The steps of management are:
  1. Weight reduction.
  2. Cessation of smoking and avoidance of alcohol.
  3. Continuous nasal positive airway pressure (CPAP) delivered by a nasal mask is advised for obstructive sleep apnoea even if apnoea/hypopnoea index is in mild range (5–15 sec). Usually CPAP is given when apnoea/hypopnoea index is high (>15).
  4. Domiciliary oxygen therapy.
  5. Respiratory stimulants may be helpful and include theophylline, acetazolamide and medroxyprogestrone acetate (10–20 mg every 8 hour).
  6. **Surgery:** It includes tracheostomy, linguoplasty, mandibular advancement, remodelling of uvula by laser, tonsillectomy and uvulopalatopharyngoplasty is the most common employed procedure.
  7. Atrial overdriving pacing to overcome the enhanced vagal tone so as to prevent apnoea.

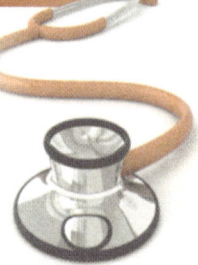

80 Superior Mediastinum Compression

INSTRUCTION

Examine the patient's chest

SALIENT FEATURES

- Puffiness of face and breathlessness

HISTORY

Ask about the following:

- Cough, fever, night sweets
- Dyspnea, chest discomfort, wheezes
- Puffiness of face
- Hoarseness of voice or stridor
- Dysphagia
- Hiccough
- Visual disturbances (blackouts), headache, alteration in consciousness (Raised intracranial pressure).

EXAMINATION

General Physical Examination

- There is suffusion of face and chemosis of conjunctivae (Fig. 80.1)
- Cyanosis is present (in this case)
- Neck veins are engorged with absent pulsations (present). JVP is raised (in this case)
- Cervical lymph nodes may be enlarged and palpable
- Pupils are normal (No Horner's syndrome)
- No pedal edema (in this case)

Chest Examination

- Neck veins are engorged over upper chest (Fig. 80.1)
- There is widening of the dullness of mediastinum
- Heart is normal

Examination of Abdomen

- No lymph node enlargement

PROVISIONAL DIAGNOSIS

The provisional diagnosis is superior mediastinal compression (lesion) caused by tubercular lymphadenitis (etiology). Patient is distressed with bovine cough (functional status).

QUESTIONS AND ANSWERS

Q.   What are the points in favor of your diagnosis?
Ans: 1. Suffusion of face and chemosis of conjunctivae
      2. Puffiness of face (rounded face)
      3. Engorged neck veins with absent pulsations
      4. JVP is raised
      5. Prominent and engorged veins over upper part of chest
      6. Hoarseness of voice
      7. Widening of mediastinal dullness

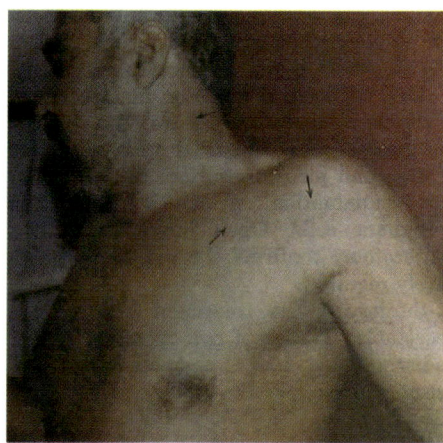

Fig. 80.1: Superior vena cava syndrome due to mediastinal compression. Note the puffiness of face (side of face visible), distended, non-pulsatile neck veins (←) and distended veins over the chest (indicated by arrows).

Q. What conditions will you keep mind in such a case?

Ans: All the conditions that produce puffiness of face will come into differential diagnosis.
- Pericardial effusion/constrictive pericarditis
- Cardiomyopathy (restrictive, dilated)
- CHF due to any cause
- Cor pulmonale
- Valvular heart diseases

Q. Comment on the neck veins.

Ans: 1. The neck veins are dilated, engorged and tortuous, full up to the angle of mandible
2. No visible venous pulsations
3. JVP is raised beyond measurement (beyond neck)
4. Hepatojugular reflux is positive
5. There is no inspiratory collapse of jugular vein

Q. What are the boundaries of superior mediastinum. Name the structures present in it.

Ans: Superior mediastinum is an area bounded above by thoracic inlet, below by the upper part of heart and vessels, anteriorly by sternum and posteriorly by spines. It contains lymph nodes, thymus, aortic arch, trachea, superior vena cava, esophagus and connective tissue.

Q. What are the causes of superior mediastinal compression?

Ans: • Bronchogenic carcinoma.
• Mediastinal lymphadenopathy e.g. tuberculosis, lymphoma, leukemia.
• Retrosternal goitre.
• Aortic aneurysm.
• Oesophageal carcinoma.
• Mediastinal fibrosis/mediastinitis.
• Pneumomediastinum.

Q. What is the mechanism of dilation of veins in superior mediastinal compression?

Ans: In superior mediastinal compression, there is obstruction to the blood flow to superior vena cava, hence, the veins that drain into superior vena cava, now opens into inferior vena cava or azygos vein, hence neck veins above the nipple become prominent due to formation of venous collaterals between superior and inferior vena cava.

Q. Name the structures involved and the resulting symptoms and signs in superior mediastinal compression.

Ans: They are tabulated (Table 80.1).

Table 80.1: Structures involved and resulting symptoms and signs

Structure compressed	Symptoms and signs
i. **Trachea**	Respiratory distress, stridor, cough
ii. **Esophagus**	Dysphagia (solids and liquids)
iii. **Bronchus**	It is usually not involved except in bronchogenic carcinoma, producing collapse of the lung
iv. **Nerves**	
– Recurrent laryngeal	Hoarseness of voice, bovine cough, stridor
– Phrenic	Breathlessness and hic-cough
– Cervical sympathetic	Horner's syndrome
v. **Vessels**	
– Superior vena cava	Suffused and puffy face, visual disturbances, headache, alteration in consciousness, prominent engorged neck veins without pulsations, chemosis
– Azygos vein	Right sided pleural effusion
– Lymphatics	Non-pitting edema of upper thorax, chylothorax

Q. What is inferior vena caval compression (IVC) syndrome?

Ans: Compression or obstruction of inferior vena cava occurs due to ascites, tumors of the abdomen or pelvis, pregnant uterus, thrombosis extending from pelvic veins, membraneous obstruction, oral contraceptives use and myeloproliferative disorders. The clinical picture resulting from IVC obstruction includes.
• Edema (pitting) of legs with dilated veins over the legs.
• Collateral veins are seen over the abdomen, flanks and back.
• Direction of blood flow in abdominal veins is "below upwards".
• Ascites.
• Chronic venous ulcer and staining of ankles in chronic cases.
• Signs of portal hypertension (post-hepatic) if venous obstruction is above the joining of hepatic veins.

Q. What is pneumomediastinum?

Ans: Pneumomediastinum means collection of air into the mediastinal space.
The causes are:
1. *Alveolar rupture with dissection of air into the mediastinum:*
   • Acute severe asthma
   • *Pneumocystis carinii* pneumonia

2. *Perforation of esophagus, trachea or bronchi:*
   - Aspiration of a foreign body.
   - Severe straining during coughing or vomiting in children. Weight lifting and glass blowing may also predispose to it.
   - Manipulation (iatrogenic).
   - Blunt trauma to the chest.
3. *Dissection of air from the neck or abdomen into the mediastinum:*
   - Blunt trauma to neck.
   - Difficult parturition.
   - Perforation of a hollow viscus and collection of air into retroperitoneal space and then dissection into mediastinum.

Clinical signs:
- Subcutaneous emphysema in supra-sternal notch with pain and dyspnea.
- *Hamman's mediastinal sign* — a crunching sound synchronous with heart beat is best heard in left lateral decubitus position on compression of mediastinum with palm of the hand.
- Chest X-ray shows air column parallel to heart and aorta, best seen in lateral film.

Q. How will you investigate such a case?

Ans: The investigations are as follows:
1. *TLC, DLC* for tuberculosis, lymphoma and leukemia.
2. *Chest X-ray (PA view)* to identify the anatomical site of tumor and its effects, i.e.
   - Mediastinal widening (Fig. 80.2)
   - Collapse or atelectasis
   - Malignancy lung
   - Pleural effusion
   - Raised hemidiaphragm (phrenic nerve palsy)
   - Rarely pericardial effusion.
3. *Sputum* for AFB and malignant cells.
4. *FNAC or excision biopsy* of palpable lymph node (scalene node, Virchow's gland or any other node).
5. *Pleural fluid* aspiration and pleural biopsy.
6. *Barium swallow* for esophageal compression.
7. *CT scan of thorax or lung scan or thyroid scan.*

Q. How would you manage this case?

Ans: 1. I.V fursemide to relieve venous congestion and oedema.
2. Depending on the cause, antitubercular, antileukemic or anticancer chemotherapy.
3. Mediastinal irradiation for cancer, if it be the cause.
4. Mechanical thrombectomy with an Amplatz thrombectomy device.

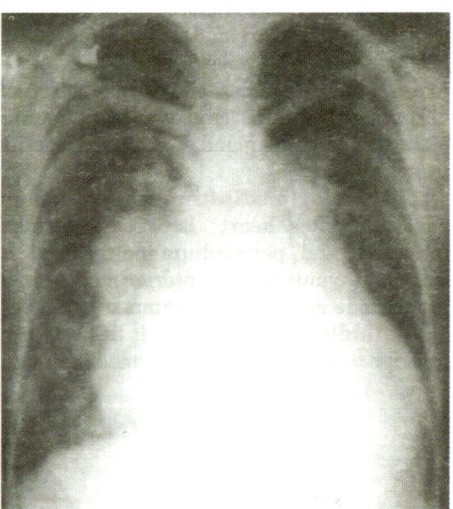

Fig. 80.2: Widening of mediastinum due to bilateral lymph nodes enlargement with pericardial effusion, could be due to tuberculosis or sarcoidosis (Note: This X-ray is not of the index patient)

81

Pulmonary Eosinophilia Syndrome

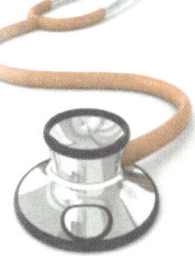

INSTRUCTION

- Examine the patient's chest

SALIENT FEATURES

- Cough, fever, dyspnoea and eosinophilia

HISTORY

Ask the following:

- Note the age, sex and place of residence
- Duration of fever, cough and breathlessness
- Onset of symptoms (acute, subacute, chronic)
- History of hemoptysis, pain chest
- Nature of cough (dry, productive)
- History of allergy, asthma or any allergic skin condition
- History of expulsion of worms (roundworm)
- History of neck swelling (lymph nodes) or an abdominal mass (liver or/and spleen enlargement)
- Drug history, i.e. the drugs being taken or had been taken in the past
- History of vasculitis
- *Past history* of similar episodes, asthma or atopy or drugs known to produce it
- *Family history* of asthma, skin allergy or atopy

EXAMINATION

General Physical Examination

- Patient is afebrile
- Respiratory rate is increased
- Blood pressure is normal
- *Nose:* No polyp, no septal deviation
- *Neck:* No lymphadenopathy
- *Hands and fingers:* No evidence of vasculitis
- No edema feet

Chest Examination

Inspection

- Chest is bilaterally symmetrical
- Movements and expansion of chest normal
- There is tachypnea

Palpation

- Expansion of chest is normal
- Vocal fremitus is normal and equal on both the sides

Percussion

- Percussion note is normal and equal on both the sides
- Cardiac dullness and liver dullness are intact

Auscultation

- Normal vesicular breathing with prolongation of expiration
- Wheezes and rhonchi are audible throughout the chest. There are diffuse coarse crackles on both sides of the chest

Abdominal Examination

- Palpate for liver and splenic enlargement

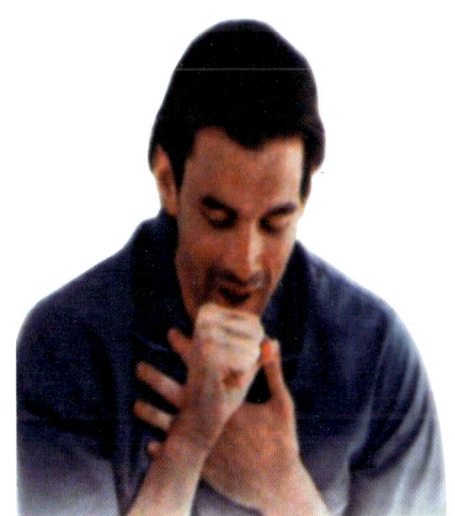

Fig. 81.1: Patient complains of dry cough with tightness of chest

PROVISIONAL DIAGNOSIS

The patient has symptoms and signs suggestive of asthmatic bronchitis (lesion) with blood eosinophilia the cause of which is to be found out (idiopathic). Patient is distressed with repeated episodes of cough and wheezing (functional status).

QUESTIONS AND ANSWERS

Q. **Enumerate the points in favor of your diagnosis?**

Ans: 1. Symptom of cough, fever, dyspnea of insidious onset
2. Repeated episodes of wheezing
3. Chest examination reveals wheezing rales and crackles all over the chest
4. Blood eosinophilia

Q. **What is normal eosinophil count?**

Ans: Normal eosinophil count is up to 4% of total leukocyte count. The maximum eosinophil count will be 440/μL.

Q. **What is eosinophilia?**

Ans: Eosinophil count more than 4% of total leukocyte count is considered as eosinophilia.

Q. **What are the causes of eosinophilia?**

Ans: The causes are grouped as under:

1. *Parasitic infections*	Strongyloidiasis, hookworm disease, schistosomiasis, ascariasis, *Wuchereria bancrofti* or *B. malayi*.
2. *Allergic conditions*	(a) Hay fever, asthma (b) Drugs: (iodides, aspirin, sulphonamide) (c) Aspergillosis
3. *Skin disorders*	Eczema, psoriasis, dermatitis herpetiformis
4. *Tumors*	Myeloproliferative disorders, lymphoma
5. *Collagen vascular disorders*	Rheumatoid arthritis, polyarteritis nodosa, SLE (systemic lupus erythematosus)
6. *Hypereosinophilic syndromes*	(a) Loeffler's syndrome due to nematodes (b) idiopathic
7. *Miscellaneous*	Sarcoidosis, Addison's disease

Q. **How would you classify pulmonary eosinophilia?**

Ans: Pulmonary eosinophilia may be extrinsic or intrinsic due to lung involvement (Table 81.1).

Table 81.1: The classification of pulmonary eosinophilia

1. Extrinsic
- Helminths (ascaris, toxicara, filaria)
- Drug (nitrofurantoin, paraminosalicylic sulphadiazine, imipramine, chlorpropamide
- Fungi (*Aspergillus fumigatus*)

2. Intrinsic
- Eosinophilic pneumonia
- Hypereosinophilic syndrome
- Churg-Strauss syndrome
- Polyarteritis nodosa

Q. **What is the differential diagnosis in your case?**

Ans: Read Table 81.2.

Q. **What do you understand by the term pulmonary eosinophilia?**

Ans: The term includes disorders in which the lesion in the lungs produce radiological abnormality associated with blood eosinophilia. The pulmonary eosinophilia may be extrinsic (cause lies outside the lungs) or intrinsic (cause lies within the lungs).

Q. **Name the parasites causing eosinophilia.**

Ans: Read the question on causes of eosinophilia.

Q. **Name the drugs causing eosinophilia.**

Ans: Read the question on causes of eosinophilia.

Q. **What is Loeffler's syndrome?**

Ans: It is a benign idiopathic acute eosinophilic pneumonia characterised by migratory pulmonary infiltrates with minimum pulmonary symptoms such as cough, fever, dyspnea. Some parasitic infestation such as *Strongyloides stercoralis, ancylostoma, toxicara, ascariasis* are associated with Loeffler's syndrome or eosinophilic pneumonia.

Q. **What is hypereosinophilic syndrome?**

Ans: The syndrome is characterised by peripheral blood eosinophilia (over 1500 eosinophilis per cubic millimeter) for 6 months or longer and lack of evidence for parasitic, allergic or other known cause of eosinophilia. It produces multisystem organs dysfunction. The hallmark of the disease is tissue infiltration by mature eosinophilis; and there is blood and bone marrow eosinophilia. The organs affected are heart, lungs, liver, spleen, skin and nervous system.

Q. **What is Churg-Strauss syndrome?**

Ans: It is also called allergic angitis with granulomatosis. It is multisystem vasculitic disorder which involves skin and nervous system in addition to lungs. Kidney involvement is

Table 81.2: Differential diagnosis of eosinophilia syndrome

Diseases	Symptoms	Blood eosinophils	Multisystem involvement	Duration	Outcome
Cryptogenic (simple or prolonged) pulmonary eosinophilia	Mild to moderate	10–20%	None	One month to few months	Good
Asthmatic bronchopulmonary eosinophilia	Moderate to severe	5–20%	None	Years	Fairs
Tropical pulmonary eosinophilia	Moderate	>20%	None	Years	Fair
Hypereosinophilic syndrome	Severe	20–50%	Always	Months/years	Poor/Fair
Polyarteritis nodosa	Severe	>20%	Always	Months/years	Poor/Fair

uncommon. The disorder involves persons of any age with family history of asthma. The clinical features consist of fever, malaise, anorexia, weight loss, severe asthmatic attacks and pulmonary infiltrates on X-ray. There is peripheral blood eosinophilia (1000 or more cells per cubic millimeter). ANCA is usually positive.

Q. What is tropical pulmonary eosinophilia (TPE) syndrome?

Ans: It is characterised by the presence of hypereosinophilia, circulating filarial antibodies, microfilariae in tissues, but not in the blood and a chronic clinical course that can be terminated with specific antifilarial treatment.

Q. What is pathogenesis of TPE?

Ans: Patients with tropical pulmonary eosinophilia lack IgG blocking antibodies against the circulating microfilariae. Microfilariae are removed from the peripheral circulation and trapped in various tissue sites by an IgG dependent cell mediated effector mechanism. Antigens are released when the parasites are destroyed which initiate an immediate type I (IgE mediated) hypersensitivity reaction. The peripheral eosinophilia occurs due to this reaction which progresses further to granuloma formation and fibrosis.

Q. What are the characteristics of TPE syndrome?

Ans: The characteristics are:

I. Clinical
- Chronic paroxysmal cough, low grade fever, weight loss, nocturnal bronchospasm.

II. Radiological
- Miliary pulmonary infiltrates or mottled opacities in the middle and lower lung fields on X-ray.

III. Pulmonary function
- Restrictive lung defect on pulmonary function tests.

Q. What are the pathogens causing allergic (asthmatic) bronchopulmonary eosinophilia?

Ans: 1. *Aspergillus fumigatus* (common)
2. *Candida albican* (rare)

Q. What are the diagnosis criteria for TPE?

Ans: The criteria include:
1. Suggestive clinical picture, i.e. fever, dry cough, episodic wheezing and rales, dyspnea with or without hemoptysis
2. History of prolonged stay in an endemic area
3. Lack of microfilariae in blood both in day and night samples
4. Peripheral blood eosinophilia in excess of 3000 cells/ml
5. High titres filarial antibodies
6. Reticular nodular shadows in both the lungs on X-ray
7. Clinical response to diethylcarbamazine

Q. Name the drug used in the treatment of TPE.

Ans: Diethylcarbamazine 4–6 mg/kg three times a day for 2–3 weeks along with corticosteroids.

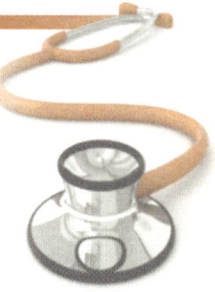

82

Graves' Disease

INSTRUCTION

• Examine the patient and determine the thyroid status of this patient

SALIENT FEATURES

• Anxious looking and restless patient

HISTORY

Ask for the following:
• Record the chief complaints in chronological order and describe them in details
• Ask for any restlessness, irritability, nervousness, insomnia, fatigue, behavior change and hyper-excitability
• Ask for weight loss, increased appetite, nausea, vomiting and diarrhea (frequency of stools)
• Ask for palpitation, breathlessness, heat intolerance and perspiration
• Ask for menstrual irregularity especially oligomenorrhea, loss of libido, gynecomastia, etc.
• Ask for proximal muscle weakness (difficulty in climbing stairs) or periodic paralysis (intermittent paralysis)
• Family history of thyroid disease
• Drug history

EXAMINATION

General Physical Examination
Face: Look at the face for perspiration, staring look, exophthalmos, loss of frowning or wrinkling (present)

Eyes: Check for eye signs of thyrotoxicosis, e.g. lid lag, lid retraction, exophthalmos [proptosis (Fig. 82.1)] ophthalmoplegia, loss of accommodation. Look for scars of previous tarsorrhaphy.

Neck: Examine the neck for thyroid enlargement (Fig. 82.1). Describe the size, shape, measurement, palpate thyroid for smooth texture or nodularity and auscultate for bruit. Examine the neck veins for JVP.
• Examine the neck for previous thyroidectomy scar.

Hands: Look at the hands for tremors, clubbing, moistness, perspiration, warmth, palmar erythema. Shake hands with the patient to note sweaty palms (present).

Feet: Examine feet for edema and legs for pretibial myxoedema. (Pinkish-brownish dermal plaques/hyperkeratosis over both shins).

Vitals: Record the pulse (for AF), BP (wide pulse pressure present) temperature and respiration.

CVS Examination
• Inspect the apex beat and look for cardiac enlargement.
• Palpate the apex beat (hyperkinetic in this case), define its location and other characters.
• Percuss the heart for cardiomegaly.
• Auscultate the heart for tachycardia, irregular heart beats, heart sounds including third heart sound, murmurs (s) or any other abnormal sound or rub.

Respiratory System
• Examine for crackles and rales for LVF.

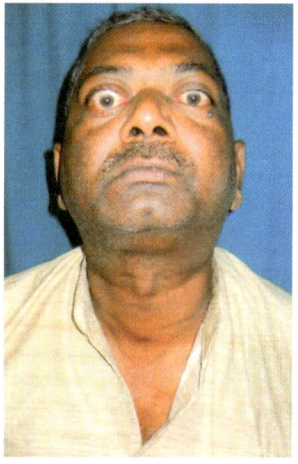

Fig. 82.1: Graves' disease

Nervous System

- Higher mental function testing for psychosis
- Abnormal movements, e.g. tremors (present), choreoathetosis
- Examine for peripheral neuropathy, proximal myopathy, etc.
- Reflexes: There is hyperreflexia (in this patient).

Tell the examiner

- That you would like to investigate the patient for thyroid receptors stimulating antibodies (TRAbs) and thyroid hormone assay for thyroid status.

PROVISIONAL DIAGNOSIS

This young patient (picture inset) has diffuse toxic goitre (lesion) due to Graves' disease (etiology). He is in fast atrial fibrillation. His functional thyroid status is *hyperthyroid*.

QUESTIONS AND ANSWERS

Q. What are points in favor of your diagnosis?

Ans:
1. A young patient with staring look, perspitation, sweaty palms
2. There is exophthalmos with eye signs of thyrotoxicosis
3. There is tachycardia and fast atrial fibrillation
4. Tremors on out stretched hands. Hyperreflexia is present
5. Heart has tic-tac sounds

Q. How do you define thyrotoxicosis and hyperthyroidism?

Ans: Thyrotoxicosis implies a state of hyperthyroidism in which the thyroid hormone is toxic to the tissues producing clinical features, while hyperthyroidism simply implies excessive thyroid function. However, both are not synonymous, yet are used interchangeably.

Q. What is the prevalence of hyperthyroidism?

Ans: The prevalence is about 0.2% in adult population.

Q. What is Graves' disease? What are its components?

Ans: It is an autoimmune disorder characterized by (i) hyperthyroidism, (ii) diffuse toxic goiter, (iii) ophthalmopathy, (iv) dermopathy (pretibial myxedema) and (v) thyroid acropachy (clubbing of fingers).

Q. What are the causes of thyrotoxicosis or hyperthyroidism?

Ans: Causes of thyrotoxicosis are:
  I. *Thyroidal (primary)*

1. Graves disease,
2. Multinodular toxic goitre (MNG),
3. Solitary toxic nodule,
4. Thyroiditis (Hashimotos, postpartum),
5. Iodine induced,
6. Excess thyroid hormone intake (iatrogenic/factitious) and
7. Drug-induced (amiodarone, radioactive contrast media)

II. *Extra-thyroidal (secondary)*
1. Pituitary or excess TSH secretion
2. Hypothalamus (TRH secretion—rare)
3. Hydatiform moles, strauma ovarii.

Q. How can hyperthyroidism present in old age?

Ans: The hyperthyroidism can present in the elderly with atrial fibrillation and these patients usually lack other symptoms and signs of thyrotoxicosis, this is known as apathetic hyperthyroidism. Low serum TSH is an independent risk factor for atrial fibrillation in elderly.

Q. What are the causes of low TSH?

Ans:
- Subclinical hyperthyroidism
- Overt hyperthyroidism
- First trimester of pregnancy
- Medications, e.g. dopamine, steroids
- Non-thyroidal illness with low free T4

Q. What are the pathological changes in thyroid in Graves' disease?

Ans: There is lymphocytic infiltration without follicular destruction of thyroid.

Q. What is the pathogenesis of Graves' ophthalmopathy?

Ans: There is development of autoimmunity due to failure of T cells to recognise TSH receptors. As a result the antibodies formed in turn, stimulate the TSH receptors on the thyroid as well as in the orbit leading to proliferation of thyroid follicular cells and fibroblasts in the orbit. In addition, γ-interferon and TNF initiate the tissue changes in ophthalmopathy of Graves' disease.

Q. What is amiodarone-induced hyperthyroidism?

Ans: Amiodarone, an iodine-containing antiarrhythmic drug can induce hyperthyroidism either by increasing circulating interleukins 6 which causes thyroid stimulation or by an increase in thyroid hormone synthesis. It is common in iodine-deficient areas and in patients with multinodular goitre and presence of thyroid antibodies. It poorly responds to treatment. Even in resistant cases, thyroidectomy has to be done.

Q. Name other autoimmune diseases associated with thyrotoxicosis.

Ans: These are:
- Diabetes mellitus (type I)
- Hyperparathyroidism
- Chronic active hepatitis
- Autoimmune hemolytic anemia

Q. What is subclinical hyperthyroidism?

Ans: In this condition, the serum T_3 and T_4 are either normal or lie in the upper limit of their respective reference range and the serum TSH is undetectable. This combination is found in patients with nodular goiter. These patients are at increased risk of over hyperthyroidism, atrial fibrillation and osteoporosis, hence, the consensus view is to treat such cases with antithyroids or ^{131}I.

Q. Name the hyperthyroid conditions with low iodine uptake.

Ans: 1. Thyroiditis (de Quervain's, postpartum)
2. Thyroid malignancy
3. Ovarian tumor (strauma ovarii)

Q. What are the treatment modalities available for hyperthyroidism.

Ans: • Drug treatment
- Subtotal thyroidectomy
- Radioactive iodine therapy

Q. Which drugs are used in thyrotoxicosis?

Ans: • Carbimazole
- Methimazole
- Propylthiouracil

Q. Which drug is safest in pregnancy?

Ans: Propylthiouracil. Now a days, it is considered safe during first trimester only, can be changed during 2nd and 3rd trimester.

Q. What are the disadvantages of drug treatment in thyrotoxicosis?

Ans: • High rate of relapse once treatment is withdrawn
- Troublesome hypersensitivity reaction
- Rarely life-threatening agranulocytosis and hepatitis may occur

Q. What are the indications of radioiodine therapy in thyrotoxicosis?

Ans: • Graves' disease with large goiter and relapse on treatment
- Multinodular goiter
- Toxic adenoma
- Ablation therapy in those with severe manifestations such as heart failure, AF or psychosis

Q. What are the contraindications of radioiodine in thyrotoxicosis?

Ans: • Breast-feeding and pregnancy
- Allergy to iodine
- Patients having urinary incontinence

Q. Does thyrotoxicosis affect bone?

Ans: Yes, it causes osteoporosis.

Q. What is the effect of iodine on thyroid status?

Ans: It may cause transient hypothyroidism (*Wolff-Chaikoff effect*) or hyperthyroidism (*Jod-Basedow effect*).

Q. What are the indications of subtotal thyroidectomy?

Ans: • Large goiter
- Patient's preference
- Drug noncompliance
- Disease relapse on drug withdrawal
- Young patients who want to raise their family

Q. What are the disadvantages of surgery?

Ans: • It is cumbersome and painful procedure
- Chances of injury to the surrounding tissue (parathyroid glands and recurrent laryngeal nerve) in the neck in less skilled hands
- Risks of anaesthesia

Q. Do the chances of development of cancer in Graves' disease increase?

Ans: No. There is no evidence to suggest that chances of cancer increase during Graves' disease.

Q. What precautions would you advise to the patients who have received radio-iodine therapy?

Ans: 1. *Avoid close contact*. Patient is advised to avoid close contact with people during journeys, at places of entertainment and at work for at least 2 weeks. Avoid contact with children and pregnant women for one month.
2. Exacerbation of symptoms or severe palpitation may be felt by the patient for 2–3 weeks, if the patient was not controlled (euthyroid) prior to treatment.
3. *Regular follow up*. Patient is advised to come for regular follow-up to determine the thyroid status (hyperthyroid/hypothyroid).
4. Advise the patient to use contraceptive method for 4 months to avoid pregnancy.
5. Discontinue digitalis for AF if patient is already taking as atrial fibrillation is likely to disappear after therapy.

Q. If a patient of thyrotoxicosis develops sudden weakness of muscles following a large oral carbohydrates meal or IV dextrose, what condition will come to your mind?

Ans: Hypokalemic periodic paralysis due to shift of K^+ into the cells by glucose in a patient with hyperthyroidism.

Q. What are the complications of hyperthyroidism?

Ans: They are:

1. Precipitation of angina (in a patient with IHD) CHF and digitalis toxicity in patients with valvular heart disease receiving digitalis
2. Cardiac arrhythmias (atrial fibrillation is the most common)
3. Thyrotoxic myopathy (proximal muscle weakness)
4. Thyrotoxic hypokalemic periodic paralysis
5. Thyrotoxic crisis/thyroid storm
6. Malabsorption syndrome
7. Osteoporosis

Q. How would you investigate the patient? Which is the best laboratory test for diagnosis and which is best to monitor response to therapy?

Ans: 1. *Measurement of radioactive iodine uptake.* It is increased.

2. *Thyroid hormones.* The total or free T_3 and T_4 are increased while TSH is decreased in primary thyrotoxicosis (Graves' disease), while all the three hormones are increased in secondary (pituitary or ectopic) thyrotoxicosis.

3. *Ultrasound of thyroid* will demonstrate either the diffuse (Graves' disease) or nodular goitre (rare in Graves' disease)

4. *Thyroid scan.* A radionuclide scan of thyroid either by ^{131}I or ^{99m}Tc will demonstrate functioning thyroid tissue. It will show diffuse increased uptake in Graves' disease.

5. *Antithyroid antibodies.* Antithyroid antibodies are detected in Graves' disease and Hashimoto's thyroiditis. TRAb antibodies and TPO antibodies are raised in Graves' disease.

Note: TSH measurement in serum is the best laboratory test to diagnose hyperthyroidism. Low TSH <0.1 mIU/L confirms the diagnosis in presence of raised FT_3 and FT_4. Plasma T_4 is used to monitor the treatment because TSH level remain suppressed until the patient become euthyroid.

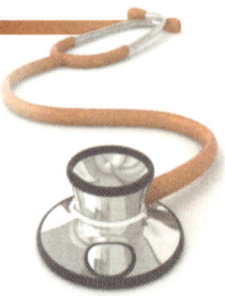

83

Exophthalmos (Proptosis)

INSTRUCTION

- Perform the general physical examination

SALIENT FEATURES

- A frightened man with prominent eyeballs

HISTORY

Ask for the following:
- Obtain the history of thyrotoxicosis (read Graves' disease), eye disorders, etc.
- Ask history of smoking (exophthalmos is more common in smokers than non-smokers)
- History of diplopia, irritation of eyes

EXAMINATION

General Physical Examination
- A staring look, widely opened eyeballs (Fig. 83.1) wide palpebral fissures and absence of wrinkling over forehead (present in this case)
- Prominent eye balls (see figure inset)
- Look for proptosis by looking at the patient's eyes by standing behind (present)
- The whole cornea is visible (positive Dalrymple's sign in this case)
- The lower sclera is also visible (in this case)
- Look for *lid lag sign*, i.e. ask the patient to look straight first. Now ask the patient to follow your

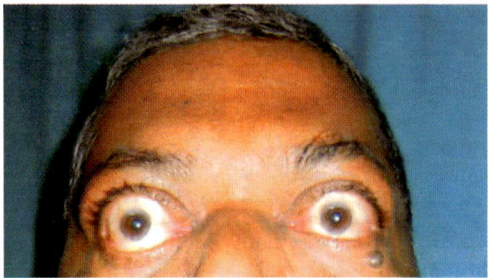

Fig. 83.1: Exophthalmos

finger which is moved along the arc of the circle from a point above the forehead to a point below the nose. Observe the movement of the upper lid which lags behind that of eyeball called **Von Graefe's sign** (lid-lag sign present). Patient must be suitably relaxed before eliciting this sign.
- Check the movements of the eyeball for ophthalmoplegia
- See the condition of cornea (ulcer, opacity)
- Now look for five important signs of exophthalmose and comment on them.
  1. Swelling of eyelid
  2. Redness of eyelid
  3. Chemosis
  4. Conjunctival redness
  5. Inflammation of the plica or caruncle
- Last of all, look for
  - Signs of thyrotoxicosis (fast pulse rate, tachycardia tremors, sweating, etc.)
  - Goitre (enlargement of thyroid)
  - Auscultate for bruit
  - Post-thyroidectomy scar, scars of tarssorhaphy

PROVISIONAL DIAGNOSIS

The patient has bilateral exophthalmos with external ophthalmoplegia (lesion) due to thyrotoxicosis (etiology). Patient is on treatment and thyroid status is euthyroid (functional status).

QUESTIONS AND ANSWERS

Q. How would you calculate the clinical activity score in Graves' ophthalmopathy?
Ans: The clinical activity score (CAS) is calculated according to presence or absence of seven characteristics:
   1. Spontaneous retrobulbar pain
   2. Pain on eye movements
   3. Redness of eyelids

4. Redness of conjunctiva
5. Swelling of the eyelids
6. Chemosis of the conjunctiva
7. Swelling of plica or caruncle

Note: The score ranges from 0 to 7, with 0–2 characteristics indicating inactive Graves' ophthalmopathy and 3 to 7 score indicate active Graves' ophthalmopathy. This score is useful for clinical assessment of severity but is not useful for monitoring the treatment response.

Q. What is your differential diagnosis?

Ans: **Ocular myasthenia gravis** which is also common in Graves' disease is to be differentiated by mild selective eye involvement and raised AChR–Ab and a thymoma is present in 9% cases.

Q. How would you class the eye signs in thyroid disease?

Ans: Many scoring systems have been used to gauge the extent and severity of orbital changes in Graves' disease. As a mnemonic, the NOSPECS scheme is used to class the eye signs as follows:

0 = **N**o sign or symptom
1 = **O**nly sign (lid lag or retraction), no symptoms
2 = **S**oft tissue involvement (pretibial myxedema)
3 = **P**roptosis (>22 mm)
4 = **E**xtraocular muscle involvement (diplopia)
5 = **C**orneal involvement
6 = **S**ight loss

Q. How would you assess proptosis?

Ans: It is assessed by *Hertel's exophthalmometer* (>20 mm is considered as an exophthalmos).

Q. What are the eye signs of thyrotoxicosis?

Ans: The various eye signs are:

Von Graefe's: Upper lid lag

Joffroy's: Absence of wrinkling on forehead when asked to look upwards with face inclined downward

Gilford's: Non-retraction of upper lid manually

Loclur's: Stare look

Naffziger's: Protrusion from superciliary ridge

Dalrymple's: Visible upper sclera

Moebius: Failure to converge eyeballs

Ballet sign: Weakness of one of extraocular muscle

Jendrassik's sign: Paralysis of extraocular muscles

Stellwags: Stare look, infrequent blinking, widening of palpebral fissure

Rosenbach's sign: Tremors of closed eyelids

N.B Read the signs and their method of demonstration in Clinical Methods in Medicine by Dr SN Chugh.

Q. What is the pathogenesis of lid lag?

Ans: • Sympathetic stimulation leads to overactivity of Muller's muscles supplied by it
• Myopathy of inferior rectus muscle results in overaction of superior rectus and levator muscles
• Restrictive myopathy of levator palpebral superioris.

Q. What is euthyroid Graves' disease?

Ans: The patient has Graves' ophthalmopathy but clinically and biochemically he/she is euthyroid. A TSH-stimulating test by administration of TRH will show a flat response.

Q. Does Graves' ophthalmopathy occur in any other condition?

Ans: Yes, rarely it can occur in amiodarone–induced thyrotoxicosis (1%).

Q. How would you investigate this patient?

Ans: • Measurement of thyroid hormones, i.e. FT_3, FT_4 and TSH
• Thyroid antibodies
• USG of thyroid

Q. How would you manage Graves' ophthalmopathy?

Ans: • *Severe Graves' ophthalmopathy* should be treated with corticosteroids, orbital irradiation and plasma exchange to prevent visual loss. If there is no improvement within 2–3 days, surgical orbital decompression should be attempted. Rituximab has been successfully used in moderate to severe steroid–resistant cases.

• *Moderate ophthalmopathy.* It is treated symptomatically. It improves within 2–3 yrs with treatment in most of the cases:

i. Considerable number of patients improve with symptomatic measures:
— Elevation of the head at night
— Diuretics to reduce retrobulbar oedema
— Use of tinted glasses for protection of eye from the sun, wind and foreign bodies

ii. Corneal dryness, grittiness and pain is treated by instillation of methylcellulose eye drops during the day and a lubricating ointment at night

iii. Lateral tarrsorhaphy for exposure keratitis. In extreme cases, surgical closure of lower lid may be performed

iv. Worsening ophthalmopathy is treated by steroids, orbital irradiation and orbital decompression

v. Patient is advised to stop smoking

vi. Cosmetic eyelid surgery can be undertaken

Q.   How would you investigate unilateral exophthalmos?

Ans: 1. Ophthalmological consultation for local disease

2. Ultrasonography of the orbit

3. Thyroid function tests

4. CT scan of the orbit

Q.   What is the role of radioiodine treatment in thyroid ophthalmopathy? How would you prepare the patient for it?

Ans:
- Radioiodine treatment should be avoided in patients with active or severe ophthalmopathy because of risk of exacerbation of pre-existing thyroid eye disease. These patients preferably should be controlled with antithyroid drugs. Radioiodine may be used in presence of mild eye disease but adjuvant steroids must be given.
- Smoking should be prohibited during radioactive treatment.
- Radioiodine treatment in uncontrolled hyperthyroidism may exacerbate the eye symptoms, hence, patient must be rendered erythroid before radioiodine treatment. These patients after treatment must be closely monitored for thyroid status because these patients may remain hyperthyroid or become hypothyroid or remain euthyroid.

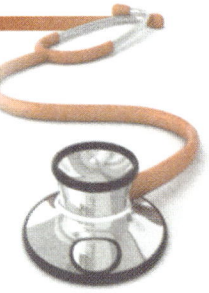

84

Pretibial Myxedema

INSTRUCTION

- Inspect the patient's legs. Perform relevant examination

SALIENT FEATURES

- Patient is a case of Graves' disease

HISTORY

- Look for all the symptoms and signs of thyrotoxicosis (present) because it is a component of Graves' disease
- History of drug treatment or radioiodine

EXAMINATION

General Physical Examination

- Look at the legs. Red thickened swelling over the shins (*peaud's orange appearance*) with nonpitting oedema is present (Fig. 84.1).

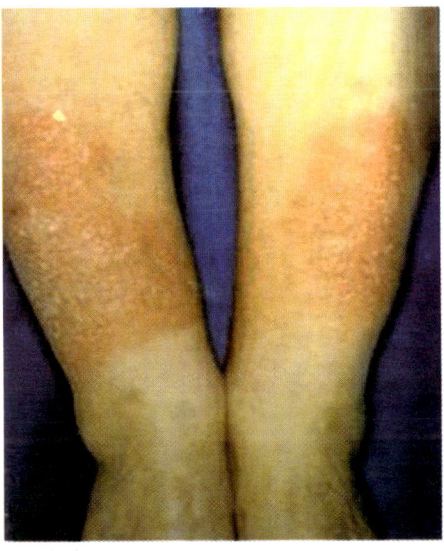

Fig. 84.1: Pretibial myxedema

- Now examine other components of Graves' disease i.e.,
  - i. Examine hands for palmer erythema, warm sweaty palms, thyroid acropachy and tremors
  - ii. Look at the neck for thyroid enlargement (goitre) or thyroidectomy scar
  - iii. Auscultate over the thyroid for bruit (present)
  - iv. Look at the eyes for exophthalmose
  - v. Examine the pulse for tachycardia or atrial fibrillation

Remember: Thyroid dermopathy and ophthalmopathy are associated with and one may follow the other in Graves' disease.

PROVISIONAL DIAGNOSIS

The clinical diagnosis of skin lesion is pretibial myxedema (lesion), caused by Grave's disease (etiology). The functional thyroid status is hyperthyroidism.

QUESTIONS AND ANSWERS

Q. How would you justify the diagnosis of pretibial myxedema?

Ans:
  i. Pretibial myxedema is a late manifestation of Graves' disease.
  ii. The site of skin changes, i.e. over the anterior and lateral aspects of the lower leg in front of tibia.
  iii. The typical skin change is noninflamed, indurated, pink or purple color plaque giving an "orange-skin" appearance.
  iv. Presence of ophthalmopathy

Q. What are the various types of pretibial myxedema?

Ans:
  1. *Nonpitting edema* accompanied by hyperkeratosis, pigmentation and pinkish, brownish red or yellow discoloration

2. *Plaque form* consisting of raised, discrete or confluent plaques
3. *Nodular form* characterized by formation of nodules

Q.   What is the pathogenesis of pretibial myxedema?

Ans: Exact cause is unknown, but it is considered autoimmune in origin because:

   i. Presence of high serum concentrations of TSH receptor antibodies

   ii. TSH receptors in the connective tissue are stimulated by an immune system.

   iii. Both humoral and cellular immune responses play a role. These immune mechanisms stimulate the fibroblasts and produce large amounts of glycosaminoglycans which get deposited over pretibial region under the influence of mechanical factors and dependent position.

Q.   What is histopathology of a skin lesion in pretibial myxedema?

Ans: There is accumulation of glycosaminoglycans and increase in mucinous material staining with PAS (periodic-acid-schiff) with resultant connective tissue fibre separation and lymphoid infiltration into the skin.

Q.   What is incidence of pretibial myxedema in thyrotoxicosis?

Ans: It occurs in 3% cases of patients with Graves' disease. It is common in those patients who have high levels of thyroid stimulating antibodies and in those with severe Graves' ophthalmopathy.

Q.   What investigations would you like to perform?

Ans: Thyroid function tests, i.e. FT_3, FT_4 and TSH.

Q.   What is the treatment of these lesions?

Ans: These are treated by:

   1. Intralesional steroids
   2. Plasmapheresis
   3. Cytotoxic therapy
   4. Octreotide

Warning: Surgical excision should be avoided because surgical scars may aggravate dermopathy and precipitate recurrence.

85

Multinodular Goiter

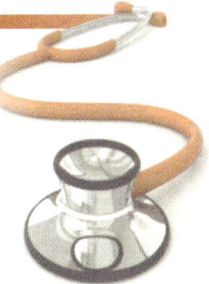

INSTRUCTION

- Examine the neck of the patient and perform relevant examination

SALIENT FEATURES

- Large neck swelling

HISTORY

Ask about the following:

- Onset and progression of the swelling. Acute painful enlargement indicates bleeding in the thyroid nodule
- Compressive symptoms, i.e hoarseness of voice (compression of recurrent laryngeal nerve), stridor (compression of trachea)
- Suffusion of face while raising the arm above the head. This suggests substernal goitre.
- History of dysphagia (esophageal compression)
- Ask about deafness (Pendred's syndrome)
- Ask about symptoms of hyperthyroidism (multinodular goitre) or hypothyroidism (Hashimoto's thyroiditis)
- Family history suggestive of thyroid cancer

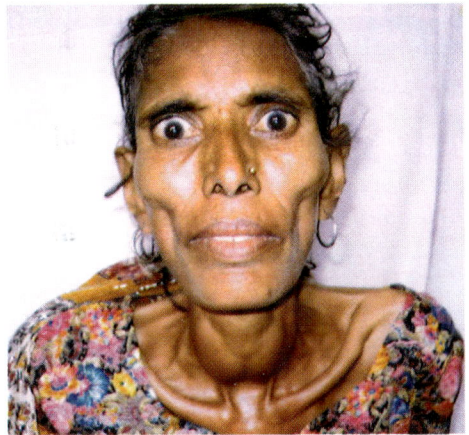

Fig. 85.1: Multinodular goitre

EXAMINATION

General Physical Examination

- Patient is middle aged elderly
- Look at the thyroid by standing in front of the patient. Palpate the thyroid and describe the characteristics of goitre, i.e. *grade, irregularity of surface. Palpate* the thyroid by standing behind the patient. Define its characteristics, i.e. texture, nodularity, tenderness, movement with deglutition. This patient has multiple nontender, firm nodules. *Ausculate* for arterial bruit
- Examine the neck for lymph nodes (malignancy thyroid)
- Examine for signs of thyrotoxicosis (present) or hypothyroidism (read hypothyroidism)
- Examine the pulse and CVS for atrial fibrillation (AF is present in this case)
- Examine for substernal goitre by asking the patient to look upwards and look for suffusion of the face

PROVISIONAL DIAGNOSIS

The middle aged female has multinodular goitre with no substernal extension (lesion), the cause of which has to be found out. The thyroid status is hyperthyroidism with atrial fibrillation (AF).

QUESTIONS AND ANSWERS

Q. What is differential diagnosis?
Ans: The other condition that comes to one's mind is **multinodular thyroid carcinoma.** In this condition, regional lymph nodes get enlarged.

Q. Can multinodular goitre be nontoxic?
Ans: Yes, nontoxic multinodular goitre is common in women, occurs commonly in iodine-deficient areas (hilly areas). It grows slowly and slowly, produces compressive symptoms (stridor, dysphagia, hoarseness, suffusion of face, etc.) with no toxic symptoms.

Q.   What is the status of thyroid in MNG?

Ans: MNG progresses to thyrotoxicosis; once thyrotoxicosis is produced, it becomes permanent with no spontaneous remissions. The thyroid nodules become autonomous. This is the reason that antithyroid drug therapy is not effective in MNG on long-term basis.

Q.   What do you understand by the term hot or cold nodule?

Ans: The hot and cold nodules are the terms used during RAIU studies and thyroid scanning. The *'hot nodule'* is the focal area of increased uptake while *'cold nodule'* is the area of decreased uptake.

The hot nodule indicates hyperactivity of that area while cold nodule is non-functioning area.

Q.   How would you investigate such a case?

Ans: Investigations to be performed are:

1. *Measurement of thyroid hormones* (FT_3, FT_4) and TSH to know the thyroid functional status
2. *Ultrasonography* to confirm the nodularity of thyroid which will differentiate it from diffuse goitre of Graves' disease. USG also defines whether nodules are solid or cystic
3. *Radioisotope scanning* to know whether nodules are hot or cold. Simultaneously radioactive iodine uptake can be calculated to confirm thyrotoxicosis
4. *FNAC* of a nodule for malignancy
5. *CT/MRI* to explore substernal extension
6. *Antithyroid antibodies* and *calcitonin* (if patient has family history of medullary carcinoma of thyroid or MEN-II syndrome)

Q.   How would you treat such a case?

Ans: I. *Symptomatic treatment*
  • Betablockers for hyperthyroidism/ thyrotoxicosis
  • Anticoagulants for AF

II. *Curative treatment*
1. Radioiodine treatment is permanent treatment of choice in this case. Sub-

total thyroidectomy is an alternative permanent therapy.

Q.   What factors would you keep in mind before referring the patient for radioiodine?

Ans: • Age and sex
  • Diagnosis and severity of hyperthyroidism
  • Presence of eye signs
  • Whether patient is controlled on drug or not. Determine the response to treatment
  • Availability of the facility
  • Patient desire to conceive or pregnancy
  • Patient willingness
  • Presence of other medical conditions

Q.   What are the treatment modalities available for toxic MNG?

Ans: • *Antithyroid drugs.* They are used for short-term basis before surgery and before and after radio-iodine treatment in elderly. The toxicity in MNG is permanent and spontaneous remissions are remote, therefore, drug therapy is ineffective on long-term basis and usually associated with adverse effects of drugs.
  • *Surgery (Subtotal or total thyroidectomy).* It is a definite treatment for MNG and preferred for patients with large goitre. The disadvantages are surgical mortality and morbidity, removal of parathyroid gland/ tissue, postoperative hypothyroidism (too much removal), persistence of hyperthyroidism or recurrence of hyperthyroidism.
  • *Radioiodine ablation.* It is treatment option for elderly, for patients who are desirous of having or completing the family and patients with cardiopulmonary disease. The disadvantage includes risks of hypothyroidism, cancer and radiation injury.
  • Betablockers

Q.   What are indications of treatment of nontoxic MNG?

Ans: The treatment is indicated:
  • In presence of compressive symptoms
  • When goitre is retrosternal or there is intrathoracic extension of goitre
  • For cosmetic reasons.

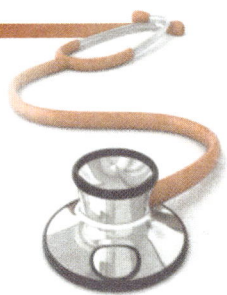

86

Hashimoto's Thyroiditis

INSTRUCTION

- Examine the neck
- Determine the thyroid functional status

SALIENT FEATURES

- Swelling neck

HISTORY

Ask about the following:

- History of fever, sore throat, myalgia, body pains
- History of childhood rubella infection
- History of deafness in the family (*Pendred's syndrome*)
- Any history of other autoimmune disease, i.e. diabetes, Addison's disease, pernicious anemia and vitiligo
- History of pregnancy or delivery (*postpartum thyroiditis*)
- Ask for symptoms of thyroid overactivity and underactivity
- History of depression
- History of drug intake (lithium) or of iodine and its compounds

EXAMINATION

General Physical Examination

- *Look* at the thyroid and define its characteristics
- *Palpate* the thyroid by standing behind as already discussed. Define the various characteristics of thyroid as discussed in the examination of MNG
- Examination the patient for signs of hypothyroidism
- Examine pulse for slow rate or bradycardia
- Examine CVS, joints, skin and GI tract for any other associated autoimmune disease

PROVISIONAL DIAGNOSIS

The provisional diagnosis is Hashimoto's thyroiditis (lesion) due to autoimmune origin (etiology). She is in euthyroid state (functional status).

QUESTIONS AND ANSWERS

Q. What are points in favor of your diagnosis?
Ans:
- A young 24 yrs female (figure inset)
- History of pain in the neck, myalgia headache and fever
- Diffuse enlargement of thyroid which is firm and tender
- No signs of hypo or hyperthyroid at presentation (recent goitre)
- TPO antibodies are present in higher titres on investigations.

Q. Which single investigation would confirm the diagnosis?
Ans: FNAC/biopsy of thyroid.

Q. What is differential diagnosis?
Ans: All other conditions producing nontoxic goitre come into differential diagnosis. The causes of nontoxic goitre are:
1. Diffuse nontoxic goitre
2. Iodine deficiency goitre
3. Multinodular nontoxic goitre

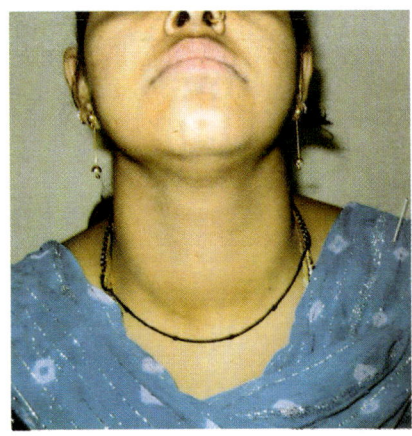

Fig. 86.1: Hashimoto's thyroiditis

Table 86.1: Differentiation between two common diffuse goitres

Features	Simple diffuse goitre	Goitre due to Hashimoto's thyroiditis
Age	Common in young girls (15 – 25 yrs) or during pregnancy	Common in young females (20 – 50 yrs)
Thyroid enlargement	Mild, tends to be noticed by friends and relatives	Large, visible from distance
Goitre	Soft, nontender	Firm, tender
Prevalence	Endemic or sporadic	Sporadic
Symptoms	Asymptomatic or there is a tight sensation in neck, patient seeks medical attention from asthetic point of view	Pain radiating to jaw or neck, increased during swallowing, coughing and neck movements.
Cause	Suboptimal dietary iodine intake and minor degrees of dyshormogenesis	Autoimmune disease, may be associated with other autoimmune conditions. Patient may be euthyroid; 25% cases are hypothyroid at presentation, others become later on.
Thyroid status	Normal	
		Initially, there may be transient
Thyroid antibodies (TPO antibodies)	Negative	thyrotoxicosis in some patient positive (95% cases)

4. Thyroiditis (de Quervaine thyroiditis and postpartum)
5. Malignancy of thyroid

Q. **What are the causes of goitre with hypothyroidism?**

Ans:
- Hashimoto's thyroiditis
- Amiodarone or lithium induced goitre with hypothyroidism
- Dyshormonogenesis (*Pendred's syndrome*)
- Postpartum thyroiditis
- Malignancy of thyroid

Q. **Could it be just a simple diffuse goitre?**

Ans: The differences between two common goitres are given in Table 86.1.

Q. **What are the causes of goitrous hyperthyroidism?**

Ans:
- Graves' disease
- Solitary toxic nodular goitre
- Multinodular toxic goitre
- Thyroiditis (de Quervain) with transient thyrotoxicosis

Q. **What is pathogenesis of Hashimoto's thyroiditis?**

Ans: It is an autoimmune thyroiditis. What triggers an autoimmunity is still unknown. Viral infection, genetic and environmental factors are presumed triggering factors. The autoimmune basis of the disease is because of:
- Strong association with HLA–DR_3, DR_4 and DR_5, support genetic predisposition
- Association with other autoimmune disorders, e.g. type I DM, pernicious

anaemia, vitiligo, Addison's disease, cardiac disease, biliary cirrhosis, etc.
- Presence of thyroglobulin and TPO antibodies (marker of autoimmunity)
- Lymphocytic infiltration on histology of thyroid

Q. **How does Hashimoto's thyroiditis differ from viral (de Quervain) thyroiditis?**

Ans: The differences are given in Table 86.2.

Table 86.2: Distinction between subacute thyroiditis and Hashimoto's thyroiditis

de Quervain thyroiditis	Hashimoto's thyroiditis
• Subacute onset	Chronic onset
• Common in young and middle aged women	Middle and old aged women, common in postpartum females
• Caused by viral infection (H/o upper respiratory infection)	An autoimmune disorder
• Goitre is small may be tender or nontender	Tender large goitre
• Antithyroid antibodies are absent	Antithyroid antibodies (Anti-Tg and Anti-TPO present)
• *Biopsy.* Granulomatous or grant cell thyroiditis	Lymphocytic thyroiditis
• Patient may have transient hyperthyroidism	It mostly transforms and progresses to hypothyroidism

Q. **What is postpartum thyroiditis?**

Ans: It is painless thyroid enlargement noted within 6 months of pregnancy. It is also considered to be due to autoimmunity (autoimmue disorder) triggered by accumulation of fetal cells in the maternal thyroid during pregnancy, a condition called *micro-chimerism*. Women in whom *postpartum thyroid* develops have a 70% chance of recurrence after subsequent pregnancies. It occurs in women who have high levels of antithyroid antibodies in the first trimester of pregnancy or immediately after delivery.

These women have asymptomatic goitre with low to normal T3 and T4 and mildly elevated TSH. The diagnosis confirmed by low RAIU and lymphocytic thyroiditis on histopathology.

Transient hyperthyroidism or hypothyroidism and hyperthyroidism followed by hypothyroidism have been reported in 5–10% cases, otherwise most of the patients are euthyroid.

Q. How would you investigate a case of thyroiditis?

Ans: 1. *Complete WBC count* (for leukocytosis), ESR (raised) and C-reactive protein (present)
2. *Antithyroid antibodies* (Anti-Tg and Anti-TPO) are diagnostic in 90–95%. They are present in higher titres in this case.
3. *RAIU studies.* Usually these studies are not required and not performed. RAIU is low in thyroiditis
4. *Thyroid function tests* (T_3, T_4, TSH). They are initially normal indicating euthyroid status. Subsequently, the thyroid hormones levels fall and TSH gets raised indicating hypothyroid status.
5. *FNAC:* In case of doubt, FNAC biopsy may be undertaken to confirm the diagnosis.

Q. What are the histological changes in Hashimoto's thyroiditis?

Ans: The changes are:
   i. Marked lymphocytic infiltration of thyroid follicles
   ii. Atrophy of thyroid follicles
   iii. Oxyphil metaplasia, follicular cell hyperplasia
   iv. Absence of colloid

   v. Mild to moderate fibrosis. Severe fibrosis indicates atrophic thyroiditis—a cause of hypothyroidism. The goitre disappears with atrophy.

Q. How would you treat a case of thyroiditis?

Ans: • Betablockers are used if thyroiditis is associated with hyperthyroidism
• Thyroxine therapy is used to treat hypothyroidism and to suppress TSH, so that goitre shrinks in size. The usual dose of thyroxine is 100 – 200 µg/day.

Q. What is Hashitoxicosis?

Ans: Hyperthyroidism may develop in patients with Hashimoto thyroiditis either due to the emergence of Graves' disease or due to transient release of stored hormone by inflammatory cellular infiltration in the thyroid, a condition called hashitoxicosis.

Q. What are the effects of Hashimoto's thyroiditis on pregnancy?

Ans: The effects are:
1. Increased risk of spontaneous miscarriages in the first trimester
2. Hashitoxicosis (hyperthyroidism) may develop during pregnancy. It is called painless postpartum thyroiditis when it occurs in women after delivery.

Q. What is Reidel thyroiditis?

Ans: It is invasive thyroiditis involving commonly middle and old aged females and producing asymmetric enlargement of thyroid. The thyroid is stony hard due to idiopathic fibrosis and there is invasion of surrounding structures. It is a part and parcel of multifocal systemic fibrosis syndrome.

Q. What is sick euthyroid syndrome?

Ans: It is a biochemical abnormality in which thyroid hormones and TSH are abnormal in the absence of thyroid disease. The syndrome is seen in acute severe/critical illness and is attributed to hormonal changes induced by cytokines released in acute illness. The low levels of T_3 (T_4 and TSH normal), low levels of both T_3 and T_4 (free T_3 free T_4 are normal) and increased or decreased levels of TSH due to fluctuations in T_3 and T_4 have been described.

87

Cushing's Syndrome

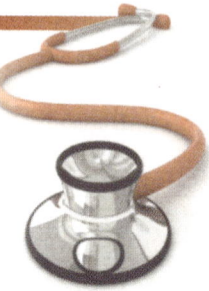

INSTRUCTION

- Examine the patient

SALIENT FEATURES

- Moon facies, central obesity

HISTORY

Ask for the following:
- Onset of symptoms
- History of steroid therapy
- Weight gain
- Excessive hair growth (hirsutism)
- Acne over face (pimples over face)
- History of easy bruisability
- Weakness of proximal muscles, difficulty in climbing stairs
- Loss of libido, menstrual irregularity
- Depression, sleep disturbances, emotional change (euphoria)
- Back pain, history of trauma
- There is history of fracture and left leg bone in this patient (not shown)

EXAMINATION

General Physical Examination
- Patient face is moon-shaped, red [plethoric (Fig. 87.1)]
- Look at the mouth for thrush
- Look for buffalo hump at the back e.g (nape of neck present)
- Look at central (truncal) obesity (present). Skin over the abdomen is thin
- Look for pink striae over abdomen (present), look for bruises
- Look for redistribution of fat, more in the centre than peripheral (present in this case)
- Weakness of shoulder and hip girdle muscle (proximal myopathy) is present. Difficulty in rising from sitting position (history is present, could not be demonstrated due to fracture of left leg)

- There is fracture of left lower limb which is plastered. Look for kyphoscoliosis, vertebral collapse
- Record BP (high in this case)

Systemic Examination
- There is no evidence of asthma, rheumatic arthritis, SLE and nephrotic syndrome

PROVISIONAL DIAGNOSIS

The provisional diagnosis of this patient (picture inset) is Cushing's syndrome (lesion) the cause of which may be adrenal hyperplasia or may be idiopathic (etiology). He is at risk of infection and bony fractures.

Q. **What would you examine further if you are asked to do so?**

Ans: Tell the examiner that:
  i. You would like to examine *urine for glucose*
  ii. *Visual fields* for pituitary adenoma
  iii. *Fundus examination* for optic atrophy, papilledema, changes of hypertension and diabetes

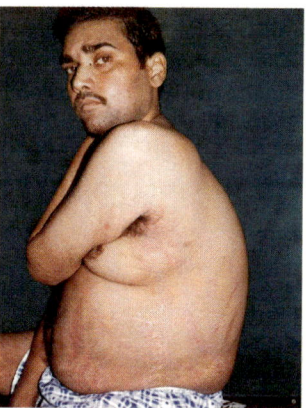

Fig. 87.1: Cushing's syndrome

QUESTIONS AND ANSWERS

Q. Enumerate the points in favour of your diagnosis?

Ans: 1. Moon (rounded) face with red (plethoric) cheeks
2. Buffalo hump, truncal (central) obesity, pink striae over the abdomen
3. Proximal limb myopathy
4. Hypertension
5. Osteoporosis (fracture of the left lower limb)

Q. What is pseudocushing's syndrome?

Ans: Pseudocushing means some abnormalities in steroid output without involvement of pituitary-adrenal axis. It includes certain conditions such as (i) obesity, (ii) chronic alcoholism, (iii) depression and (iv) acute illness of any type which share abnormalities in steroid output, modestly elevated urine cortisol, blunted circadian rhythm of cortisol level (absent diurnal variation of plasma cortisol) and positive overnight dexamethasone suppression test similar to cushing's syndrome, but these tests return to normal with withdrawl of alcohol or improvement in emotional status.

Q. What are the causes of moon-like face?

Ans: 1. Cushing's syndrome
2. Nephrotic syndrome, nephritic syndrome
3. Myxedema (hypothyroidism)
4. Angioneurotic oedema
5. Superior mediastinum compression
6. Superior vena cava syndrome
7. Pseudocushing syndrome

Q. Name the abdominal striae.

Ans: The striae are named as follows:
- *Silvery white striae/striae gravidarum* due to pregnancy or following delivery
- *Pink striae* due to Cushing's syndrome or steroid excess
- *Striae Ignou* due to heat or hot water bottle
- *Striae alba* (white striae) due to stretching of abdominal wall.

Q. What is Cushing's disease and what is Cushing's syndrome?

Ans: *Cushing's disease* is increased production of steroids by adrenals secondary to excess of pituitary ACTH.

Cushing's syndrome is excess of steroids from any cause including steroid therapy.

Q. What are the characteristics of Cushing's syndrome due to ectopic ACTH production (paraneoplastic)?

Ans: The features are:
- Acute onset of symptoms
- Moon facies and abdominal striae are less common
- Hyperpigmentation
- Hypertension and edema are more common
- Hypokalemic alkalosis is a characteristic feature
- The diagnosis is confirmed by markedly elevated ACTH level (>300 ng/L)

Q. What are the common causes of Cushing's syndrome?

Ans: The common causes are:
1. Iatrogenic (steroid or ACTH use)
2. Pituitary adenoma (Cushing's disease)
3. Adrenal adenoma, adrenal hyperplasia
4. Adrenal carcinoma
5. Ectopic ACTH production (small-cell carcinoma lung)

Q. How will you investigate a case with Cushing's syndrome?

Ans: Investigations are:
1. *Blood examination* for eosinopenia and neutrophilia.
2. *Serum sodium* (hypernatraemia), K^+ (hypokalemia) and pH (alkalosis).
3. *24-hour urinary free cortisol*: This is most direct and reliable index of cortisol secretion. It may be increased.
4. *Glucose tolerance test* may show impaired tolerance or diabetes (20%).
5. *X-ray skull and spine:* X-ray skull may show enlargement of pituitary fossa if a pituitary tumor is suspected to be the cause. X-ray spines may show cord-fish vertebrae or fish-mouth appearance of intervertebral disk spaces.
6. *CT scan abdomen* for adrenals (adenoma or carcinoma) if adrenal is the cause.
7. *Plasma cortisol level elevated:* There is loss of circadian rhythm.
8. *Plasma ACTH levels:* They are high in ectopic ACTH production, may be normal to high in pituitary tumor. Pituitary radiography and MRI gadolinium enhancement confirms the diagnosis of pituitary tumor.
9. *Dexamethasone suppression test:* There is no suppression of cortisol secretion in Cushing's syndrome whereas high dose dexamethasone (2 mg 6 hourly for 48 hrs)

suppresses at least 50% of urinary steroid secretion.

10. *Metyrapone test:* It differentiates between ACTH dependent Cushing's disease (exaggerated response) and non-ACTH dependent Cushing syndrome (no response).

11. *Corticotrophin releasing hormone (CRH) test* is helpful in distinguishing pituitary led Cushing's disease from ectopic ACTH production.

Q. What is the pathogenesis of truncal obesity in Cushing's syndrome?

Ans: It is due to redistribution of fat to central part under the effect of glucocorticoids.

Q. Name the hormones secreted by adrenal cortex

Ans: The hormones secreted by adrenal cortex are:

1. *Glucocorticoids,* e.g. cortisol
2. *Mineralocorticoids,* e.g. aldosterone
3. *Adrenal androgens,* e.g. androgens.

Q. What are endocrinal causes of obesity?

Ans: • Cushing syndrome
• Hypothyroidism
• Hypogonadism (e.g. Frohlich's syndrome, Laurence-Moon-Biedl syndrome, Prader-Willi syndrome)

• Type 2 diabetes
• Following pregnancy and postpartum

Q. How would you manage Cushing's syndrome?

Ans: *For Cushing's disease*
• Trans-sphenoidal microadenalectomy, pituitary irradiation, total bilateral adrenalectomy

For Adrenal tumor
• Surgical resection
• Mitotane therapy
• Resection of recurrent tumor

For Ectopic ACTH tumor
• Surgical resection of tumor

For exogenous corticoids (iatrogenic syndrome)
• Taper off corticosteroid

Q. What is Nelson's syndrome?

Ans: This is characterized by increased ACTH production, hyperpigmentation and erosion of sella turcica due to development of chromophobe adenoma in patients with Cushing's disease who have undergone bilateral adrenalectomy. This syndrome will not occur if pituitary has also been irradiated after bilateral adrenalectomy.

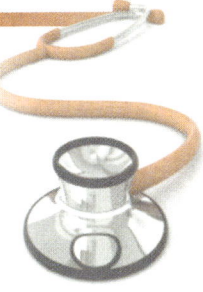

88

Addison's Disease

INSTRUCTION

- Examine the patient

SALIENT FEATURES

- Mature looks, sunken cheeks and pigmented tongue and mucous membrane.

HISTORY

Ask for the following:

- History of dizziness and syncope
- History of skin pigmentation
- Ask history of fatigue, weakness, apathy, anorexia, nausea, vomiting, weight loss, abdo-minal pain and diarrhea (present)
- History of depression
- History of delivery and postpartum hemorrhage
- History of cessation of lactation after delivery
- History of adrenalectomy or adrenal irradiation

EXAMINATION

General Physical Examination

Thin built, emaciated female with flabby muscles

- Look for pigmentation at different sites, i.e.
  — Creases of palm
  — Compare the pigmentation with your own hand
  — Mouth (mucous membranes) and lips (inner surface) (Fig. 88.1)
  — Covered areas such as nipples, areas under belts, straps and collar rings
- Look for vitiligo
- Look for signs of vitamins and nutrients deficiencies
- Take blood pressure in sitting and standing position for postural hypotension (BP is low in this case, i.e. 90/60 mmHg)
- Look for sparse, axillary and pubic hairs and breast atrophy (present)
- Look for scar of adrenectomy on the abdomen

PROVISIONAL DIAGNOSIS

The provisional diagnosis of this patient is Addison's disease (lesion) caused probably by autoimmune adrenal insufficiency (etiology). Patient feels undue weakness.

QUESTIONS AND ANSWERS

Q. **What are the points in favour of your diagnosis?**

Ans: 1. A young female with gradual onset of symptoms
2. Emaciation, thin built and flabby muscles.
3. Triad of weakness, postural hypotension and pigmentation of skin and sun exposed areas
4. Mucous membrane pigmentation
5. Frequent diarrhoeas and signs of vitamins and nutrient deficiencies and weight loss

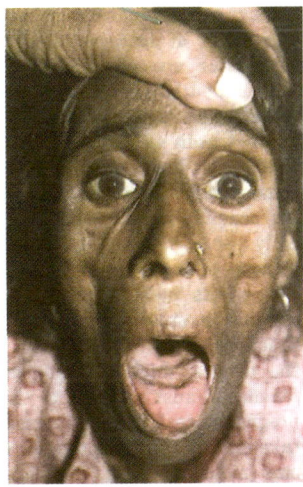

Fig. 88.1: Skin and mucous membrane pigmentation in Addison's disease

6. Low blood pressure (90/60 mmHg)

7. Sparse axillary and pubic hair

Q. What do you understand by the term Addison's disease?

Ans: Deficiency/insufficiency of adrenocortical hormones is called *Addison's disease*. It can be primary or secondary.

Primary Addison's disease indicates adrenal involvement with high ACTH levels due to feedback mechanism.

Secondary Addison's disease means involvement of either pituitary (hypopituitarism) or hypothalamus with decreased ACTH levels.

Q. What are the causes of Addison's disease?

Ans: The causes are:

I. *Common*

- Autoimmune or idiopathic (90%)
- Congenital adrenal hyperplasia
- Pituitary necrosis (Sheehan's syndrome)
- MEN Type I, II syndromes
- Tuberculosis, fungal infections, (histoplasmosis, coccidioidomycosis, etc.) involving adrenals
- Bilateral adrenalectomy

II. *Rare*

- Metastatic tumors (bilateral)
- Amyloidosis, sarcoidosis
- Waterhouse-Friderichsen's syndrome, Adrenal hemorrhage in meningococcal disease
- Hemochromatosis
- Adrenal infarction

Q. What are polyglandular syndromes?

Ans: These are autoimmune syndromes involving multiple endocrine glands and are grouped as MEN–syndromes, type I and II.

MEN Type I (Werner's syndrome). It is characterised by neoplasia of parathyroid, pituitary and pancreas

MEN Type II (Medullary thyroid carcinoma, pheochromocytoma *plus* other neoplasia).

Nipple syndrome: It consists of medullary thyroid carcinoma, pheochromocytoma, parathyroid carcinoma.

Mucosal neuroma syndrome: It includes medullary thyroid carcinoma, pheochromocytoma, mucosal and gastrointestinal neuromas, marfanoid features.

Q. What is the size of heart in Addison's disease?

Ans: It is small.

Q. What other autoimmune disease are associated with Addison's disease?

Ans:
- Graves' disease
- Hashimoto's thyroiditis
- Primary ovarian failure
- Pernicious anemia

Q. Mention some common causes of hyperpigmentation.

Ans: Read hyperpigmentation as a full case disussion.

Q. What is Schmidt's syndrome?

Ans: It is a combination of Addison's disease and hypothyroidism.

Q. How would you investigate such a case?

Ans: The investigations are done to confirm the diagnosis and to find out the cause whether primary or secondary. The preliminary investigations are:

1. *Full blood count* for lymphocytosis and eosinophilia
2. *Serum electrolytes* for hyponatremia, hyperkalemia, hypercalcemia and hyperchloremic acidosis
- *Blood sugar* for hypoglycemia
- *ACTH and cortisol levels* (morning and evening). In Addison's disease, ACTH levels are elevated (>300 ng/l)
- *Adrenal autoantibodies* (21 hydroxylase autoantibodies are elevated)
- *Radiology* (chest X-ray, X-ray abdomen for adrenal calcification)
- *CT scan of adrenals*

Q. Name the adrenal hormones deficient in Addison's disease? What are their effects?

Ans:
1. There is deficiency of glucocorticoids which produces weakness, fatigue and low blood sugar
2. Deficiency of mineralocorticoid in Addison's disease produces hypotension, hyponatraemia and hyperkalemia.
3. Deficiency of androgens produces features of hypogonadism

Q. Which singlemost investigation helps in differentiating primary from the secondary Addison's disease?

Ans: ACTH levels (i.e high in primary and low in secondary Addison's disease)

Q. What is the cause of postural hypotension in your case?

Ans: Low mineralocorticoids (aldosterone) levels.

Q. What is the cause of pigmentation in this case?

Ans: High ACTH levels associated with high MSH levels.

Q. What is the cause of low blood sugar in Addison's disease?

Ans: Low levels of glucocorticoids.

Q. How would you treat autoimmune Addison's disease?

Ans:
1. Replacement of steroids (prednisolone 5 mg in the morning and 2.5 mg at night), adjust the dose to achieve desired levels of serum cortisol and clinical well being of the patient
2. For postural hypotension, administer mineralocorticoid (fludrocortisone 0.025 to 0.15 mg at night) and adjust the dose
3. Advise regular follow up with cortisol levels every 6 months. During follow up record BP (standing and lying down) and monitor electrolytes
4. Advise the patient to increase the dose during stress, i.e. dental procedure, UTI or minor surgery
5. Advise the patient that treatment is life long, therefore, he/she must keep injection of hydrocortisone at home for emergency.

Q. How would you treat adrenal crisis?

Ans: Read Textbook of Emergency Medicine by Prof SN Chugh.

Q. What is risk of anaesthesia in such patients?

Ans: They should not be given general anaesthesia because of risk of precipitation of hypotension and adrenal crisis. They can be operated under local anaesthesia only.

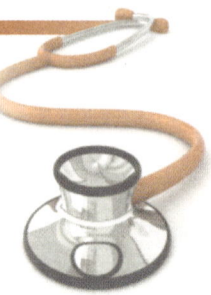

89

Gynecomastia

INSTRUCTION

- Look at the patient chest
- Perform appropriate examination

SALIENT FEATURES

- Female like breasts in a male

HISTORY

Ask for the following:

- Age of onset
- History of thyroid or renal disease
- History of drug intake, e.g. estrogens, digoxin, spironolactone, cimetidine, methyldopa, alkylating agents, clomiphene
- History of mumps, castration or prostatic cancer in old
- Ask whether the breasts are painful or tender on self palpation
- History of tuberculosis, debiliating illness, cirrhosis of liver

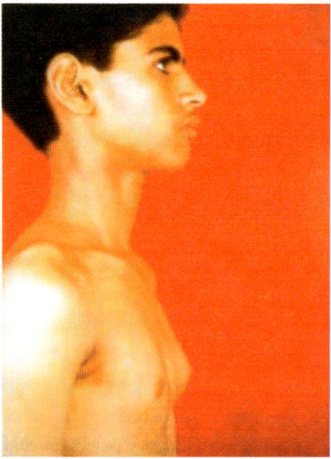

Fig. 89.1: Gynecomastia. A young adolescent male with bilateral gynecomastia

EXAMINATION

Examination of Breasts

- *Inspection.* The breast are enlarged bilaterally (Fig. 89.1). Look at secondary sexual characters, e.g. axillary and pubic hair. Look for distented neck veins, suffusion of face (for superior mediastinal compression). Look for skin lesions of leprosy (hypoanaesthetic patches)
- *Palpation.* Proceed as follows:
  Ask the patient to lie flat comfortably on his back with hands clasped below the head. Palpate the breast with thumb and fingers separated over the breast. Now try to approximate the fingers from either side of the breast slowly. In patients with true gynecomastia a circular disc/mount/ring of tissue is felt around the nipple-areolar region which is rubbery or firm in consistency, confirms the presence of glandular tissue (present). There is no such disc of tissue in pseudogynecomastia

Examine Both Testes for Size and Consistency.

- Hypogonadism occurs in Klinefelter's syndrome

PROVISIONAL DIAGNOSIS

- Patient has bilateral gynecomastia (lesion) due to spironolactone (diuretic) therapy (etiology). It is painful and distressing (functional status)

QUESTIONS AND ANSWERS

Q. **What would you like to examine further if you are asked to do so?**
Ans: Tell the examiner that you would look for other stigmatas of cirrhosis of the liver, signs of superior mediastinal compression, tuberculosis and leprosy.

Q. **What do you understand by gynecomastia?**
Ans: The enlargement of breast in the male like that of female is called *gynecomastia*.

Q. Why do you say it true gynecomastia not pseudogynecomastia?

Ans: On palpation of the breast, glandular tissue is being felt which is hard and tender, confirms the diagnosis of true gynecomastia.

Q. What are the causes of gynecomastia?

Ans: I. *Pathological*
- Klinefelter's syndrome (testicular failure)
- Neoplasm (oestrogen producing tumor)
- Cirrhosis of the liver
- Thyrotoxicosis
- Renal failure
- Starvation/refeeding
- Neoplasms (bronchogenic carcinoma, testicular carcinoma, hepatoma)
- Drug-induced (spironolactone is the most common)
- Idiopathic

II. *Physiological*
- New born
- Adolescent
- Old age

Q. Name the drugs causing gynecomastia?

Ans: Read the history of drug intake in this case.

Q. What are the causes of pseudogynecomastia?

Ans: Causes are:
- Fat deposition
- Neoplasm
- Neurofibromatosis
- Factitious

Q. How would you investigate such a patient?

Ans: Investigations done are mainly to find out the cause, i.e.
1. *Chest X-ray* for bronchogenic carcinoma or metastasis
2. *Plasma human chorionic gonadotrophin (hCG)* — detectable levels indicate testicular tumor or lung or liver neoplasm
3. *Plasma testosterone and luteinising hormone (LH)* for the diagnosis of hypogonadism (Klinefelter's syndrome, etc.)

4. *Serum oestradiol* usually normal
5. *Other hormones,* e.g.
   - Serum prolactin
   - Serum T_3, T_4, TSH for thyrotoxicosis
6. *Chromosomal analysis* for Klinefelter's syndrome

Q. How will you treat a case with gynecomastia?

Ans: Treatment of gynecomastia is:
- Find out the underlying cause and treat it, i.e. treatment of leprosy, hepatocellular failure. If drug is the cause, withdraw it.
- Pubertal gynecomastia is painless, self-limiting and disappears within 2 years.
- Therapy is indicated if gynecomastia in an adult causes pain, embarrassment and emotional discomfort.
- Medical therapy with testosterone is indicated in androgen deficiency. Anti-estrogen therapy with tamoxifen (2 mg/day) is indicated if estrogen excess is the cause.
- Surgery (simple mastectomy or liposuction) is indicated if medical therapy fails or gynecomastia shows continued growth or for cosmetic and psychological reasons.

Q. What are the causes of feminization?

Ans:
- This is due to either an excess of estrogens in male or an imbalance between free estrogen and androgens resulting in excess free estrogen.
- Estrogens producing tumors
- Increased levels of estrogens as a result of cirrhosis of liver
- Increased extraglandular estrogens production (ectopic estrogen production)
- Relative increase in ratio of estrogens to androgens, e.g. testicular failure
- Drugs (oestradiol and estrone)

Q. What is mammoplasia?

Ans: It is soft gynecomastia that occurs following oestrogen therapy.

90

Hypopituitarism

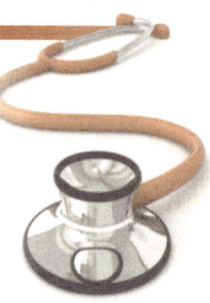

INSTRUCTION

- Perform general physical examination of the patient

SALIENT FEATURES

- Postpartum female with sunken cheeks and absent lactation (picture inset)

HISTORY

Ask about the following:

- History of shaving in males (frequency)
- Impotence in males (hypogonadism)
- Amenorrhoea, postpartum hemorrhage in female (*Sheehan's syndrome*)
- History of radiation, e.g. proton–beam radiation
- History of surgery on pituitary gland

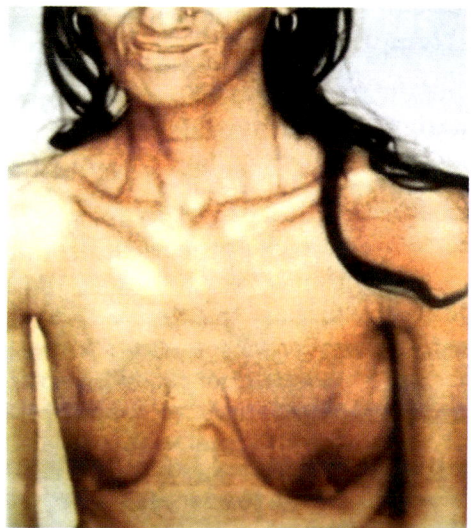

Fig. 90.1: Hypopituitarism. A young female presented with sunken cheeks, breast atrophy following post-partum bleeding (Sheehan's syndrome—postpartum pituitary necrosis)

- History of tuberculosis, sarcoidosis, hemochromatosis

EXAMINATION

General Physical Examination

- The patient is pale with soft shiny skin
- Loss of axillary and pubic hair (hair are scanty)
- Breast atrophy in females (Absence of lactation present)
- BP is low (postural hypotension present)
  Eyes: Test the visual fields (bitemporal hemianopia may be present)
- Examine the fundus for optic atrophy
- *Genitalia* in males for hypogonadism

PROVISIONAL DIAGNOSIS

- The female patient has soft skin and scanty pubic and axillary hair with breast atrophy (lesion) caused by hypopituitarism (cause) due to postpartum pituitary necrosis following postpartum hemorrhage. She is nonlactating mother (functional status).

QUESTIONS AND ANSWERS

Q. **What are the points in favour of your diagnosis?**

Ans:
- A young postpartum female
- Absence of or scanty pubic and axillary hair. Thin built with sunken cheeks, soft shiny skin
- Absence of lactation following delivery
- Breast atrophy
- Low blood pressure
- Debility and muscle wasting (flabby muscles)

Q. **What do you mean by hypopituitarism?**

Ans: Deficiency of one or more pituitary hormones irrespective of its cause is called *hypopituitarism*. It may be primary (pituitary involvement) or secondary (hypothalamic involvement)

Q. What are common causes of hypopituitarism?

Ans: 1. Tumors (pituitary adenoma, craniopharyngioma)
2. Postpartum pituitary necrosis (*Sheehan's syndrome*)
3. Surgical removal of the pituitary or irradiation
4. Autoimmune hypophysitis
5. Metastatic tumors, granulomas (tuberculosis, sarcoidosis, histiocytosis and haemochromatosis)

Q. What hormones secretion is chiefly affected and in which order?

Ans: The hormones are affected in the following order.
  i. Growth hormone (somatotrophs secretion)
  ii. FSH and LH secretion (gonadotrophs secretion)
  iii. TSH (thyrotrophs secretion)
  iv. ACTH (corticotrophs secretion)
  v. Last of all antidiuretic hormone secretion is affected

Q. How would you investigate such a case?

Ans: • *Hemogram* for anaemia
  • *Serum sodium* for dilutional hyponatremia
  • *Fasting blood glucose* may be low
  • *Measurement of pituitary hormones*, i.e. gonadotropins (LH, FSH), TSH, ACTH and GH are usually low
  • *Serum testosterone, estradiol, T_3, T_4* and *cortisol* are usually also low
  • *Pituitary stimulation tests*, e.g. TRH stimulation test, tetracosactrin test, insulin hypoglycarmia test and LHRH stimulation tests have no effect.
  • *X-ray of pituitary fossa* for a space occupying lesion
  • *MRI* provides excellent evidence of parasellar lesions
  • *Perimetry* for visual fields (there may be visual field defects if a tumor is suspected)

Q. What is Houssay phenomenon?

Ans: A diminishing insulin requirement by diabetics may be a sign of hypopituitarism with fall in secretion of GH and ACTH (both are diabetogenic hormones). This phenomenon is called *Houssay phenomenon*. Based on this phenomenon diabetes in acromegaly may improve with pituitary surgery or octreotide therapy.

Q. How would you treat such patients?

Ans: These patients are treated with life-long replacement of thyroid, adrenal and gonadotrophic hormones.

91

Down Syndrome

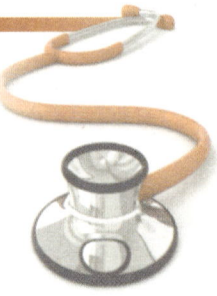

INSTRUCTION

- Examine the patient
- Perform relevant systemic examination

SALIENT FEATURES

- A single crease over the palm (Fig. 91.1), idiotic face

HISTORY

Ask for the following:

- Ask the mother at what age she delivered the child. Down syndrome is common in deliveries occurring in later age groups > 35 yrs of age.
- Education status of the child (mental retardation). How does he perform in school?
- Symptoms of hypothyroidism

EXAMINATION

General Physical Examination

- *Nose:* Look for depression of bridge of the nose
- *Ears:* Look for low-set ears
- *Eyes:* Look for epicanthal folds. Look at the iris for Brush field shots and yellow speckles, cataract, squint
- *Hands:* Look at the hands (Fig. 91.1) for;
  - Single palmar crease (*simian crease* present)
  - Clinodactyly (hypoplasia of middle phalanx of little finger resulting in incurving of it, Fig. 91.1)
  - Missing of one crease in little finger

Examine feet for:

- *Sandle gap,* e.g. increased gap between first and second toe
- Single longitudinal crease in the sole

Systemic Examination

- *CVS* for signs of mitral regurgitation (endocardial cushion defect) and ASD (atrial septal defect) of ostium primum type

- *CNS examination* for IQ (Intelligent Quotient) and mental status
- *Thyroid examination* for hypothyroidism

Note: Tell the examiner, that you would like to check thyroid antibodies.

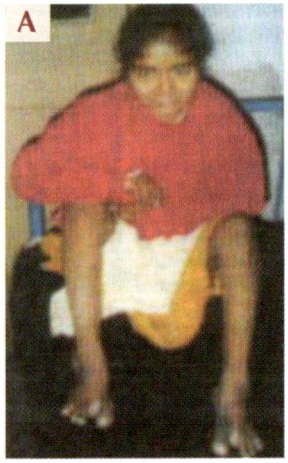

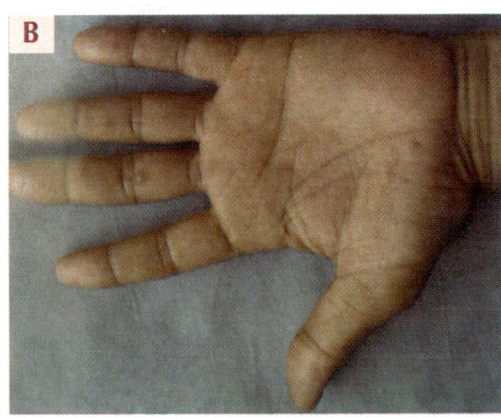

Fig. 91.1: Down's syndrome. (A) Patient with clinodactyly; (B) A single palmar crease

PROVISIONAL DIAGNOSIS

The patient is dwarf and has a single palmar crease with large ears and a systolic murmur in the heart, probably has Down syndrome (lesion) as a result of chromosomal defect, i.e. trisomy 21 (etiology) and has reduced life expectancy (functional status).

QUESTIONS AND ANSWERS

Q. **What are the points in favour of your diagnosis in this case?**

Ans: 1. Depression of nose, low set ears (mongoloid face)
2. Syndactyly, single palmer crease
3. Evidence of mitral regurgitation (endocardial cushion defect).
4. Low IQ (mental retardation)

Q. **What is Down syndrome?**

Ans: *Down's syndrome* is a chromosomal disorder characterised by trisomy 21 (chromosome 21 is present in triplicate) as a result of nondysjunction during meiosis.

Q. **What are characteristics of Mongoloid facies?**

Ans: *Mongol facies (mongolism) comprises of*:
- Microcephaly
- Upward slanting eyes with epicanthal folds
- Small, low-set ears
- Depressed bridge of the small nose
- Widely-set eyes (hypertelorism)
- Open mouth, fissured protruding tongue (macroglossia)
- High arched palate and small teeth
- Idiotic face, mental retardation (low IQ)

Q. **Is pregnancy possible in Down syndrome?**

Ans: It is possible only in mosaic individuals with a normal 46 XX cell line (45XO/46XX).

Q. **Which maternal serum markers are used for prenatal screening of Down syndrome?**

Ans:
- Serum α-fetoprotein
- Chorionic gonadotropin
- Estriol

Q. **What complications can occur in Down syndrome?**

Ans: I. Increased chances of acute leukemias
II. Alzheimer type presenile dementia which is the cause of reduced life expectancy
III. Atlantoaxial subluxation
IV. Duodenal/jejunal/biliary atresia

Q. **What are the chromosomal abnormalities in this condition?**

Ans:
- Trisomy 21 (common)
- Mosaicism (46XY/47XY)

Q. **What are underlying genetic defect?**

Ans:
- Nondysjunction
- De novo translocation
- Familial translocation (translocation of the long arm of chromosome 21 to another acrocentric chromosome, e.g. 22 or 14.

Q. **What would you advise to a pregnant women who want to confirm whether fetus has Down syndrome or not?**

Ans: Chorionic-villus sampling at 10–12 weeks for chromosomal analysis.

or

Amniocentesis at 15 and 20 weeks for chromosomal analysis.

92

Turner's Syndrome

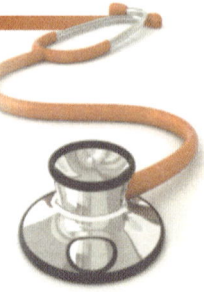

INSTRUCTION

- Look at the patient
- Perform relevant systemic examination

SALIENT FEATURES
- Short necked female.

HISTORY

General Physical Examination
- Examine the patient's look (immature facies), neck [webbed short neck (Fig. 92.1), hairline low (Fig. 92.1B)].
- Short stature (patient is dwarf)
- Examine chin (receding), and ears (low set)
- Look at eyes for double eyelashes, epicanthal folds, strabismus
- Flat (shield shaped) chest with wide separation of nipples (present)
- Multiple pigmented nevi
- Short 4th metacarpal

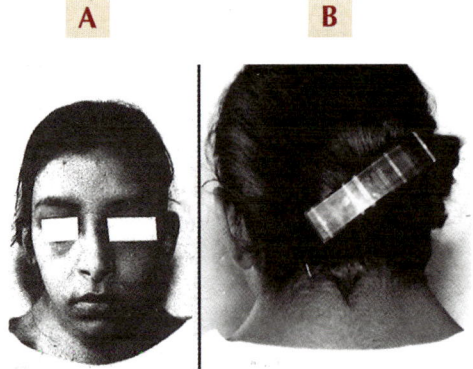

Fig. 92.1: Turner's syndrome. (A) Short webbed receding chin; (B) Low hairline. The female has flat chest with failure of sexual maturation, short stature, and cubitus valgus

- Examine extremities for swelling (lympho-edema)
- History of primary ammenorrhea (present)

Systemic Examination
- Palpate the pulses for radiofemoral delay (coarctation of aorta) and aortic stenosis.
- Examine the genitalia for infantalism
- Look for signs of hypothyroidism
- CVS examination for aortic stenosis (bicuspid aortic valve)

PROVISIONAL DIAGNOSIS

The patient has Turner's syndrome (lesion) which is a chromosomal defect (monosomy – 45XO). She has menstrual disturbance and skeletal abnormalities (functional status).

QUESTIONS AND ANSWERS

Q. **What are points in favor of your diagnosis?**
Ans: 1. A young female
2. A short webbed neck, low hair line, receding chin
3. Flat chest, nondevelopment of secondary sexual character. History of primary amenorrhea
4. Skeletal abnormality (cubitus valgus)
5. Genitalia infantalism.

Q. **What are features of Turner's syndrome?**
Ans: It is X-linked disorder characterized by monosomy X (45XO) and affects the females. The features of this syndrome are:
- Short stature, short webbed neck, low-hairline on the back, receding chin and low-set ears (Fig. 92.1)
- Primary amenorrhea
- Poorly developed secondary sexual characters
- Shield breast (flat breast)
- Cubitus valgus (increased carrying angle)

- Short 4th metacarpal or metatarsal
- Coarctation of aorta/aortic stenosis
- Peripheral lymphedema (hands and feet)
- Nail hypoplasia, epicanthal folds, double eyelashes, multiple pigmented nevi

Q. **What is cardiac abnormality in your case?**

Ans: Clinically, no cardiac abnormality is detectable in this case.

Q. **What do you understand by a neck web (webbed neck)?**

Ans: It means either a fan-like fold of skin extending from shoulder to the neck or an abnormal splaying out of the trapezius.

Q. **Name cardiovascular diseases associated with webbed neck?**

Ans: • Noonan's syndrome (ASD)
- Ullrich's syndrome with pulmonary stenosis

Q. **What is karyotype in Turner's syndrome?**

Ans: Karyotype is 45 XO. Other variants include 46X (with abnormal X), 45 XO/46XX mosaics and 45XO/46XY mosaics.

Q. **What are the renal abnormalities in Turner's syndrome?**

Ans: 1. Horse-shoe kidney
2. Hydronephrosis

Q. **Is pregnancy possible in Turner's syndrome?**

Ans: As there is primary amenorrhoea and sexual infantalism in these cases, hence, chances of pregnancy are remote.
However, in Turner's mosaic who have normal 46XX line with sufficient ovarian follicles to initiate pubertal changes and ovulation can have pregnancy subsequently.

Q. **What do you understand by Turner's mosaics?**

Ans: Turner's mosaics may have 46X (with other abnormal X), 45, XO/XX mosaic and 45, XO/XY mosacis. Although, it is a single chromosomal disorder but > 95% of the foetuses are aborted. Only, Turner's mosaics with 45XO/46XX cell line with sufficient follicles can sustain pregnancy as already discussed.

93

Klinefelter's Syndrome

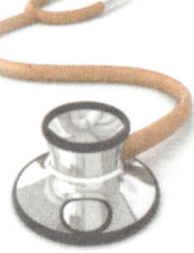

INSTRUCTION

Examine the patient including genitalia

SALIENT FEATURES

- Gynecomastia, small testes, scanty pubic hair

HISTORY

Ask for the following:

- History of bilateral breasts enlargement (present)
- History of small testes, lack of beard (present)
- Is he mentally normal/subnormal? Ask how does he perform in the school/college?
- If married, ask about sexual history including fertility. Does he has any issue?
- Ask about the sense of smell/altered smell (anosmia is a feature of hypogonadotrophic hypogonadism, Klinefelter's syndrome (hyper-gonadotrophic hypogonadism).

EXAMINATION

General Physical Examination

- *Face:* Immature face with vacant look and lack of beard (present).
- *Body habitus.* Measure upper and lower segment. In Klinefelter's syndrome lower segment is > upper segment.
- *Examine the breasts.* There is gynecomastia (Fig. 93.1) in Klinefelter's syndrome (Read examination of gynecomastia as a separate case discussion)
- Test the *mental IQ*
- *Examine the testes,* i.e. size, texture or consistency (Fig. 93.1).

PROVISIONAL DIAGNOSIS

The patient has Klinefelter's syndrome (lesion) due to chromosomal defect (aetiology). Patient is infertile (functional status).

QUESTIONS AND ANSWERS

Q. What are the points in favour of your diagnosis?

Ans:
1. A young male with enuchoidism (lack of androgenisation)
2. Body habitus (LS > US)
3. Immature face, lack of beard
4. Bilateral gynecomastia, small firm testes and scanty pubic hair
5. Obesity
6. Femine voice

Q. What is the phenotype in Klinefelter's syndrome?

Ans: They are phenotypically male.

Q. What is Klinefelter's triad?

Ans: Enuchoidism, gynecomastia and hypo-gonadism in a male constitute a Klinefelter's triad.

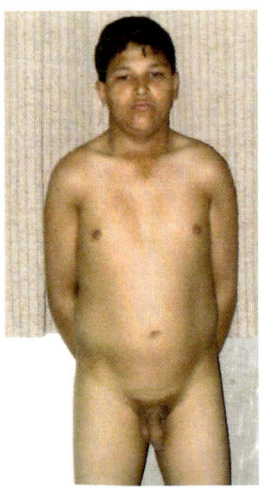

Fig. 93.1: Klinefelter's syndrome. Note bilateral gynecomastia, testes scanty pubic hair, smaller size of penis and enuchoidism

Q. What happens to gonadotrophins in Klinefelter's syndrome?

Ans: They are raised, hence, hypogonadism is hypergonadotrophic (primary testicular)

Q. Enumerate the characteristic features of Klinefelter's syndrome?

Ans:
1. Enuchoidism
2. Lower segment > upper segment (body habitus)
3. Lack of sexual characters, i.e. lack of axillary and pubic hair, small testes and azoospermia
4. Phenotype is male
5. Voice is feminine
6. Mentally clear, but sometimes subnormal

Q. What is the most common Karyotype in Klinefelter's syndrome?

Ans: The most common karyotype is 47/XXY (80%) which results from non-dysfunction of sex chromosomes at meiosis during gametogenesis in one of the parents.

Q. Are patients of Klinefelter's syndrome fertile?

Ans: Classical cases of Klinefelter's syndrome are infertile. However, some men having chromosomal mosaicism (46, XXY/47,XXX) are fertile called mosatic Klinefelter's. Mosaic forms result from chromosomal mitotic nondysjunction within the zygote and occurs in 10% cases.

Q. How would you investigate Klinefelter's syndrome?

Ans:
- *Plasma gonadotrophins levels*: FSH levels are persistently high in hypergonodotrophic hypogonadism.
- *Plasma testosterone levels*: They are low.
- *Plasma estradiol levels*: They are raised.
- *Chromosome analysis*: It shows two or more X-chromosomes and one or more Y-chromosome.

Q. What is the genetic defect in Klinefelter's Syndrome?

Ans: There is excess of DAX1 gene in Klinefelter's syndrome which encodes a number of nuclear proteins that inhibit testicular differentiation.

94

Marfan's Syndrome

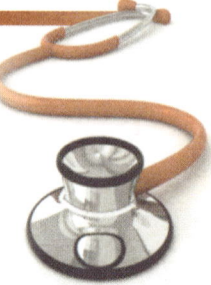

INSTRUCTION

- Have a look at the patient
- Examine cardiovascular system

SALIENT FEATURES

A thin tall person (tall stature)

HISTORY

Ask about family history of tall stature (present)

EXAMINATION

General Physical Examination

1. *Examine height and arm span*: Patient is tall, has disproportionately long and thin extremities. Arm span is more than height on measurement (Fig. 94.1).
   - *Head*: Head is long (dolichocephalic, narrow face, high-arched palate, body proportions, i.e. lower segment > upper segment, fingers, i.e. long slender finger called arachnodactyly (present).

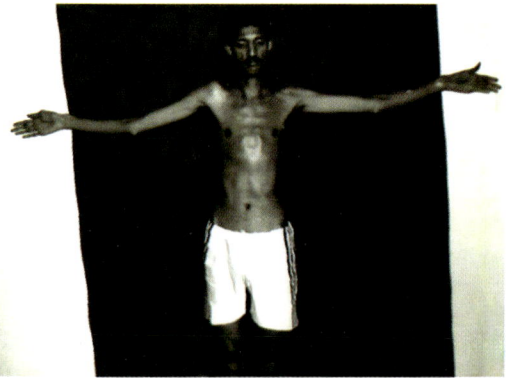

Fig. 94.1: Marfan's syndrome. Note tall stature on measurement. Height is 6'–1½"; Arm span 6'–6"; upper segment 31½"; Lower segment 42"; Ratio 0.75

- Hyperextensible joints and laxity of ligaments leading to recurrent dislocation of hip and femoral and inguinal hernias.
- *Steinberg's sign or thumb protrusion sign* in which the thumb when apposed across the palm protrudes beyond the ulnar border of the hand (positive in this case)
- *Wrist-sign* the thumb and little finger overlap when elapsed around the opposite wrist.
- Tell the examiner that you would like to see X-rays of hands for metacarpal index > 8 (the average ratio of lengths/breadth of last 4 metacarpals from 2nd to 5th as seen on X-ray).

Examination of Eyes

- Ectopia lentis—upward bilateral dislocation of lens, may be seen on slit lamp examination
- Myopia with blue sclera
- Squint, nystagmus
- Iridodonesis may be seen

Systemic Examination

CVS Examination for

- Mitral valve prolapse (signs of MR present)
- Dissecting aneurysm of aorta
- Aortic regurgitation
- Conduction abnormalities
- Congestive heart failure

Examination of Chest for

- Pectus excavatum
- Cystic lung disease

Examination of Spine

- Scoliosis and kyphosis

PROVISIONAL DIAGNOSIS

The musculoskeletal features are suggestive of Marfan's syndrome. In addition, patient has mitral valve prolapse without heart failure (functional cardiac status).

QUESTIONS AND ANSWERS

Q. **What is Marfan's syndrome? What are its characteristic features? What is Marfan's habitus?**

Ans: Marfan's syndrome (Fig. 94.1) is an autosomal dominant disorder characterized by two of the three (a triad) abnormalities:
1. Musculoskeletal (tall stature, lower segment > upper arm span > height, arachnodactyly, etc.)
2. Ocular (ectopia lentis, iridodonesis)
3. Cardiovascular (MR or AR, aortic dissection)

Marfan's habitus refers to presence of some of skeletal abnormalities without other features of Marfan's syndrome.

Q. **What are the diagnostic criteria for Marfan's syndrome? Does your case fit into the criteria.**

Ans: The diagnostic criteria are:
I. Positive family history with two systems involvement out of three systems.
II. If no positive family history, then skeletal features *plus* involvement of two other systems and one of the major criteria, ectopia lentis, aortic root dilation or aortic dissection and lumbosacral duct ectasia on CT/MRI.

Yes, my case fits into the diagnosis because of positive family history, musculoskeletal manifestation and mitral regurgitation.

Q. **What are the causes of arachnodactyly?**

Ans: 1. Marfan's syndrome
2. Congenital contractual arachnodactyly
3. Homocystinuria

Q. **What are ocular manifestations of Marfan's syndrome?**

Ans: Read the examination of eyes in this case

Q. **What is the differential diagnosis of Marfan's syndrome?**

Ans: The only condition in which skeletal manifestations of Marfan's syndrome are present is homocysteinuria which has to be differentiated. Presence of ectopia lentis with downward displacement of lens, mental retardation and homocystein in urine differentiates homocysteinuria from Marfan's syndrome.

Q. **What is the basic defect in Marfan's syndrome?**

Ans: Being a heritable (autosomal dominant) disorder of connective tissues the basic defect lies in gene mutation of single allele of the fibrillin gene (FBNI).

Q. **Is eunuchoidism a feature of Marfan's syndrome?**

Ans: No, eunuchoidism refers to androgen deficiency leading to tall stature. The patients with Marfan's syndrome have normal sex characters and sexual development.

Q. **What are the cardiovascular manifestations of Marfan's syndrome?**

Ans: Read examination of CVS in this case

Q. **What are the pulmonary manifestations of Marfan's syndrome?**

Ans: • Associated cystic lung disease
• Spontaneous pneumothorax

Q. **What are the complications of pregnancy in women with Marfan's syndrome?**

Ans: • Early premature abortion
• Maternal death from aortic dissection. Pregnancy is not dangerous when aortic root diameter is < 40 mm.

Q. **What is the cause of death in Marfan's syndrome?**

Ans: Cardiovascular complication (aortic dissection or congestive heart failure due to aortic regurgitation).

Q. **What would you advise the patient of Marfan's syndrome with cardiovascular manifestations?**

Ans: • Annual echocardiography to measure aortic diameter and mitral valve function
• Long-term beta-blockers to retard the progression of aortic root dilatation
• Prophylaxis against infective endocarditis
• Prophylactic replacement of the aortic root with a composite graft when the diameter reaches 50 – 55 mm (normal < 40 mm)

Q. **What are the features of homocysteinuria?**

Ans: Following are the features:
• It is a genetic disorder inherited as autosomal recessive
• There is reduced activity of the enzyme–cystathionine beta synthetase
• Mental retardation
• Osteoporosis is common
• Ectopia lentis with displacement of lens downward (in Marfan's, lens is displaced upwards), glaucoma and impaired visual acquity may result
• Thrombotic episodes may occur
• Plasma methionine and homocysteine are raised and cysteine is low. The cyanide-nitroprusside test is positive.

95

Tall Stature

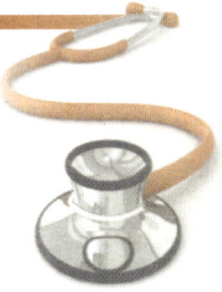

INSTRUCTION

- Examine the patient

SALIENT FEATURES

- Tall stature (Fig. 95.1)

HISTORY

Ask for the following:

- Age of the patient
- Height of the patient
- Family history of tall stature (constitutionally tall)
- Built of the patient (thin built in Marfan's syndrome, Kallmann's syndrome, thick and stout built in gigantism and acromegaly)
- Infertility, if person is married
- Any mental subnormality
- History of decreased or loss of smell (anosmia)

EXAMINATION

General Physical Examination

Proceed to examine the case as follows:

- Note the age (prepubertal or post-pubertal) and total height of the patient
- Measure both the upper and lower segments
- Measure the arm span and deduce the arm span with total height

I. *If lower segment (pubis to heel) is equal or more than upper segment (crown to pubis), then look for;*
   1. Marfanoid features (Marfan's syndrome), i.e. arachanodactyly (spidery fingers) confirmed by thumb protrusion sign or wrist sign, hypermobility of the joints, eyes for iridodonesis (ectopia lentis), high arched heart for valvular regurgitation (MR and AR)
   2. Features for Klinefelter's syndrome , i.e. lack of beard and scanty pubic hair, female voice, gynecomastia, small atrophic testes and infertility

   3. Features of acromegaly / gigantism, i.e. large head, prognathism, large tongue, thick stout built, short stubby fingers, large feet, etc.
   4. Features of Kallmann's syndrome, i.e. tall stature, thin built, small testes and anosmia.

II. *If upper segments is > lower segment, then*
   - Look for the features of precocious puberty of adrenal virilization.

N.B Never forget to examine primary and secondary sexual characters in a patient with tall stature. There is corollary that the longer the person, the more are chances of infertility.

PROVISIONAL DIAGNOSIS

- Tall stature with hypogonadism and anosmia (lesion) suggest the diagnosis of Kallmann's syndrome (aetiology). The patient is mentally disturbed infertile (functional status)

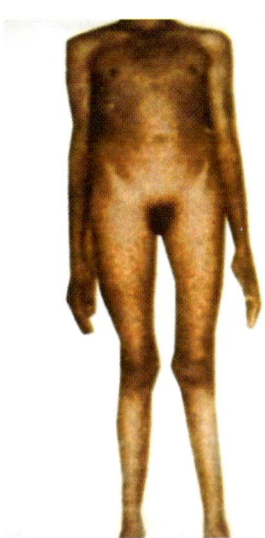

Fig. 95.1: Tall stature. A patient with hypogonadotropic hypogonadism—Kallmann's syndrome

QUESTIONS AND ANSWERS

Q.   What is stature?

Ans: Stature means total height from crown to heel. Tall stature means height above 97th percentile of normal population of same age and sex.

Q.   What is Kallmann's syndrome?

Ans: It is a congenital disorder inherited as an X-linked recessive trait, characterised by prepubertal hypogonadotropic hypogonadism (low testosterone, low LH and FSH levels) due to GnRH deficiency associated with eunuchoidism, small testes, scanty pubic hair (Fig. 95.1) and anosmia (loss of smell) as a result of defect in the developing olfactory tract. In some cases, cerebellar dysfunction, cleft palate and congenital deafness are present (not present in this case). Cryptorchidism may occur.

Q.   What are the causes of tall stature?

Ans: These are:
- Constitutional
- Racial
- Marfan's syndrome
- Klinefelter's and Reifenstein's syndromes
- Gigantism, acromegaly
- Hypogonadotrophic hypogonadism (*Kallmann's syndrome, Frohlich's syndrome*)
- Homocysteinuria
- Congenital contractural arachnodactyly
- Supermales (XYY) and superfemales (triple X)

Q.   What is eunuchoidism?

Ans: Leydig cell failure (loss of androgens or testosterone prior to puberty) results in hypogonadism, delayed sexual maturation and tall stature due to *nonclosure* of the epiphyses—a condition called *eunuchoidism*, which in addition includes infantilism, i.e. scanty distribution of both poor muscle mass.

In common sense, androgens loss implies eunuchoidism.

Q.   What do you understand by the proportion? What are different body parts in tall stature?

Ans: Body proportion means ratio of upper (vertex to pubis) to lower segment (pubic-heel) which is normally 0.93 in adults because of long legs than trunk. The different body proportion stature are:

1. The upper segment is equal to lower (1 : 1) in:
   - Gigantism
   - Kallmann's syndrome
   - Frohlich's syndrome
   - Constitutional cause

2. Lower segment > upper segment
   - Marfan's syndrome
   - Klinefelter's syndrome
   - Hypogonadism
   - Homocysteinuria

3. Upper segment > lower segment
   - Precocious puberty
   - Adrenal cortical tumors

96

Hypoparathyroidism

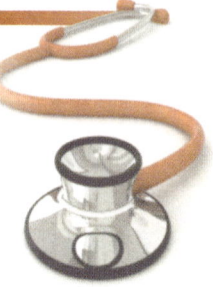

INSTRUCTION

- Look at the patient's hands
- Perform relevant examination

SALIENT FEATURES

- Complains of intermittent painless carpopedal spasms (Figure inset)

HISTORY

Ask about the following:

- History of thyroid surgery (present) because hypoparathyroidism is common following thyroid surgery
- Paresthesias of hands, toes and circumoral regions (These are common presenting features of hypoparathyroidism)
- History of muscle cramping, laryngeal stridor, convulsions, carpopedal spasms involving hands and feet will also be asked (This is main complaint of this patient)

EXAMINATION

General Physical Examination

- Examine the hands and feet for carpopedal spasms (Fig. 96.1). There is spasm of the hands, fingers are extended except at metacarpophalangeal joints and thumb is adducted. The feet also show spasms.
- If spontaneous spasm is not evident but there is history of carpopedal spasms then, perform **Chvostek's sign** (Tap over the facial nerve in front of tragus of the ear and look for facial spasms) or **Trousseau's sign** (Inflate the BP cuff just above the systolic BP of the patient for 3 minutes and look for carpopedal spasms) (present Fig. 96.1B)
- Look into the mouth for any evidence of oral candidiasis (*Candida endocrinopathy*)
- Check for any scar of thyroid surgery (scar of thyroid surgery present)
- Look at the finger nails for candidiasis/fungal infection
- Look for cataracts (cataract is common in hypoparathyroidism)

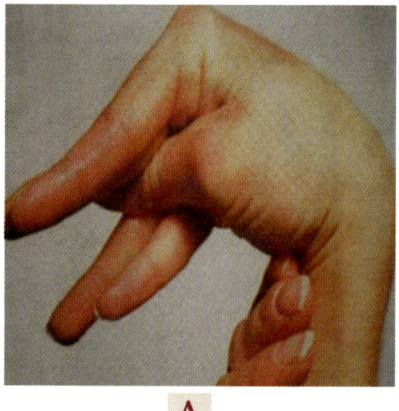

A

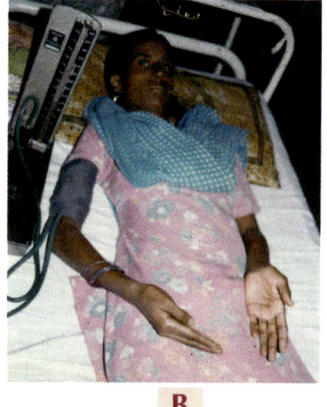

B

Fig. 96.1: Spontaneous carpopedal spasm in tetany. (A) Note the main D' accoucher's or obstetrician's hand; (B) A patient with hypoparathyroidism showing provoked carpopedal spasms (Trousseau's sign)

PROVISIONAL DIAGNOSIS

• The patient has carpopedal spasm (lesion) caused by hypoparathyroidism as a complication of thyroid surgery (aetiology). There is hypocalcemia, i.e. low ionised calcium (functional status).

QUESTIONS AND ANSWERS

Q. **What are points in favor of hypoparathyroidism in your case?**

Ans: 1. History of thyroid surgery and presence of a scar over thyroid region.
2. History of paraesthesias of hands, toes and circumoral region
3. Painless intermittent, carpopedal spasms
4. Positive Trousseau's sign.

Q. **What other condition would you keep in mind in this case?**

Ans: Pseudohypoparathyroidism (read Table 96.1)

Table 96.1: True vs pseudohypoparathyroidism

Idiopathic hypoparathyroidism	Pseudohypoparathyroidism
• Usually acquired	• Congenital
• PTH levels are low	• PTH levels are high
• Autoimmunity plays a role in some cases	• Non-responsiveness to PTH either due to receptor post-receptor defect
• Besides tetany, other features include epilepsy, psychosis, cataract, calcification of basal ganglia and papilledema	• Besides tetany, other features include skeletal and developmental abnormalities such as short stature, short 4th and 5th metacarpal or metatarsals (*Albright's syndrome or Albright's hereditary osteodystrophy*)

Q. **What do you understand by carpopedal spasms?**

Ans: Low ionized calcium results in carpal spasms (there is extension of interphalangeal joints and adduction and flexion of metacarpophalangeal joints with adduction of the thumb) and pedal spasms.

Q. **Does the patient has spasms or cramps? What is the difference between the two?**

Ans: The only difference is that cramps are painful while spasms are painless.

Q. **What are the common causes of hypoparathyroidism?**

Ans: The common causes are:

A. PTH absent

i. Hereditary hypoparathyroidism—DiGeorge syndrome, candidiasis endocrinopathy and familial autoimmune polyglandular deficiency syndrome
ii. Acquired hypoparathyroidism, e.g. parathyroidectomy or irradiation damage
iii. Hypomagnesemia due to any cause

B. PTH ineffective

i. *Chronic renal failure*
ii. *Vit. D deficiency*, e.g. rickets, osteomalacia, drug-induced (phenytoin)
iii. *Vit. D resistance*
— Vit. D resistant rickets (type II)
— Intestinal malabsorption
vi. *Pseudohypoparathyroidism*, e.g. Albright's syndrome

C. PTH overwhelmed

i. Severe, acute hyperphosphatemia
• Tumor lysis
• Acute renal failure
• Rhabdomyolysis

Q. **What are the common causes of hypocalcemia?**

Ans: 1. Hypoparathyroidism or pseudohypoparathyroidism
2. Rickets, osteomalacia (vit. D deficiency)
3. Chronic renal failure
4. Chronic diarrhea, malabsorption syndrome
5. Hyperphosphatemia due to any cause, e.g. tumour lysis, ARF
6. Acute pancreatitis.

Q. **What are causes of transient hypocalcemia?**

Ans: Transient hypocalcemia does not produce tetany, occurs due to: Severe sepsis, Burns, ARF, Repeated transfusions with citrated blood and Medications such as protamine, heparin, dilantin and glucagon

Q. **Does the low calcium levels are always associated with tetany?**

Ans: No. Total low calcium is not associated with tetany because ionised calcium may be normal in such a case. Low ionised calcium irrespective of calcium levels is associated with tetany.

Q. **What are the causes of tetany?**

Ans: Tetany occurs due to low ionised calcium, hypokalemia, hypomagnesemia and alkalosis. The causes are:

I. *Hypocalcemia*
• Malabsorption
• Rickets and osteomalacia
• Hypoparathyroidism
• Chronic renal failure (usually tetany is prepare acidosis

- Acute pancreatitis
- Drugs, e.g. dilantin (Phenytoin)

II. *Hypomagnesemia*

III. *Alkalosis and hypokalemia.*
- Repeated prolonged vomiting
- Excessive intake of alkali
- Hysterical hyperventilation
- Primary hyperaldosteronism
- Acute anion load

Q. **What is normal ionised serum calcium level? How would you define hypo- and hyper-calcemia?**

Ans: Normal ionised calcium is 1.1–1.4 mmol/L 4.4–5.6 mg/dl)

Usually **hypocalcemia** is said to be present when serum calcium is <8.5 mg/dl (normal 9–10.5 mg%). On the other hand **hyper-calcemia** is said to be present when calcium levels are >11.0 mg/dl.

Q. **How would you collect blood sample for calcium?**

Ans: Blood sample for calcium should be taken without the help of compression of the arm or tourniquet, otherwise false reading will be obtained.

Q. **What are the factors that affect serum calcium levels? How would you correct calcium levels in these condition?**

Ans:
- *Albumin concentration:* Low albumin concentration lowers the serum total calcium levels, hence it has to be corrected by a formula as follows;
  – For 1 gm/dl fall in serum albumin you add 0.8 mg to calcium level
- *Serum immunoglobulin:* Fall in serum immunoglobulins also lowers the serum total calcium. Algorithm for correction is
  – For 1 gm/dl fall in serum immu-noglobulin you add 0.5 mg/dl to calcium
- Acidosis also alters ionized calcium by reducing its association with proteins.

Q. **What is latent tetany?**

Ans: The absence of symptoms and signs of tetany in a patient with hypocalcemia is called *latent tetany*. The tetany becomes manifest on provocative tests.

(i) **Trousseau's sign** (Fig. 96.1B). Raising the BP above systolic level by inflation of sphygmomanometer cuff produces characteristic carpal spasms within 3–5 minutes

(ii) **Chvostek's sign.** A tap at facial nerve at the angle of jaw produces twitching of facial muscles.

Q. **How would you investigate a patient of tetany?**

Ans:
- *Blood biochemistry*, i.e. potassium, cal-cium, magnesium, phosphate, alkaline phosphate, urea and creatinine
- *Blood pH*
- *Blood PTH* and 1–25 dihydroxy cho-lecalciferol levels
- *Urinary excretion of calcium*
- *X-ray skull* for basal ganglia calcification
- *ECG for QT* prolongation which predis-poses to arrhythmias

Q. **How does hyperventilation lead to tetany?**

Ans: Hyperventilation occurring frequently or if prolonged leads to tetany by producing alkalosis due to washing out of CO_2.

Q. **How will you treat tetany?**

Ans: The steps of treatment are:
1. *Treatment of hypocalcemia* by calcium gluconate (10% 20 ml I.M or I.V) followed by oral supplementation of calcium and vitamin D analog. If not relieved by calcium, potassium and magnesium may be tried.

2. *Treatment of alkalosis*
   - Withdraw the alkalies if it has been the cause
   - Isotonic saline IV if vomiting is the cause
   - Inhalation of 5% CO_2 in oxygen if hyperventilation is the cause
   - Psychotherapy for hysterical hyper-ventilation.

Q. **What is pseudohypoparathyroidism? What is pseudopseudohypoparathyroidism?**

Ans: *Pseudohypoparathyroidism:* It is a heritable or congenital disorder characterised by tissue resistance to the effects of PTH.

In pseudohypoparathyroidism, in addition to symptoms and signs of hypoparathyroidism, there are distinct skeletal and development defects — a characteristic phenotype termed as 'Albright hereditary osteodystrophy'.

Pseudopseudohypoparathyroidism: A familial disorders in which skeletal and developmental defect are present without signs of hypoparathyroidism. PTH level is normal, but there is resistance to its effects.

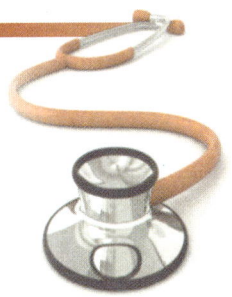

97

Acromegaly and Gigantism

INSTRUCTION

- Examine the patient's face and hands
- Perform relevant examination

SALIENT FEATURES

- Giant looking female (Fig. 97.1)
- Tall giant male (Fig. 97.2)

HISTORY

Ask for the following:

- Ask about the height of the patient
- Ask about the history of change in size of the shoes or tightness of rings or size of the hat/cap
- Ask about excessive sweating
- Ask for headache, visual field defects, paresthesia in hands and feet

- Ask about any menstrual irregularity in females or impotence in male
- Any history of dyspnea
- Any history of arthritis
- Any change in acral parts or face

EXAMINATION

General Physical Examination

1. First of all, *shake the hands* with the patient and note the moist hands. Note the tall stature in gigantism (Fig. 97.2).
2. Now look at the *hands*, i.e. note the large size of hands or square shape hand with short and wide fingers (Figs 97.1 and 97.2). There is thick skin of hands. Volume of the hand is increased (in both the case).
3. Look at the *face* and note the following:

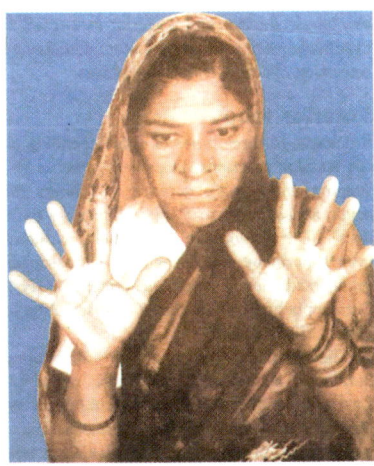

Fig. 97.1: Acromegaly in a female. Features are:
1. Acromegalic face, i.e. broad thick nose, thickening of skin, prominent eyebrows, coarsening of facial features.
2. Prognathism (elongation and widening of mandible).
3. Spade-like hands with short, thick stout fingers.

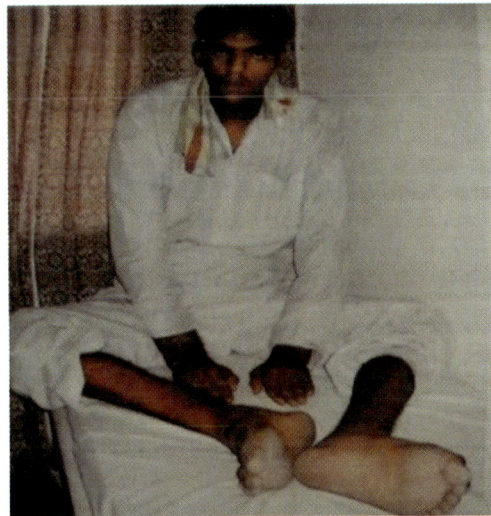

Fig. 97.2: Gigantism. Note the height of patient (8 feet 2 inches). The hands and feet are large. The built is stout

- Prognathism [protruding jaw (Fig. 97.1)], thick lips, large tongue, large incisors, elongated face, prominent sinuses (frontal and maxillary) prominent supraorbital ridges and large nose.
4. Examine the eye and neck (for goiter)
5. Check the teeth and note the malocclusion and splaying of the teeth (interdental separation).

Systemic Examination

- *Chest* for heart enlargement. Take BP
- *Abdomen* for hepatosplenomegaly
- *Joints* for osteoarthritis and chondrocalcinosis
- *Spine* for kyphosis
- Tell the examiner that you would like to look for bitemporal hemianopia on visual field and optic atrophy on fundus examination
- Test for deafness (audiometry).

PROVISIONAL DIAGNOSIS

- The first patient has features suggestive of acromegaly and second patient has gigantism (lesion) the cause of which may be a pituitary tumor. Both the patients are disturbed due to coarse facial features and large acral parts (functional status)

QUESTIONS AND ANSWERS

Q. **What are the points in favor of your diagnosis?**
Ans: 1. Acromegalic or gigantic face (e.g. broad thick nose, thickening of skin, prominent eyebrows,
2. Tall stature in gigantism
3. Prognathism, macrosomia, macroglossia.
4. Large acral parts (e.g. large spade-like hands and feet) and head (hat-size) are present in both the cases
5. Excessive perspiration and increasing headache (present in both)
6. Visual field defect (bitemporal hemianopia)
7. Second patient had early onset of symptoms than the first

Q. **Which physical findings suggest a pituitary tumor?**
Ans: • Bitemporal hemianopia
• Headache

Q. **What bedside test would you like to perform?**
Ans: • Urine for glycosuria
• Blood sugar for IGT and diabetes

Q. **Which pituitary tumors can lead to acromegaly or gigantism?**
Ans: • GH secreting pituitary adenoma
• Prolactinoma

Q. **Name the diseases caused by GH excess?**
Ans: 1. *Gigantism* due to excess of GH in prepubertal age group (before fusion of metaphysis) (Fig. 97.2)
2. *Acromegaly* due to excess of GH in postpubertal age groups (after fusion of metaphysis)
3. *Gigantic acromegaly* — A combination of both (GH is secreted in excess in prepubertal age which continues in postpubertal age).

Q. **What are the actions of GH?**
Ans: 1. GH induces protein synthesis, nitrogen retention and impairs glucose tolerance by antagonising insulin action (insulin antagonist)
2. It stimulates lipolysis leading to increased fatty acid levels, enhanced lean body mass and omental fat mass.
3. It promotes Na, K and water retention
4. It stimulates linear bone growth

Q. **What are the neurological manifestation of acromegaly or gigantism?**
Ans: Neurological manifestations are as follows:
A. *Cranial nerve palsy*
1. *Optic nerve.* Pressure on the optic chiasma leads to bitemporal hemianopia (common), compression of optic nerve leads to blindness due to optic atrophy.
2. *Paralysis of 3rd, 4th and 6th nerves* and external ophthalmoplegia.
3. *VIIIth nerve* involvement leads to deafness.
B. *Peripheral nerve compression*
- Carpal tunnel syndrome (median nerve compression).

Q. **How can you assess the activity in acromegaly and gigantism?**
Ans: Acromegaly or gigantism is assessed for its activity as follows:
- Increasing sizes of the gloves, rings and shoes
- Ill–fitting of previous dentures
- Excessive perspiration and increasing headache
- Increasing visual loss
- Excessive sebum production
- Serial photographs of the patient may reveal progressive macrosomia
- Biochemical evidence of raised GH and somatomedian C levels

Q. **What are the complications or sequale of acromegaly or gigantism?**
Ans: • Cardiomegaly and heart failure
• Hypertension

- Impaired glucose tolerance
- Arthritis of hip, knee and spine
- Hypopituitarism
- Visual field defects
- Carpal tunnel syndrome
- Spinal canal stenosis

Q. Which drug is used to control the activity in acromegaly or gigantism?

Ans: Octreotide or lanreotide—a somatostatin analogue.

Q. How will you investigate such a patient?

Ans: The investigations are given in Table 97.1.

Q. What is the treatment of acromegaly or gigantism?

Ans: Following are the treatment methods:

1. *Medical:* Bromocriptine, a long-acting dopamine agonist may be used to lower the GH levels in active disease. The dose is 15–30 mg/day in divided doses, starting at a low dose of 2.5 mg/day and then gradually increasing it. Side effects include nausea, vomiting, postural hypotension, constipation and dyskinesia.

   Now a days a somatostatin analog, i.e. octreotide is used subcutaneously three times a day.

2. *Surgical:* Removal of adenoma by transsphenoidal route is preferred mode of surgery for compressive symptoms.

3. *Radiotherapy:* Pituitary is irradiated externally by gamma rays or by accelerated proton beam (linear accelerator) or internally by implanting rods of yttrium (radioactive isotope) into the pituitary gland.

Table 97.1: Investigations for acromegaly/gigantism

Tests	*Results*
Basal GH or serum IgF – 1 (insulin like growth factor I levels)	High
Prolactin level	High (in 30%)
Glucose tolerance suppression test by 75 g glucose	There is either no suppression or failure of suppression ($<1\mu L$) or paradoxical rise of GH
X-ray skull for pituitary fossa	There may be enlargement of pituitary fossa with destruction of clinoid processes
X-ray heel pad thickness	Increased (>22 mm)
X-ray sinuses	Large and widened sinuses
Visual fields	Bitemporal hemianopia or scotoma
CT scan	A small or large hypodense microadenoma may be seen

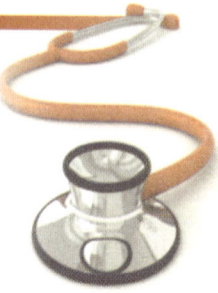

98

Pituitary Dwarfism

INSTRUCTION

- Examine 18-year girl

SALIENT FEATURES

- Short stature

HISTORY

Ask for the following:

Take the natal (prenatal, intranatal and postnatal), the family and personal history as follows:

1. *Prenatal history:* Ascertain the following:
   - Age of mother at conception
   - Exposure to smoking and alcohol
   - TORCH infection (Toxoplasmosis CMV, Herpes)
   - Exposure to irradiation
   - Any chronic illness during pregnancy
   - Any thyroid disorder during pregnancy
   - Exposure to drug (e.g. phenytoin)

2. *Intranatal*
   - Duration of gestation, e.g. prematurity
   - Nature of delivery, e.g. vaginal delivery or cesarean section
   - Birth weight
   - Birth asphyxia, cry after birth
   - Persistence of neonatal jaundice

3. *Postnatal*
   - Development of milestones (normal or delayed)
   - Height gain in a year
   - History of chronic or recurrent illness

4. *Family history*
   - Parent's height, e.g. mother and father
   - Height of the siblings
   - Any family history of growth delay
   - Constitutional growth delay

5. *Personal history*
   - Dietary history—caloric intake, foods taken
   - Protein and calcium intake
   - Scholastic performance
   - Relationship with peers

EXAMINATION

General Physical Examination

- Measure height (Fig. 98.1) and weight (obese). Measure upper as well as lower body segments.
- Measure body proportions
- Assess mental function
- Look for features of hypothyroidism, hypogonadism
- Sexual functions if patient is married

PROVISIONAL DIAGNOSIS

The patient has obesity, dwarfism and hypogonadism (lesion) due to hypopituitarism (etiology).

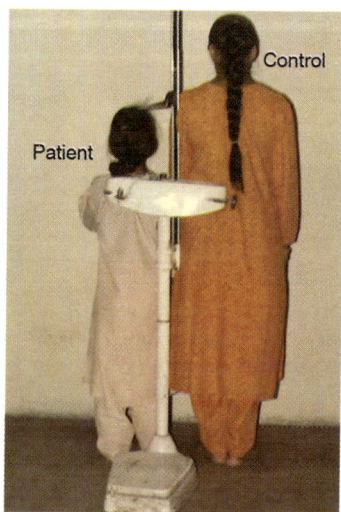

Fig. 98.1: Pituitary dwarfism. An 18-year-old female pituitary dwarf compared with age and sex matched control

Table 98.1: Differential conditions for short stature

Causes	Clinical features
GH deficiency	Chubby child, frontal bossing, central obesity, high pitched voice, midline defects
Hypothyroidism (cretinism)	Read the clinical feature in case disenssion on hypothyroidism
Cushing's syndrome	Moon face, central obesity, striae, hypertension, camel hump, hirsutism (Read Cushing syndrome)
Pseudohypoparathyroidism	Moon facies and obesity, short metacarpals and metatarsals, mental retardation, tetany, epileptic convulsions, basal ganglia calfication
Rickets	Craniotabes, widened wrist joint, rickety rosary, Harrison's sulcus, genu valgum, scoliosis, lordosis, kyphosis, protuberant abdomen
Down's syndrome (Trisomy 21)	Read the clinical features of Down's syndrome – separate case
Noonan's syndrome	Phenotype characteristics of Turner's syndrome, microphallus and delayed puberty are common
Achondroplasia (premature fusion)	Normal mental and sexual development, short limbs (shortened proximal extremities), large head with saddle nose, normal sized trunk, lumbar lordosis or kyphoscoliosis. They are seen as jokers in circus
Prader-Willi syndrome	Hypotonia, obesity, hypogonadism, mental deficiency, small hands and feet with growth retardation
Laurence-Moon-Biedl syndrome	Obesity, hypogonadism, mental retardation, polydactyly and retinitis pigmentosa
Chronic Renal failure	History of chronic kidney disease in childhood, puffiness of face, oedema feet, anaemia, hypertension, renal osteodystrophy
Constitutional delay	Positive family history, normal milestones, no other cause of dwarfism
Coeliac disease	History of chronic diarrhoea/malabsorption, sensitivity to gluten-rich diet, deficiency of vitamins and nutrients (Read it as a separate case discussion).

QUESTIONS AND ANSWERS

Q. How do you define dwarfism and short stature?

Ans: *Dwarfism* means short stature, where the height of a person is much below the prescribed normal height in relation to his/her chronological age and sex. Short stature is defined as height of the child >2.5 SD below the mean for chronological age, or the growth velocity that falls below 5th percentile on the growth velocity curve. Dwarfism means height below 3rd percentile of normal population of same age and sex.

Q. What is differential diagnosis of dwarfism?

Ans: Read Table 98.1 for causes and differential features

Q. What are the different body proportions in dwarfism?

Ans: 1. *The upper segment and lower segment are equal.* The causes are: Hereditary, constitutional dwarfism and hypopituitarism.

2. *The upper segment is more than lower segment.* The causes are: achondroplasia and hypothyroidism (cretinism, juvenile hypothyroidism)

3. *Upper segment is less than lower segment in spinal deformities.*

Q. How would you investigate such a case?

Ans: The tests and their significance are listed in Table. 98.2

Table 98.2: Investigations for short stature

Tests	For
Complete hemogram	Anemia (chronic infection, worm infestation)
ESR	Inflammatory bowel disease, tuberculosis
Urine pH,	Renal tubular acidosis (RTA)
Ca^{++}, PO_4^{+++} and alkaline phosphatase	Hypoparathyroidism, metabolic bone disease
Stool for ova and cysts	Intestinal infestation (hook worm, giardiasis)
Blood urea, nitrogen, SGOT and SGPT	Renal and liver disease
Radiology (X-ray skull and hands)	Bone age and pituitary fossa assessment
Thyroid function tests	Primary and secondary hypothyroidism
Chromosomal karyotyping	Gonadal dysgenesis
GH level and provocative test	GH deficiency

Q.   How will you treat dwarfism?

Ans: Correction of primary medical disorder is the treatment of choice for growth failure. The GH or IGF-1 therapy can improve the growth of the child, but complete gain of the height may not be possible without correction of the underlying cause.

- *Treatment of constitutional delay of growth and adolescence (CDGA).* This condition is a normal variant in which children have short stature with normal growth rate during childhood. They have delayed puberty and attenuated pubertal growth rate. The GH is normal or low for the skeletal age, but lower than normal for chronological age. The final height remains lower than predicted height in this group. These cases can be managed after careful assessment with sex steroids for few months. In girls, low dose estrogen may be used. The bone age acceleration does not occur with this therapy.

- *Treatment of GH failure:* GH can be used in growth hormone deficiency and even non-growth hormone deficient short statured children.

  The dose of human GH (recombinant) is 0.175 to 0.35 mg/kg/week subcutaneously, preferably at bed time for 6–7 weeks. The growth accelerates from 3–4 cm/yr to 10–12 cm/yr in first year. It slows down in 2nd year of therapy. Treatment is continued till target height is achieved and then dose adjusted so that growth of child is maintained to >4 cm/yr. The side effects of the therapy is development of leukaemia and intra-cranial tumor.

- *Treatment of short stature due to other causes:* GH has been used with growth failure not due to GH deficiency with some success. It is indicated in children with dwarfism (>2.5 SD below the mean of age) who do not have GH deficiency. Many of these children show short-term increase in growth rate in response to GH therapy, but whether their final target height will be achieved or not has no been established.

Q.   What are the features of achondroplasia (Read case discussion on achondroplasia)?

Ans: Read the differential diagnosis of dwarfism (Table 98.1).

Q.   What is gene defect in achondroplasia (Read achondroplasia as a case)?

Ans: It is inherited as an autosomal dominant trait with complete penetrance, mutation of the fibroblast growth factor receptor 3 (FGFR–3) gene on chromosome 4.

99

Hypothyroidism

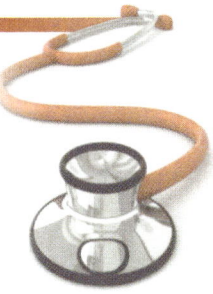

INSTRUCTION

- Take detailed history and perform relevant examination

SALIENT FEATURES

- Recent weight gain, tiredness, constipation and menstrual irregularities (Figure in set)

HISTORY

Ask for the following:

- Onset of symptoms and their progression
- History of recent weight gain, change in appearance and voice, malaise, tiredness and slowness of activity (present)
- History of cold intolerance (present), change in mood or behavior disturbance and deafness
- History of arthralgia, myalgia, dryness of skin and decreased sweating
- History of menstrual irregularity (present), poor libido and sterlity
- History of anorexia and constipation (present)
- History of delayed milestones, slow mentation or mental insufficiency in a child
- History of infertility, depression, muscle cramps and dementia
- History of radioiodine therapy for Graves' disease or medications (e.g. lithium, amiodarone, contrast agents, iodine containing expectorants
- Family history of thyroid disorder, DM, Addison's disease, etc.

EXAMINATION

General Physical Examination (GPE)

- *Face*. Note puffiness or periorbital edema, coarse thick facial appearance, rounded face, peaches and cream complexion (Fig.99.1)
- Eyes for xanthelasma, loss of outer third of eyebrows
- *Tongue*. Large protruding (macroglossia)
- *Lips:* thick, hoarseness of voice (present)

- Neck examination for JVP, thyroid enlargement and lymph node, scar of thyroidectomy
- Pulse (slow pulse present), BP (high in this case), temp, and respiration
- *Skin*. Note the texture, dryness and coarse (toad-like skin present)
- *Hair*. The hair are sparse, thin and brittle in hypothyroidism (present)
- *Hands*. Dry cold hands (present), thick skin, creases of palm prominent (present), carpal tunnel syndrome
- *Feet*. Note dryness and nonpitting edema (present)

Systemic Examination

CVS Examination

- Examine the heart for evidence of CHF and pericardial effusion.

Examination of Abdomen

- For adynamic ileus and any organ enlargement.

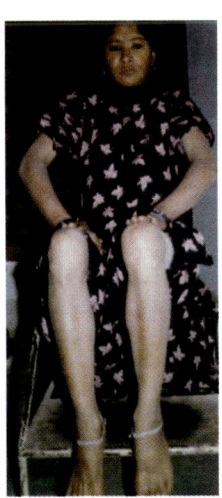

Fig. 99.1: Adult hypothyroidism

Nervous System

- Higher function for mental insufficiency
- VIII nerve examination for deafness
- Motor system for myopathy (proximal), myotonia and for delayed reflexes (present)
- Sensory system for peripheral neuropathy, carpal tunnel syndrome

Respiratory System

- Chest wall is thick with decreased and slow movements

PROVISIONAL DIAGNOSIS

The patient has features suggestive of hypothyroidism (lesion) the cause of which has to be found out. She is at present in uncontrolled state inspite of treatment (functional status)

QUESTIONS AND ANSWERS

Q. **What are points in favor of your diagnosis?**
Ans: 1. Coarse facial features, periorbital oedema, peaches and cream complexion
2. Large tongue, thick lips, toad like skin, sparse and thin hair, hoarseness of voice
3. Dry cold hands, prominent creases of palm
4. Non pitting pedal oedema
5. Slow pulse rate (bradycardia), hypertension (BP 160/100 mmHg)
6. Delayed tendon reflexes (ankle jerks)
7. Thick chest wall with slow movements

Q. **What is hypothyroidism?**
Ans: *Hypothyroidism* is a clinical condition reflecting hypofunctioning of thyroid gland, characterized by low levels of circulating thyroid hormones. It is called *primary* when the cause of it lies in the thyroid gland itself. It becomes *secondary* when hypothyroidism occurs due to disease of anterior pituitary or hypothalamus.

Q. **What are the cardiovascular manifestations of hypothyroidism?**
Ans: • Slow pulse rate (bradycardia)
• Hypertension
• Hypercholesterolemia (xanthelasma)
• Pericarditis and pericardial effusion
• Precipitation of angina and coronary artery disease
• Cardiomyopathy (diminished cardiac output and cardiac failure)
• Low voltage graph on ECG

Q. **What are the neurological manitestations of hypothyroidism?**
Ans: 1. Delayed relaxation of ankle jerks
2. Peripheral neuropathy, carpal tunnel syndrome
3. Myxoedema madness, myxoedema coma
4. Pseudodementia
5. Deafness to higher tones
6. Hoffmann syndrome (muscle aches with myotonia)
7. Proximal myopathy

Q. **What is subclinical hypothyroidism?**
Ans: *Subclinical hypothyroidism* means biochemical evidence of hypothyroidism (low to normal T_3 and T_4 but raised TSH) without any symptoms of hypothyroidism (asymptomatic hypothyroidism). The causes of subclinical hypothyroidism are same as described under transient hypothyroidism. It may persist for many years. Treatment with replacement therapy with small dose of thyroxine is indicated.

Q. **What are the causes of hypothyroidism?**
Ans: • Idiopathic (autoimmunity is the cause)
• Hashimoto's thyroiditis
• Iodine deficiency
• Drug-induced (PAS, phenylbutazone, lithium, iodides)
• Dyshormogenesis
• Following surgery or ^{131}I therapy
• Thyroiditis (postpartum)
• *Maternally transmitted* (iodides, antithyroid drugs, TRABs antibodies)

Q. **What is thyroid status in Hashimoto's thyroiditis?**
Ans: Read Case No. 86

Q. **What is best clinical sign of hypothyroidism?**
Ans: Delayed ankle jerks

Q. **How would you record delayed ankle jerks?**
Ans: Photomotogram

Q. **What is the the cause of delayed relaxation of jerks in hypothyroidism?**
Ans: The exact cause is unknown. It is probably due to decreased and slow muscle metabolism leading to slow activation.

Q. **What is Pendred's syndrome?**
Ans: It is genetically determined syndrome (autosomal inheritance) consisting of a combination of dyshormonogenetic goitre, mental retardation and nerve deafness. The dyshormogenesis is due to deficiency of intrathyroidal peroxidase enzyme.

Q. **What is the relation between iodine and hypothyroidism?**

Ans: Both iodine deficiency and iodine excess can produce hypothyroidism.

Iodine when taken for prolonged period (*iodine excess*) in the form of expectorants containing potassium iodine or use of amiodarone (contains a significant amount of iodine) may cause goitrous hypothyroidism by inhibiting the release of thyroid hormones. This is common in patients with underlying autoimmune thyroiditis.

Iodine deficiency in certain parts of the world especially Himalayas, produces endemic goiter (>70% of the population is affected). Most of the patients usually are euthyroid and have normal or raised TSH levels. In general, more severe is iodine deficiency, the greater is the incidence of hypothyroidism.

Q. **How will you diagnose hypothyroidism?**

Ans: The diagnosis is made on the basis of:
1. Clinical manifestations
2. Investigations

The investigations are done to confirm the diagnosis, to differentiate between primary and secondary hypothyroidism, for follow-up of treatment and to monitor the response. The TSH levels are used to monitor the response to treatment (Table 99.1).

Table 99.1: Thyroid hormone levels in various forms of hypothyroidism

Hormone	Primary	Secondary	Subclinical
T_3	Low	Low	Normal (lower limit of normal)
T_4	Low	Low	Normal (lower limit of normal)
TSH	High	Low	Slightly high

Q. **What are the other diagnostic tests for hypothyroidism?**

Ans:
- *Serum cholesterol* is high (hypercholesterolemia)
- *ECG* may show bradycardia, low voltage graph and ST-T changes
- *Blood examination* may reveal anemia (usually normocytic or macrocytic)
- *Thyroid peroxidase antibodies* (TPO) help to find out the cause of hypothyroidism.

Their presence indicate autoimmune thyroiditis as the cause of hypothyroidism
- *X-ray chest.* It may be normal or may show cardiomegaly due to pericardial effusion–common in primary rather than secondary hypothyroidism.

Q. **What is the best diagnostic test for hypothyroidism?**

Ans: Elevated TSH level

Q. **What are the causes of raised TSH?**

Ans:
- Subclinical hypothyroidism
- Overt hypothyroidism
- Medications, such as lithium and amiodarone
- Recovery from hypothyroxinemia of non-thyroidal disorders.
- Iodine deficiency goitre
- Puberty goitre

Q. **How would you treat hypothyroidism?**

Ans: *Oral thyroxine replacement* is given for life long. Therapeutic dose varies from 50 to 200 µg/day taken as a single dose empty stomach and adjustments are made once in 3 weeks. The dose is adjusted depending on the clinical response and suppression of TSH levels.

Lack of response indicates poor compliance, an underlying psychiatric abnormalities or an associated autoimmune disease (e.g. Addison's disease).

Q. **What precaution would you take while prescribing thyroxine in elderly?**

Ans: Rapid T_4 replacement in elderly may precipitate angina and myocardial infarction, hence, starting dose of thyroxine in elderly should be low (25 µg/day).

Q. **What are the complications of myxedema?**

Ans: Complications arise as a result of infiltration of myxomatous tissue into various other structures, especially in primary myxoedema.
1. *CVS*, e.g. pericardial effusion, restrictive cardiomyopathy, conduction disturbances
2. *Respiratory.* Cor pulmonale, type 2 respiratory failure
3. *Myxedematous* madness and myxoedema coma
4. *Entrapement neutropathy* (Carpal Tunnel syndrome)

100

Hirsutism

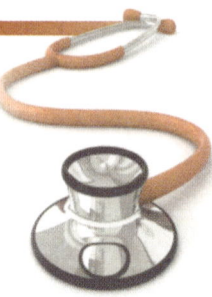

INSTRUCTION

- Look at the young female patient and perform relevant examination

SALIENT FEATURES

- Facial hair growth in a female patient (picture inset)

HISTORY

Ask the following:

- Age of the patient
- Rate of progression of hirsutism
- History of thinning of scalp hair and deepening of voice
- History of obesity
- Drug history (corticosteroids, androgens, phenytoin, minoxidil, diazoxide, cyclosporine)
- Menstrual history, i.e. oligomenorrhea, infertility, acne, seborrhea and voice change (present in this case) and suggest polycystic ovarian diseases an important case of hirsutism
- Family history (familial)

EXAMINATION

General Physical Examination

- Examine the excessive growth of hair over the following sites:
- i. The chin (Fig. 100.1), sternum, upper abdomen and upper back

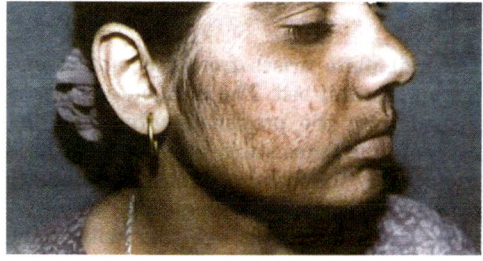

Fig. 100.1: Hirsutism (Idiopathic)

ii. Terminal hair (excessive normal hair growth) can be seen normally in females on the arms, legs, periareolar area and tinea alba
- Record the BP
- Look for the features of Cushing's syndrome
- Look for the signs of virilization (receding hair line, muscular built, breast atrophy and clitoromegaly).

PROVISIONAL DIAGNOSIS

The female patient has hirsutism (lesion) caused by polycystic ovarian disease (cause) and patient is socially and cosmetically disturbed (functional status).

QUESTIONS AND ANSWERS

Q. Enumerate the points in favor of your diagnosis?

Ans: 1. Primary amenorrhea
2. Married for the last 5 yrs but no issue (infertility)
3. Hirsutism and acne
4. Mild obesity

Q. Which investigation would support your diagnosis?

Ans: Ultrasonography of ovaries showing polycystic ovaries.

Q. What do you mean by hirsutism?

Ans: Hirsutism is defined as a male pattern of hair growth in women.

Q. What is the significance of menstrual history in this case?

Ans: If menstruation is normal, it indicates that there is no increase in testosterone production. However, if menstruation is abnormal, then the cause of hirsutism is polycystic ovarian disease (PCOD).

Q. What are the causes of hirsutism?

Ans: Causes are:
1. Cushing's syndrome
2. Adrenal tumors

3. Polycystic ovarian syndrome
4. Drug induced
5. Familial
6. Acromegaly
7. Ovarian tumors
8. Congenital adrenal hyperplasia
9. Idiopathic

Q. What do you understand by the term virilization and defeminisation?

Ans: Androgens are responsible for differential hair distribution in women. *Virilization* means androgens excess in women. It causes deepening of voice, temporal balding, acne, greasy skin, clitoromegaly, hirsutism and increased muscle mass. Therefore, hirsutism can be *without virilization, or with virilization* leading to diminishing female characters, e.g. decrease in breast size, loss of female body contours, amenorrhea called *defeminisation*.

Q. What are the sources of androgens in females?

Ans: Androgens in women are derived both from ovaries and adrenals, as well as, from peripheral conversion, hence, cause of hirsutism lies either in the ovaries or adrenals.

Q. What is polycystic ovarian disease?

Ans: Polycystic ovarian disease, a severe form of which is called *Stein-Leventhal syndrome* is characterised by multiple ovarian cysts and excessive androgen production from the ovaries and adrenals.

The clinical features are:
- Symptoms onset immediate after menarche
- Ammenorrhea/oligomenorrhea
- Hirsutism or acne
- Obesity
- Mild virilization in severe cases
- Insulin resistance associated with menstrual irregularity, hypertension and hyperlipidemia
- The diagnosis is confirmed by typical ultrasonic findings and raised LH with normal or low FSH with LH : FSH ratio >3:1.

Q. What is pathophysiology of PCOD?

Ans: It is due to an abnormality of pulsatile secretion of GnRH (gonodotrophin-releasing hormone) causing increased leutinizing hormone (LH) and follicle stimulating hormone (FSH) secretion. This results in hyperplasia of the ovarian theca cells leading to multiple follicular cysts formation and excessive androgen production and ovulation.

Q. What is the relationship of body weight and hirsutism?

Ans: Hirsute women are more likely to be obese (PCOD). Thus weight reduction must be priority in treating overweight women with hirsutism.

Q. What are the other conditions associated with insulin resistance?

Ans: Besides polycystic ovarian disease, the other conditions are:
- Obesity
- Lipodystrophies
- Ataxia-telangiectasia
- Werner's syndrome
- Alstrome syndrome
- Pineal hyperplasia syndrome

Q. How metabolism of glucose is affected by PCOD?

Ans: PCOD is associated with insulin resistance and hyperinsulinemia which results in impaired glucose tolerance. The site of insulin resistance is skeletal muscles and adipose tissue and there is no hepatic resistance.

Q. What is the treatment of impaired glucose tolerance (IGT) in PCOD?

Ans:
- Life style modifications and weight reduction
- Insulin sensitizers, e.g. metformin, pioglitazone (thiazolidinedione derivative)

Q. What is the role of testosterone in hirsutism?

Ans: Testosterone is the most potent androgen and is directly derived from ovarian secretion and peripheral conversion of androstenedione. 98% of testosterone is bound and only 2% is free which can enter the target cells to produce androgen effect. In the skin, it is converted to dihydrotestosterone (DHT) which stimulates the hair follicles and cause hirsutism.

Q. How would you investigate such a case?

Ans: Following investigations are done:
1. *Serum androgens.* Dehydroepiandrosterone (DHEAS) > 8000 ng/ml and serum testostosterone >2 ng/ml suggest adrenal neoplasm or congenital adrenal hyperplasia.
2. *Other hormones assay*, e.g. TSH, ACTH, cortisol, prolactin. A short ACTH stimulation test may be performed if needed for congenital adrenal hyperplasia.
3. *LH and FSH and their ratio*. The LH: FSH ratio >3:1 suggest polycystic ovarian disease.

4. *Glucose tolerance test (GTT) and insulin* levels for polycystic ovarian disease. This would help to establish insulin resistance that occurs in polycystic ovarian disease.

5. *USG* of ovaries for polycystic disease (10 or more ovarian cysts >2 mm in diameter, increased ovarian stroma and a thickened capsule suggest polycystic ovarian disease).

6. *Laparoscopy* and *biopsy* of the ovary for ovarian neoplasm.

7. *CT scan* of adrenals for adrenal tumor.

Q. How will you proceed to treat such a case?

Ans: The treatment is as follows:

1. In case it is drug-induced, stop the offending drug. If it is due to a tumor, surgical removal is indicated.

2. Adrenal steroidogenic defects are treated with glucocorticoids to suppress excess ACTH and inhibit adrenal androgen secretion.

3. In idiopathic cases and in polycystic ovarian disease both cosmetic treatment (concealment or removal of hair from exposed skin areas) and suppression of androgen production or antagonism of its action by antiandrogens, e.g. cyproterone, flutamide, spironolactone, cimetidine and 5-alpha-reductase inhibitor (finasteride). GNRH analogs (leuprolide, nafarelin) have been found useful.

4. Local treatment, e.g. shaving, epilation, laser-assisted epilation, waxing, electrolysis or bleaching.

Q. Name the few drugs that produce hirsutism?

Ans: The drugs are:
- Phenytoin
- Androgens
- Psoralens
- Oral contraceptives
- Diazoxide
- Minoxidil

Q. What is adrenal virilization in females? What is its commonest cause?

Ans: Adrenal androgens excess resulting from excessive production of dehydroepiandrosterone and androstenedione get converted into testosterone and lead to virilization, hirsutism, acne and oligomenorrhea.

Congenital adrenal hyperplasia is the most common cause of virilization in a female. It is characterized by excess of androgens with low or normal levels of glucocorticoids and mineralocorticoids.

101

Obesity

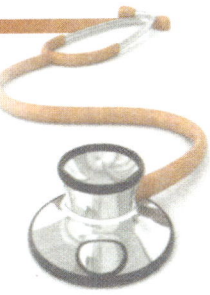

INSTRUCTION

- Look at the patient
- Perform relevant examination

SALIENT FEATURES

- An obese young man

HISTORY

Ask for the following:

- Age of the patient
- Full dietary history pertaining to eating habits and pattern
- History of sleep apnoea, day-time snoring somnolence or insomnia (obesity-hypoventilation syndrome)
- History of hypertension, diabetes, dyslipidaemia (metabolic syndrome), joints problem, etc. (obesity related disease)
- History of retrosternal discomfort or pain especially during lying down (gastroesophageal reflux disease), angina (CV risk), dyspnoea (respiratory problem)
- History of biliary/abdominal colic (gallstones), jaundice (cancer of gallbladder and biliary system)
- History of genital (endometrial) and breast cancer in females
- *Family history* of obesity
- History of colorectal, prostate and renal cancer
- *Drug history*, e.g. ask the history of drugs known to produce obesity

EXAMINATION

General Physical Examination

- Moon-like round face (pseudocushing face)
- Skin is shiny, glossy and contains lot of sub-cutaneous fat resulting in redundant folds of skin (Fig. 101.1)
- BP is high (hypertension present)
- Measure height and weight and calculate BMI (35 kg/m² in this case)

- Measure hip/waist circumference and midarm circumference (increased)
- Examine the joints (knee joints for crepitus due to osteoarthritis)
- Look for signs of Cushing's syndrome, hypo-thyroidism, polycystic ovarian disease (females)

Systemic Examination

- *Cardiovascular system* for hypertensive cardiac involvement/CHF
- *Abdominal examination* for cancer of abdominal organs, i.e. palpation of gallbladder, colon, rectum, prostate and kidneys
- *Respiratory system* for pickwickian syndrome
- *Joints examination* for osteoarthritis

PROVISIONAL DIAGNOSIS

The young patient has 80 kg weight and his BMI is 35 kg/m², hence, he is obese (lesion) probably due to genetic origin (cause). In addition, patient has hypertension impaired glucose tolerance and osteoarthritis (functional status).

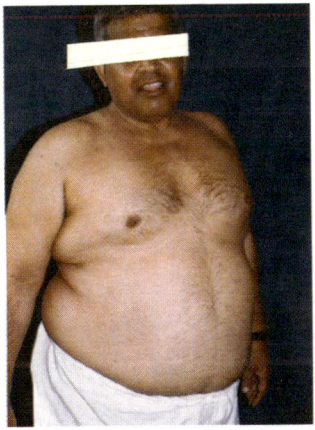

Fig. 101.1: Obesity (BMI > 35 kg/m²). Note the protuberant abdomen, thick hanging skin folds and prominence of hips and nape of the neck

QUESTIONS AND ANSWERS

Q. How do you define obesity?
Ans: Obesity is defined as an excess of body fat and body mass index (BMI) is an indirect parameter of fat assessment, hence BMI ≥ 30 kg/m² is considered as obesity.

Q. What do you understand by the term BMI? How do you calculate it?
Ans: It is a measure to determine the excess body fat. It is calculated by dividing the body weight (kg) by height (m²),

$$BMI = \frac{Body\ weight\ in\ kg}{Height\ in\ meters^2 (m^2)}$$

hence, is expressed as kg/m².

Q. How did WHO classified obesity based on BMI?
Ans: WHO and National Institute of Health (NIH) define normal BMI as 18.5 – 24.9 kg/m².
Overweight is defined as BMI as 25 – 29.9 kg/m². Obesity is designated when BMI is ≥ 30 kg/m². The various classes of obesity are given in Box-I.

Box I: WHO and NIH classification of overweight and obesity

Class	BMI (kg/m²)	Risk of comorbidities
Normal	18.5–24.9	—
Overweight	25–29.9	Mildly increase
Obese	≥30	— do —
• Class I	30–34.9	Moderate
• Class II	35–39.9	Severe (5 – 10 times risk)
• Class III	≥40	Very severe (10 times risk)

Q. What is morbid obesity?
Ans: Class III obesity with BMI > 40 kg/m² is called *morbid obesity* and is associated with 10-fold increase in the mortality rate.

Q. How common is obesity?
Ans: Obesity a health problem, is becoming more prevalent and common in all the countries of the world particularly in USA.
Current USA survey data demonstrate that 68% of Americans are overweight and 33.8% are obese. Women are more obese than men and African-American and Mexican-American women are more obese than whites.

Q. What are the adverse health consequences of obesity?
Ans: Obesity is associated with significant increase in both morbidity and mortality. A large number of health problems are associated

with obesity. The most common adverse consequences of obesity are:

I. *Cardiovascular consequences*
   • Coronary artery disease
   • Hypertension
II. *Respiratory consequences*
   • Pickwickian syndrome (obesity with hypoventilation)
   • Obstructive sleep apnoea
   • Infections
III. *Metabolic consequences*
   • Type 2 DM, impaired glucose tolerance (IGT)
   • Insulin resistance
   • Hyperlipidemia
   • Hyperuricemia and gout
IV. *Gastrointestinal consequences*
   • Gall stones
   • Gastroesophageal reflux
   • Colorectal cancer
V. *Blood related*
   • Polycythaemia
VI. *Predisposition to genitourinary cancer,* e.g. cancer of prostate, kidney, uterus, breast and ovary
VII. *Miscellaneous*
   • Increased foetal death if mother is obese.

Q. Name some obesity related syndromes?
Ans: • Cushing's syndrome
   • Pickwickian syndrome
   • Metabolic syndrome
   • Frohlich's syndrome
   • Laurence-Moon-Biedle syndrome
   • Prader-Willi syndrome
   • Alstrom syndrome

Q. What are the two phenotypes of obesity?
Ans: 1. Abdominal/central obesity called *android (apple shaped)*
   2. Generalised obesity (*gynaecoid or pear shaped*)

Q. Which obesity pattern is dangerous?
Ans: Central obesity (truncal obesity) is more dangerous than generalised as it is associated with premature CAD and cardiovascular risks.

Q. How would you assess/evaluate obesity?
Ans: The parameters of obesity are:
   1. Calculation of *BMI* (> 30 kg/m²)
   2. *Triceps skinfold thickness* by spring loaded calipers. The thickness > 20 mm in man and > 30 mm in women indicate obesity

3. *Abdominal girth/circumference* (i.e. more than 102 cm in men and > 88 cm in women suggest obesity)

4. *Waist-hip ratio* (e.g. > 1.0 in men and > 0.85 in women indicate obesity)

Q. **How fat can act as an endocrine gland?**

Ans: Adipose tissue secretes many hormones:
1. Leptin: It encodes the adipose specific gene and regulates body weight
2. Adiponectin
3. Resistin

Q. **What are the mechanisms of pathogenesis of obesity?**

Ans: It is complex and produced by interactions of following factors:
i. Genetic
ii. Behavioral
iii. Psychosocial
iv. Others (unidentified)

The mechanisms involved are:
i. Insensitivity to leptin
ii. Hyperphagia induced by neuro-peptide Y
iii. Deficiency or inaction of anorexigenic hypothalamic neuropeptides
iv. Inaction of insulin (insulin resistance) and glucocorticoids
v. Mutation in the gene for nuclear PPAR-γ (perioxisome proliferator activated receptor-γ) accelerates differentiation of adipocytes, hence, may cause obesity

Q. **Name the adiposogenic drugs?**

Ans:
- Steroids
- Oral contraceptives
- Phenothiazines (antipsychotics)
- Insulin
- Antidepressants
- Betablockers
- Oral hypoglycaemics
- Anticonvulsants
- Antihistamines
- Pitzotifen

Q. **How would you define metabolic syndrome?**

Ans: Metabolic syndrome is a cluster of several risk factors and is characterised by obesity, insulin resistence, hyperlipidemia and hypertension.

Q. **What are the WHO diagnostic criteria for metabolic syndrome?**

Ans:
1. Central obesity (i.e. BMI > 30 kg/m², waist hip ratio > 1 in men > 0.85 in women)
2. Triglycerides > 150 mg/dl
3. HDL cholesterol (men < 35 mg% and women < 39 mg%)
4. Blood pressure > 140/90 mm Hg
5. Fasting glucose > 110 mg%
6. Microalbuminuria

Note: Diagnosis is made when 3 or more risk factors mentioned above are present.

Q. **How would you manage obesity?**

Ans:
I. *Life style modifications*
- Weight reduction by hypocaloric, vitamin rich, high rouphage diet
- Exercise (graded weight reducing exercises)
- Avoidance of alcohol and smoking

II. *Behaviour modification and social support*

III. *Drugs*
- Sibutramine (serotonin-norepinephrine reuptake inhibitor) reduces appetite and results in weight loss of about 5%.
- *Orlistat.* It inhibits the absorption of dietary fat.
- *Rimonabant* (a selective block of cannabinoid receptor) also result in 5% weight reduction.

IV. *Bariatric surgery*
- *Gastric banding* and vertical (gleeve) gastrectomy.
- *Roux-en-Y gastric bypass.* It is popular gastrojejunostomy procedure, is considered as a *gold standard* because of its effectiveness and durability.
- *Wiring of the Jaws.* This is rarely done.
- *Biliopancreatic* is also a diversion procedure, limits absorption and includes vertical gastrectomy.

Q. **What is the link between obesity and diabetes?**

Ans: The link between obesity and diabetes is insulin resistance. Fat cells release fatty acids and tumor necrosis factor-α which cause insulin resistance. Leptin on the other hand causes insulin sensitivity.

Resistin (a hormone secreted by fat cell) produces insulin resistance.

Q. **Name the drug which overcome insulin resistance.**

Ans:
1. Biguanides
2. Thiazolidinediones derivatives

102

Diabetic Foot

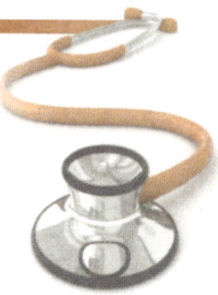

INSTRUCTION

- Examine the neurological system of lower limbs

SALIENT FEATURES

- Non healing ulcer on plantar surface of great toe of right foot

HISTORY

Ask for the following:

- History of polyuria, polydipsia and polyphagia
- History of pain, numbness, tingling and paraes-thesias
- Intermittent claudication during walking
- Rest pain (present)
- History of wearing ill-fitted shoes
- History of blistering or previous history of foot ulcer
- History of puffiness of face, oedema legs/feet
- History of delayed healing of the wound (present)
- History of IHD, hypertension
- History of visual disturbance, change in glasses

EXAMINATION

General Physical Examination

- Foot is cold to touch (present)
- The skin over the foot is shiny and thin (atrophic) with scanty hair
- There is an amputated stump of big toe with flattening of the arch of the foot.
- There is large foot ulcer on the planter surface of the amputated great toe (Fig. 102.1) which is painful
- Peripheral pulses, e.g. dorsalis pedis and posterior tibial artery pulses are weak (in this case)

Neurological Examination

- There is sensory loss (pain, touch, temperature, position sense and sense of vibration) involving the feet and legs (peripheral neuropathy present)
- There is loss of bilateral ankle jerks. Planters are not elicitable (motor component of neuropathy)

- Motor system examination shows calf and foot muscles wasting with hypotonia.
- Gait. Patient feels difficulty in walking due to foot ulcer
- No evidence of autonomic disturbance

PROVISIONAL DIAGNOSIS

The patient has features of ischemic and neuro-pathic foot (lesion) produced by diabetes mellitus (aetiology). There is difficulty in walking due to planter ulcer (functional status).

QUESTIONS AND ANSWERS

Q. What is a diabetic foot?

Ans: Diabetic foot comprises of following three components:
1. *Vasculopathy* (involvement of small and large vessels of the foot)
2. *Neuropathy* (loss of sensation)
3. *Secondary infection*

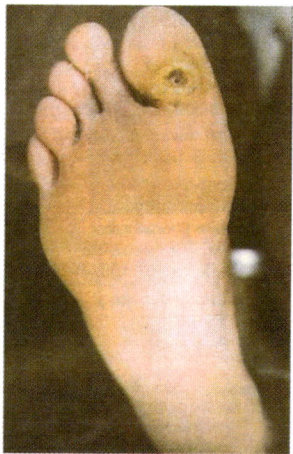

Fig. 102.1: Diabetic foot. A large ulcer is present on the sole at the base of big toe

Q. What are the characteristic clinical manifestations of diabetic foot?

Ans: Symptoms and signs are enumerated in the Box I

Box I: Clinical features of diabetic foot	
Symptoms	*Signs*
• None	• Ulcer
• Pain, numbness, paraesthesias	• Sepsis, abscess
	• Osteomyelitis
• Claudication	• Loss of the arch of foot
• Rest pain	• Gangrene
	• Charcot joint
	• Loss of toes

Q. What are the causes of neuropathic ulcers?

Ans: Following are the causes of neuropathic foot or neuropathic ulcer. They have already been listed in charcot's joint.

1. Sensory neuropathy
2. Tabes dorsalis
3. Leprosy
4. Amyloidosis
5. Porphyria
6. Subacute combined degeneration

Q. What is pathogenesis of a diabetic foot?

Ans: The denervation of the small muscles of foot results in clawing of toes and displacement of the metatarsal foot pads anteriorly. These changes combined with joints and connective tissue changes alter the biomechanics of the foot with loss of foot arch and increased plantar pressure. Therefore, the triad of *decreased pain threshold, abnormally high foot pressures* and *repetitive stresses* lead to foot ulceration in high pressure areas. Vascular changes in the small and large vessels lead to ischemia of foot and may result in gangrene.

Q. What is neuropathy disability score? What is its significance?

Ans: The neuropathy disability score is based on the impairment of sensation and reflexes. The scale is measured over score of 10 (5 for each foot). A score of ≥ 6/10 is indicative of foot ulceration.

Sensation	Result and Score	
1. Vibration sense tested by 128 Hz great toe	*Normal*	0
	Abnormal	1
2. Temperature test over dorsum of foot	*Normal* (can distinguish hot and cold)	0
	Abnormal	1
3. Pinprick sensation over great toe	*Normal* (can distinguish sharpness and lack of sharpness)	0
	Abnormal	1
4. Achilles reflex	Present	0
	Present with reinforcement	1
	Absent	2

A maximum of 5 points can be scored on each foot

Q. How would you test cutaneous sensory perception? What is its significance?

Ans: Cutaneous sensory perception is assessed by monofilaments. Normal individuals can feel the 4.17 monofilament (–1 g linear pressure) patient who can not feel 5.07 monofilament (–10 g of linear pressure) are considered to have lost sensations.

A seven fold increase in risk of ulceration is associated in patients who are insensitive to 5.07 monofilaments.

Q. How would you manage diabetic foot?

Ans:
- Debridement of necrotic tissue and antiseptic dressing daily
- Control of hyperglycemia with insulin
- Antibiotics for infection
- Removal of weight bearing and friction from ulcerated area, e.g. avoid crutches, use appropriate foot wear
- Patient education. Avoid smoking and alcohol, inspect foot daily for blisters. Do not walk bare-footed. Avoid tight shoes, cut toe nails across
- Chiropody
- Surgical and orthopedic consultation

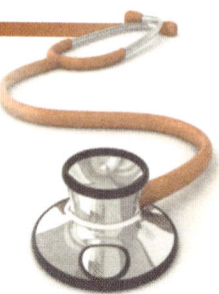

103

Type 1 DM

INSTRUCTION

- Examine the patient

SALIENT FEATURES

- Loss of weight more than 10 kg over a period of one month (Fig. 103.1)

HISTORY

Ask for the following:

- Age of the patient
- History of polyuria, polydipsia and polyphagia (present)
- Weakness and weight loss (present)
- Diminution of vision or visual disturbance (retinopathy)
- History of numbness, tingling in the hands and feet (neuropathy)
- Fever, night sweats
- Repeated infections (chest, urinary tract, GI tract)
- Oedema feet or legs (nephropathy)
- History of white spots on shoes (glycosuria)
- Positive *family history* may or may not be present
- *Post history* of disturbed consciousness or hospital admissions (present)

EXAMINATION

General Physical Examination

- A young adult (18 yrs male)
- Thin, lean and emaciated (Fig. 103.1)
- Significant weight loss (present)
- Loss of body fat (bony rib cage is prominent, clavicles are also prominent)
- Thin extremities (present)
- Insulin injection marks over the abdomen
- Eyes for visual loss, cataract, styes or eye infection
- Skin for boils, carbuncles, wound, ulcer, etc.

Systemic Examination

- *Neurological examination* for peripheral and autonomic neuropathy
- *Cardiovascular system examination* for hypertension and IHD.

- *Fundus examination* for retinopathy
- *Renal system examination* for UTI, nephropathy and calculi

PROVISIONAL DIAGNOSIS

A thin lean young adult type I diabetes mellitus (lesion) idiopathic or genetic in origin (aetiology). Patient is predisposed to frequent ketoacidosis (functional status).

QUESTIONS AND ANSWERS

Q. What is the diagnostic clinical triad of type 1 DM?

Ans: *Polyuria, polydipsia* and *polyphagia* leading to significant weight loss and weakness constitute a diagnostic clinical triad.

Q. How would you confirm your diagnosis by the bedside?

Ans: • Urine examination for sugar, proteins and ketone bodies
- Blood glucose by bedside glucometer (Fig. 103.1)

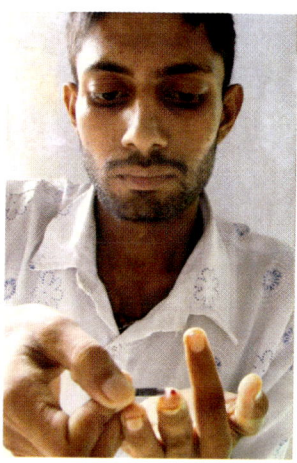

Fig. 103.1: Type 1 DM doing self monitoring of glucose

Q.   What are prediabetic states?

Ans: • Impaired fasting glucose (IFG)

• Impaired glucose tolerance (IGT)

Q.   What is pathogenesis of type 1 diabetes?

Ans: It is considered as an autoimmune disorder due to following reasons;

• HLA linkage

• Its association with other autoimmune disorders

• Lymphocytic infiltration of beta cells of pancreas

• Circulating anti-insulin antibodies

• Recurrence of beta cells destruction in pancreas

Q.   What is role of genetics in type 1 DM?

Ans: Genetic susceptibility is a major determinant while environmental factors act as trigger to initiate autoimmune destruction of beta cells of the pancreas. The genetic predisposition is HLA linked class II genes at D locus (DR_3 and D_4) on short arm of chromosome 6. Immunological response results in production of class II beta cell specific molecules which play a role in autoimmune destruction. Beta cell mass declines, insulin secretion becomes progressively impaired although normal glucose tolerance is maintained. The rate of decline of beta cell mass varies with some patients progressing rapidly to clinical diabetes, while other evolving slowly. Features of diabetes will appear once > 80% of beta cells have been destroyed. At this point, residual functional existing beta cells are insufficient in number to maintain glucose tolerance. Thus, there is a transition period between impaired glucose tolerance and frank diabetes. After the onset of type IA diabetes, there is *"honey-moon"* period of 1 to 2 years during which glycemic control is achieved with modest dose of insulin or rarely, insulin is not required. This is a transient or fleeting phase.

Q.   What are the differences between type 1 and type 2 DM?

Ans: Read Table 103.1.

Q.   What is glycosylated hemoglobin? What is its significance?

Ans: The hemoglobin (Hb) gets glycosylated due to formation of a covalent bond between glucose molecule and β-chain of hemoglobin. Glycosylated Hb is related to prevailing glucose concentration, hence, hyperglycemia and its excursions lead to increased glycosylation. Glycoslylated Hb is expressed as percentage of normal hemoglobin (4–6% depending on the technique of measurement).

It is a parameter of diagnosis (> 6.5% indicates DM) as well as long-term control, (i.e. past 6 weeks) of DM because it is an index of blood glucose concentration over the average life of the hemoglobin molecule (e.g. approx 6 weeks). Its higher values reflect various grades of control of DM. The target value of glycosylated Hb ($HbAI_c$) for control of diabetes is < 7%, so as to retard or delay the onset of complications.

Q.   What is diabetic retinopathy? What are ocular fundi changes in DM?

Ans: This is discussed as a case report of fundus examination.

Q.   What are the clinical presentations of type 1 DM?

Ans: 1. Type 1 diabetics may present with symptom triad of polyuria, polydipsia and polyphagia

Features	Type 1	Type 2
Table 103.1: General clinical characteristics of type 1 and type 2 DM		
1. Gene locus	Chromosome 6	Chromosome 11
2. Age of onset	< 30 years	> 30 years
3. Onset of symptoms	Rapid	Slow
4. Body weight	Thin, lean	Normal weight or obese
5. Duration of symptoms	Weeks	Months or years
6. Presenting features	Polyuria, polydipsia polyphagia, weight loss	Present with different complications, e.g. nephropathy, IHD, HT, CVA, infections, neuropathy
7. Ketonuria (ketoacidosis)	Present	Absent
8. Complications at the time of diagnosis	Absent or occasional	Present (10 – 20%)
9. Family history	Negative	Positive
10. Plasma insulin	Low or absent	Normal to high
11. Choice of treatment	Insulin	Oral hypoglycemics
12. Mortality if untreated	High	Low

2. They may be present as diabetic keto-acidosis
3. They may present with microvascular complications, retinopathy, neuropathy and nephropathy
4. They may present with repeated infections (skin, urinary tract) or delayed wound healing
5. May remain asymptomatic, detected on routine urine examination for any other purpose, i.e. medical examination

Q.   How do you diagnose DM?
Ans: Read Table 103.2.

Q.   What are the indications of insulin in DM?
Ans: • Type 1 DM
  • Type 2 DM with complications or OHA failure
  • Gestational diabetes
  • Diabetic ketoacidosis
  • Diabetics undergoing surgery or procedure.

Q.   What are the complications of insulin therapy?
Ans: • Insulin lipoatrophy/lipodystrophy
  • Insulin tumefaction
  • Insulin induced hypoglycemia
  • Insulin resistance

Q.   What is whipple triad for hypoglycemia?
Ans: • Symptoms and signs suggestive of hypoglycemia
  • Documentation of hypoglycemia
  • Reversal of hypoglycemia with administration of glucose

Q.   How do you define hypoglycemia? At which blood glucose levels do the symptoms appear?
Ans: Hypoglycemia is defined as blood glucose levels below the lower limit of the normal, i.e. <70 mg%

There is a great degree of variation among individuals in awareness of symptoms of hypoglycemia in diabetes. Some patients may feel symptoms when blood sugar is <70 mg%, while others may not appreciate the symptoms even when blood glucose is <55 mg%. The exact level is difficult to define. However majority of patients are symptomatic at <55 mg of blood glucose level.

Q.   What are the symptoms and signs of hypoglycemia?
Ans: The symptoms and signs are:
1. *CVS,* e.g. palpitation, tachycardia and anxiety cardiac arrhythmias
2. *CNS,* e.g. tremors, confusion, headache, tiredness, difficulty in concentration, incoordination, slurred speech, drowsiness, convulsions and plantar extensors
3. *GI tract,* e.g. nausea and vomiting
4. *Skin,* e.g. sweating and hypothermia

Q.   What are the common causes of hypoglycemia?
Ans: The common causes in adults are:
  I. *Fasting hyperglycemia*
    • Pancreatic β-cell tumor
    • Overadministration of insulin or OHA
  II. *Postprandial hypoglycemia*
    • Alimentary
    • Noninsulinoma (non-islet tumor) hypoglycemia syndrome
    • Functional
    • Autoimmune hypoglycemia
  III. *Alcohol related hypoglycemia*
  IV. *Factitious hypoglycemia*
  V. *Hypoglycemia due to insulin receptor antibodies*
  VI. *Drug-induced hypoglycemia*

Note: Students are further advised to remain prepared for more questions on insulins (types, mode of administration, dosage schedule, etc.)

Table 103.2: American Diabetic Association (1997, 2010) criteria endorsed by WHO (1998) for diagnosis of diabetes or other related conditions

Condition	HbAIC (%)	Venous plasma glucose concentration in mg% (mmol/L)	
		Fasting	Postprandial (2 hr GTT)
Normal	4–6.0	<110 (6.1)	<140 (7.3)
Diabetes	≥6.5	>126	>200
		Or	
		Symptoms of diabetes plus random blood sugar ≥ 200 mg% (11.1 mmol/l)	
Impaired fasting glycemia		110–126 (6.1–7.0)	<140 (7.8)
Impaired glucose tolerance	6–6.5	<126 (7.0)	≥140 but <200 (7.8–11.1)

Note: 2 hours GTT means following 75 glucose load. Venous blood glucose concentration is lower than capillary blood. Whole blood glucose is lower than plasma because RBC contain little glucose.

104

Type 2 DM

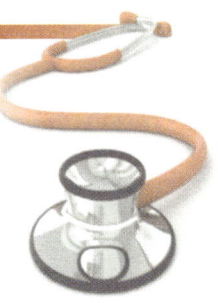

INSTRUCTION

- Examine the patient

SALIENT FEATURES

- Diabetes with oedema feet

HISTORY

Ask for the following:

- Age at onset of symptoms
- Obesity (increased BMI), metabolic syndrome
- History of polyuria, polyphagia and polydipsia
- History of weakness and fatigue
- History of visual disturbances and changes in refraction (retinopathy)
- History of pruritus vulvae, menstrual irregularity and infertility
- History of dyspnea, orthopnea and PND
- History of cough, hemoptysis, pain chest and night sweats
- Dysuria, pyuria, burning micturition, increased frequency of micturition
- Edema feet and legs (present)
- Paraesthesias, sensory loss, motor deficit (monoplegia, paraplegia, hemiplegia), facial asymmetry, deafness, mental features and disturbance in consciousness
- Ask for symptoms of hypoglycemia
- Drug treatment being taken or taken in the past
- Dietary history
- History of smoking, alcohol and physical inactivity
- History of infection of skin (fungal, bacterial)

EXAMINATION

General Physical Examination

- Calculate BMI, and examine fat distribution
- *Mouth* for candidiasis, ulceration, sepsis
- *Dental* hygiene, sepsis
- *Facial* puffiness (present)
- *Eyes* for infection, xanthelasma (present)

- *Ear* for discharge, infection (otitis media), deafness
- *Neck* for JVP, lymph nodes enlargement and carotid pulsations
- Record pulse, BP (high in this case), temperature and respiration
- Examine the *hands* for Dupuytren's contracture, chiroarthropathy, carpal tunnel syndrome, trigger finger, muscle wasting
- Examine *legs* for lipoidica dystrophica diabeticorum
- Examine *feet* for oedema (present), diabetic foot
- Palpate all the *peripheral pulses* for pulsations

Systemic Examination

- *Cardiovascular system* for cardiomegaly, CHF and murmurs
- *Respiratory system* for bacterial or fungal lung infection
- *CNS* for peripheral neuropathy, mononeuritis or mononeuritis multiplex and cranial nerve palsies
- *Genital examination* for vulvitis, vaginitis, etc.

PROVISIONAL DIAGNOSIS

The adult obese patient has hypertension, oedema feet, puffiness of face and xanthelasma due to chronic kidney disease (lesion) caused by diabetic nephropathy (aetiology). Patient is likely to develop chronic renal failure (functional status).

Q. What is stage of nephropathy in your case?
Ans: Stage III due to presence of features of nephrotic syndrome without features of CRF

QUESTIONS AND ANSWERS

Q. How do the patients with type 2 DM clinically present?
Ans: These patients present to different specialities or super specialities with features which arise as a result of complications. The organs/systems involvement and their presenting features are as follows:

Organ/system affected	Clinical presentation
• Eye	• Recurrent styes, chalazion, uveitis (hypopyon), frequent change of glasses due to error of refraction, visual impairment due to premature development of cataract or retinopathy
• Urinary tract	• Urinary tract infections, acute pyclitis or pyelonephritis, nephrotic syndrome
• GI tract	• Chronic diarrhea, malabsorption, gastroparesis (dilatation of stomach)
• Genital tract	• Females present with pruritus vulvae, vaginal discharge, menstrual irregularities, recurrent abortions, infertility, etc.
• Cardiovascular	• Ischemic heart disease, hypertension, peripheral vascular disease (cold extremities, absent peripheral pulses, gangrene or diabetic foot)
• Nervous	• Peripheral neuritis (tingling sensations in the extremities with numbness) symptoms of autoimmune neuropathy (Table 104.1), cerebral ischemic episodes and strokes
• Skin	• Multiple boils, carbuncles, abscesses, non-healing wounds, mucocutaneous candidiasis
• Respiratory	• Pneumonias, lung-abscess, tuberculosis, etc.

Remember: These features actually constitute the organ involvement (complications) due to type 2 DM.

Table 104.1: Classification of DM based on etiology

I **Primay**
- **Type 1 diabetes mellitus** (beta-cell destruction with absolute insulin deficiency)
  A. Immune-mediated
  B. Unknown mechanism (idiopathic)
- **Type 2 DM** (either due to insulin resistance with relative insulin deficiency or insulin secretion defect with insulin resistance)

II **Other specific types of diabetes**
  A. *Genetic defect of beta-cell function leading to gene mutation*
   - MODY I [(hepatocyte nuclear transcription factor (HNF-4-alpha)]
   - MODY 2 (Glucokinase). MODY 3 (HNF-1-alpha)
     MODY 4 (insulin promotor factor), MODY 5 (HNF-1-beta), MODY 6 (Neuro DI)
   - Proinsulin or insulin conversion
  B. *Genetic defect in insulin action*
   - Type I insulin resistance
   - Lipodystrophy syndromes
  C. *Pancreatic diabetes* (pancreatitis, hemochromatosis, cystic fibrosis)
  D. *Endocrinopathies* (acromegaly, Cushing's syndrome, thyrotoxicosis, pheochromocytoma)
  E. *Drug and chemical induced*
  F. *Other genetic syndromes*, e.g. Down's and Klinefelter's syndrome, DIDMOAD (diabetes insipidus, DM, optic atrophy and deafness) Turner's syndrome, hereditary ataxia, Huntington's chorea, Laurence-Moon-Biedl and dystrophic myotonia

III **Gestational diabetes mellitus** (GDM)

Q. How would you classify diabetes?
Ans: Read Table 104.1.

Q. What are the clinical stages and time course of diabetic nephropathy?
Ans: The clinical stages and their time course is as follows:
1. *Stage of microalbuminuria* (incipient nephropathy). It takes 5 years for its appearance
2. *Overt proteinuria* (non-nephrotic range). It takes 5–10 years for development
3. *Nephrotic syndrome* (Fig. 104.1). It takes 5–10 years for development

4. *Renal failure/insufficiency*	Both these stages take
5. *End stage renal disease (ESRD)*	10–15 years for their development

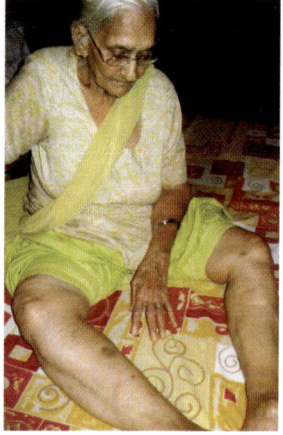

Fig. 104.1: Type 2 DM

Q. Why dose of insulin decreases in diabetic nephropathy?

Ans: It is due to:

- Excretion of insulin binding antibodies with albumin in urine
- Decreased degradation of insulin
- CRF tends to impair neoglucogenesis

Q. What is microalbuminuria? What is its significance?

Ans: Microalbuminuria is defined as:

i. Loss of < 300 mg of albumin in urine over 24 hrs

ii. Albumin excretion rate in urine is 20 μg/min

It indicates early diabetic nephropathy, i.e. stage I from which nephropathy can be reversed with tight metabolic control.

Q. What are the chronic or long term complications of DM?

Ans: Read Table 104.2.

Table 104.2: Chronic or long-term complications of DM

I. **Vascular**
   A. *Microvascular*
      i. Eye disease, e.g. Retinopathy, Macular edema
      ii. Neuropathy, e.g. sensory, motor, mixed, autonomic (Table 104.3)
      iii. Nephropathy
   B. *Macrovascular*
      - Coronary artery disease
      - Peripheral vascular disease
      - Cerebrovascular disease
      - Diabetic foot (Fig. 102.1)
      - Hypertension

II. **Others/nonvascular**
   - Gastrointestinal, e.g. gastroparesis, diarrhoea
   - Genitourinary (nephropathy (Fig. 104.1) UTI/sexual dysfunction)
   - Dermatologic
   - Infections/pressure sore
   - Cataracts
   - Glaucoma

Q. What are the pathogenic mechanisms for complications of DM?

Ans: All these mechanisms lead to endothelial dysfunction and development of vascular complications.

- Activation of polyol pathway
- Formation of advanced glycation end products (AGEs) leading to endothelial dysfunction
- Activation of protein kinase C second messenger system
- Oxidative stress

Q. What are the various neurological complications in DM? How do you manage them?

Ans: 1. **Somatic**
      a. Symmetric sensory and distal (large fiber, small fiber, mixed type)
      b. Asymmetric, motor, proximal (diabetic amyotrophy)

2. **Mononeuropathy**
   - Mononeuritis or cranial polyneuritis
   - Mononeuritis multiplex (entrapment of ulnar, median and popliteal nerves)

Q. What are the autonomic disturbances in diabetes?

Ans: Read Table 104.3.

Table 104.3: Autonomic disturbances in diabetes mellitus

a. *Cardiovascular*, e.g.
   - Postural hypotension, resting tachycardia, fixed heart rate

b. *Gastrointestinal*, e.g.
   - Oesophageal atony, gastroparesis, intestinal paresis (colonic atony)

c. *Genitourinary*, e.g.
   - Impotence, urinary incontinence, bladder atony

d. *Pseudomotor plus vasomotor*, e.g.
   - Gustatory sweating or anhydrosis

e. *Eyes*, e.g.
   - Dilatation of pupils

Q. What are the parameters used to control DM?

Ans: Parameters of control are:

i. Blood sugar, e.g.
   Female < 126 mg% PP < 200 mg%

ii. Serum lipids
   HDL Male > 40 mg/dl and Female > 60 mg/dl LDL < 100 mg/dl
   Triglycerides < 150 mg/dl

iii. HbAlc (glycosylated Hb)
   - < 7% with a check once in 3 months

Q. What are the factors which push a controlled patient of diabetes into the uncontrolled state or coma?

Ans:
- Acute illness, infection, sepsis
- Acute catastrophic event, e.g. MI, stroke
- Hemodialysis or any other procedure

Q.   What are the GI complications of DM?

Ans: Gastrointestinal complications in DM are:

- Candidiasis or fungal infections of oral cavity (an opportunistic infection)
- Diabetic esophageal hypomotility and gastroparesis
- Chronic gastritis
- Diabetic enteropathy
- Pancreatitis (chromic) causing steatorrhea
- Hepatomegaly (fatty infiltration)
- Acalculous cholecystitis

Q.   What do you understand by the term insulin sensitizers? Name them. What are their advantages?

Ans: Insulin sensitizers are the drugs which lower the blood sugar in type 2 DM by sensitizing the insulin receptors to insulin, hence, overcome insulin resistance and hyper-insulinemia in type 2 DM. They are:

- Biguanides, e.g. *metformin*
- Thiazolidinedione derivatives, e.g. rosiglitazone, pioglitazone

Advantages are:

- Hypoglycemia is rare as compared to insulin secretagogues, e.g. sulphonylureas
- They lower the blood lipid
- They lower the mortality and morbidity
- They can be used to lower blood sugar in patients with impaired glucose tolerance (IGT)

Q.   What are the key points (Do's and Don'ts) in the management of type 2 DM?

Ans: The Do's and Don'ts are tabulated in Table 104.4.

Q.   How will you investigate a case with DM?

Ans: The various investigations done are:

1. *Blood*
   - TLC, DLC, ESR for an evidence of infection
   - Sugar (fasting and PP) for diagnosis and monitoring of diabetes
   - HbAlc (glycosylated Hb) for diagnosis and long-term management of diabetes
   - Serum lipids for hyperlipidemia–a common finding in DM
2. *Urine examination* for specific gravity, pus cells, RBCs, proteins, sugar, casts and culture and sensitivity
3. *ECG* for diagnosis of silent myocardial infarction or hypertension
4. *Chest X-ray* for pulmonary tuberculosis, fungal infections, cardiomegaly
5. *Fundus examination* for diabetic retinopathy
6. Other investigations depending on the system involved

	Do's	Don'ts
Diet	Eat a balanced diet Eat fiber rich foods	Avoid consumption of sweetened beverages, fried foods, alcohol, red-meat, honey, jaggery, sugar and bakery products
	Consume small, frequent meals	Do not skip your meal
Exercise	Exercise should be low to moderate in intensity	Do not exercise if your blood sugar values are low or high and diabetes is not under control
	Consult you doctor before starting any exercise	Do not exercise on an empty stomach
	Remeber to walk and exercise daily Keep sugar or something sweet, e.g. candy, to avoid low blood sugar levels	
Foot	Keep your feet clean, warm and dry Change daily clean, soft socks and wear well fitting shoes	Do not use alcohol based solutions. It makes your feet dry Never walk barefooted
	Examine your shoes daily for cracks, pebbles, nails and other irregularities	Never apply heat of any kind to your feet Do not cut corns or calluses yourself
Eye	Consult your doctor if you have pain in your eyes	Do not neglect any infection in your eyes
	Have an yearly eye examination done by your doctor	

Table 104.4: Do's and Don'ts in the management of type 2 DM

Adapted from 2004 clinical practice recommendations by ADA

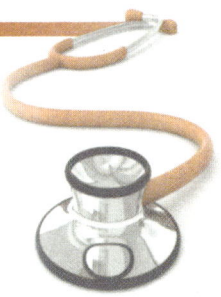

105

Galactorrhea

INSTRUCTION

- Examine the patient

SALIENT FEATURES

- Wetting of brassier with milk in nonlactating mother

HISTORY

Ask about the following:

- Is she a lactating mother? Yes or No (in this case)
- History of stress, pregnancy, wetting of brassier during walking (present)
- History of headache, blurring vision, polyuria, polydipsia (craniopharyngioma)
- Hypothyroidism
- Drug history, e.g. phenothiazines, antidepressants, antiemetics, antihypertensive (reserpine, methyldopa)
- Oral contraceptive
- Primary amenorrhea (polycystic ovary disease)
- History of wearing tight brassier

EXAMINATION

Examination of Breasts

- Patient has spontaneous milk discharge from the breast (Fig. 105.1)
- Breasts are not heavy (she is non lactating mother of two children)

PROVISIONAL DIAGNOSIS

The patient has non lactating galactorrhea as a result of hyperprolactinemia (lesion) caused by some drug (etiology). She wets her brasser's during brist walking and running (functional status).

QUESTIONS AND ANSWERS

Q. What do you understand by the term galactorrhea?

Ans: Milk discharge in nonlactating mother is called *galactorrhea*.

Q. What are the causes of galactorrhea?

Ans: Galactorrhea invariably is either due to hyperprolactinemia or due to increased sensitivity to prolactin or due to local irritation of breasts. The causes are:

I. *Galactorrhea due to pathological causes (hyperprolactinemia)*
  - *Pituitary tumor*, e.g. prolactinoma, craniopharyngioma, mixed pituitary tumor, non-functioning tumor
  - *Drug-induced*, e.g. phenothiazines, antidepressants, antiemetic (domperidone, metoclopramide) antihypertensive (reserpine, methyldopa), oral contraceptive pill, etc.
  - *Chest wall irritation* due to any cause
  - *Acromegaly*
  - *Cirrhosis*
  - *Hypothyroidism*
  - *Polycystic ovarian disease*

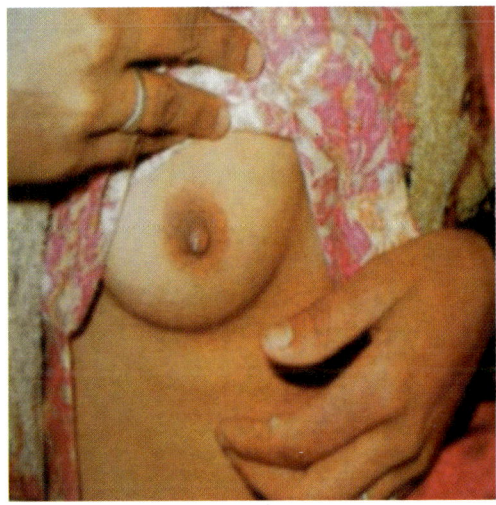

Fig. 105.1: Galactorrhea

II. *Galactorrhea due to physiological causes*
- Stress, pregnancy, puerperium lactation, sleep, coitus, exercise.

Q. What are the clinical manifestations or prolactinoma?

Ans: The clinical manifestations are:

I. *In males*
- Loss of libido, impotence, visual field defects, headache
- Prepubertal hypogonadism

II. *In females*
- A. *Married:* Galactorrhea and amenorrhoea, sometimes oligomenorrhea, infertility, headache
- B. *Unmarried girls:* Hypogonadism, delayed onset of puberty

III. *Irrespective of Sex*
- Long term disease may lead to osteoporosis.

Q. How would you investigate this case?

Ans: Investigations to be done are:

I. *Basal prolactin levels.* They may be raised above 500 mIU/L (normal level is ≤ 300 mIU/L)

II. *Visual field defect*

III. *X-ray skull for pituitary fossa.* There may be enlargement of sella turcica and destruction of anterior clinoid processes in large macroadenoma of pituitary

IV. *Pituitary hormones.* There may be low levels of other pituitary hormones

V. *MRI* will confirm the space occupying lesion

Q. How would you treat it?

Ans:
- Find out the cause and treat it. If local irritation is the cause, ask the patient to wear loose clothes. If drug is the cause, it must be stopped
- If prolactinoma is the cause, then there are three modes of treatment:

  i. *Medical treatment with bromocriptine, cabergoline, quinagolin or pergolide.* All these drugs are dopamine agonists, lower the basal prolactin levels with return of gonadal functions

  ii. If macroadenoma is found on investigations, then it should be surgically removed

  iii. Radiotherapy by external irradiation may be needed to stop the regrowth of microadenoma after medical therapy or after surgical removal.

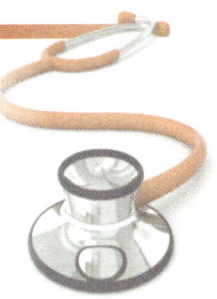

106 Ptosis and Horner's Syndrome

INSTRUCTION

Examine the cranial nerves of the patient

SALIENT FEATURES

- Patient complains of double vision

HISTORY

Ask for the following:

- Is there absence of sweating on one side of the face?
- History of migraine (hemicranial headache)
- History of cervical sympathectomy
- History of lung cancer
- History of diabetes (present), hypertension

EXAMINATION

General Physical Examination

- Look for ptosis (complete, incomplete). Is ptosis unilateral or bilateral? Ptosis is present on left side (Fig. 106.1)

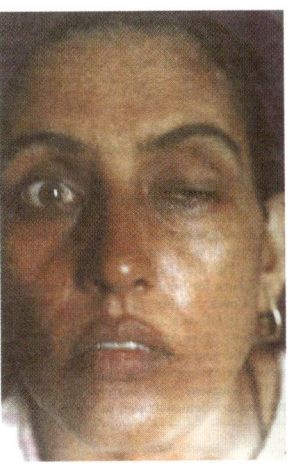

Fig. 106.1: Left third nerve palsy

- Look at the size of pupil, is it dilated (Horner's syndrome) or constricted (third nerve palsy)?
- Are the extraocular muscles involved (third nerve involvement in this case)
- Is the ball sunken, (enophthalmos), normal or prominent?
- Is the light reflex intact?
- Look for scar of cervical sympathectomy (Horner's syndrome)
- Examine the neck for cervical lymph nodes or pancoast tumor (dullness at supraclavicular area (apex of lung)
- Palpate the trachea for tracheal shift (pancoast tumor)
- Aneurysm of aorta or carotids (expansile pulsations)
- Examine the hands for clubbing, (Pancoast tumor) for pain sensation and small muscle wasting (syringomyelia)

Neurological Examination

- All other cranial nerves except 3rd are normal
- Nervous system for motor or sensory involvement

PROVISIONAL DIAGNOSIS

A diabetic patient developed ptosis on left side (lesion) due to third nerve palsy (aetiology). The diabetic status is controlled (functional status).

QUESTIONS AND ANSWERS

Q. Why do you say third nerve palsy?
Ans: All the signs of 3rd nerve palsy are present, i.e.
  - Unilateral ptosis (left side)
  - Dilated pupil slowly or incompletely reacting to light (e.g. paralysis of constrictor of pupil) on left side.
  - Paralysis of accommodation (paralysis of ciliary muscle).

- Paralysis of the movement due to weakness of muscles supplied by 3rd nerve.
- Position of the eye is down and out called paralytic squint (4th and 6th clinical nerves are intact).
- Diplopia on lateral gaze.

Q. What are the ocular muscles supplied by 3rd nerve? How would yout test them?

Ans: • Superior and inferior recti
- Medial rectus
- Inferior oblique

Q. How would you test superior oblique muscle?

Ans: Superior oblique is supplied by trochlear (4th cranial) nerve which intorts the eye (SIN). Tilt the head of the patient to same side — the affected eye will intort if 4th nerve (superior oblique) is intact.

Q. Name few common causes of third cranial nerve paralysis.

Ans: • Hypertension
- Multiple sclerosis
- Trauma
- Ophthalmoplegic migraine
- Tumor (parasellar neoplasm), meningioma, carcinoma at base of skull
- Diabetes
- Aneurysm of posterior communicating artery (painful ophthalmoplegia)
- Encephalitis, basal meningitis
- Collagen vascular disorders

Q. When would you suspect a lesion of third nerve nucleus?

Ans: It is suspected under two conditions:
  i. Unilateral third nerve palsy with contralateral superior rectus palsy and bilateral partial ptosis.
  ii. Bilateral third nerve palsy (with or without internal ophthalmoplegia associated with spared elevator function).

Q. What are the causes of ptosis?

Ans: The causes are:

Unilateral ptosis	Bilateral ptosis
• Third nerve palsy	• Myasthenia gravis (common)
• Horner's syndrome	• Dystrophic myotonia
• Myasthenia gravis (sometimes)	• Ocular or oculopharyngeal myopathy
• Congenital	• Mitochondrial dystrophy
• Idiopathic	• Tabes dorsalis
• Cyst/tumor over the upper lid (local cause)	• Congenital
	• Bilateral Horner's syndrome (Syringomyelia)
	• Snake bite (Scorpion bite)

Q. What is the difference between ptosis and pseudoptosis?

Ans: Read Clinical Methods in Medicine by Prof SN Chugh.

Q. How would you test third nerve?

Ans: Read Clinical Methods in Medicine by Prof SN Chugh.

CASE NO. 2 HORNER'S SYNDROME

INSTRUCTION

Examine the eyes of this patient

SALIENT FEATURES, HISTORY and, **EXAMINATION** are same as discussed case No. 1

PROVISIONAL DIAGNOSIS

The patient has pseudoptosis (lesion) on left side produced by Horner's syndrome, congenital in origin (etiology).

Q. Enumerate the points in favor of your diagnosis.

Ans: • Unilateral ptosis called *pseudoptosis*
- Meosis (left side)
- No squint/diplopia
- Sunken eyeball (enophthalmos)
- Loss of sweating and ciliospinal reflex on left side

QUESTIONS AND ANSWERS

Q. What are the features of Horner's syndrome? How does it differ from 3rd nerve palsy?

Ans: It is due to involvement of cervical sympathetic trunk. Its characteristics and differentiating features are given below.

Horner's syndrome (Fig. 106.2)	Third cranial nerve palsy (Fig. 106.1)
• Incomplete ptosis (pseudoptosis)	Complete ptosis
• No squint, no diplopia	Squint and diplopia present
• Eyeball is in center	It is deviated down and out
• Meosis	Mydriasis
• Loss of sweating	No loss of sweating
• Light reflex intact	Light reflex lost
• Eyeball sunken (enophthalmos)	Normal eyeball
• Ciliospinal reflex lost	Intact
• No extraocular muscle paralysis	Extraocular muscle paralysis present

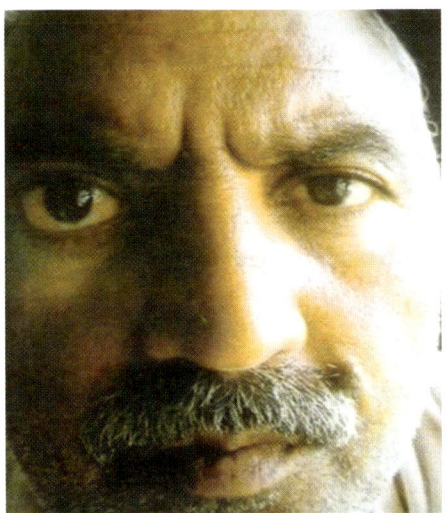

Fig. 106.2: Horner's syndrome. There is pseudoptosis

Q. What is the aetiology of Horner's syndrome? Name few common conditions which produce Horner's syndrome.

Ans: The syndrome is caused by involvement of the sympathetic pathways which extend from the sympathetic nucleus and travels through brain stem and spinal cord (from C_8 to T_1/T_2) to the sympathetic chain, stellate ganglion and cervical (carotid) sympathetic plexus. The causes are:

1. Midbrain involvement, e.g. vascular lesion, demyelination.
2. Lateral medullary syndrome.
3. Cavernous sinus thrombosis.
4. Involvement of cervical sympathetic by
   - Enlarged lymph nodes
   - Aortic/carotid aneurysm
   - Pancoast's tumor (squamous cell carcinoma of lung)
   - Cervical sympathectomy

Q. What is the pathway of oculosympathetic fibres (reflex arc)?

Ans: 1. First order neuron descends from the hypothalamus to thoracic spinal cord without decussation.
2. The second order neurons exit from cervicothoracic spines, e.g. $C_8/T_1/T_2$ to enter the sympathetic chain around the subclavian artery which ascend to the bifurcation of carotid artery.
3. Third order neurons travel along the sympathetic chain around internal carotid

artery to innervate the Muller's muscle (smooth muscles) of the eyelids and along the external carotid to innervate the facial sweat glands.

Q. How would you decide whether lesion is above or below the superior cervical ganglion in the neck?

Ans: It is decided based on the features given below

Test	Above superior ganglion	Below the superior ganglion
Sweating	No effect on sweating	Sweating is lost over the entire neck, arm and upper trunk. Lesions in the lower neck affect sweating only over the entire face
Cocaine 4% in both eyes	• Dilates the normal pupil	Dilates both pupils
Adrenaline (1 : 1000)	• No effect on normal eye	• No effect on both eyes

Q. Why do you say it congenital?
Ans: • Ptosis since childhood passing into adulthood
• Eye ball is central
• Presence of heterochromia
• Isolated partial pseudoptosis

Q. Which eye muscles get involved in Horner's syndrome?
Ans: Muller's muscles (smooth muscles of the eye).

Q. What is congenital Horner's syndrome?
Ans: Congenital Horner's syndrome has heterochromia of iris in addition to other features of Horner's syndrome.

Q. Which feature differentiates the central from peripheral lesion in Horner's syndrome?
Ans: Sweating is lost over entire half of head, arm and upper trunk in central lesion.

Q. What is the cause of intermittent ptosis?
Ans: Migraine

Q. What is the difference between supranuclear and infranuclear 3rd, 4th and 6th nerve palsies.
Ans: Supranuclear palsies of 3rd, 4th and 6th nerves produce gaze paralysis while infranuclear palsy produces paralysis of extraocular muscles and reflex activity of the eye.

Q.   Name the movements of eyes and muscles involved.

Ans:

Movements	Muscle	Cranial nerve
Adduction	Medial rectus	3rd cranial
Abduction	Lateral rectus	6th cranial
Extortion of abducted eye	Inferior rectus	3rd cranial
Depression of adducted eye	Inferior rectus	3rd cranial
Extortion of adducted eye	Inferior oblique	3rd cranial
Depression and intortion the adducted eye	Superior oblique	4th cranial

Syndrome	Features	Site of lesion
Weber's Syndrome	• Ipsilateral 3rd nerve • Contralateral hemiplegia	Midbrain
Benedict's Syndrome	• Ipsilateral 3rd nerve palsy • Contralateral involuntary movements	Red nucleus in midbrain
Claude's Syndrome	• Ipsilateral 3rd nerve • Contralateral ataxia, tremors	Both red nucleus and 3rd nerve in midbrain

Q.   Name the syndromes associated with 3rd cranial nerve paralysis.

Ans: It can easily be remembered by the word WBC (Weber's, Benedict's and Claude's) syndrome

Q.   Name the condition when eyeball is fixed (no movement).

Ans: Paralysis of all the three cranial nerves (3rd, 4th and 6th).

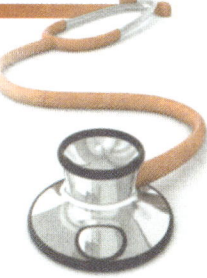

107 Seventh Cranial Nerve (Bell's) Palsy

INSTRUCTION

- Examine the cranial nerves of this patient

SALIENT FEATURES

- Facial asymmetry

HISTORY

Ask for the following:

1. Onset whether acute followed by worsening over the next day (Bell's palsy).
2. Pain preceding or accompanying the weakness (Bell's palsy).
3. Time of paralysis. Paralysis occurs in the morning in most of the cases.
4. Difficult in closing the eye and watering of the eye (present).
5. Ask asymmetry of the face as face is pulled to one side (present).
6. Drooling of the saliva and repeated clearing of the mouth with handkerchief (present).
7. Disturbance of taste (involvement of fibers of chorda tympani).
8. Watering of the eyes (lacrimation)
9. Hyperacusis (involvement of the nerve to stapedius).
10. History of diplopia

EXAMINATION

Examination of Face

- There is asymmetry of face (Fig. 107.1). There is drooping of angle of the mouth on left side.
- Loss of facial expression (expressionless face).

Cranial Nerve Examination

- Patient is not able to close the left eye tightly when asked to do so (Fig. 107.1). Secondly, the closed eye on the left side can be opened easily without much resistance.
- Palpebral tissue on the left side is wide (present).

- Nasolabial fold is flattened at rest and when asked to clench the teeth (present).
- On clenching of the teeth, the left angle of mouth does not get elevated (present).
- Bell's phenomenon is positive (in this case).
- Patient cannot wrinkle her forehead when asked to do (present).

Now look for the cause of 7th nerve palsy as follows:

1. Look at the external auditory meatus for vesicles/scars of herpes vesicles/scars of zoster (*Ramsay Hunt syndrome*)
2. Look for parotid enlargement (mixed parotid tumour, mumps)
3. Examine the taste from anterior two third of the tongue (chorda tympani)
4. Check the hearing for hyperacusis (nerve to stapedius)
- Elicit mastoid tenderness. Examine the ear for discharge and look at the tympanic membrane for perforation.

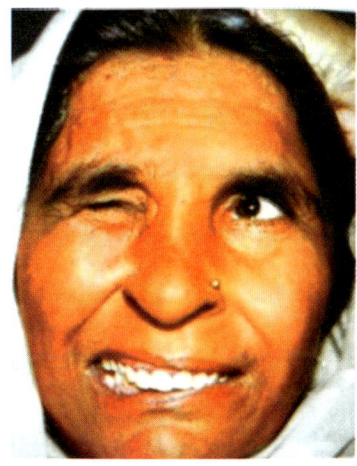

Fig. 107.1: Bell's palsy (idiopathic 7th cranial nerve infranuclear paralysis on left side)

PROVISIONAL DIAGNOSIS

All the above features suggest facial nerve palsy (lesion) due to idiopathic origin called Bell's palsy (aetiology). Patient is distressed due to facial asymmetry (functional status).

QUESTIONS AND ANSWERS

Q. What is Bell's palsy?

Ans: It is an acute infranuclear (LMN type) palsy of 7th cranial (facial) nerve involving all the muscles of face. The cause is unknown (idiopathic) though a viral etiology is suspected. The lesion is nonsuppurative inflammation or edema of the nerve at the level of stylomastoid foramen, hence, lacrimation and taste sensation are not reduced. Hyperacusis does not occur.

Q. What is Bell's phenomenon?

Ans: An attempt to close the involved eye by the patient with Bell's palsy producing rolling of the eyeball upwards, is called *Bell's phenomenon*.

Q. What is the difference between UMN and LMN VII nerve palsy?

Ans: In upper motor neuron paralysis of VII nerve, the upper face (patient can make wrinkles) escapes because of bilateral innervation. In LMN, the whole one half of the face is involved. In UMN, emotional disturbance occur not in LMN.

Q. How facial palsy is graded?

Ans: *House Brackman* grading is as follows:

    Grade I Normal

           II Mild dysfunction (slight weakness, normal symmetry)

         III Moderate dysfunction characterised by obvious weakness and incomplete eye closure

        IV Moderately severe dysfunction (full-fledged clinical picture with facial asymmetry)

          V Severe dysfunction, barely perceptible movements visible, asymmetry at rest

        VI Complete paralysis

Q. What are the causes of unilateral facial nerve palsy?

Ans: Common causes of unilateral 7th nerve palsy

UMN palsy	LMN paralysis
• CVA (stroke hemiplegia)	• Bell's (idiopathic) palsy
• Neoplasm	• Herpes zoster (Ramsay Hunt syndrome)
• Multiple sclerosis	• Cerebellopontine angle tumor
	• Otitis media
	• Parotid tumor
	• Poliomyelitis (old)
	• Guillain-Barre syndrome (cranial polyneuritis)
	• Skull fracture/injury

Q. What are the causes of bilateral facial palsy?

Ans: Causes of bilateral facial palsy (facial diplegia) are divided into UMN and LMN paralysis as follows:

Bilateral palsy

  I. *Supranuclear (UMN paralysis)*
- Cerebral atherosclerosis (common)
- Double hemiplegia
- Pseudobulbar palsy

  II. *Infranuclear and nuclear (LMN paralysis)*
- Acute Guillain-Barré syndrome (most common)
- Leprosy
- Sarcoidosis (common)
- Leukemia or lymphoma, Lyme disease
- Forceps delivery
- Bilateral Bell's palsy
- Bilateral otitis media
- Myasthenia gravis
- Melkerson-Rosenthal syndrome (a triad of recurrent facial paralysis, recurrent facial oedema and plication of tongue)

Q. How will you localize the lesion in infranuclear 7th cranial nerve paralysis?

Ans: In a lower motor neuron facial paralysis, it is important to obtain a history of diplopia, lacrimation, hyperacusis and taste sensation to localise the level of the lesion (*see* Table 107.1).

Q. What is Ramsay Hunt syndrome?

Ans: It is herpetic infection of geniculate ganglion. It is characterised by:
- Fever with headache and bodyache
- Herpetic vesicles/rash on the tympanic membrane, external auditory meatus and pinna.
- Loss of taste in anterior two-thirds of the tongue
- Hyperacusis on the affected side
- LMN type of ipsilateral facial nerve palsy

Q. Is facial nerve a motor or a sensory or a mixed nerve?

Ans: It is a mixed nerve. Motor part supplies all muscles concerned with facial expression and

Table 107.1: Localization of lesion in facial nerve paralysis

Site of lesion	Features
A. Stylomastoid foramen (Bell's palsy)	A. Paralysis of all muscles of facial expression only
B. Facial canal (chorda tympani branch is involved)	B. Features described above (A) plus loss of taste sensation from anterior two-thirds of tongue
C. A higher lesion in facial canal (nerve to stapedius is damaged)	C. Features described above in A plus hyperacusis
D. Geniculate ganglion	D. In addition to features of A, there is loss of lacrimation and salivation. 8th nerve may also be involved
E. In pons	E. 6th and 7th cranial nerve palsy (Millard-Gubler syndrome)
F. Cerebellopontine angle	F. The facial nerve, 8th cranial nerve and nervus intermedius involved

the stapedius muscle; sensory part which is small, carries sensation of taste from the anterior two-thirds of the tongue and cutaneous impulses from the anterior wall of the external auditory meatus/canal.

Q.   What are the branches of facial nerve?

Ans: • *Motor branches* supply to muscles of face after exit from the stylomastoid foramen.
  • *Secretory nerve*, i.e. greater superficial petrosal nerve supplies lacrimal, nasal and parotid glands.
  • *Chorda tympani* supplies taste to anterior two-thirds of the tongue, submaxillary and submandibular glands.

Q.   How will you diagnose bilateral UMN type of 7th nerve paralysis?

Ans: In bilateral supranuclear palsy, the upper part of face is not spared (i.e. total face is paralysed), hence, there will be:
  • Mask like face
  • Emotion preserved
  • Exaggerated jaw jerk
  • Absence of Bell's phenomenon
  • Glabellar tap is positive

  • Double hemiplegia (long tracts signs on both the sides)

Q.   What are the complications of Bell's palsy?

Ans: Following are the complications:
  • Exposure keratitis and corneal ulceration
  • Hemifacial spasms
  • Crocodile tears
  • Social stigma

Q.   What is the relationship between diabetes and Bell's palsy?

Ans: Diabetes and impaired glucose tolerance are commonly associated with Bell's palsy.

Q.   What is Mobius' syndrome?

Ans: It consists of congenital bilateral facial palsy associated with 3rd and 6th nerve palsies.

Q.   What are crocodile tears?

Ans: Watering of the eye (lacrimation) on the paralysed side during chewing is called *"Crocodile tears"*. These are due to aberrant re-innervation of the lacrimal gland by fibers originally meant for the salivary gland.

Q.   What is mimic facial nerve palsy?

Ans: Mimic palsy refers to preservation of voluntary movements, but the emotional movements are lost. This is seen in frontal lobe lesion.

Q.   What is hemifacial spasm?

Ans: Hemifacial spasm is characterized by the narrowing of the palpebral fissure on the affected side and pulling of the angle of the mouth due to contraction of facial muscles. The spasms may be post-paralytic or "essential". The pathogenesis is compression of the facial nerve by loops of cerebellar arteries or by AVM (arteriovenous malformation), or aneurysm or a cerebellopontine angle tumor.

Q.   How will you manage a case with Bell's palsy?

Ans: Management of Bell's palsy includes:
  1. NSAIDs for inflammation and relief of pain.
  2. A short course of steroids is given to reduce edema around the nerve.
  3. Acyclovir plus prednisolone is more effective in improving volitional muscle activity and in preventing partial nerve degeneration as compared to prednisolone treatment.
  4. Physiotherapy: Massage, electrical stimulation, splint to prevent drooping of the lower part of the face.

5. Protection of the eye with lubricating eyedrops and a patch during sleep.
6. If no improvement occurs with in 6 weeks, the surgical decompression at the stylomastoid foramen is advised.
7. Facial exercises in front of a mirror.

Q.   What is facial synkinesis? Name few examples.

Ans: Facial dyskinesis means that attempts to move one group of facial muscle result in contractions of other associated facial muscles. It is due to aberrant anatomical innervation of facial nerve during regeneration. For examples:

1. *Crocodile tears* may occurs during eating due to innervation of lacrimal glands by the fibers originally connected with muscles of the face.
2. Closure of the eyelid on the affected side causes retraction of the mouth. This occurs when fibres originally connected with orbicularis oculus innervate the orbicularis oris.
3. Opening of jaw may cause closure of the eyes called Jaw-Winking.

Q.   What reflexes would you test for facial nerve?

Ans: Corneal reflex, palmomental reflex, sucking reflex.

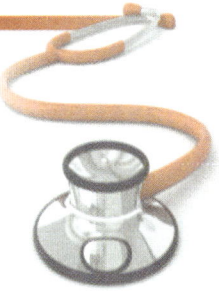

108 Sixth Cranial Nerve Palsy

INSTRUCTION

Examine the patient's cranial nerves

SALIENT FEATURES

- History of diplopia

HISTORY

Ask for the following:

- Diplopia. Does it occurs in all directions of gaze except away from the affected side?
- Rotation of head towards paralysed side.
- Closure of the eye to prevent diplopia.
- History of loss of hearing, diabetes and hypertension.

EXAMINATION

General Physical Examination

- Record the pulse and B.P.

Cranial Nerve Examination

- First and second cranial nerves are normal
- Third, fourth, fifth cranial nerves normal
- The eye is deviated medially and there is failure of lateral movement (Fig. 108.1)

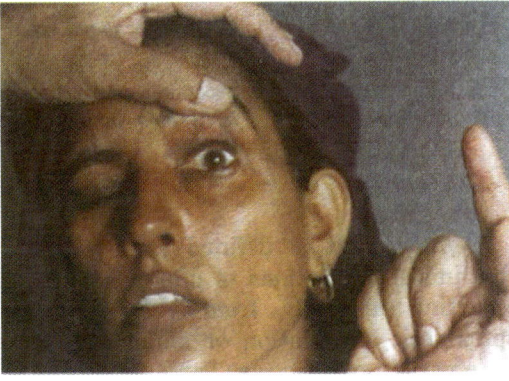

Fig. 108.1: Left sixth nerve palsy

- The double vision (diplopia) is maximum (present) when patient is asked to look towards the affected side
- The two images are placed parallel to each other and separated in the horizontal plane
- On covering the affected eye, the actual image disappears in this case (actual image is produced by the affected eye)
- Test for hearing and corneal sensation
- From 7th to XII th cranial nerves are also normal

PROVISIONAL DIAGNOSIS

The patient has left 6th cranial nerve (abducent nerve) palsy (lesion) cause by diabetes mellitus (aetiology). Patient is upset due to diplopia (functional status)

QUESTIONS AND ANSWERS

Q. What are the points in favor of your diagnosis?

Ans:
- History of diplopia on attempting to look at the left side
- Failure of lateral movement on attempted abduction on the involved side
- History of diabetes (uncontrolled state)

Q. What are the common causes of 6th nerve palsy?

Ans: Causes are:
- Hypertension
- Diabetes
- Multiple sclerosis
- Encephalitis
- Raised intracranial pressure (false localizing sign)
- Basal meningitis
- Acoustic neuroma, nasopharyngeal carcinoma

Q. What is the course of 6th cranial nerve in the brain?

Ans: The course is lengthy, that is the reason that it is involved in raised intracranial pressure.

After its origin in the pons, it comes out at lower border of pons, then passes upwards over the apex of the petrous temporal bone and joins 3rd and 4th cranial nerves in cavernous sinus. It enters along with 3rd and 4th nerves into the orbit through superior orbital fissure.

It can be involved:
- In the pons (nuclear lesion)
- Outside the pons (infranuclear lesion) at lower pons, at petrous temporal bone, in cavernous sinus and in the orbit.

Q. **Where is the nucleus of 6th cranial nerve? What is its relation with 7th nerve?**

Ans: Nucleus lies in the pons. The fibres of the 6th cranial nerve hook around the 7th cranial nerve nucleus in the lower pons.

Q. **Name the structures that lie in close proximity to 6th cranial nerve nucleus and its fascicles?**

Ans:
- Facial and trigeminal nerves (5th, 6th and 7th nerve nuclei lie in pons)
- Pyramidal tract (corticospinal tracts)
- Median longitudinal fasciculus (MLF)
- Parapontine reticular formation.

Q. **What is Gradinego's syndrome?**

Ans: It involves 5th, 6th cranial nerves and greater superficial petrosal nerve due to inflammation of the tip of temporal bone. It is characterized by:
- Unilateral 6th nerve palsy
- Pain in distribution of first division of 5th cranial nerve
- Excessive lacrimation

Q. **What are the causes of nuclear involvement of 6th cranial nerve?**

Ans: As the 6th cranial nerve nucleus lies in the pons in relation to other structures, hence, nuclear involvement is associated with involvement of other structures also.

1. *Raymond's syndrome*
   - Ipsilateral 6th nerve paralysis
   - Contralateral paresis of extremities

2. *Millard-Gubler syndrome*
   - Ipsilateral 6th nerve paralysis
   - Contralateral hemiplegia (crossed hemiplegia)

3. *Foville's syndrome*
   - All features of Millard-Gubler syndrome
   - Paralysis/palsy of lateral conjugate gaze.

Q. **Name other syndrome associated with 6th cranial nerve involvement.**

Ans: *Mobius syndrome* (Read third nerve palsy)
Gebhardt'syndrome
- Bilateral 6th nerve palsy

Q. **What is Tolosa-Hunt syndrome?**

Ans: It has been attributed to inflammation of cavernous sinus and is characterized by:
- Unilateral recurrent pain in retroorbital region
- Extraocular muscles paralysis (3rd, 4th and 6th cranial nerve involvement)
- 5th cranial nerve involvement

Q. **How would you investigate such a case?**

Ans:
1. Urine and blood sugar for diabetes
2. X-ray of skull including orbit
3. CT scan/MRI brain for encephalitis or meningitis or any other vascular lesion and for raised ICP
4. Audiometry for hearing loss

109

Hydrocephalus and Raised Intracranial Pressure (ICP)

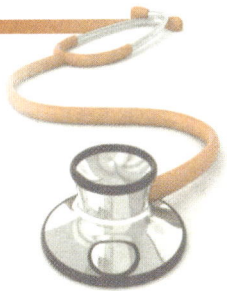

INSTRUCTION

- Perform neurological examination

SALIENT FEATURES

- Large head in an adolescent male

HISTORY

Ask for the following:

- Age of the patient.
- Onset and progression of symptoms.
- Symptoms of raised intracranial tension, i.e. headache, vomiting (projectile), speech disturbance, visual disturbance.
- Any disturbance in the level of consciousness.
- History of fever, headache, vomiting, convulsions, etc. (meningitis, encephalitis, abscess).
- History of delivery or postpartum state.
- Head injury.
- History of drug intake.

EXAMINATION

General Physical Examination

- Eyes are rotated upwards (Fig. 109.1)
- Fundus examination shows papilloedema (in this case)
- Pulse is 64/min regular
- BP = 140/90 mm Hg
- No ear discharge/mastoid tenderness (optic hydrocephalus)
- No signs of vitamin deficiency or hypervitaminosis (A)

Neurological Examination

- Head circumference is large (more than normal) (Fig. 109.1)
- Third and 6th cranial nerves are normal
- Neck rigidity, kernig's signs (negative)
- Tendon reflexes (normal)

Other System Examination

- No evidence of hypoparathyroidism

PROVISIONAL DIAGNOSIS

The patient has raised intracranial tension (lesion), the cause of which is to be found out or may be benign (aetiology). There is no visual disturbance and net neurological deficit (functional status).

QUESTIONS AND ANSWERS

Q. What are the points in favor of your diagnosis?

Ans:
- Large head circumference.
- Headache, vomiting and papilloedema.
- Eyes are deviated upwards (sun-rising sign).
- Presence of false of localising signs

Q. What do you mean by hydrocephalus?

Ans: The term *hydrocephalus* (*hydro* means excess of water, *cephalus* means head) implies dilatation of the ventricles of brain due to excessive accumulation of CSF. It may be associated with raised, normal or low ICP. Raised ICP with hydrocephalus is called *hypertensive hydrocephalus*.

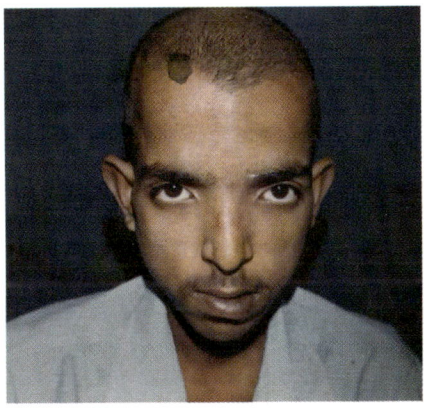

Fig. 109.1: A patient with raised intracranial pressure

Q. **What do you understand by the term raised intracranial pressure? How would you measure ICP?**

Ans: Normal intracranial pressure within cranial cavity measured indirectly is 5 – 10 mm Hg. Any ICP above 15 mm Hg is taken as *raised intracranial pressure.*

Nowadays, ICP can be measured directly by devices implanted in the lateral ventricle or intraparenchymal placement.

Q. **What are the causes of hydrocephalus and Raised ICP?**

Ans: I. *Congenital causes*
- Arnold-Chiari malformation
- Aqueductal stenosis
- Dandy-Walker syndrome
- Agenesis of arachnoid villi

II. *Acquired causes*
- Encephalitis, meningitis, cerebral abscess
- Hemorrhage (cerebral, subarachnoid, hypertensive)
- Brain tumors (craniopharyngioma, astrocytoma)
- Dural sinus thrombosis
- Neurocysticercosis

III. *Idiopathic*
- Benign raised ICP

Q. **What is benign raised intracranial tension?**

Ans: The term benign or idiopathic raised intracranial pressure is used to signify increased intracranial pressure (ICP) produced by diffuse swelling of brain and characterized by a triad of symptoms (*headache, vomiting, papilledema*) and dilated ventricular system (Fig. 109.2). The CSF pressure is raised, but

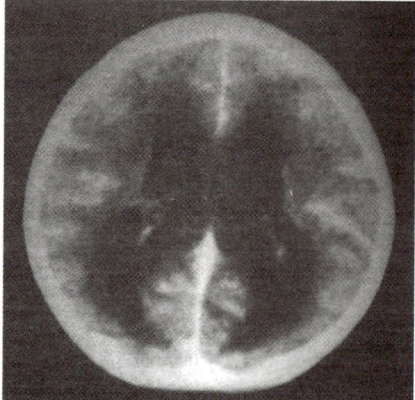

Fig. 109.2: The CT scan shows dilatation of ventricular system without any demonstrable cause

CSF analysis is normal. Neuroimaging is normal except dilated ventricles. The other terms used for this condition are:
- Otitic hydrocephalus
- Pseudotumor cerebri
- Serous meningitis

N.B Benign intracranial hypertension is diagnosed by exclusion of all other causes that produce raised ICP.

Q. **What are the conditions associated with benign ICP?**

Ans:
- Hypervitaminosis A
- Hypoparathyroidism
- Prolonged steroid therapy
- Addison's disease
- Severe anemia
- Pregnancy
- Middle-aged female with obesity
- Drug-induced, e.g. tetracyclines, ampicillin, amphotericin B and ciprofloxacin.

Q. **What do you understand by the term false localizing signs?**

Ans: These are signs which do not have localizing value, often bilateral but can be unilateral, occur in raised ICP called *false localizing signs*. These are:
- Bilateral or unilateral 6th nerve palsy
- Bilateral or unilateral 3rd nerve palsy (pupillary changes)
- Bilateral plantar extensor responses
- Bilateral mild cerebellar dysfunction
- Mild endocranial dysfunction

Q. **What are the consequences of raised ICP?**

Ans:
- Compression of cerebral hemisphere due to dilated ventricular system leading to false localising signs (bilateral plantars extensor, convulsion, etc.).
- Herniation syndromes.

Q. **What do you mean by herniation? What are the various types of herniation?**

Ans: Herniation means protrusion of a part of the brain. It may be supratentorial, transtentorial and infratentorial.

Types of herniation

i. *Supratentorial (Uncus herniation).* It is characterised by (i) Contralateral hemiparesis (direct compression of crus cerebri) or ipsilateral hemiparesis by contralateral crus cerebri against the tentorium, (ii) pupillary dilatation and (iii) paresis of extraocular muscles.

ii. *Infratentorial (cerebellar tonsillar herniation).* Increased ICP in infratentorial compartment results in tonsillar coning compressing the medulla oblongata resulting in respiratory irregularities or distress and cardiovascular arrest.

iii. *Transtentorial central herniation* in which brainstem protrudes through the tentorium resulting in:

- Occipital headache, neck rigidity
- Decorticate posturing
- Bradycardia and hypertension
- Bilateral plantar extensor responses
- Dilated and fixed pupils
- Brain death

Q. How would you investigate this case?

Ans: Following investigations will be done:

1. *X-ray skull:* It may reveal sutural diastasis (separation of sutures) in infants, thinning and increased convolutional markings (*Silver-beaten appearance*) in adolescents and adults.
2. *CT scan:* It reveals dilatation of ventricular system, cortical thinning, effacement of cisterns, an underlying lesion (Fig. 109.3) and periventricular lucency and compression of ventricle (s).

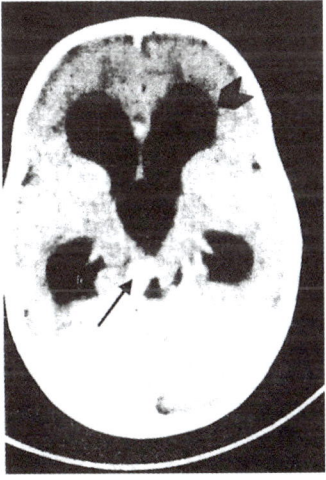

Fig. 109.3: CT scan showing dilated ventricular system. The (↑) arrow indicates the causative lesion

3. *MRI:* It can differentiate between vasogenic and cytopathic cerebral edema seen in patients with raised ICP and predicts response to shunts.
4. *Measurement of ICP:* It confirms the diagnosis. Ventriculography and pneumoencephalography are not performed now-a-days.

Q. What is normal pressure hydrocephalus or occult hydrocephalus?

Ans: A syndrome of dilated ventricles with normal intracranial pressure associated with a triad of symptoms, i.e. dementia, ataxia and urinary incontinence in older persons is called normal *pressure hydrocephalus*. This is actually a misnomer. It is a communicating hydrocephalus in which CSF hemodynamics compromise and result in normal pressure. Though, it may be seen in patients with head injury, hypertensive hemorrhage or meningitis, but in majority of cases no cause is identified.

Q. What is the treatment of raised ICP or hydrocephalus?

Ans: Following treatments are advocated:

1. The *drug therapy* to reduce the ICP include:
   - Mannitol (20%), e.g. 100 ml I.V 4–6 hourly
   - Glycerol (10%), e.g. 1.2 g/kg over 4 hours
   - Dexamethasone (10–20 mg/day I.V in divided doses).
   - Furosemide, e.g. 20–40 mg I.V
   - Acetazolamide (50–75 mg/kg/day) orally.
2. *Shunt surgery*
   The various shunts performed are:
   - Ventriculoperitoneal shunt (commonly used)
   - Endoscopic third ventriculostomy
   - Endoscopic placement of a stent in cerebral aqueduct in aqueductal stenosis.
3. *Repeated lumbar puncture* in a patient with benign raised intracranial pressure may be helpful to reduce ICP.

110

Parkinsonism

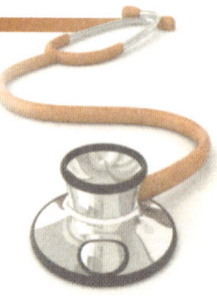

INSTRUCTION

Examine the patient in detail

SALIENT FEATURES

- Slow walking and slowness of activity

HISTORY

Ask for the following:

- History of involuntary movements (present)
- Difficulty in rising up from the chair and initiation of movements (present)
- Poverty of movements, difficulty in swallowing, writing and drooling of saliva.
- Difficulty in turning in bed
- History of change in voice
- Pain and stiffness of muscles
- Imbalance and difficulty in maintaining posture
- History of smoking
- Family history of the disease

To find all the cause, ask for the following:

1. History of excessive tea and coffee (Those who take less caffeine are at increased risk of the disease, i.e. caffeine is protective).
2. History of exposure to dust, manganese, carbon disulphide, carbon monoxide.
3. History of drugs.
4. History of herbal medicines, i.e. sedative kava and Indian snoke root, Rauwafia serpentina.
5. History of head injury, encephalitis, hypertension, CVA.
6. History of use of MPTD (Methyl-phenyl-tetra-hydropyridine) for recreational purposes.

EXAMINATION

General Physical Examination

- *Posture*—Stooped posture (Fig. 110.1)
- *Face:* Expressionless, mask-like face (fixed stare, infrequent blinking and no wrinkles present)
- *Mouth:* Drooling of saliva from the angles of the mouth

- *Hands:* Pin-rolling movements
- *Head:* For seborrhoea
- *BP* for postural hypotension (i.e. Shy-Dragger syndrome, levodopa therapy).

Neurological Examination

- Check for anosmia
- *Examine tone.* Increased tone (Cog-wheel rigidity characteristic of parkinsonism is present).
- *Gait:* Short-shuffling-fascinating gait (describe the gait in detail)
- *Glabellar tap.* Elicit it by tapping the forehead above the bridge of the nose repeatedly about 2 – 3 times/sec. In normal person, blinking stops after few taps, but in parkinsonism, blinking occur continuously with each tap called *Myerson's sign* (present).
- *Speech.* There is dysarthria (present).
- *Jerks* may be normal (in this case), slow or exaggerated.

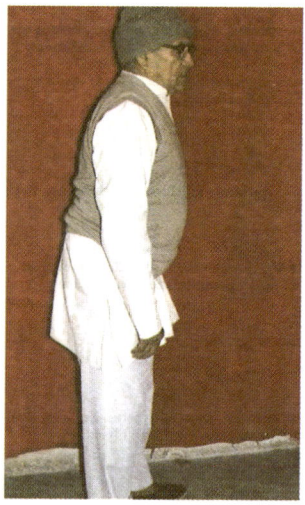

Fig. 110.1: Fastinant gait. Note the characteristic stooped posture. Patient walks with poor arms swinging

PROVISIONAL DIAGNOSIS

The patient has Parkinson's disease (lesion), the cause of which is to be found out (Idiopathic). The patient is disturbed by the tremors and bradykinesia (functional status).

QUESTIONS AND ANSWERS

Q. What are the points in favor of your diagnosis?

Ans: The points in favor of diagnosis are:
- A stooped posture
- Mask-like face
- Slowness of activity (bradykinesia)
- Resting tremors
- Rigidity (Cog-wheel type)
- Monotonus speech
- Fascinating gait
- Glabellar sign positive

Q. What are your other possibilities?

Ans: The other conditions that come in differential diagnosis are:

1. *Essential tremors:* Absence of other features of parkinsonism, bilateral presence of tremors, which have higher, frequency and show postural dependency and abolition of tremors with alcohol favor this diagnosis.
2. *Wilson's disease*: Read it as a separate case roport.
3. **Huntingtion's disease:** Read chorea.
4. *Neurotoxin-induced parkinsonism,* e.g. carbon monoxide and manganese poisoning.

Q. What is mask-like face? What are its causes?

Ans: It is an expressionless face with:
- Fixed stare, infrequent blinking
- No wrinkles

Causes are:

- Parkinsonism
- Hypothyroidism
- Dementia, depression
- Myasthenia and myopathy involving facial muscles of expression
- Scleroderma
- Pseudobulbar palsy

Q. What is parkinsonism? What is parkinsonian plus syndrome?

Ans: Parkinsonism is a movement disorder due to involvement of extrapyramidal system (basal ganglia) and is characterized by tremors, rigidity, akinesia or bradykinesia and postural disturbances. This is also called *akinetic* (loss or paucity of movements) *rigid* (rigidity) *syndrome.*

Parkinsonism plus syndrome refers to parkinsonism plus *bulbar palsy* (progressive supranuclear palsy), *multiple system atrophies,* e.g. olivopontocerebellar degeneration and *primary autonomic failure* (Shy-Drager syndrome).

Q. What is rigidity, plasticity and Gagenhalten phenomenon?

Ans: *Rigidity* means hypertonia affecting agonistic and antagonistic muscles equally. It is present throughout the range of passive movement; when continuous and smooth, it is called *leadpipe rigidity* and when intermittent it is termed as *'cog-wheel' rigidity*. It is commonly seen in extrapyramidal disease, Wilson's disease and Crutzfeld-Jacob disease.

Spasticity refers to hypertonia of clasp-knife type which is maximum at the beginning of movement and then suddenly decreases as passive movement is continued. It is seen in flexors of the upper limbs and extensors of lower limbs (antigravity muscles). It indicates pyramidal lesion.

Gragenhalten or paratonia refers to variable tone which becomes worse as the patient relaxes, seen in catatonia, dementia and CO-poisoning.

Q. What are the causes of parkinsonism?

Ans: The causes are:

1. Idiopathic Parkinson's disease
2. Secondary parkinsonism is due to:
   - *Viral infection,* e.g. encephalitis lethargica, Japanese B encephalitis, Creutzefeldt-Jacob disease, subacute sclerosing panencephalitis.
   - *Drug induced* (Chlorpromazine, metoclopramide perchloperazine, etc).
   - *Toxins,* e.g. manganese, MPTP (1-methyl-4-phenyl tetrahydropyridine), carbon disulphide.
   - *Hypoxia,* e.g. carbon monoxide.
   - *Vascular,* e.g. atherosclerotic.
   - *Metabolic,* e.g. Wilson's disease, hypopara thyrodism.
   - *Head injury,* e.g. Punch-drunk syndrome.
   - *Brain tumors* (They cause hemiparkinsonism).

Q. What is festinating gait of parkinsonism?

Ans: It comprises:
- Slow movements
- Narrow-based gait

- Short shuffling steps taken rapidly as if patient is chasing his/her centre of gravity
- Stooped posture with head-tilting forward (Fig. 110.1)
- Sometimes, the feet may appear to be glued to the floor, so called *freezing phenomenon*
- The fall is characteristic like a telegraph pole. There is tendency to frequent forward falls due to postural instability.
- There is propulsion (*push test*) and retropulsion (*pull test*). The patient starts walking forward and backward when pushed or pulled.
- There is infrequent swinging of the arms during walking.

Q. What autonomic disturbances occur in parkinsonism?

Ans: The common features of autonomic disturbance in parkinsonism are:
- Constipation
- Feeling of cold
- Frequency of micturition
- Postural edema
- Nocturia
- Impotence
- Excessive salivation and drooling of saliva from the mouth
- Orthostatic hypotension

Autonomic disturbances are common and early in Shy-Dragger syndrome.

Q. What are the eye signs in parkinsonism?

Ans:
- Fixed stare, widened palpebral fissure
- Infrequent blinking
- Reflex blepharospasm
- Oculogyric crisis was seen in postencephalitic variety. It is now rare.

Q. Name the components of extrapyramidal system and disease caused by them.

Ans:

Name	Disease
Caudate nucleus	Chorea
Subthalamic nucleus	Hemiballismus
Putamen	Athetosis
Globus pallidus	Parkinsonism

Q. What is freezing phenomenon?

Ans: Freezing of gait momentarily occurs commonly at the onset of locomotion (Start hesitation), when attempting to change direction or turn around and upon entering a narrow space such as doorway. It is a feature of more advanced disease due to involvement of locus ceruleus.

Q. How is severity of parkinsonism disease graded?

Ans: The gross Parkinson's disease is graded into five stages as follows:
Stage I: Newly diagnosed disease or mild disease.
Stages II and III: Moderate to moderately severe disease.
Stages IV and V: Advanced disease.

Q. What is the role of genetics in familial Parkinson's disease?

Ans: Parkinson's disease (PD) is the most common example of a family of neurodegenerative disorders characterized by a neuronal accumulation of the presynaptic protein α-synuclein. It is transmitted in autosomal manner (both autosomal dominant and autosomal recessive).

Q. What is "wheel chair sign" in parkinsonism?

Ans: Patients with advanced disease and on-off motor fluctuations require a wheel-chair when 'off' and no chair when 'on' (are seen to walk about and sometimes pushing the chair). These patients are rarely permanently disabled (wheel chair bound).

Q. What are the changes in higher mental functions in parkinsonism?

Ans: Following changes can be observed:
- Emotional lability (e.g. spontaneous laughter is common in manganese poisoning)
- Depression—mask-like face and mood disturbance
- Anxiety
- Frontal lobe dysfunction
- Dementia in uncommon

Q. What are the drugs available for treatment of parkinsonism?

Ans: *First line dopaminergic agents:*
I. *Levodopa (1500 – 6000 mg/day)*
   The various combinations of L-dopa are:
   - Carbidopa plus/revodopa (25/100, 10/100, 25/250). Dose is 300–1000 mg of L-dopa/day
   - Benserazide/levodopa (25/100, 12.5/50). Dose is 600–800 mg of L-dopa/day
   - Controlled release carbidopa/levodopa (50/200). Dose is 200–800 mg/day

   Dopamine agonists
   - Bromocryptine (5 – 10 mg/day)
   - Pergolide (0.1 – 0.2 mg/day)
   - Non ergot (pramipexole, ropinirole)

II. *Second line alternatives:*

Amantidine (100 – 200 mg/day)

Anticholinergics

- Trihexyphenidyl (4 – 8 mg/day)
- Benztropine (1 – 1.5 mg/day)

Antihistamines

- Diphenhydramine (50 – 100 mg/day)
- Orphenadrine (150 – 200 mg/day)

MAO-B inhibitor

- Selegiline (5 – 10 mg/day)

Q.   What is the golden rule for the use of anti-parkinsonian drugs?

Ans: "Start low and go slow".

Q.   What is type of speech in parkinsonism?

Ans: The voice becomes soft (hypophonic), mono-tonous and stuttering. The speech is rapid than normal. In advanced cases, speech is reduced to muttering. Dribbling of saliva is common.

Q.   What do you understand by 'drug holidays' in L-dopa therapy?

Ans: Drug holiday means discontinuation of therapy for few days. It was practiced previously in L-doapa therapy because it was claimed to enhance the efficacy of treatment when it was resumed. This is now considered as dangerous and is of doubtful value.

Q.   What is Shy-Drager syndrome?

Ans: It is called *Parkinsonism plus syndrome* and includes:

- *Parkinsonism.* (rest tremors gait and postural abnormality).
- *Autonomic disturbance* (dysautonomia), e.g. orthostatic hypotension, sphincter disturbance and impotence.
- In addition, patients may have *laryngeal stridor* and *pyramidal features*.

Q.   What are the causes of slowness of movements?

Ans: Causes include parkinsonism, hypothyroi-dism and depression.

Q.   Name the agents tried to delay the progression of the disease?

Ans: 1. Selegiline in DATATOP study showed beneficial results, its metabolite des-methyl selegiline is under trial
2. Coenzyme Q10—an antioxidant
3. Dopamine agonists

4. Nitric oxide synthetase inhibitors
5. Antiapoptotic agents
6. Minocycline—a tetracycline

Q.   Mention some newer drugs in treatment of parkinsonism.

Ans: 1. *Dopamine agonists*, e.g. cabergoline, ropinirole, pramipexole.
2. *Inhibitor of catechol O-methyl-trans-ferase (COMT)*, e.g. entacapone, tolca pone. They are known as levodopa aug-mentations because they increase "on" time and reduce the duration of the "off" time and thus allow reduction of daily dose of L-dopa.
3. *Inhibitors of glutamate receptors*, e.g. CPP (3, 6-carboxy piprazin-4-yl propyl-l-phosphonate), lamotrigine.
4. *GM-I ganglioside*, e.g. There is experi-mental evidence that when monkeys were treated with this drug from cow's brain, their motor function returned to normal.

Q.   What is the role of fetal tissue in Parkinson's disease?

Ans: Animal experiments have suggested that transplantation of fetal dopaminergic neurons can survive and restore neurological func-tion. Trials are on to determine whether fetal graft can improve motor functions in patients with Parkinson's disease. Fetal ventral mesencephalic tissue is implanted in patient's postcommissural putamen.

Q.   What are the indications of stereotactic surgery in Parkinson's disease?

Ans: Indications are:

- Severe tremors
- Levodopa-induced dyskinesia or levodopa failure
- Advanced Parkinson's disease (Stages IV and V)
- Akinetic-rigid syndrome.

Q.   Name some heredodegenerative parkin-sonian disorders.

Ans: 1. *Hallervorder-Spatz disease* (dementia, choreoathetosis, dystonia, retinitis pig-mentosa).
2. *Fahr's disease* (Chorea, dementia pali-lalia).
3. *Olivopontocerebellar* and *spinocere-bellar degeneration*.

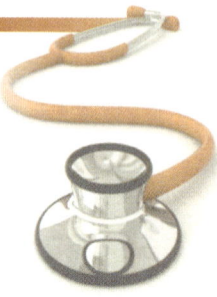

111

Tremors

INSTRUCTION

- Look at the hands of the patient
- Perform relevant systems examination

SALIENT FEATURES

- Patient has involuntary movements of hands

HISTORY

Ask for the following:

- Do tremors occur at rest or during action (cerebellar disease)?
- Does patient complain of uneasiness due to presence of involuntary movements?
- Disturbance during normal activities, i.e. combing, holding the glass, etc.
- History of thyrotoxicosis (tachycardia, sweating, enlarged thyroid, etc.)
- Effect of emotion (makes the tremors worse) and sleep (relieves tremors) on parkinsonism and alcohol relieves benign essential tremors
- History of alcoholism
- History of drug intake, e.g. beta-stimulants
- Occupational exposure to mercury (hatters shake)
- Family history is positive (benign essential tremors run in families)

EXAMINATION

General Physical Examination

It is done for tremors and their demonstration, i.e.

1. *Tremors,* e.g. fine, more than 10/sec occur in liver disease, benign essential tremors, anxiety and thyrotoxicosis; while coarse tremors occur in cerebellar disease, parkinsonism (Fig. 111.1), may be drug induced.
2. *Effect of posture.* Demonstrate action tremors (holding something in hands) and resting tremors
3. Demonstrate the tremors on outstretched hands and widely separated fingers [Flapping tremors (Fig. 111.2)].

4. *Intention tremors* (Ask the patient to touch the tip of nose with the fingers, if tremors occur when patient approaches the nose are called intension tremors).
5. Postural tremors more in the arms than legs occur in neuropathy.
6. Examine handwriting
7. Look for signs of *sympathetic overactivity*, i.e. tachycardia, sweating, etc. for anxiety.

Systemic Examination

It is done to find out the cause, i.e.

   I. Examination of *thyroid* and signs of thyrotoxicosis.
  II. *Cardiovascular system* for hypertension (pheochromocytomas).
 III. *Neurological examination for Cerebellar signs* for cerebellar disease (intention tremors present or past-pointing sign is positive).

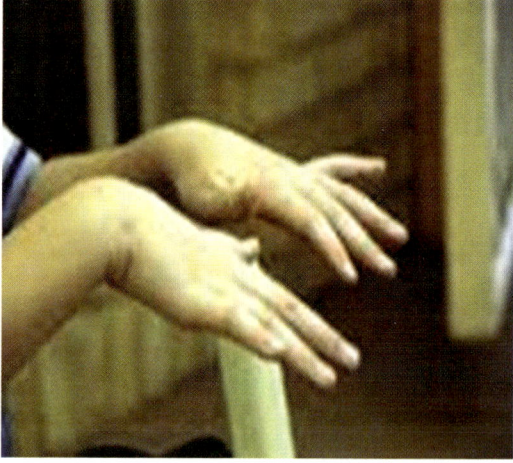

Fig. 111.1: Tremors. A patient with resting tremors

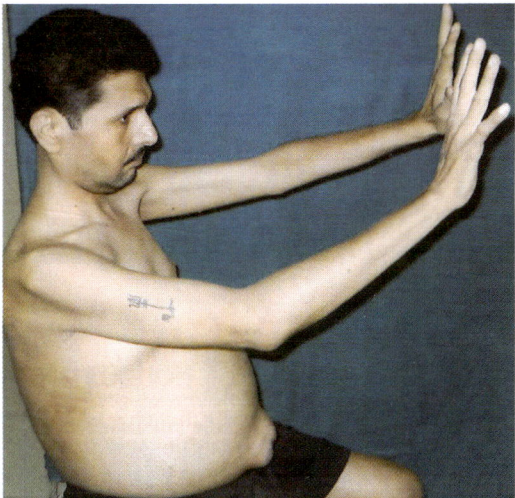

Fig. 111.2: Demonstration of flapping tremors in a patient with cirrhosis of the liver

PROVISIONAL DIAGNOSIS

A young male presented with tremors, fine in nature, relieved by alcohol (lesion), the cause has to be found out (idiopathic or benign essential tremors).

QUESTIONS AND ANSWERS

Q.   What do you understand by the term benign essential tremors?

Ans: These are fine tremors which run in the families, are relieved by intake of alcohol.

Q.   What are the causes of tremors?

Ans: I. *Causes of fine tremors*
- Anxiety, thyrotoxicosis, pheochromocytoma
- Benign essential tremors (idiopathic)
- Flapping tremors due to hepatic disease, uraemia, respiratory insufficiency, raised intracranial pressure
- Drug-induced

II. *Coarse tremors*
- Cerebellar disease • Multiple sclerosis
- Parkinsonism   • Senile

Q.   What are fine and coarse tremors?

Ans: *Fine tremors* have more frequency (7–10/sec), but less amplitude. They may or may not be visible, but can be demonstrated.
Coarse tremors have less frequency (4–5/sec), but more amplitude.

Q.   How do you define tremors?

Ans: These are involuntary (unintended) rhythmical oscillatory movements about a joint or a groups of joints produced by alternating contractions and relaxations of group of muscles.

Q.   How would you classify tremors?

Ans: They are classified as follows:
I. *Resting tremors*, e.g. Parkinsonism, senility
II. *Action tremors/kinetic tremors/postural tremors* (It is brought on outstretched arms and hands)
- Anxiety, thyrotoxicosis, pheochromocytoma, alcohol, drugs
- Syphilis
III. *Intention-tremors* (aggravated by voluntary acts), e.g.
- Cerebellar disease
IV. *Flapping tremors* (asterixis), e.g. hepatic encephalopathy, uraemia, respiratory failure, raised intracranial pressure
V. *Tremor from neuropathy.* These are postural tremors, involves arms more than legs.

Q.   Name the various involuntary movements.

Ans: These are:
- Tremor   • Chorea
- Athetosis   • Hemiballismus
- Myoclonus   • Dyskinesia
- Dystonia   • Fasciculation
- Torticollis

Q.   Name the drugs associated with tremors.

Ans: Drugs are associated with tremors in two ways:
I. *Drugs-induced tremors*
- Beta-agonists (salbutamol, terbutaline), caffeine, theophylline, lithium, antidepressants, serotonin reuptake inhibitors, neuroleptics, valproate, etc.
II. *Tremors associated with drug withdrawl*
- Alcohol (delirium tremons)
- Benzodiazepines, barbiturates, opiates (CNS depressants)

Q.   How would you investigate the patient with tremors?

Ans: Investigations are directed to find out the cause, i.e.
1. *Thyroid function test* for thyrotoxicosis
2. *MRI/PET scan* for cerebellar diseases
3. *Liver function tests* and serum copper for Wilson's disease and cirrhosis liver

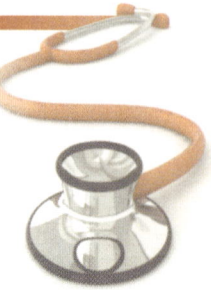

112

Chorea and Athetosis

INSTRUCTION

- Look at the patient. Describe the movements
- Perform neurological examination

SALIENT FEATURES

- Patient has involuntary movements

HISTORY

Ask for the following:

- Ask the history of sore throat in adults especially in females for *Sydenham's chorea* (*St Vitus dance*) in rheumatic fever
- Ask for such a disease in the family, or history of demention, i.e. *Huntington's chorea*
- Take a history of oral contraceptive use in young woman or recent pregnancy (*chorea gravidarum*)
- Ask for drug history, e.g. lithium, phenothiazine.
- History of fever, convulsions, stroke or systemic illness
- Ask for history of liver disease (*Wilson's disease*)
- History of restlessness, fidgeting
- History of dropping objects from hands

EXAMINATION

Neurological Examination

- Check higher mental function for dementia or mental retardation.
- Describe the movements of the upper limbs as irregular jerking, wide-flunging, ill-sustained, non repetitive quasi-purposive movements (Fig. 112.1).
- Ask the patient to hold an object (glass of water). There is tendency to drop the objects (present).
- Demonstrate inability to maintain posture. Ask the patient to hold outstretched upper limbs in front of him/her. He/she can no longer hold the limbs, i.e. there is spontaneous deviation of the limbs (Fig. 112.2).
- *Reptile tongue.* Ask the patient to protrude the tongue and keep it in that position. Patient is

unable to hold the tongue, takes it back with rapid (reptile) speed.

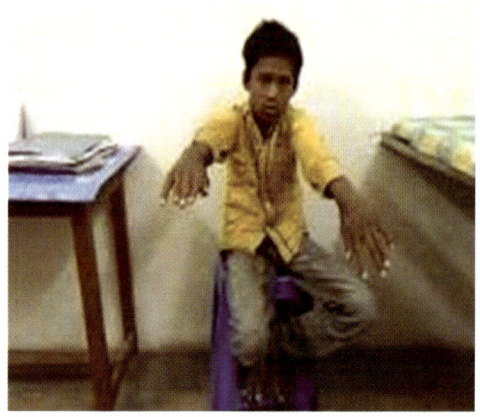

A

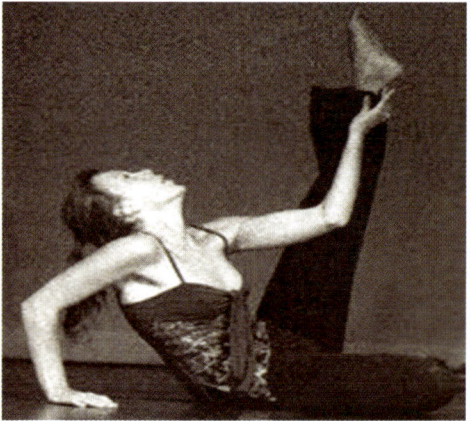

B

Fig. 112.1: (A) Sydenham's Chorea; (B) Dancing movements of chorea

- *Pronator sign.* There is pronation of the forearms with hands opposing each other, when patient is asked to raise both upper limbs above the head.
- *Waxing and Waning of the grip (milkmaid's grip).* Ask the patient to squeeze your fingers with the hand. A squeezing and relaxing motion occurs.
- *Dinner-fork deformity.* Ask the patient to outstretch the hands and spread the fingers. He/she adopts a characteristic posture, i.e. hyperextended limb with hyperpronation of forearms, flexion of wrist, extension of metacarpophalangeal joints with separation of fingers called dinner-fork deformity (present).
- *Check the tone of muscles.* There is hypotonia.
- *Check the tendon Jerks.* They are pendular.

PROVISIONAL DIAGNOSIS

The young patient (picture inset Fig. 112.1A) has dancing movements due to Sydenham's chorea (lesion/disease) caused by streptococcal sore throat/rheumatic fever (aetiology) and the condition is self-limiting (functional status).

Q. **What are the points in favour of Sydenham's chorea?**

Ans: 1. Dancing movement (all characteristics of choreiform movements are present) in a young patient (an adolescent)
2. Hypotonia
3. Pendular jerks
4. No family history
5. No mental retardation
6. All the signs of chorea, e.g. spontaneous deviation of limbs, pronator signs, reptile tongue and waxing and waning grip are present.

QUESTIONS AND ANSWERS

Q. **What are the causes of chorea?**

Ans: 1. *Hereditary,* e.g. Huntington's chorea, ataxia telangiectasia and Wilson's disease
2. *Sydenham's chorea,* chorea gravidarum (rheumatic chorea)
3. *Postencephalitic chorea*
4. SLE
5. Following stroke
6. Idiopathic hypoparathyroidism
7. Kernicterus in children
8. Drugs and toxin-induced, e.g. oral contraceptives, lithium the phenothiazines.

Q. **What are the cardinal features of chorea?**

Ans: Cardinal features are:
1. *Pronator sign*

2. *Waxing and wanning of the grip called "milkmaid's" grip or milking sign.*
3. *Dinner-fork deformity.*
4. *Hypotonia and instability.* It is elicited by:
   - *Pendular knee jerk* or hung-up reflex (a choreic movement is superimposed on a tendon jerk).
   - *Lizard or reptile tongue.*

Q. **How will you diagnose chorea?**

Ans: The diagnosis of chorea is clinical. Perform all the signs described above.

    The simplest way to diagnose chorea is to ask the patient to raise the arms above the head with hands facing each other (Fig. 112.2). If chorea is present, the patient will tend to pronate the arms and rapid jerky movements of upper limbs will appear.

Q. **What is the site of lesion in chorea?**

Ans: Caudate nucleus.

Q. **What is hemichorea?**

Ans: Choreic movements limited to one half of the body is called *hemichorea, can occur in patients with stroke.*

    N.B Usually chorea is a bilateral disease.

Q. **What is "pure chorea"?**

Ans: Pure chorea means isolated rheumatic chorea when other rheumatic manifestations (*Jones major criteria*) are not seen. This is due to the fact that chorea is a delayed or late manifestation of rheumatic fever when carditis, arthritis and other rheumatic features either have not appeared or have disappeared.

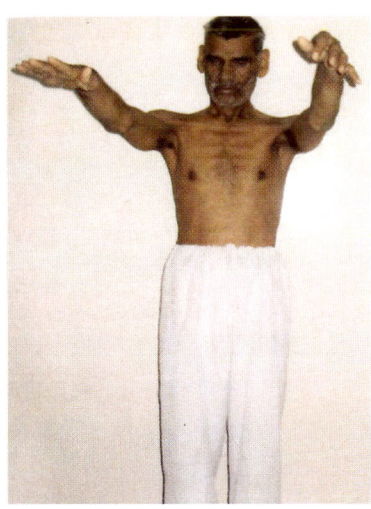

Fig. 112.2: Huntington's chorea

Q. What is chorea gravidarum?

Ans: It is actually rheumatic chorea manifesting during pregnancy or postpartum period.

Q. What are the conditions that produce irregular, rapid jerky movements of limbs?

Ans: Read Clinical Methods by Prof. SN Chugh.

Q. What are the differences between Syndenham's chorea and Huntington's chorea?

Ans: The differences are:

Syndenham's Chorea (Fig. 112.1)	Huntington's Chorea (Fig. 112.2)
1. Occurs in young age (5 – 15 yrs)	Occurs in middle age (around 40 yrs)
2. Acquired (Rheumatic in origin	Hereditary (autosomal dominant)
3. Mental retardation absent	Mental retardation is a characteristic feature
4. Other Jone's criteria features may be present (carditis)	No associated feature
5. Non-progressive	Progressive
6. Recurrences are common. Chorea gravidarum is an example	Nonrecurrent
7. Can be generalised or hemichorea	Usually generalised
8. No family history	Positive family history

Q. What are the characteristic features of Huntington's chorea?

Ans: Read the differences between two common choreas above.

Q. What is the genetics of Huntington's chorea?

Ans: It is an autosomal dominant disorder associated with random repetition of CAG. In Huntington's disease the greater the number of CAG repeats, the earlier is the onset of the disease. The protein product for gene is called *huntingtin*.

Q. What is the role of assessing CAG expansion in Huntington's chorea?

Ans: Assessment of CAG expansion allows assessment of genetic risk without DNA analysis.

Q. What is the treatment of Huntington's chorea?

Ans: • Clozapine, risperidone and olanzapine are better tolerated drugs for behavioural disturbance.
• Tetrabenazine, haloperidol may be used to control dyskinesia.

Q. What is the treatment of Syndenham's chorea?

Ans: The drugs blocking the dopamine receptors such as phenothiazines or haloperidol are used to control chorea and any behavioural disturbances.

Q. What is athetosis? How will you differentiate if from chorea?

Ans: *Athetosis* means instability of posture. It is defined as slow, sinuous writhing, involuntary movements involving the wrist, fingers and ankle (peripheral parts of a limb). The lesion is in the putamen. Its differentiation from chorea is given in Table 112.1.

Table 112.1: Chorea vs Athetosis

Features	Chorea	Athetosis
1. Site of lesion	Caudate nucleus	Putamen
2. Prevalence	Common	Uncommon
3. Tone	Decreased	Increased
4. Movements	Rapid, continuous, uninterrupted and quasipurposive	Slow and sinuous writhing movements, i.e. extension and supination of the arm with alternating flexion and extension of fingers
5. Effect of excitement	Increased	No effect
6. Parts involved	Proximal more than distal	Distal parts involved more than proximal
7. Tongue	Lizard tongue	Chewing tongue
8. Deep tendon jerks	Pendular to hung-up	Normal

113

Hemiballismus

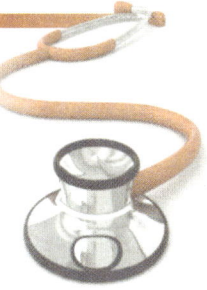

INSTRUCTION

- Examine the nervous system

SALIENT FEATURES

- Patient has involuntary movements

HISTORY

Ask about the following:

- Onset and progression
- Symptoms of cardiovascular (valvular) disease, e.g. dyspnea, palpitation, cough and hemoptysis
- History of stroke (patient had an acute stroke)
- History of irregular heart beats or missed beats
- History of myocardial infarction

EXAMINATION

General Physical Examination

- Examine pulse for irregularity (atrial fibrillation)
- Describe the movement as irregular unilateral flinging involuntary movement of the proximal upper limb (right) (Fig. 113.1)

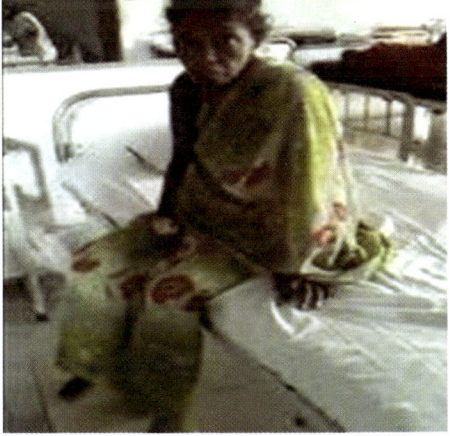

Fig. 113.1: Hemiballismus

Systemic Examination

- *Examine cardiovascular system* for valvular lesion or myocardial disease which predispose to thromboembolism
- *Examine CNS* for any tumor, abscess or multiple sclerosis or stroke (present)

PROVISIONAL DIAGNOSIS

The patient has hemiballismus (lesion) caused by stroke (aetiology) and has severe exhaustion (functional status).

QUESTIONS AND ANSWERS

Q. Where is the site of lesion?
Ans: Contralateral subthalamic nucleus of Luys and its afferent or efferent pathways.

Q. What are the causes?
Ans:
- Congenital
- Acquired
- Vascular lesions, e.g. embolic stroke or hypertensive lacunar infarct
- Rarely tumor, abscess and multiple sclerosis.

Q. What is ataxic hemiballismus syndrome?
Ans: It is a clinical manifestation of lacunar infarct in contralateral subthalamic nucleus.

Q. How would you investigate?
Ans: Investigations are done to find out the cause.
1. *ECG for* atrial fibrillation
2. *Echocardiogram* for valvular lesion and clot in atrium/ventricle (source of embolism)
3. *MRI of the brain* for lacunar infarct

Q. What is the prognosis?
Ans: As in majority of the patient, it is caused by a small infarct, hence, recovery occur within 4–6 weeks. Prognosis is good.

Q.   What is the effect of hemiballismus?

Ans: Patient of hemiballismus is prone to injuries, exhaustion and dehydration.

Q.   What is the treatment of this condition?

Ans: 1. Tetrabenazine (interfers with storage of biogenic amines), haloperidol, levetiracetam, clonazepam are beneficial.

2. In intractable cases, contralateral pallidotomy or thalamotomy can be highly effective.

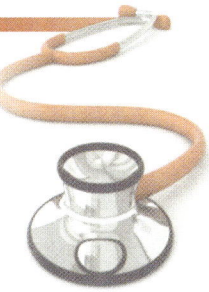

114

Myoclonus

INSTRUCTION

- Examine the nervous system

SALIENT FEATURES

- Jerking movements

HISTORY

Ask for the following:

- Onset of symptoms and their progression
- Headache, malaise, weight loss, ill-defined pains, sleep disturbance and fatigue
- Higher mental function disturbances, e.g. impaired judgement, memory loss, lack of concentration, etc.
- Visual disturbance (blurred vision, diminished visual acuity)
- Cerebellar deficit, e.g. gait abnormality, ataxia
- Extrapyramidal symptoms, e.g. rigidity, parkinsonian features and choreoathetosis
- Pyramidal weakness (quadriplegia)
- Seizures, sensory and motor disturbance
- Myoclonic jerks (present)

EXAMINATION

Neurological Examination

- Higher mental function (intellect, memory) impaired

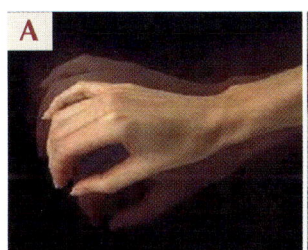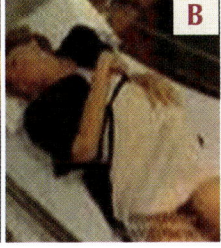

Fig. 114.1: Myoclonus. (A) Movement; (B) Patient with myoclonic jerks

- Cranial nerves are normal
- Cerebellar functions normal
- Speech is normal

Motor System

- There is myoclonic jerks involving the upper limbs (Fig. 114.1). There is no associated convulsions/seizures
- There is hypertonia
- Jerks are exaggerated and plantars are extensor

Sensory System is normal

PROVISIONAL DIAGNOSIS

An old woman (60 yrs) has slow onset and progressive dementia, myoclonus and pyramidal signs (lesion) due to prion disease probably Creutzfeldt-Jakob disease (etiology) and is incapacitated (functional status).

Q. What are and points in favor of your diagnosis?

Ans:
- An old woman
- Slow onset, progressive course
- A constellation of dementia, myoclonus and pyramidal tract involvement

QUESTIONS AND ANSWERS

Q. What is myoclonus? What are its common causes?

Ans: *Myoclonus* (Fig. 114.1A) is rapid, irregular jerky movements of a limb due to contraction of a single muscle or a group of muscles. They occur spontaneously at rest, in response to sensory stimuli or voluntary movements. The common *causes* are:

- *Cerebral hypoxia* (posthypoxic intention myoclonus)
- *Lipid-storage disease*
- *Encephalitis or Creutzfeldt-Jacob disease*

- *Metabolic encephalopathies*, e.g. liver cell failure, renal failure, respiratory failure, electrolyte imbalance, etc.
- A feature of myoclonic epilepsy
- Neurosyphilis

Q.   What is differential diagnosis?

Ans: Many conditions that may mimic Creutzfeldt-Jakob disease (CJD) are:

1. *Alzheimer's disease (AD)*. Myoclonus is rare. Motor and visual dysfunction donot occur
2. Neurosyphilis
3. Cryptococcal meningitis
4. Adult onset leukodystrophies
5. Myoclonic epilepsy with lafora bodies
6. Anoxic encephalopathies, subacute sclerosing panencephalitis, herpes simplex encephalitis, Hashimoto's encephalopathy
7. AIDS–dementia complex

Q.   What do you understand by the term prion? What are the common prion diseases?

Ans: Prions are infections proteins that cause degeneration of the central nervous system.

   Prion diseases are disorders of protein conformation and the most common of which in humans is called *Creutzfeldt- Jakob disease* and *kuru*. Few patients (10 – 15%) have familial (inherited) prion diseases such as *familial CJD* (fCJD), *Gerstmann-Straussler-Scheinker* (GSS) *disease* and *fatal familial insomnia*.

Q.   How prion diseases are transmitted?

Ans: In addition to heredofamilial transmission, prion diseases are also infections and transmittable. Iatrogenic Creutzfeldt-Jakob Disease (CJD) is transmitted through:

- Corneal transplantation

- Contaminated electron encephalogram electrode implantation
- Surgical procedures (accidental inoculation of prions)
- Duramater grafts
- Human growth hormone and pituitary hormone therapy.

Q.   What are the pathological Hallmarks of CJD?

Ans: 1. Spongiform degeneration and astrocytic gliosis.
2. Amyloid plaques are uncommonly seen.

Q.   How would you investigate this patient?

Ans: 1. *EEG*. It is useful in late stage of the disease when high-voltage triphasic and polyphasic sharp discharges are seen.
2. *CSF*. It is usually normal, but protein elevation may occur. The stress protein 14-3-3 is elevated in CSF of some patients with CJD.
3. *CT/MRI* scan may show increased intensity in the basal ganglia with T_2 or diffusion–weight imaging.
4. *Measurement of Pr P^{SC} by immunoassay* is extremely sensitive and quantitative method and is useful for both postmortum and antemortum detection of prions.
5. *Sequencing of PRNP gene*. The identification of a mutation in PRNP gene sequence suggests familial prion disease
6. *Brain biopsy*.

Q.   How would you decontaminate CJD prions?

Ans: Autoclaving at higher temperature (132°C) for 5 hours or treatment with 2N NaOH for several hours is recommended for sterilization of prions.

Q.   Which drug is used in the treatment of CJD?

Ans: Quinacrine

115

Facial Dyskinesia/ Facial Dystonia

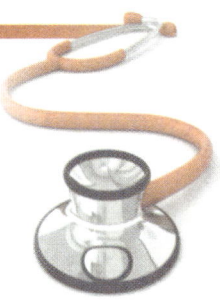

INSTRUCTION

- Look at the patient. Describe the movement. Perform relevant examination

SALIENT FEATURES

- Abnormal facial movements

HISTORY

Ask the followings:

- Onset and duration of abnormal movements.
- Removal of teeth and its duration (how long the patient has been edentulous).
- *Drug history.* Ask about the use of levodopa, phenothiazines (present) and other antipsychotics.
- Does patient has psychiatric illness (psychosis present) for which he is being treated?

EXAMINATION

- The patient has smaking and chewing movements of the lips, jaw and involuntary protruding tongue movements
- Patient is not edentulous

PROVISIONAL DIAGNOSIS

Patient has orofacial dyskinesia or dystonia (lesion) caused by phenothiazine toxicity (aetiology) and is in considerable distress.

QUESTIONS AND ANSWERS

Q. **What is dyskinesia?**

Ans: Dyskinesia is an involuntary repetitive movement disorder due to intermittent or sustained muscle contractions. These are of many types and also called *focal dystonias.*

Q. **What is Meige syndrome?**

Ans: A combination of blepharospasm, oromandibular and cranial dystonia is called *Meige syndrome.* There is spastic dysarthria (spasmodic dysphonia) due to involvement of throat and respiratory muscles. Neck muscles are invariably involved. In fact it is facial and jaw dystonia.

Q. **What is tardive dyskinesia?**

Ans: It is a drug-induced dystonia which appears long after discontinuation of the drug therapy. It is characterised by rapid repetitive, non-random, stereotyped movements involving the lips, tongue and jaw.

Q. **Name few other focal dystonias.**

Ans: 1. *Blepharospasm.* It is frequent opening and closing of the eyes.

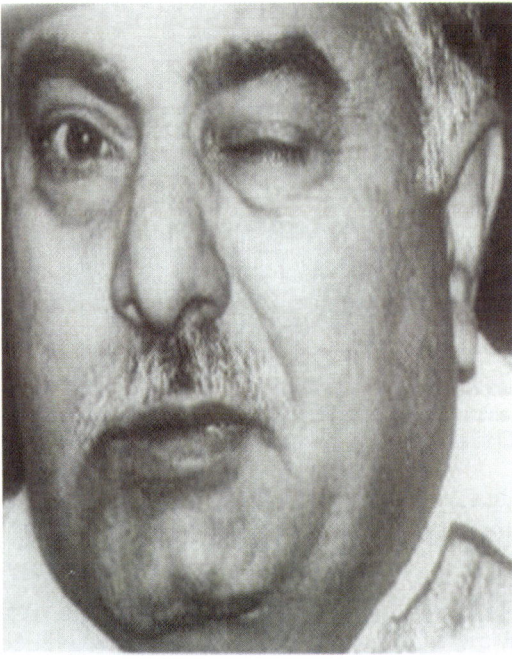

Fig. 115.1: Facial dyskinesia/Facial dystonia

2. *Spasmodic torticollis* (wry neck). It is frequent turning of the neck to one side.

3. *Laryngeal dystonia* (spasmodic dysphonia) is characterised by strained and discontinuous quality of voice due to involuntary closure of the vocal cords.

4. *Writer's cramp or musician cramps.* These are task-specific focal dystonias that affect hand and forearm during specific activity, i.e. writing or typing (writer's cramps) or playing the musical instrument/piano (*musician cramps*).

Q.   How would you treat it?

Ans: I. *Drugs.* Anticholinergics, e.g. benzodiazepine, baclofen and tetrabenazine have been used, but are less effective.

II. *Botulinum toxin.* An injection of botulinum toxin into jaw muscles results in improvement in chewing and speech in majority of the patients.

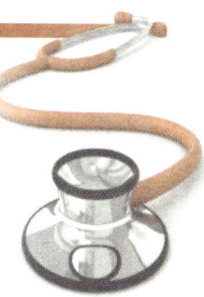

116

Torsion Dystonia

INSTRUCTION

- Examine the patient

SALIENT FEATURES

- Abnormal posturing of limbs

HISTORY

Ask the following:

- Age of onset and course
- Difficult labor, birth injury/trauma
- Kernicterus
- History of intake of neuroleptics for psychiatric illness

EXAMINATION

Neurological Examination

- Examine the posture [limbs are adopting abnormal posture (Fig. 116.1)]
- Spasmodic movements of head and neck
- Blepharospasm

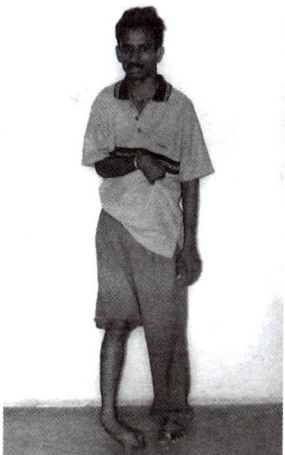

Fig. 116.1: Torsion dystonia

- Facial movements, smacking movements, for opening and closing of the mouth
- Torticollis
- History of seizures
- Examine higher mental functions (normal in this case)
- Examine pyramidal and extrapyramidal systems to exclude other causes of dystonia

PROVISIONAL DIAGNOSIS

In view of a characteristic abnormal posture of the limbs, patient has torsion dystonia (lesion) which could be idiopathic (etiology). Patient is profoundly disabled (functional status).

QUESTIONS AND ANSWERS

Q. **What are the points in favor of your diagnosis?**

Ans:
- Normal labor and normal developmental milestones
- Age of onset of symptoms during childhood
- Persistence of symptoms and signs
- Increased tone of the limb muscles
- Torsion of body due to axial muscle involvement
- A characteristic and abnormal posture
- Positive family history

Q. **What do you mean by idiopathic torsion dystonia (oppenheim's dystonia)?**

Ans: Idiopathic torsion dystonia can occur sporadically or on a hereditary basis (autosomal dominant or recessive and X-linked transmission). Symptoms begin in childhood or later and persist throughout life.

Q. **What is inheritance of dystonia?**

Ans: One responsible gene located at chromosome 9(9q 34) named DYT1 involving its mutations through DYT3 are responsible for autosomal dominant, autosomal recessive and X-linked causes of dystonias called *primary dystonias*.

Q. **What are other causes of dystonias?**

Ans: 1. *Perinatal anoxia, birth trauma, kernicterus* are common causes of dystonia occurring before the age of 5 yrs. These children have seizures and mental retardation.

2. *Cerebral palsy* [choreoathetoid movements, mental retardation, epilepsy and pyramidal signs may also be present (Fig. 116.2)].

3. *Wilson's disease.*

4. *Huntington's disease.*

5. *Parkinsonism and dystonia* following post encephalitis lethargica.

6. *Neuroleptic drugs* therapy.

7. *Toxic exposure to manganese, cyanide* and *nitropropionic acid.*

Q. **What are focal torsion dystonias?**

Ans: 1. *Cervical dystonia:* There is combined head rotation and backward head deviation.

2. *Blepharospasm:* There is involuntary eye closure with facial grimacing.

3. *Oromandibular dystonia* (involuntary jaw opening).

4. Lower limb dystonia (involuntary ankle inversion and toe flexion, Fig. 116.2).

5. *Upper limb dystonia (writer's cramps*

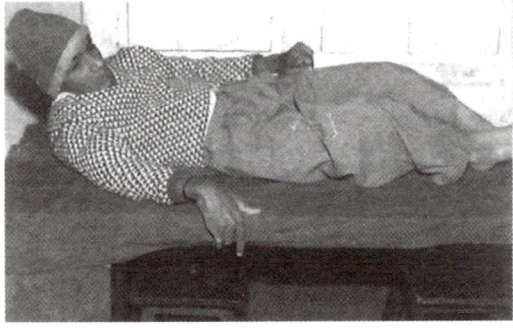

Fig. 116.2: Cerebral palsy. A child presented with mental ratardation, spasticity and scissoring gait. There is dystonic posturing

and musician's cramps). There is flexion dystonia of the wrist and digits when the patient is writing or playing musical instrument.

Q. **How would you treat idiopathic torsion dystonia?**

Ans: 1. *Drug therapy,* e.g. levodopa, diazepam, baclofen, carbamazepine, amantadine or anticholinergic are occasionally effective as idiopathic torsion dystonia is refractory to medical treatment.

2. *Pallidal deep brain stimulation* is helpful in medically refractory cases.

3. *Stereotactic thalamotomy* is sometimes useful in predominantly unilateral dystonia.

Q. **Name dystonia plus syndrome.**

Ans: 1. Dopamine-responsive dystonia.

2. Myoclonic dystonia which is usually alcohol-responsive.

Q. **What is dopamine-responsive dystonia?**

Ans: Dopamine-responsive dystonia (DRD) is an inherited disorder (now classified as DVTS) that results in dopamine deficiency in the basal ganglia unaccompanied by neuronal degeneration. As the name suggests, it improves in a sustained manner with orally administered dopaminergic therapy.

Two biochemical pathway defects described are:

1. Autosomal dominant guanosine triphosphate cyclohydralase 1 (GTPCH1) deficiency.

2. Autosomal recessive tyrosine hydroxylase deficiency.

GTPCH1 is the rate limiting enzyme which has a central role as a cofactor in the synthesis of biogenic amine dopamine, in the metabolism of phenylalanine to tyrosine and in the production of the serotonin precursor–5HT. Because of incomplete penetrance and high rates of sporadic mutation in genes, many patients have no positive family history.

117

Jugular Foramen Syndrome

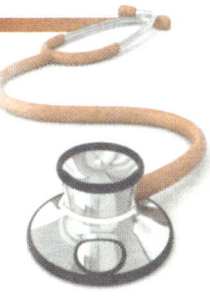

INSTRUCTION

- Examine the cranial nerves

SALIENT FEATURES

- Difficulty in speech

HISTORY

Ask the following:

- Hoarseness of voice (vocal cord paralysis)
- Speech—nasal or bleating character of speech (soft palate involvement)
- Dysphagia and nasal regurgitation (IX and X involvement present)
- Frequent aspiration of food or fluid and sensation of choking (IX and X involvement)
- Difficulty in raising the shoulders (present)
- Wasting of tongue (noticed by the dentist)
- Pain in and around the ear (IX and X nerve carry sensations from this area)
- Headache
- Drooping of the upper lid (Horner's syndrome)

EXAMINATION

Test IX, X and XI cranial nerves (Read clinical method's by Prof SN Chugh)

Testing of IX and X cranial nerves

A. Unilateral IX and X cranial nerve paralysis:

- Decreased/Sluggish movements of the palate on the involved side occur when patient is asked to say 'aah' (present)
- Gag reflex is absent on the involve side
- Test the sensation over the tonsillar, palatal and posterior pharyngeal wall with a swab. Also test the sensations over the posterior third of the tongue. In IX and X cranial nerve palsy, sensations are lost in these areas (present).
- Test the speech: It is blurred and has nasal twang or bleating character in unilateral IX and X nerves

palsy (present).
- Bovine, cough: Ask the patient to cough. There is nasal/bovine nature of the cough.

Testing of IX cranial nerve

- There is flattening of the shoulder on the affected side (present).
- Ask the patient to shrug the shoulder against resistance. Patient cannot do so on the affected side.
- Notice the wasting of sternomastoid on the involved side (present).
- Ask the patient to move the chin to one side against resistance. Due to weakness of sterno-mastoid, patient is unable to move the chin to healthy side.

Testing of XII cranial nerve

- Look for the wasting and deviation of the tongue to the side involved.
- Ask the patient to move the tongue. In XII nerve paralysis, patient neither can protrude the tongue nor can move the tongue from side to side. (XII nerve is not involved in this case).
- All other cranial nerves are normal

PROVISIONAL DIAGNOSIS

Patient has a combination of IX, X and XI cranial nerves palsy due to jugular foramen syndrome (lesion) caused by nasopharyngeal carcinoma (aetiology). Patient has severe dysphagia and require ryle's tube feeding (functional status).

QUESTIONS AND ANSWERS

Q. **Where is jugular foramen located?**

Ans: It is a foramen located at the base of skull between the lateral part of occipital bone and the petrous part of temporal bone (Fig. 117.1A) on each side.

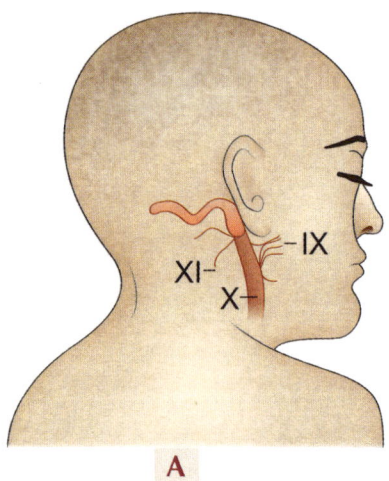

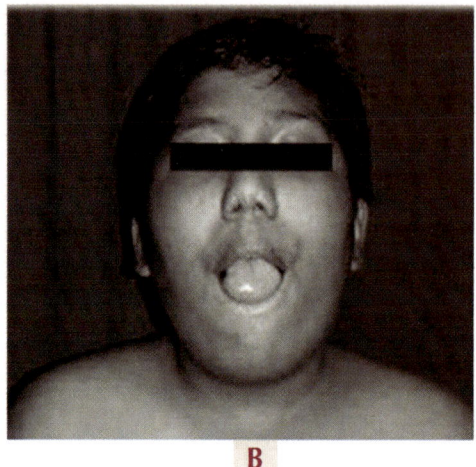

A   **B**

Fig. 117.1: Jugular foramen syndrome. (A) Diagrammatic illustration of contents of jugular foramen syndrome; (B) A patient

Q.   Name the cranial nerves that pass through jugular foramen.

Ans: The ninth, tenth and eleventh cranial nerves.

Q.   What are the common causes of jugular foramen syndrome?

Ans: 1. Carcinoma of nasopharynx
2. Fracture of the base of skull
3. Jugular foramen neoplasm (glomus jugular paraganglioma)
4. Basal meningitis
5. Neurofibroma involving the cranial nerves
6. Paget's disease
7. Jugular vein thrombosis
8. Metastases at the base of brain

Q.   Enumerate the syndromes involving lower cranial nerves.

Ans: They are given in Table 117.1.

Table 117.1: Common syndromes involving the lower cranial nerves			
Syndrome	*Nerves involved*	*Site of lesion*	*Causes*
Vernet	IX, X and XI	Jugular foramen inside the skull	Pharyngeal carcinoma, fracture of base of skull, basal meningitis, glomus jugular paraganglioma and Paget's disease
Collet-Sicard	IX, X, XI and XII	Jugular foramen outside the skull	—same as above—
Villaret	IX, X, XI, XII and Horner's syndrome	Posterior retropharyngeal space	—same as above—

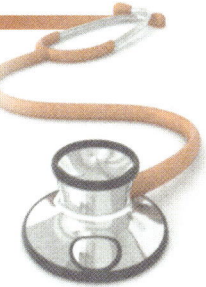

118

Cerebellar Ataxia

INSTRUCTION

- Examine the nervous system of the patient.

SALIENT FEATURES

- Complains of frequent falls on one side.

HISTORY

Ask for the following:

- History of falls (present), wide-based gait, clumsiness and difficulty with fine coordinated movements (cerebellar disease)
- History of tremors. Intention tremors occur in cerebellar disease
- Waxing and waning symptoms of ataxia (multiple sclerosis as the cause)
- History of CVA (stroke) for brainstem infarction as the cause
- Drugs toxicity, e.g. phenytoin, alcohol, lead poisoning
- History of hypothyroidism
- History of intracranial tumor or false localizing symptoms and signs for posterior fossa tumor
- Family history
- History of birth defect

EXAMINATION

General Physical Examination

- Patient stands with wide-based gait and tends to fall on one side (Fig. 118.1)
- Nodding of head may be present (absent in this case)
- Horizontal Nystagmus with fast component to the side of lesion (right side in this case)
- Bone deformity, e.g. kyphoscoliosis pes cavus
- Pulse, BP normal
- Ear—No ear discharge
- Fundus examination for optic atrophy
- Look for the signs of hypothyroidism

Neurological Examination

- Higher functions are normal (in this case)

- Cranial nerves (normal)
- Speech, e.g. dysarthria (Staccato or scanning speech present)
- Gait is abnormal, ataxic (present)
- *Cerebellar function tests;*

A. *Signs of incoordination in the upper limbs*

i. *Intention tremors:* The tremors appear as the patient approaches his/her target/goal. For example, ask the patient to touch his/her nose with index finger, the tremors appear as nose is approached (present).

ii. *Finger nose test:* This is a useful test (positive on the side involved).

iii. *Finger to finger test:* In cerebellar disease, there will be pastpointing (past-pointing is positive).

iv. *Dysmetria:* Movements during finger-nose testing is imprecise in force, direction and distance (present).

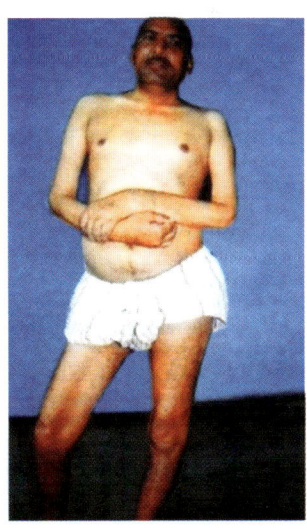

Fig. 118.1: Cerebellar ataxia. Note the unsteadiness during standing

v. *Dyssynergia:* Movements involving more than one joints are broken into parts (present).

vi. *Dysdiadochokinesia:* Impairment of rapid alternating movements (right side in this case).

vii. *Rebound phenomenon:* Inability to arrest strong contractions on sudden removal of resistance.

B. *Signs of incoordination in lower limbs*

- *Knee-heel test* (positive on the right side).
- *Tandem walking* (heel-to-toe walking). Patient sways on the right side involved.
- *Romberg's sign:* Patient sways to the side involved when he/she stands with eyes open with feet together (negative in this case).
- *Abnormal gait:* Patient sways or tends to fall to the side involved while walking (Fig. inset).

Motor System Examination

- Hypotonia of all the four limbs (present).
- Tendon jerks are pendular due to hypotonia (present).
- Romberg's sign (negative).

PROVISIONAL DIAGNOSIS

Patient has all features of cerebellar disease on right side (lesion) due to multiple sclerosis (aetiology). Patient is markedly ataxic (functional status).

QUESTIONS AND ANSWERS

Q. **What is classical triad of cerebellar disease?**
Ans: It is denoted by three 'A'
- Ataxia, Atonia (hyptotonia), Asthenia.

Q. **What are the functions of cerebellum?**
Ans: It maintains:
- Tone, posture and equilibrium
- Coordination of movements

Q. **What do you mean by the term ataxia?**
Ans: Ataxia does not merely mean gait impairment, but has following symptoms and signs:
1. Gait impairment
2. Scanning speech
3. Visual disturbance due to nystagmus
4. Incoordination of hands and feet
5. Tremors

Q. **What are the various cerebellar signs?**
Ans: Read the 'clinical methods' by Prof. SN Chugh. However, these signs have been discussed during examination of this case.

Q. **What are the causes of cerebellar ataxia?**
Ans: *A. With Unilateral Signs*
- *Vascular*, e.g. cerebellar hemorrhage, infarction or subdural hematoma.
- *Infection*, e.g. cerebellar abscess.

- *Neoplasm*, e.g. glioma and metastatic tumor in the posterior fossa.
- *Demyelinating*, e.g. multiple sclerosis, AIDS related multifocal leukoencephalopathy.
- *Congenital*, e.g. Dandy-Walker syndrome, Arnold-Chiari malformation.

B. *With Bilateral Signs*
- Hereditary (Friedreich's ataxia)
- Alcoholism and phenytoin toxicity
- Post-infections, acute cerebellitis
- Paraneoplastic syndrome
- Hypothyroidism

Q. **How would you localise the cerebellar signs?**
Ans: They are localised as follows:

Sign	Localisation
• Gait ataxia	Anterior lobe involvement
• Truncal ataxia (drunken gait, titubation)	Vermis of cerebellum
• Limb ataxia	Cerebellar hemispheres

Q. **What other condition comes into differential diagnosis of unilateral ataxia?**
Ans: **Vertiginous ataxia:** Ataxia associated with vestibular nerve or labyrinthine disease (labrinthitis) is mainly a disorder of gait associated with significant degree of dizziness, lightheadness or the perception of movement.

Q. **Which investigation would you like to perform in this case?**
Ans: *MRI brain* for cerebellum involvement.

Q. **What are the various types of ataxia?**
Ans: Ataxia is a movement disorder. A movement needs coordination of cortex, cerebellum, the reflex arc and impulses from the eyes, ears (labyrinth) and cervical spine. Hence, ataxia is of following types:
1. Cerebellar (read the causes).
2. Sensory
3. Labyrinthine or vertiginous ataxia, e.g. labyrinthitis, Meniere's disease and streptomycin induced.
4. *Central* (lesion lies in the medulla).
5. Miscellaneous, e.g. ataxia due to severe muscular weakness and hypotonia.

Q. **What are the causes of sensory ataxia?**
Ans: 1. Peripheral neuropathy
2. Subacute combined degeneration
3. Tabes dorsalis
4. Sensory cortical lesion

N.B Read this question again in Friedreich's ataxia case discussion.

119

Friedreich's Ataxia

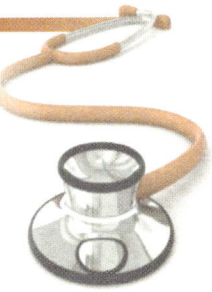

INSTRUCTION

* Examine the nervous system of the patient

SALIENT FEATURES

* Unable to stand due to severe ataxia

HISTORY

Ask for the following:

* Onset of symptoms and progress of the disease
* History of wide-based gait and frequent falls (present)
* History of stroke (brainstem infarction)
* Ask about the drug history, e.g. phenytoin or alcoholism, lead poisoning and solvent abuse
* History of fever, sore throat, vaccination, immunisation (multiple sclerosis)
* History of hypothyroidism
* Symptoms and signs of lung cancer (cough hemoptysis, hoarseness of voice, chest discomfort)
* Family history is positive in this case

* Bony deformities, e.g. pes cavus, kyphoscoliosis
* Birth defect (congenital malformation at the level of foramen magnum)

EXAMINATION

General Physical Examination

* Look for jerky nystagmus (present)
* Examine ears for chronic otitis media or ear infection
* Eyes for optic atrophy (multiple sclerosis)
* Kyphoscoliosis and pes cavus are present (Fig. 119.1)

Systemic Examination

Neurological Examination

* Perform all the cerebellar signs. They are positive on both the sides in this case.
* Motor system examination reveals hypotonia, pendular/diminished jerks and plantars extensor (present).
* Sensory system is for posterior column sensation, e.g. loss of sense of position and vibration (present).

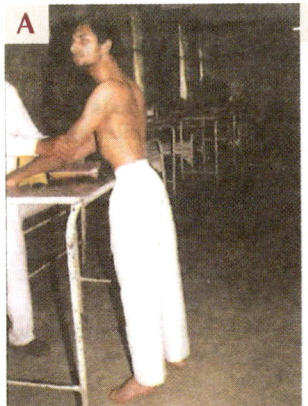
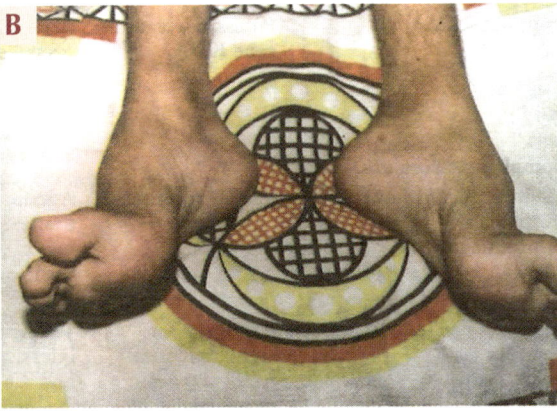

Fig. 119.1: Friedreich's ataxia. (A) Patient with Friedreich's ataxia is unable to stand due to severe disease is being supported on the cardiac table; (B) Pes cavus in the same patient

- *Gait:* Patient has ataxic gait, tends to fall on both sides. He is unable to stand without support (Fig. 119.1).
- *Speech*—dysarthria (present).

Endocrinal Examination

- Look for the signs of hypothyroidism (read hypothyroidism)

Examination of Lungs

- Look for signs of bronchogenic carcinoma

PROVISIONAL DIAGNOSIS

The young man has progressive bilateral cerebellar involvement (lesion) due to Friedreich's ataxia a heredofamilial disease (etiology). Patient has severe ataxia (functional status).

Q. **What are the points in favor of your diagnosis?**

Ans:
- Slow onset and progressive symptoms and signs in a young patient.
- Jerky nystagmus and optic atrophy
- Dysarthria
- Diminished or loss of lower limb reflexes
- Loss of sense of vibration and position
- Plantars are extensors
- Presence of pes cavus and kyphoscoliosis
- Negative Romberg's sign

QUESTIONS AND ANSWERS

Q. **What is differential diagnosis?**

Ans:
1. All 22 genotypes of spinocerebellar ataxia (SCAI-22). Although the clinical manifestations and neuropathological findings of cerebellar disease dominate in these SCA families but many gradations are observed from pure purely cerebellar features to mixed cerebellar and brainstem features, cerebellar and basal ganglia involvement and spinal cord or peripheral nerves disease. Rarely dementia may be present clinical picture may be homogeneous or heterogeneous within families. The SCAI to 22 include dentatorubropallidoluysian atrophy (DRPLA) and are caused by CAG triplet repeat expansions in different genes.
2. **Sensory ataxia**
3. **Vertiginous ataxia**
4. **Proximal myopathy of lower limbs** sometimes resembles cerebellar ataxia. Weakness of proximal muscles of leg, positive Gower's sign, absent reflexes favor the diagnosis of proximal myopathy.

5. **Hysterical:** These patients are anxious and careful. They become ataxic when they are asked to walk or stand (e.g. when they are being observed). There is astasia abasia. They neither have reduced muscle power nor any sensory loss. They can move the limbs and can perform all the movements (signs of cerebellum function) very well without any incoordination, but when asked to walk (tendem walking) they become ataxic.
6. **Ataxia telangiectasia**

Q. **What is Friedreich's ataxia?**

Ans: It is heredofamilial ataxia (autosomal recessive) characterized by progressive degeneration of dorsal root ganglia, spinocerebellar tracts, corticospinal tracts and Purkinje cells of cerebellum.

Q. **What are the diagnostic criteria for Friedreich's ataxia?**

Ans: Read Table 119.1.

Table 119.1: Diagnostic criteria for Friedreich's ataxia (FA)

Essential criteria

- Progressive ataxia
- Young age (< 25 years)
- Extensor plantar responses
- Absent ankle and knee jerks
- Dysarthria (after 5 years of onset of symptoms)
- Motor nerve conduction velocity > 40 m/sec in upper limbs with small or absent sensory action potential

Additional criteria (present in 2/3rd patients)

- Pyramidal weakness in lower limbs
- Distal loss of joint position and vibration sense in lower limbs
- Scoliosis
- Abnormal ECG (wide spread T wave inversion and ventricular hypertrophy)

Other supportive features (present in < 50% patients)

- Nystagmus, optic atrophy
- Pes cavus
- Distal weakness and wasting
- Diabetes
- Deafness

Q. **What are the causes of absent ankle jerk with extensor plantars response?**

Ans: Following are the causes:
- Friedreich's ataxia
- Tabes dorsalis
- Nutritional deficiency of B1 and B12 with ataxia
- Paraneoplastic syndrome
- Motor neuron disease

- Combined conus medullaris and cauda equina syndrome (Cord-cauda) and subacute combined degeneration of spinal cord
- Peripheral neuropathy in a patient with stroke
- Hypothyroidism

Q. What are the neurological involvements in Friedreich's ataxia?

Ans:
- Posterior root ganglion
- Degeneration of peripheral sensory fibers
- Involvement of posterior and lateral columns

Q. What are the features of central (vermis) cerebellar lesion?

Ans: Following are the features:
- Head nodding (titubation)
- Truncal ataxia
- Positive heel-to-toe gait (tandem gait)
- Difficulty in sitting, rising from a chair, standing and walking. There is unsteadiness and swaying during these activities.

Q. What is genetics in Friedreich's ataxia?

Ans: It is the most common inherited ataxia accounting >80% cases of all hereditary ataxias. It is inherited in an autosomal recessive manner. The chromosome involved is number 9. The mutant gene is *frataxin*, expanded *GAA triplet repeats*. There is point mutation of frataxin in this ataxia.

Q. Why are tendon reflexes absent even though plantars are extensor in Friendreich's ataxia?

Ans: It is due to combined involvement of pyramidal tracts and peripheral nerves (asymptomatic) in this syndrome.

Q. If you are allowed to choose one investigation to confirm your diagnosis, which would you choose and why?

Ans: Magnetic resonance imaging (MRI) is the best test to evaluate soft tissue lesion such degeneration of tracts.

Q. Which vitamin abnormality is associated with Friedreich's ataxia?

Ans: Vitamin E (α-tocopherol).

Q. What is sensory ataxia? What are its causes? What is Romberg's sign?

Ans: Sensory ataxia results from defective proprioceptive sensations (posterior column involvement), hence, does not occur with eyes open, as sense of position is compensated by open eyes. Thus, sensory ataxia manifests or gets increased when the eyes are closed.

Causes: Sense of proprioception is affected by lesions of peripheral nerves, sensory root, posterior column and postcentral gyrus in parietal lobe, hence causes are:

1. *Lesion of peripheral nerves*, e.g. neuropathy due to any cause.
2. *Sensory root lesion*, e.g. tabes dorsalis, radiculopathy (disk prolapse).
3. *Posterior column involvement*, e.g. multiple sclerosis, syringomyelia and intramedullary compression.
4. *Parietal lobe lesion* (sensory cortex involvement), e.g. vascular lesion or a tumor.

Q. What are the differences between cerebellar and sensory ataxia?

Ans: Sensory ataxia is differentiated from cerebellar ataxia (See Table 119.2).

Romberg's Sign. It is a sign of sensory ataxia. It is said to be positive if a person can stand without swaying when eyes are open, but tends to sway when eyes are closed.

It is negative in cerebellar lesions and Friedreich's ataxia, as person tends to sway with eyes open as well as closed.

N.B False positive Romberg's sign may occur in hysteria.

Table 119.2: Distinction between sensory and cerebellar ataxia

Features	Sensory ataxia	Cerebellar ataxia
Muscle power	Diminished	Normal
Deep tendon reflexes	Lost	Pendular or hung-up
Cerebellar signs	Absent	Present
Posterior column sensations	Lost	Preserved
Plantar reflex	Lost	Extensor response or normal
Charcoat joint and trophic changes	Present	Absent
Romberg's sign	Positive	Negative
Gait	High-steppage or stamping gait	Broad-based gait
Common causes	Tabes dorsalis and peripheral neuropathy, etc.	Friedreich's ataxia, multiple sclerosis etc.

Q.   What is vertiginous ataxia?

Ans: Vertiginous (labyrinthine) ataxia is a disorder of gait associated with vertigo, dizziness and light headedness. The causes of labyrinthine ataxia are due to involvement of labyrinth:

- Acute labyrinthitis
- Meniere's disease
- Vestibular neuronitis
- Streptomycin-induced

Vertiginous ataxia resembles cerebellar ataxia except that vertigo and dizziness accompany the former but not the later.

Labyrinthine ataxia also occurs more when the eyes are open than when the eyes are closed. Romberg's sign is negative.

Q.   Name the ataxias in which Romberg's sign is negative.

Ans:
- Cerebellar ataxia, friedreich's ataxia
- Vertiginous ataxia
- Labyrinthine ataxia

Q.   What is ataxia telangiectasia (Louis-Barr syndrome)?

Ans: It is an inherited ataxia due to defect in ATN gene, presents in first decade of life, is characterized by

- Cerebellar ataxia similar to Friedreich's ataxia, hence, is to be differentiated. It is characterized by
- Ö Nystagmus
- Ö Progressive telangiectatic lesion
- Ö Thymic hyperplasia with defective cellular and humoral immunity
- Ö Recurrent pulmonary infections
- Ö Sometimes, neoplasia of lymphatic and reticuloendothelial system may develop (e.g. lymphoma, leukemia)

Q.   How do you classify inherited ataxias?

Ans: A genomic classification has now largely superseded previous one base on clinical expression alone as follows:

1. *Autosomal dominant ataxias*
   - SCA 1 to 22 types
   - Episodic ataxias type 1 and 2
2. *Autosomal recessive ataxias*
   - Friedreich's ataxias
   - Ataxia telangiectasia
   - Spinocerebellar ataxia with neuropathy

It is very difficult to describe genomic classification (Read textbooks)

Q.   What do you understand by episodic ataxias?

Ans: Both types of episodic ataxia type 1 (potassium channel gone defect) and type 2 (voltage-dependant calcium channel defect) are auto-somal dominant characterized by episodes of ataxia lasting for minutes (type 1) or lays (type 2) are provoked by startle, exercise, stress, fatigue with transient cerebellar signs (type 1) or progressive cerebellar signs (type 2). They respond either to phenytoin (type 1) or acetazolamide (type 2)

Q.   What is treatment of Friedreich's ataxia?

Ans: It is an inheritable disorder, hence, there is no definite treatment. Identification of an at-risk person's genotype, together with appropriate family and genetic counseling can reduce the incidence of these cerebellar ataxia in future generations.

Q.   What are the treatable causes of ataxia?

Ans:
- Treatable ataxias include;
- Ataxia with antigliadin antibodies and malabsorption may improve with gluten-free diet and steroids.
- Vitamin E deficiency must be explored and treated if co-exists.
- Drug (phenytoin) and alcohol must be stopped, if being used.
- Hypothyroidism must be explored and treated, if found.

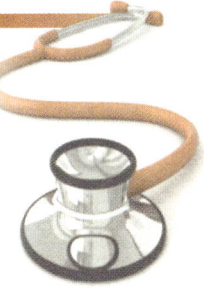

120

Jerky Nystagmus

INSTRUCTION

- Examine the patient's eyes
- Perform neurological examination

SALIENT FEATURES

- Jerking of the eyes

HISTORY

Ask for the following:

- Age of onset and progression
- Ataxia, frequent falls, dysarthria (cerebellar degeneration)
- Waxing and waning of symptoms (multiple sclerosis)
- Ear discharge/infection or vertigo (vestibular nystagmus)

EXAMINATION

General Physical Examination

Eyes: Patient has horizontal nystagmus with fast component to the right or left side. Now look for the vertical nystagmus.

Fundus examination for optic atrophy (present).

Neurological Examination

- Test the VIII cranial nerve for vestibular function.
- Perform all the cerebellar signs for cerebellum involvement. Cerebellar signs normal.
- Motor and sensory systems are normal.

PROVISIONAL DIAGNOSIS

The patient has jerky nystagmus (fast component to the right) with optic neuritis (lesion) caused by multiple sclerosis (etiology). There is no cerebellar or spinal cord involvement (functional status).

QUESTIONS AND ANSWERS

Q. **What is nystagmus?**

Ans: Involuntary rhythmic oscillatory movements of one or both eyes is called *nystagmus*.

Q. **What are the various types of nystagmus?**

Ans: 1. Congenital
2. Dissociated
3. Gaze-evoked
4. Vestibular

Q. **What is pendular nystagmus?**

Ans: It is characterised by the oscillations that are equal in speed and amplitude in both the directions of movement. It may be seen on central gaze when the vision is poor, as in severe refractive error or macular disease.

Q. **What do you understand by the term jerky nystagmus?**

Ans: Jerky or phasic nystagmus (Fig. 120.1) is a condition in which eye movement in one

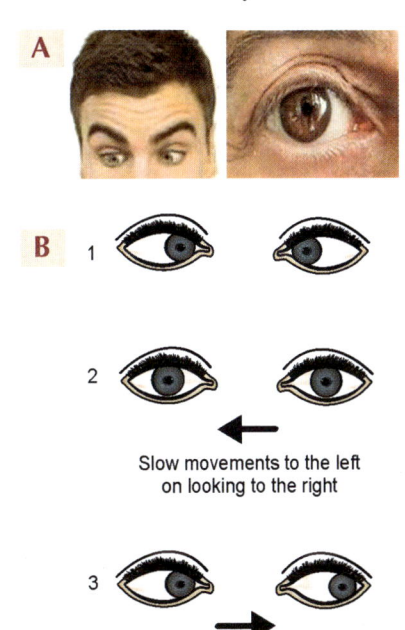

Slow movements to the left
on looking to the right

Fast component movement is to
right and to and fro on looking to the left

Fig. 120.1: Jerky nystagmus. (A) To the right; (B) To the left

direction is faster than that in the other. This is usually seen in the horizontal plane and is brought out by lateral gaze to one or both sides. It is seen with lesions of the cerebellum, vestibular apparatus or their connections in the brainstem.

Q. What is dissociated nystagmus?

Ans: Dissociated or ataxic nystagmus is irregular nystagmus in the abducting eye. It is bilateral in multiple sclerosis, brainstem tumour or Warnicke's encephalopathy. It is unilateral in vascular disease of the brainstem. It is caused by a lesion in the medial longitudinal fasciculus (which links the sixth nerve nucleus on one side to the third nerve nucleus on the other side).

Q. Where is the lesion in vestibular nystagmus?

Ans: It may be in one of the two locations:

- *Peripheral (labyrinth or vestibular nerve)*, as in labyrinthitis, Meniere syndrome, acoustic neuroma, otitis media, head injury.
- *Central* (affecting vestibular nuclei), as in stroke, multiple sclerosis, tumours, alcoholism.

Q. What do you know about 'downbeat' and 'upbeat' nystagmus?

Ans: *Downbeat nystagmus* is associated with brainstem lesions, meningoencephalitis and hypomagnesemia. *Upbeat nystagmus* is caused by lesions of the anterior vermis of the cerebellum.

Note: You may be asked about upward and downward gaze pathways.

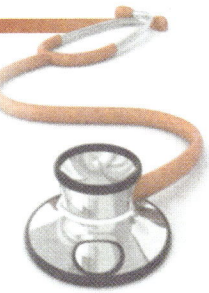

121

Dysarthria

INSTRUCTION

- Examine the speech of the patient
- Perform relevant neurological examination

SALIENT FEATURES

- Difficulty in speech

HISTORY

Ask about the following:

- Name, age, occupation and handedness
- History of dysphagia, dysphonia or hoarseness of voice, nasal regurgitation, etc. (lower cranial nerve palsy)
- History of unsteadiness, frequent falls, visual disturbance (cerebellar disease)
- History of abnormal movements, difficulty in initiation and slowness of movements, rigidity, etc. (parkinsonism)
- History of stroke, motor neuron disease, multiple sclerosis (optic atrophy, nystagmus and cerebellar ataxia)

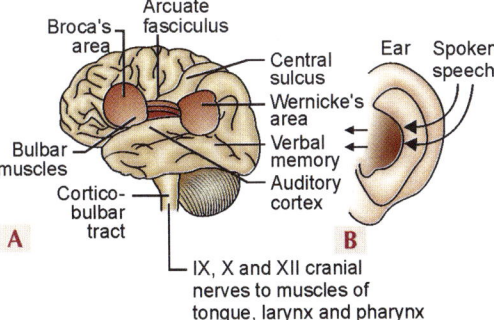

Fig. 121.1: A and B: The diagrammatic representation of main language areas and their associations and the mechanism of speech. The spoken words pass from the ear of the listener's (B) to auditory cortex (A) and then to Wernicke's area (arrows). The corticobulbar fibres supply larynx, pharynx, palate and tongue muscles, the involvement of which produce dysarthria

- Difficulty in chewing and swallowing
- History of chocking on liquids
- History of drooping of lids, fatiguability, exhaustion and muscle weakness (myasthenia gravis and ocular myopathy)

EXAMINATION

General Physical Examination

- Expressionless, mask-like face in parkinsonism
- Nystagmus for cerebellar disease, multiple sclerosis
- Ptosis (myasthenia, ocular myopathy) or pseudoptosis (Horner's syndrome)

Speech: Proceed as follows:

1. *Check for comprehension* by asking the patient to put the tongue out, shut your eyes, touch your nose, etc. Now use two-steps commands such as touch your left ear with your right hand, etc. Comprehension in this patient is normal.
2. *Check orientation to place, person, time, etc.* It is normal.
3. *Name familiar objects*, e.g. pen, pencil, coin, etc. It is normal.
4. *Check articulation.* Ask the patient to repeat the followings (Fig. 121.2):
   - British constitution
   - Artillary
   - Registrar
   - Ram Rattan
   - The speech is scanning in this case (each letter is scanned and produced slowly and in a measured fashion)

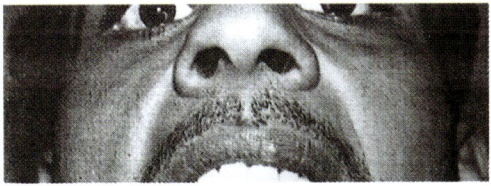

Fig. 121.2: A patient with dysarthria

- Articulation is uneven, words are slurred and there is variation in pitch and loudness.

Neurological Examination

Once, it has become clear that there is defect in articulation, proceed to examine the neurological system as follows;

(*a*) Higher mental functions in short
  - Lower cranial nerves, e.g. 8th, 9th to 12th

(*b*) *Cerebellar signs:* Perform the cerebellar signs to explore the possibility of cerebellar disease. Few signs testing the incoordination are positive in this patient. Romberg's sign is negative.

(*c*) *Test extrapyramidal system*
  - Bradykinesia/hypokinesia/akinesia
  - Rigidity
  - Tremors
  - Glabellar sign
  - Gait abnormality

There is no involvement of extrapyramidal system in this casse

PROVISIONAL DIAGNOSIS

The patient has dysarthria, i.e. scanning speech (lesion) caused by cerebellar involvement secondary to alcoholism (cause).

QUESTIONS AND ANSWERS

Q. What is dysarthria? How is it produced?

Ans: Difficulty/inability to articulate properly is called *dysarthria*.

It is produced by disarticulation of different structures, e.g. lips, tongue, pharynx, palate, larynx and expiratory muscles.

Q. How would you test different structures responsible for articulation?

Ans: How to test the articulation has been described already.

The different structures responsible for articulation are tested as follows:

1. *Lips:* Ask the patient to say "me, me, me"
2. *Tongue:* Ask the patient to say "La, La, La"
3. *Pharynx:* Ask the patient to say "kuh, gut"
4. *Palate, larynx and expiratory muscles.* Ask the patient to pronounce 'ah'

Q. What are the causes of dysarthria?

Ans:
- Stutter
- Lower cranial nerves (9th, 10th and 11th) palsy, bilateral Bell's palsy
- Pseudobulbar palsy (monotonous, high pitched speech)
- Progressive bulbar paralysis (nasal or bleating character of speech)
- Cerebellar disease, e.g. scanning or staccato speech
- Parkinsonism (slow, slurred, quiet and monotonous speech)

Q. What are the various components of speech and their disturbance?

Ans:
1. Phonation—disturbance is called *dysphonia*
2. Articulation—disturbance is called *dysarthria*
3. Language—disturbance is called *dysphasia*

122

Pseudobulbar Palsy

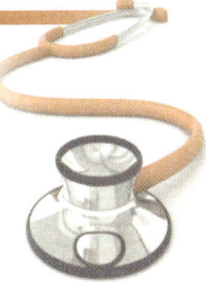

INSTRUCTION

- Examine the patient's cranial nerves
- Perform appropriate neurological examination

SALIENT FEATURES

- Patient complains of speech disturbance

HISTORY

Ask for the following:

- Difficulty in swallowing and nasal regurgitation
- Abnormal speech (dysarthria)
- Emotional changes
- Cough and chocking during swallowing
- Excessive salivation

EXAMINATION

Neurological Examination

- Higher mental function
- Emotional lability:
    i. Inappropriate laughing and crying
    ii. Irritability
    iii. Uncontrolled anger
- *Speech:* There is dysarthria with indistinct voice (Donald Dutch Speech)

Cranial Nerves Examination

- Cranial nerves from Ist to 8th are normal
- Test the lower cranial nerves
    I. *Test the IX, X and XI cranial nerves* (Read case discussion on Jugular foramen syndrome)
    II. *Testing the 12th cranial nerves*
        - Tongue is small, stiff and spastic and shrivelled up
        - The movements of the tongue are restricted (in this case)

Motor System Examination

- Increased tone bilaterally (hypertonia present)
- Tendon jerks are exaggerated (in this case)
- Planters are bilateral extensor

- Superficial reflexes are absent
- Jaw jerk is exaggerated

These signs indicate bilateral corticospinal involvement above the medulla.

PROVISIONAL DIAGNOSIS

The patient has pseudobulbar palsy (lesion) caused by bilateral cerebrovascular accident (aetiology). Patient is emotionally labile (functional status).

QUESTIONS AND ANSWERS

Q. **What are the points in favour of your diagnosis?**

Ans: *Points are:*
- Old age
- Supranuclear ninth, tenth, eleventh and twelfth nerve palsy (gag reflex, palatal reflex are present. Jaw jerk is exaggerated)
- Emotional lability
- Bilateral upper motor neuron signs

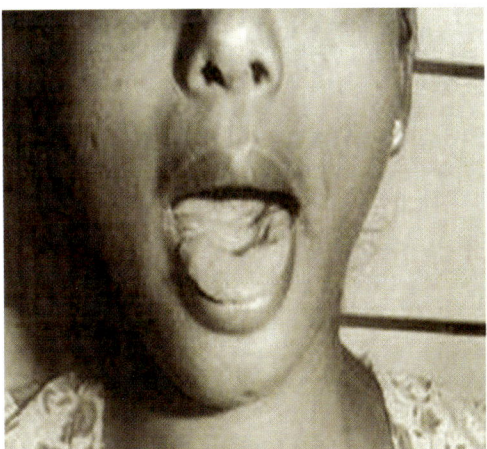

Fig. 122.1: Pseudobulbar palsy

Q.   Where is the site of lesion in pseudobulbar palsy?

Ans: Bilateral internal capsule/cortex

Q.   What are the causes of pseudobulbar palsy?

Ans: 1. Double hemiplegia (stroke)
2. Multiple sclerosis
3. Motor neuron disease
4. Creutzfeldt-Jakob disease

Q.   What are the differences between Bulbar and pseudobulbar palsy?

Ans: Read Table 122.1.

Q.   How would you manage the swallowing and speech difficulties?

Ans: The patient would usually require initial assessment by speech therapist and then appropriate speech therapy will be advised.

For swallowing difficulty, barium swallow with videofluoroscopy should be done for visualizing the swallowing. Patient is advised to take small bites of liquid/semisolid food and swallow it with gravity in sitting position.

Q.   How would you control emotional lability?

Ans: There is no specific treatment, but a combination of dextromethorphan and quinidine improves symptoms and quality of life in patients with emotional lability.

Q.   What do you mean by CADASIL?

Ans: CADASIL (cerebral autosomal dominant arteriopathy with subcortical infarcts and leukoencephalopathy) is a common heritable cause of vascular dementia and stroke in adults. These patients have early onset of stroke, increased frequency of migraine with aura and variable pattern of ischemia of white matter on MRI.

NOTCH 3 (Notch homolog 3), the gene involved in CADASIL, encodes the transmembrane receptor expressed in arterial smooth muscle cells.

Table 122.1: Difference between Bulbar and Pseudobulbar Palsy

Bulbar Palsy	Pseudobulbar Palsy
• Rare	• Common
• LMN type of paralysis of palatal, pharyngeal and tongue muscles	• UMN type of paralysis leading to loss of voluntary palatal, pharyngeal and tongue movements
• The muscles are atrophic and hypotonic	• The muscles tone is increased (spastic)
• It may be unilateral or bilateral	• It is bilateral
• Gag reflex and palatal reflex are lost	• Gag reflex and palatal reflexes are preserved
• Tongue is atrophic, motionless	• Tongue is spastic (e.g. small with poor movements)
• Dysphonia, dysphagia and dysarthria are common symptoms	• Spastic dysarthria with indistinct voice
• Nasal regurgitation prominent	• Not prominent
• Jaw jerk absent	• Jaw jerk exaggerated (a cardinal diagnostic sign)
• No emotional change	• Emotional lability (inappropriate laughing or crying)
• Site of lesion is medulla oblongata	• Site is lesion is in both cerebral hemispheres
• Causes, i.e. medullary infarction, MND, syringobulbia, myasthenia, GB syndrome, poliomyelitis, vasculitis, brainstem glioma or meningitis	• Causes, i.e. bilateral hemispherical infarction, MND, multiple sclerosis, high brainstem tumor

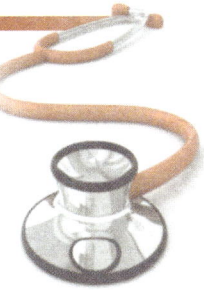

123

Bulbar Palsy

INSTRUCTION

- Examine the cranial nerves
- Perform brief relevant neurological examination

SALIENT FEATURES

- Abnormal speech, nasal regurgitation

HISTORY

The symptoms and signs of pseudobulbar and bulbar are same, hence **ask the following**:
- Nasal regurgitation and difficulty in swallowing
- Coughing and chocking on swallowing of liquids
- Difficulty in chewing
- Abnormal speech, e.g. dysarthria or drunken speech

EXAMINATION

Neurological Examination

- Higher mental functions (normal)
- Speech: normal/abnormal (in this case)
- Testing of the bulbar cranial nerves
  - I. *Ninth, tenth and eleventh*
    - Weakness of soft palate. Ask the patient to pronounce 'aah'
    - There is accumulation of saliva and vocal cord movements are absent
    - Palatal and gag reflex are absent (in this case)
  - II. *Testing of the XII cranial nerve*
    - Tongue is lying motionless in the mouth
    - On protrusion, tongue deviates to paralysed side in unilateral bulbar palsy (Fig. 123.1), lies motionless in bilateral palsy
    - Tongue is flaccid and wasted on the side involved (present)
    - Fasciculations in the tongue may be present
    - Movements of the tongue absent
  - III. *Motor System Examination*
    - There will be signs of lower motor neuron paralysis, i.e.

- Fasciculations of trunk and hands
- Absent tendon jerks
- Jaw jerk is absent

  IV. *Sensory System*
  Check for sensations especially dissociated anaesthesia (syringobulbia as a cause of bulbar paralysis)

PROVISIONAL DIAGNOSIS

The patient has progressive bulbar palsy (lesion) caused by motor neuron disease (aetiology) and has troublesome dysphagia (functional status).

QUESTIONS AND ANSWERS

Q. **What is bulbar paralysis?**
Ans: The involvement of motor nuclei of lower cranial nerves (IX to XII) leading to their paralysis is called *bulbar palsy*.

Q. **What are the characteristics of bulbar palsy?**
Ans: Read the differences between the bulbar and pseudobulbar palsy (case discussion on pseudobulbar palsy).

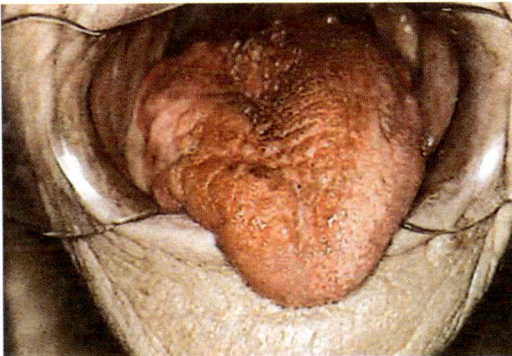

Fig. 123.1: Bulbur palsy. Note wasting of right side of tongue in unilateral bulbar palsy

Q.   What are the causes of bulbar palsy?

Ans: 1. Motor neuron disease
2. Guillain-Barre syndrome (Cranial polyneuritis)
3. Syringobulbia
4. Poliomyelitis
5. Nasopharyngeal cancer
6. Neurosyphilis
7. Neurosarcoidosis
8. Neurotuberculosis
9. Basilar meningitis

Q.   What are the causes of multiple cranial nerves palsy?

Ans: • Cranial polyneuritis (Guillain-Barre syndrome)
• Multiple sclerosis
• Motor neuron disease
• Meningitis/Meningoencephalitis
• Neurosarcoidosis

124

Myotonia Dystrophica

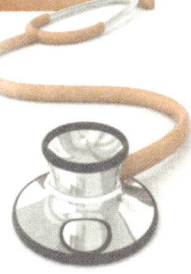

INSTRUCTION

- Examine the nervous system

SALIENT FEATURES

- Depressed look expressionless face and muscle weakness

HISTORY

Ask for the following:

- Onset is usually in middle age, i.e. 3rd or 4th decade. If the mother is carrier, then weakness manifests during infancy and progresses fast.
- Is there any difficulty in releasing the grip? Is there any difficulty in kicking the ball
- History of progressive distal muscle weakness
- History of falls (Pseudo-drop attacks) due to proximal muscles weakness
- History of dysphagia (present)
- History of impotence
- History of recurrent pulmonary infections
- History of sleep disturbance (day time sleep, but bar somnolence is common)
- History of diabetes

EXAMINATION

General Physical Examination

- Note for frontal baldness (Fig. 124.1)
- Note difficulty in opening the eye after closure
- Note the ptosis (bilateral present), cataract or any surgery for cataract
- Note expressionless face (hatchet face) and swan neck due to thinning of neck muscles (Fig. 124.1)

Neurological Examination

- Test higher mental function for IQ.
- Release of hand grip while shaking hand. Note the slow release of handgrip (present)
- Note weakness of sternomastoids. Test them
- Examine for wasting of distal muscles of upper limbs

- Elicit percussion myotonia over thenar muscles and tongue (if possible). Not the pit which slowly and slowly resolves
- Elicit deep tendon jerks. They are depressed due to hypotonia (present)

Other System Examination

- Examine the breasts for gynecomastia and testes for atrophy (present)

PROVISIONAL DIAGNOSIS

The patient has myotonia dystrophia (lesion) which is an inherited disorder (etiology). He has dysphagia and severe muscle weakness (functional status).

QUESTIONS AND ANSWERS

Q. What are the points in favor of your diagnosis?

Ans: 1. Adult patient
2. Slow onset of symptoms
3. Frontal boldness, bilateral ptosis
4. Expressionless face (hatchad face)

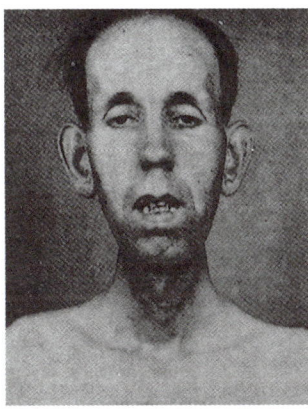

Fig. 124.1: Myotonia dystrophica. Note the frontal baldness, abnormal facial appearance and dysarthria

5. Swan-neck (wasting of neck muscles)
6. Percussion myotonia test positive
7. Testicular atrophy (hypogonadism)

Q. What is myotonia? What are its type?

Ans: Myotonia is defined as continued muscle contractions with poor relaxation after the cessation of voluntary effort. Myotonias are inherited disorders (autosomal dominant).

The inherited rare types of myotonias are:
1. Myotonia dystrophica
2. Myotonia congenital (Thomsen's disease)
3. Proximal myotonic myopathy. It is characterized by myotonia in middle aged persons with proximal muscle weakness and cataract. It is also inherited as autosomal dominant.

Q. What is inheritance of this condition?

Ans:
- Autosomal dominant inheritance
- Defect located on chromosome 19
- There is dynamic mutation with increased number of triplet repeats (AGC repeats)
- The repeat size typically increases from generation to generation providing a molecular basis for the clinical phenomenon of anticipation.

Q. Name some diseases known to be associated with increased number of triplet repeats?

Ans:
- Huntington's chorea
- Myotonic muscular dystrophy
- Spinocerebellar ataxias type 1 to 3
- Fragile syndrome
- Hereditary dentatorubral pallidoluysian atrophy (DRPLA).

Q. What are the clinical characteristics of dystrophia myotonica (mytonia dystrophica)?

Ans: It is an autosomal dominant condition characterized by:
- Late age of onset (20–50 years).
- Progressive distal muscle weakness.
- Bilateral ptosis.
- "*Hatchet-face appearance*" due to atrophy of temporalis, masseter, sternomastoid and facial muscles (Fig. 124.1).
- Dysarthria due to weakness of palatal, pharyngeal and tongue muscles.
- Myotonia can be demonstrated by percussion over the tongue, thenar eminence and wrist extensor muscles. There is delayed handgrip relaxaion.

Other features
- Frontal baldness
- Cataract (stellate)
- Mental retardation
- Cardiomyopathy and conduction defects
- Hypogonadism and small pituitary fossa
- Glucose intolerance
- Low serum IgG leading to respiratory infections
- Somnolence
- Occasionally external ophthalmoplegia.

Q. How will you demonstrate myotonia at the bed side?

Ans: The methods of demonstration are:
1. *Hand grip:* There is poor relaxation of hand grip during shaking hand with the patient.
2. *Percussion:* Percussion over the thenar eminence or tongue produces a dimple which disappears (relaxes) slowly.
3. *Slow relaxation of eye after closure:* Ask the patient to close the eyes forcibly and now ask him to open the eyes. The patient opens the eyes slower than normal.

Q. How will you investigate such a case?

Ans: Investigations are:
- *Serum CK level:* It may be normal or mildly elevated.
- *EMG (electromyography):* It is diagnostic, shows high frequency waxing and waning discharges and a myopathic pattern.
- *Muscle biopsy:* It shows type I fibers with increased numbers of central nuclei, ring fibers and sarcolemmal masses.

Q. Name the drugs useful in myotonia.

Ans: Drugs used in myotonia are:
- Phenytoin
- Quinine
- Procainamide
- Mexiletine

Q. Which myopathies produce distal weakness and wasting of muscles?

Ans:
- Myotonic dystrophy
- Welander's distal myopathy

Q. What tests would you perform on patient's sister if she asks about risks to her offspring?

Ans:
- Clinical evaluation
- Slit lamp examination for cataract
- EMG

Q. What are the characteristic EMG findings in myotonia?

Ans: Waxing and wanning of the potentials called "*dive bomber effect*". The EMG changes can be recorded in any muscle.

Q. What would you advise if patient had undergone major surgery?

Ans: These patients of dystrophic myotonia tolerate the anesthesia poorly due to impaired cardiorespiratory function, hence, they need intensive postoperative observation.

Q. How would you treat myotonia dystrophica?

Ans:
- Footdrop is controlled by caliper or moulded-foot arthroses.
- Myotonia, when disabling may respond to drugs described above
- Advanced heart block with or without syncope need pacemaker insertion.

125

Myotonia Congenital

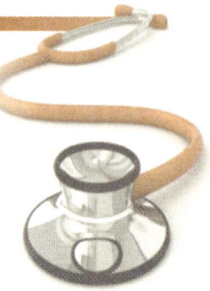

INSTRUCTION

- Examine nervous system

SALIENT FEATURES

- Difuse muscle hypertrophy (Fig. 125.1)

HISTORY

Ask for the following:

- Age of onset and progression of the disease
- Seasonal variation in the symptoms
- Family history of the disease
- Repeated respiratory infection

EXAMINATION

Neurological Examination

- Note the cry and facial muscles weakness

- Examine the muscles. There is diffuse muscles hypertrophy.
- Shake the hand with the patient (Note the relaxation of the grip) (slow relaxation Fig. 125.2).
- Elicit the warm-up phenomenon (present). Ask the patient to clinch and release your fingers repeatedly. Myotonia decreases or even vanishes completely when repeating the movements several times.

Tests

- Elicit signs of myotonia by hand grip (Fig. 125.2), percussion of thenar eminence or thighs (Fig. 125.1B) and opening the eyes after closure.
- Elicit the tendon jerks.

PROVISIONAL DIAGNOSIS

The diffuse muscle hypertrophy in a child with features of myotonia indicate myotonia congenita

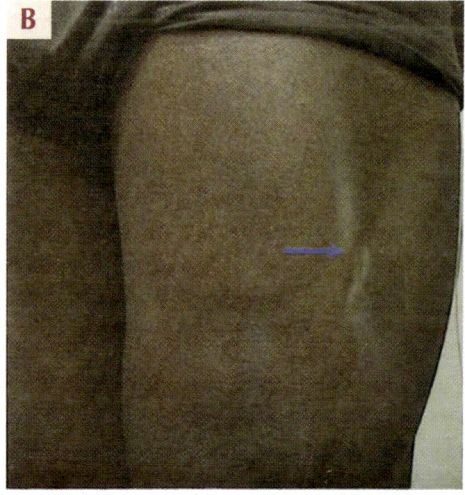

Dimple (→) after percussion of hypertrophied thigh muscles that returns to normal level slowly

Fig. 125.1: Myotonia congenita. (A) Hypertrophy of biceps and forearm muscles; (B) Percussion myotonia in thigh

(lesion) caused by autosomal dominant diseases called *Thompson's disease* (aetiology).

QUESTIONS AND ANSWERS

Q.   **What are the points in favor of your diagnosis?**

Ans: 1. An adolescent patient
2. Diffuse muscle hypertrophy since childhood
3. History of repeated chest infections during infancy
4. All the signs of myotonia (e.g slow relaxation of hand grip, percussion myotonia, disappearance of myotonia on repeated movements) are present

Q.   **What is myotonia congenita?**

Ans: This is also an autosomal dominant disorder, milder form occurs in childhood and persists throughout life. Severe form occurs in infants of affected mothers and characterised by perculiar cry, facial and bulbar muscles weakness, respiratory insufficiency and mental retardation.

This myotonia is accentuated by rest, cold and is more noticeable on starting the activity following prolonged rest. There may be diffuse hypertrophy of the muscles. Strength is well preserved. Myotonia may be apparent on shaking hands with the person.

Q.   **When does the muscle hypertrophy manifest?**

Ans: During adulthood (2nd decade Fig. 125.2).

Q.   **What is the cause of muscular hypertrophy?**

Ans: Continued isometric exercise during childhood.

Q.   **What is the life expectancy in this disease?**

Ans: Normal life expectancy.

Q.   **What is the cause of death?**

Ans: Repeated chest infections leading to respiratory failure.

Q.   **Which drugs are used for myotonia?**

Ans: Quinidine, Procainamide

Q.   **What is genetic inheritance of this disease?**

Ans: The disorder may be transmitted by autosomal dominant or recessive trait. Myotonia congenita is a specific inherited disorder of muscle membrane hyperexcitability caused by reduced chloride conductance in sarcolemma as a result of mutations of the gene encoding the skeletal muscle chloride channel CIC-I.

Q.   **Name the conditions associated with myotonia.**

Ans: 1. Myotonia dystrophica (already discussed)
2. Myotonia congenita
3. Paramyotonia (sodium channel conductance disturbance)
4. Hyperkalemic periodic paralysis with myotonia (potassium channel aggravated myotonia)
5. Drug induced myotonia, e.g. colchicine, clofibrate
6. Certain myopathies (myotubular, acid maltase deficiency)
7. Polymyositis

Q.   **How would you recognise the disease in an infant?**

Ans: It is recognised by:
1. Peculiar cry
2. Difficulty in feeding
3. Inability to reopen the eyes after face wash

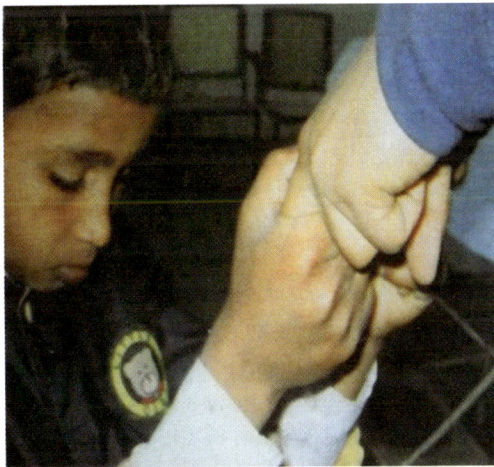

Fig. 125.2: Myotonia congenita. There is difficulty in relaxation of hand grip

126

Duchenne Muscular Dystrophy

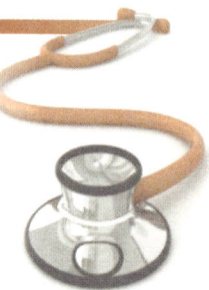

INSTRUCTION

- Examine the motor system of the patient

SALIENT FEATURES

- Difficulty in running during playing

HISTORY

Ask for the following:

- Age of onset and progression
- Difficulty in standing from the sitting position (Fig. 126.1)
- Family history
- History of dyspnea, palpitations, etc. (cardiomyopathy)
- History of mental retardation

EXAMINATION

Motor System Examination

- Test the proximal muscles for weakness (the proximal muscles involved in this case, Fig. 126.2) Gower's sign is positive.

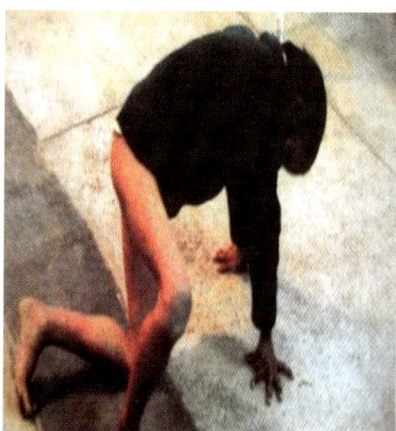

Fig. 126.1: Duchenne muscular dystrophy (positive Gower's sign)

- There is loss of tendon reflexes in the lower limbs
- Note the pseudohypertrophy of the calf, if present (Becker's muscle dystrophy). There is hypotonia inspite of increased bulk of the muscles (present).
- Kyphoscoliosis
- Facial muscle weakness, if present
- Sensory system is normal

PROVISIONAL DIAGNOSIS

This patient has primary muscular disorder, i.e. myopathy (lesion) caused by an X-linked Duchenne muscular dystrophy (etiology). Patient finds difficulty in running and playing, and routine activity (functional status).

QUESTIONS AND ANSWERS

Q. What are the points in favor of your diagnosis?
Ans:
- A young patient (fig inset)
- Slow onset and progressive weakness of legs
- Muscle bulk of the calves is increased (pseudohypertrophy of calves)
- Gower's sign is positive due to proximal muscle weakness (Fig. 126.1)
- Loss of tandon reflexes in lower limbs
- Positive family history

Q. What are the features of Duchenne muscle dystrophy not present in your case?
Ans:
- Mental retardation and cardiomyopathy
- Kyphoscoliosis, repeated chest infection

Q. What is myopathy?
Ans: Myopathy (muscular dystrophy) is defined as genetically determined primary degeneration of muscle fibers without an evidence of involvement of central or peripheral nervous system.

Q. How do you classify myopathies?
Ans: The myopathy being heredofamilial disorders are classified on the basis of inheritance as follows:

I. **X-linked**
- *Duchenne type* (severe type of pseu-dohypertrophic muscular dystrophy)
- *Becker type* (milder form with pseu-dohypertrophy)

II. **Autosomal dominant**
- *Limbs girdle* (e.g. scapulohumeral or pelvi-femoral)
- *Congenital* muscular dystrophy

III. **Autosomal dominant**
- *Facioscapulohumeral* (Landouzy-Dejerine type)
- *Scapuloperoneal*
- *Oculopharyngeal or ocular*
- *Distal myopathy*

Q. **What are the characteristic features of Duchenne type of muscular dystrophy?**

Ans: A male child may present with difficulty in climbing stairs and difficulty in getting up from sitting position (Fig. 126.1). Other features are:
- Positive family history
- Slow onset and progressive disease
- Mental retardation (may be present)
- Positive Gower's sign
- Pseudohypertrophy of the calves and atrophy of other limb muscles
- Lower limbs jerks may be normal or diminished
- Normal sensory system and sphincter control
- No fasciculations
- Waddling gait may be present

Q. **Which muscles are not involved in Duchenne muscle dystrophy?**

Ans: Facial and small muscles of hand.

Q. **What is Gower's sign? What are the conditions in which Gower's sign is positive?**

Ans: When the patient is asked to stand from lying down, he adopts a peculiar manner of rising called *Gower's rising sign or Gower's sign.* To demonstrate this sign, the patient (child) is asked to sit on the floor and then rise. In rising from the floor, the affected child gets up first on his hands and knees, brings the legs close to the arms, then "climbs up" the legs to the erect position.
Significance: This sign indicates just the proximal (pelvic girdle) muscle weakness, hence, is not specific for Duchenne muscular dystrophy (DMD). It may be present in following conditions:
- Proximal myopathy involving legs (pelvic girdle) due to any cause
- Myasthenia gravis with proximal limb muscles involvement

- Polymyositis
- Spinal muscular dystrophy
- Endocrinal myopathy

Q. **What type of cardiomyopathy occurs in Duchenne muscle dystrophy?**

Ans: Hypertrophic cardiomyopathy characterised by hypertrophy of the chambers, arrhythmias, conduction disturbance and congestive heart failure.

Q. **What is the role of skipping of antisense mediated exon in Duchenne muscle dystrophy?**

Ans: The skipping of antisense mediated exon induces dystrophin synthesis in selected patient of Duchenne myopathy. The skipping of additional exon restores the reading frame of the mRNA, allowing new production of dystrophin. The new dystrophin produced is not normal, but retains considerable function.

Q. **What is the role of stem cell transplantation in degenerative muscular disorder?**

Ans: Myogenic stem cell transplant in the experimental animals has been found effective and successful. When purified, these precursor cells were engrafted into the muscle of dystrophin–deficient mdx mice and were found to restore 94% dystrophin expression and significantly improved the muscle histology and muscle contractile function. Transplanted skeletal muscle precursors also entered the satellite cell compartment, renewed the endogenous stem cell pool and participated in subsequent rounds of injury repair.

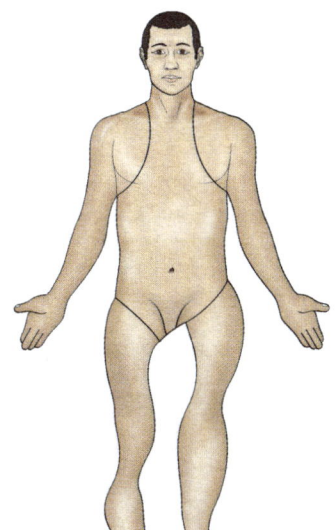

Fig. 126.2: Pattern of distribution of muscle dystrophy

127

Becker's Muscular Dystrophy

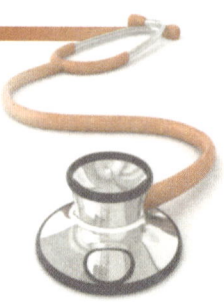

INSTRUCTION

• Examine the motor system of the patient

SALIENT FEATURES

• Progressive muscular weakness

HISTORY

Ask for the following:

• Age of onset (i.e. adult)
• Progression of the muscular weakness
• Difficulty in standing from sitting position (present)
• Family history
• Mental retardation
• Kyphoscoliosis
• Respiratory infections/involvement
• History of breathlessness/palpitations

EXAMINATION

Motor System Examination

• It is similar to Duchenne type of muscle dystrophy

PROVISIONAL DIAGNOSIS

The young patient has proximal muscle weakness (Fig. 127.1B) and pseudohypertrophy of the calves (Fig. 127.1A) caused by Becker's muscular dystrophy (etiology). The patient has mild disability and condition is usually progressive (functional status).

QUESTIONS AND ANSWERS

Q. **What are the differences between two common X-linked muscular dystrophies?**

Ans: The difference between two common X-linked muscular dystrophy, i.e. Duchenne and Becker's muscular dystrophy are listed in Table 127.1.

Q. **What are the difference between true hypertrophy and pseudohypertrophy of muscles?**

Ans: Read Table 127.2.

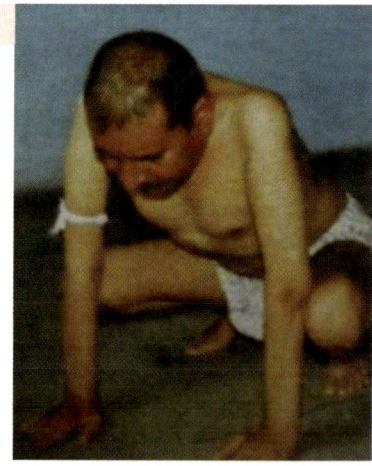

Fig. 127.1: Becker's muscular dystrophy. (A) Pseudohypertrophy of calf muscles; (B) Positive Gower's sign. Patient demonstrating this sign.

Table 127.1: Duchenne vs Becker's muscular dystrophy

	Duchenne type	Becker type
• Age of onset	• Infancy or childhood	• Adolescence or adult onset
• Severity	• Severe	• Mild
• Mental retardation	• Common	• Uncommon
• Cardiomyopathy and ECG abnormalities	• Common	• Uncommon
• Kyphoscoliosis	• Common	• Uncommon
• Respiratory involvement	• Early	• Late
• Prognosis	• Death occurs before second decade	• Death beyond second decade

Table 127.2: Pseudohypertrophy vs true hypertrophy

Pseudohypertrophy	True hypertrophy
• Muscle bulk is due to deposition of fibrofatty tissue	Muscle bulk is due to increase in muscle mass
• Muscles are doughy to feel (elasticity is lost)	Muscles are soft and elastic
• Muscles are firm and globular on contraction	Muscles are hard and globular on contraction
• The muscles are weak and hypotonic in spite of bulky size	The muscles are stronger than normal
• Muscles showing pseudohypertrophy are, calf muscles, glutei, quadriceps, deltoids and infraspinati. Tongue muscles may be involved	Muscles showing true hypertrophy include calf muscles or glutei and quadriceps. Tongue muscles not involved

Q. **What are the similarities between Duchenne and Becker's muscle dystrophy?**

Ans: Similarities are:
- Both are X-linked (mutation of dystrophin gene), progressive myopathies
- Positive family history
- Positive Gower's sign
- Presence of pseudohypertrophy
- EMG and muscle biopsy findings
- Treatment protocol similar

Q. **What are the causes of true hypertrophy of the calves muscles?**

Ans: Causes are:
- Laborers (manual hard work)
- Athletes
- Myotonia
- Cysticercosis in the muscles
- Hypertrophic musculorum vera (a rare inherited muscle disorder)

Q. **What are the causes of pseudohypertrophy of muscles?**

Ans: Causes are:
- Duchenne muscular dystrophy (DMD)
- Myxoedema (hypothyroidism)
- Glycogen storage disease
- Trichinosis

Q. **Name some other X-linked myopathy?**

Ans:
- X-linked tubular myopathy
- Emergy-Dreifuss muscular dystrophy. It presents in early childhood and is slowly progressive. Initially it has humeral-peroneal pattern of muscle involvement.

Q. **Is there any genetic difference between Duchenne and Becker's muscle dystrophy?**

Ans: No, Both Duchenne and Becker's muscular dystrophy are caused by mutation in the same gene located on the chromosome 21. Dystrophin is the muscle protein product which is absent in Duchenne dystrophy, but is reduced in amount in Becker's muscular dystrophy.

Q. **How would you confirm your diagnosis?**

Ans: Confirmation of both Duchenne and Becker's dystrophy is done by western blot analysis of muscle biopsy specimen demonstrating the abnormal or reduced dystrophin.

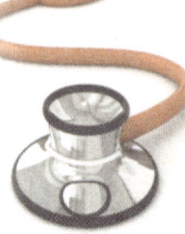

128

Fascioscapulohumeral Dystrophy

INSTRUCTION

- Examine the motor system and cranial nerves of this patient

SALIENT FEATURES

- Difficulty in putting the things on the shelf.

HISTORY

Ask for the following:

- Age of onset and pattern of muscles involvement
- Family history of such weakness
- History of weakness of shoulder muscles leading to difficulty in lifting the shoulder, coombing, difficulty to put or remove the things from shelf
- History of sleep apnoea/snoring during sleep

EXAMINATION

Cranial Nerve Examination

- All cranial nerves are normal

Motor System Examination

Following abnormalities have been noted;

- Ptosis
- Difficulty in closing the eyes
- Dull expressionless face (mask-like face) due to facial weakness
- Inability to whistle
- Inability to blow out the cheeks
- Dysarthria due to difficulty in articultation of speech

Proceed to test the muscles as follows:

1. Test the shoulder girdle muscles (Fig. 128.1). Read the clinical methods to test the muscles. Following abnormalities may be noticed.
   - Winging of the scapula (present)
   - Pectorals and trapezii are severely affected
   - Weakness of biceps and triceps (present)
   - True hypertrophy of deltoids to compensate other shoulder muscles

- Upper limb jerks, i.e. biceps and triceps are absent. Supinator jerk is present (in this case)
2. Test the Trunk muscles
   - Perform the Beevor's sign by asking the patient to raise the trunk or flex the neck in a lying down position. Note the movement of the umbilicus (Read the clinical methods by Prof. SN Chugh).

     Lower abdominal muscle are weak in this muscle dystrophy with the result, there is upward movement of the umbilicus (present).
3. Test for the hearing loss
4. Look for retinal telangiectasia

PROVISIONAL DIAGNOSIS

The patient has facial as well as shoulder girdle muscle weakness (lesion) caused by fascioscapulohumeral dystrophy (etiology). Patient finds difficulty in combing the hairs and performing other routine activites (functional status).

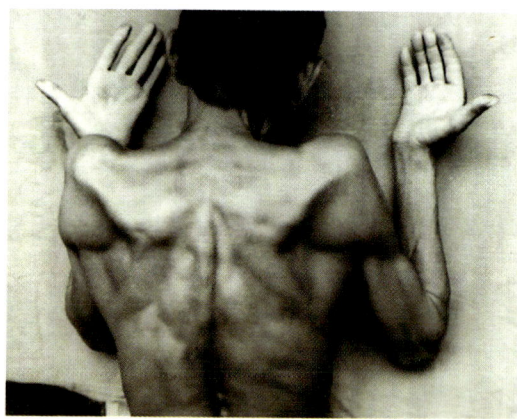

Fig. 128.1: Fascioscapulohumeral myopathy. Note the wasting of shoulder girdle muscles leading to winging of scapulae

QUESTIONS AND ANSWERS

Q. **What are the points in favor of your diagnosis?**

Ans: All the characteristics of fascioscapulohumeral myopathy are present (Read Table 128.1)

Q. **What is the mode of inheritance in this myopathy?**

Ans: It is transmitted by autosomal dominance inheritance. Both sexes are equally affected. The gene is located on the chromosome 4.

Q. **What is the age of onset of this disorder?**

Ans: Between 10 and 40 years of age.

Q. **Is there a mental retardation is this case?**

Ans: No. IQ is normal.

Q. **What are the characteristics of fascioscapulohumeral myopathy? How does it differ from limb girdle myopathy?**

Ans: The differences are given in Table 128.1:

Table 103.2: Fascioscapulohumeral vs limb girdle myopathy	
Fascioscapulohumeral myopathy	*Limb girdle myopathy*
1. *Face* is involved, e.g. ptosis, difficulty in closing the eyes, marked facial weakness leading to expressionless face with lips open. There is difficulty in whisting and puffing out the cheeks, examine all these features	1. Face is not involved
2. Neck muscles including sternomastoids are weak	2. No involvement of neck muscles
3. Shoulder girdle is weak: • Winging of the scapula • Lower pectoralis and trapezii are wasted • Wasting of triceps and biceps • True hypertrophy of deltoids to compensate other muscles • Absent biceps and triceps jerk	3. *Upper limbs:* • Biceps, brachioradialis and wrist extensors are involved • Deltoids may show pseudohypertrophy *Lower limbs:* • Initially hip flexors and glutei are weak • Wasting of quadriceps and tibialis anterior • Lateral quadriceps and calves may show hypertrophy

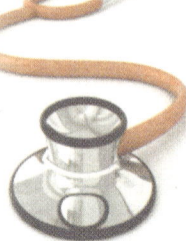

129

Proximal (Limb Girdle) Myopathy

INSTRUCTION

- Examine the motor system

SALIENT FEATURES

- Difficulty in running and playing

HISTORY

Ask for the following:

- Age of onset
- Pattern of muscles of the limbs involvement (Fig. 129.1)
- Progression of muscle weakness. Weakness may remain confined to girdle muscles for years before peripheral weakness and wasting occur
- Difficulty in running and playing (present)
- Difficulty in putting or removing the things from the shelf (present)

EXAMINATION

Motor System Examination

I. Examine upper limbs (upper girdle) muscles, i.e.

- Biceps, triceps, brachioradialis are involved late (present). Wrist extensors are involved first when the wrist is involved.
- Deltoids are spared. They may even show compensatory hypertrophy.

II. Examine lower limbs (lower girdle) muscles

- Test hip muscles. Glutei and hip flexors are weak (in this case).
- Test thigh muscles. Quadriceps and tibialis anterior are weak.
- Calves muscles may show pseudohypertrophy.
- Face is never affected.

  N.B For individual muscles testing, read "Clinical Methods in Medicine" by Prof SN Chugh

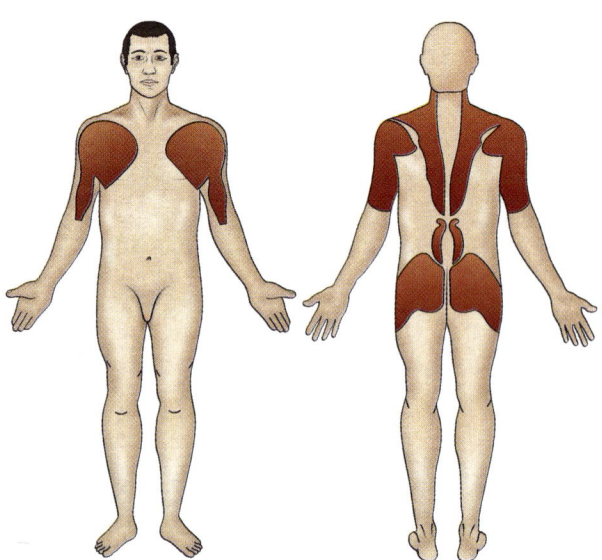

Fig. 129.1: Pattern of weakness in limb-girdle dystrophy

PROVISIONAL DIAGNOSIS

The weakness of proximal muscles of arm, shoulder, hips and legs (lesion) is caused by limbs girdle myopathy (etiology). The weakness is stationary (functional status)

QUESTIONS AND ANSWERS

Q. **What is limb girdle myopathy?**

Ans: Limb girdle myopathy transmitted as autosomal dominant or recessive inheritance, is characterized by muscle weakness of pelvic and shoulder girdle muscles (Fig. 129.1). It affects both males and females in the age group of 10–30 years. Diaphragm may be involved producing respiratory insufficiency. The disease is progressive and varies from family to family. Cardiac involvement (cardiomyopathy) may lead to CHF or arrhythmias. CK levels are elevated. EMG and muscle biopsy reveal myopathic pattern.

Q. **What is the common mode of inheritance?**

Ans: It is commonly transmitted by autosomal recessive manner. Both sexes are equally affected. Recently limb girdle myopathy has been identified to be transmitted by autosomal dominant (type 1) and autosomal recessive (type 2) manner. Many further subtypes of both recessive and dominant types have been reported. In four of limb girdle recessive myopathy, mutations affecting the sarcoglycan complex of proteins have been identified. *Dysferlin* is a sarcolemmal protein and its deficiency causes proximal and distal form of recessively inherited muscular dystrophies.

Q. **What is the age of onset?**
Ans: Between 10 and 30 years.

Q. **Is mental retardation present.**
Ans: No. IQ is normal.

Q. **Do the facial muscles involved?**
Ans: No. Face is spared.

Q. **What is the expected life span?**
Ans: Life span is normal.

Q. **How will you investigate a case of myopathy?**
Ans: Following investigations are helpful:
- *CK (creatinine kinase) enzyme serial estimation.* The levels are increased.
- *EMG* shows myopathic pattern.
- *Muscle biopsy confirm the diagnosis* by showing changes of muscle degeneration and regeneration without any cellular infiltration. There is decreased level of dystrophin in the muscles demonstrated by immunochemical staining (*Western blot*).

Q. **What are the causes of proximal muscle weakness?**
Ans: The causes of proximal muscle weakness (myopathy) are:
- Muscular dystrophies
- Collagen vascular disorders, e.g. polymyositis
- Diabetic amyotrophy
- Endocrinal myopathy, e.g. Cushing's syndrome, thyrotoxicosis
- Metabolic myopathies, e.g. hypokalemic
- Porphyria
- Guillain-Barré syndrome
- Myasthenic-myopathic syndrome
- Drug-induced, i.e. steroid, triamcinolone
- Paraneoplastic syndrome
- Osteomalacia

130

Winging of the Scapulae

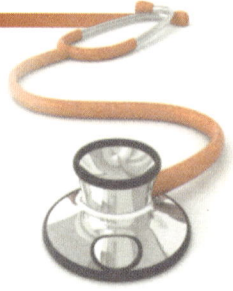

INSTRUCTION

* Look at the back of the patient. Examine the motor system.

SALIENT FEATURES

* Weakness of upper limbs

HISTORY

Ask for the following:

* Difficulty in combing, putting or removing the things from the shelf above the head
* Winging of the scapulae (scapulae are lifted off the chest) or a scapula

EXAMINATION

Motor System Examination

* Note the winging of the scapulae or a scapula
* Difficulty in raising the limbs above the head when asked to do so
* Ask the patient to push the wall with outstretched hands; check whether winging becomes prominent or not (become prominent in this case on right side)
* Test the muscles of the arms and legs to rule out muscle dystrophy

PROVISIONAL DIAGNOSIS

The patient has winging of the scapula on one side (lesion) due to palsy of the long thoracic nerve (aetiology).

QUESTIONS AND ANSWERS

Q. **What is winging of a scapula? What are its causes?**

Ans: This is lifting off the scapula from the chest when patient attempts abduction and forward movement, e.g. pressing against a wall in standing position. This is due to weakness of scapular stabilizing muscles, seen in facioscapulohumeral myopathy (*see* **Fig.** 128.1), palsy of long thoracic nerves (C5–C7) in this case (Fig. 130.1), and brachial neuritis.

Q. **Which muscles are weak to produce winging of a scapula?**

Ans: • Serratus anterior
• Trapezius

Q. **How would you differentiate winging caused by serratus anterior weakness from trapezius muscle weakness?**

Ans: In serratus anterior palsy, abduction of the arm laterally produces little winging, whereas winging is intensified due to weakness of trapezius on abduction of arm against resistance.

Q. **What do you know about brachial neuritis?**

Ans: Brachial neuritis (*neuralgic amyotrophy*) often follows an infection or surgery. Initially, patient has pain around the shoulder followed by muscular weakness affecting the shoulder girdle especially deltoid and serratus anterior producing winging of the scapula. Atrophy around the shoulder is prominent feature.

In this syndrome, more than one nerve lesion is involved. Recovery occurs over a period of a year, but may not be complete.

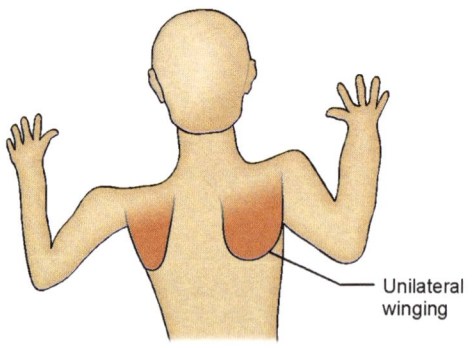

Unilateral winging

Fig. 130.1: Winging of right scapula

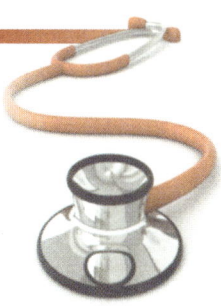

131 — Wasting of Small Muscles of Hands

INSTRUCTION

- Examine the hands of the patient (Fig. 131.1)
- Perform neurological examination

SALIENT FEATURES

- Deformities of the fingers

HISTORY

Ask for the following:

- History of painful small joints (rheumatoid arthritis)
- History of painful neck movement (cervical spondylosis)
- History of weakness of small muscles with fasciculations (flickering or twitchings inside the muscles) due to motor neuron disease
- History of sensory loss in hands (syringomyelia). Note any burn mark if patient is smoker
- Family history of such weakness (Charcot-Marie-Tooth disease)
- Ascending muscle weakness (Guillaine-Barré syndrome)
- History of upper limb trauma (bilateral median and ulnar nerve lesions)

EXAMINATION

Examination of Hands

- Look at the hands, both palm and dorsum. Note the wasting of the thenar and hypothenar muscles on the back. Note the hollowing of dorsum of hand due to wasting of dorsal interossei (Fig. 131.1)
- Look for any deformities of the fingers (present) and swelling
- Look for fasciculations. If not visible, tap the belly of the muscles to evoke them
- Check the sensations over the hands especially index and little fingers
- Test the grip of the hand for muscle strength
- Test for median and ulnar nerve compression
- Test the neck movements

- Ask the patient to perform fine movements with hands, i.e. unbuttoning clothes or ask him to write
- Palpate for the cervical ribs and palpate and compare both the radial pulses
- Look for Horner's syndrome

Examination of Limbs

- There are UMN signs in the lower limbs due to cervical compressive myelopathy

PROVISIONAL DIAGNOSIS

The patient has wasting of the small muscles of hands (Fig. 131.1) with limited cervical movements (lesion) caused by cervical compressive myelopathy (aetiology). He is unable to button his clothes (functional status).

QUESTIONS AND ANSWERS

Q. What are the causes of wasting of the small muscles of the hand (s)?

Ans: The causes are given in Table 131.1.

Table 131.1: Causes of wasting of small muscles of hand (s)

Bilateral wasting	Unilateral wasting
• Rheumatoid arthritis	• Brachial plexus injury
• Old age	• Pancoast tumor
• Cervical myelopathy	• Cervical cord lesion (Brown-Sequard's syndrome)
• Bilateral cervical ribs	• Malignant infiltration of the brachial plexus
• Motor neuron disease	of the brachial plexus
• Syringomyelia	• Thoracic outlet syndrome
• Gullain-Barre syndrome	drome
• Peripheral neuropathy	• Unilateral cervical rib
• Charcot-Marie-Tooth disease	
• Bilateral median and ulnar nerve lesions	

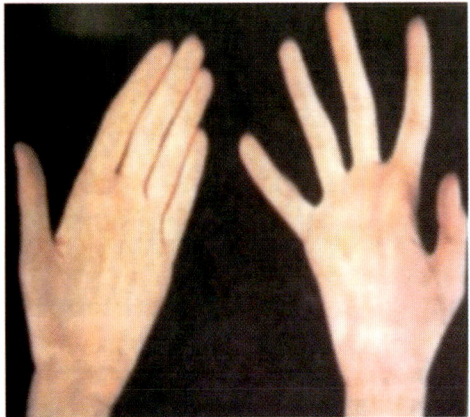

Fig. 131.1: Wasting of small muscles of hands

Q. What roots are involved in wasting of small muscles of hands?

Ans: $C_8 - T_1$

Q. What are the causes of involvement of $C_8 - T_1$ roots?

Ans: • Lesions of radial, median and ulnar nerves
• Brachial plexus trauma
• Cervical spondylosis involving $C_8 - T_1$
• Thoracic outlet syndrome
• Involvement of anterior horn cells of $C_8 - T_1$ by motor neuron disease, spinal cord tumor, syringomyelia, poliomyelitis, etc.)

Q. How do you diagnose a cervical rib clinically?

Ans: The cervical rib is suspected clinically when the patient complains of pain along the ulnar border of the hand and forearm. Examination reveals sensory loss in the distribution of T_1 with wasting of the thenar muscles. Horner's syndrome may occur. The Adson's test is positive.

Q. What is Adson's test?

Ans: *Adson's test:* This is positive in cervical rib and thoracic outlet syndrome. The examiner feels the pulse of sitting patient by standing behind the patient. Now patient is instructed to turn the head on the affected side and asked to take deep breath. The pulse either get diminished or obliterated on the side affected during this maneuver.

Q. Name the muscles of thenar and hypothenar eminence.

Ans: Following are the muscles:

Muscles of thenar eminence	Muscles of hypothenar eminence
• Abductor pollicis brevis	• Abductor digiti minimi
• Flexor pollicis brevis	• Flexor digiti minimi
• Opponens pollicis	• Opponens digiti minimi

Q. What is claw hand? What are its causes?

Ans: Read case discussion on peripheral neuropathy.
Paralysis of interossi and lumbricals produce *claw hand*.

Q. What is wrist drop?

Ans: Read case discussion on peripheral neuropathy.

Q. How will you arrive at the etiological diagnosis of wasting of small muscles of hands?

Ans: History and physical examination will help to find out the cause of wasting of small muscles of hand.
1. *History:* Wasting since childhood is common with poliomyelitis and birth injury (Klumpke's paralysis).
2. Neck pain indicates cervical spondylosis, cervical rib and intra- or extramedullary tumor.
3. Fasciculations with brisk tendon reflexes in the case described above indicate amyotrophy lateral sclerosis.
4. Symmetrical joint involvement suggests rheumatoid arthritis.
5. Trophic changes in hands occur in leprosy, syringomyelia and cervical rib.
6. Thickened ulnar nerve points towards leprosy.
7. Absence of sensory loss indicates motor neuron disease while dissociated sensory loss indicates syringomyelia.
8. Absence of upper limb tendon reflexes with UMN signs in the lower limbs indicate cervical compressive myelopathy (this case)

Q. What are the causes of distal muscle weakness?

Ans: • Distal myopathy of Grower
• Charcoat-Marie-Tooth disease
• Familial polyneuropathy or acquired polyneuropathy
• Myotonia dystrophica

132

Myasthenia Gravis

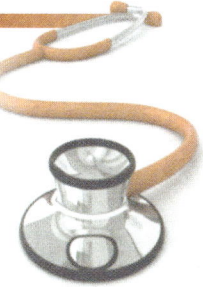

INSTRUCTION

- Examine the nervous system of the patient.

SALIENT FEATURES

- Patient complains of drooping of the eyelids in the evening.

HISTORY

Ask for the following:

- Obtain history of weakness and diplopia at the end of the day (present)
- Is muscle weakness painless and transient? Does it improve with rest and sleep (yes, in this case)?
- Obtain history in details regarding the muscles affected, i.e. difficulty in smiling, difficulty in chewing, speaking, difficulty in holding the neck for long period and difficulty in walking
- Obtain history of thyrotoxicosis, diabetes mellitus, rheumatoid arthritis, SLE and thymoma (mediastinal compression)
- History of drug, e.g. d-penicillamine

EXAMINATION

Neurological Examination

- Look at the eyes for ptosis (present)
- Check the worsening of ptosis after sustained upward gaze for one minute
- Check extraocular muscles for diplopia or squint
- Ask the patient to smile, note the characteristic snarling smile
- Speech is nasal (nasal twang)
- Ask the patient to sip some amount of water, note any nasal regurgitation
- Examine the limbs for weakness, hypotonia, decreased power and reflexes. The limb weakness is proximal and symmetric. Deep tendon reflexes are preserved (in this case)
- Examine the neck muscles. Neck extensors may be weak
- Test for sensations and coordination

PROVISIONAL DIAGNOSIS

The patient has myasthenia gravis (lesion) which is an autoimmune disorder (etiology). Patient is disturbed due to weakness and fatigue (functional status).

Q. **What are the points in favor of your diagnosis?**

Ans: 1. A young female (25 yrs) complaining of drooping of eyelids in the evening and relieved by rest
2. History of diplopia
3. Bilateral ptosis
4. Weakness and fatigue of muscles on repeated testing of the muscles and speech disturbance on asking the patient to count up to 100
5. No sensory disturbance
6. Intermittent nature of symptoms and signs
7. Tendon jerks are preserved

QUESTIONS AND ANSWERS

Q. **What is your differential diagnosis?**

Ans: Other conditions that can mimic myasthenia gravis are:

- Botulism
- Drug-induced myasthenia
- Myasthenia-myopathic syndrome (Eaton-Lambert syndrome)
- Hyperthyroidism
- Neuroasthenia
- Oculopharyngeal myopathy

Q. **What is myasthenia gravis?**

Ans: Myasthenia gravis is an autoimmune disorder of neuromuscular junctions, characterized by weakness and fatiguability of muscles worsened by repetitive use with a tendency to recover with rest and anticholinergic drugs. The underlying defect is a decrease in the number of acetylcholine receptors (AchRs) at neuromuscular junctions due to antibody mediated autoimmune attack.

Q. **What is the common age of involvement in myasthenia gravis?**

Ans: The myasthenia gravis has bimodal peaks (two peaks of involvement).

1. One peak is second and third decade chiefly involving women in this age groups.
2. Second peak is late, i.e. in 6th and 7th decades involving commonly the men.

Q. **Which groups of muscles get involved in myasthenia?**

Ans: The order of muscles involvement is as follows:

• Extraocular, bulbar, neck, limb girdle followed by distal limbs and trunk.

Q. **What is oculopharyngeal myopathy?**

Ans: It is an autosomal dominant disorder, characterised by:

• Late onset (5th or 6th decade).
• Ptosis (bilateral), external ophthalmoplegia (limitation of eye movements with sparing of pupillary reaction for light and accommodation).
• Diplopia is not a feature.
• Dysphagia resulting in pooling of secretions and repeated episodes of aspiration.

• There may be involvement of facial, neck and limb muscles (occasional).

Q. **What is neuroasthenia?**

Ans: It is a historic term used for myasthenia-like fatigue syndrome without an organic basis. These patients may present with subjective symptoms of weakness and fatigue. Muscle testing reveal "jerky release" or "give-away weakness" characteristic of nonogranic disorders. The complaint of fatigue in these patients means tiredness or apathy rather than decreasing muscle power on repeated effort.

Q. **Name the drug that can cause myasthenia?**

Ans: Penicillamine.

Q. **Name the antibiotics not to be used in infection in myasthenia gravis.**

Ans: Aminoglycosides.

Q. **Name few precipitating factors/events that can provoke myasthenia.**

Ans: • Exertion, exercise, fatigue
• Infection, change of climate
• Pregnancy, hyper and hypothyroidism
• Magnesium containing enemas
• Drugs (aminoglycosides, propranolol, morphile, barbiturate, procainamide, quinidine, etc.)

Q. **How does myasthenia differ from oculopharyngeal myopathy?**

Ans: Read Table 132.1.

Table 132.1: Myasthenia vs oculopharyngeal myopathy	
Myasthenia	*Oculopharyngeal myopathy*
1. An autoimmune disorder (anticholinergic antibodies present)	1. Heredofamilial disorder
2. Can occur in any age group	2. More common in younger age
3. Common in females	3. Occurs in both sexes
4. Defect lies in neurotransmission at neuromuscular junction	4. Defect lies in the muscles (intrinsic muscle disease)
5. Muscle weakness is intermittent, worsened by repetitive use and relieved by rest and anticholinergics	5. Weakness is stationary and may be progressive
6. Bilateral ptosis with diplopia	6. Bilateral ptosis without diplopia. Progressive external ophthalmoplegia is presenting feature
7. Exacerbations and remissions common	7. Slowly progressive disease
8. Facial muscles and muscles of mastication are commonly involved. Limb muscles are also involved	8. They are rarely or occasionally involved. Involvement of limb muscles is uncommon
9. Thymoma may be associated	9. No link with thymoma
10. Repetitive nerve stimulation (reduction in the amplitude of evoked response) and anticholinergic receptors antibodies tests are positive	10. EMG and muscle biopsy are specific for diagnosis but anticholinergic receptor antibodies are absent
11. Steroids, immunosuppressive drugs, thymomectomy, plasmapheresis and I.V immunoglobulins are therapeutic options	11. No treatment, hence, no therapeutic option

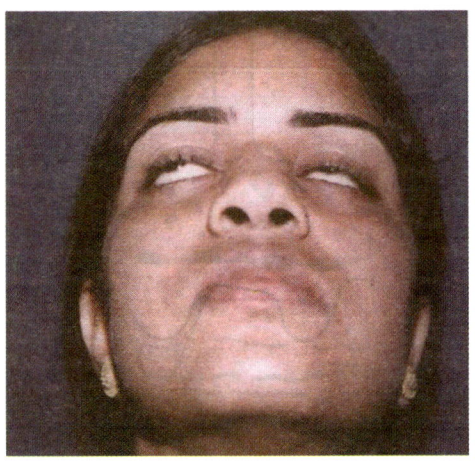

Fig. 132.1: Myasthenia gravis. A young female with my-asthenia gravis developed bilateral ptosis while talking

Q. **How would you investigate your patient?**

Ans: 1. *Therapeutic edrophonium (tensilon) test.* On edrophonium therapeutic challenge, there is reversal of myasthenia clinically (muscle strength improves)

2. *Vital capacity*

3. *CT/MRI scan of mediastinum for thymoma*

4. *Serum acetylcholine receptor antibodies* (present in 80%)

5. *Serum muscle specific tyrosine kinase antibodies*

6. *Investigations done to rule out associated diseases,* i.e.
   - T_3, T_4, TSH and antithyroid antibodies for thyrotoxicosis
   - Blood sugar (Fasting, PP) for diabetes
   - Antistriated muscle antibodies (for thymoma)
   - Antinuclear antibodies (SLE) and rheumatoid factor (for RA)
   - EMG (Electromyography) shows decremental response to tetanic nerve stimulation at 5–10 Hz and evidence of neuromuscular blockade in the form of jitter variability and blocking of motor potential in single muscle fibre EMG

Q. **How would you grade myasthenia gravis?**

Ans: The grades of myasthenia *(Osserman grading)* are:

Grade I: Ocular myasthenia (focal disease limited to eye).

Grade IIa: Mild generalised disease with slow progression. No crises. Drug responsive.

IIb: Moderate generalised myasthenia with severe skeletal and bulbar involvement. No crises. Drug response is less satisfactory.

Grade III: Acute fulminant myasthenia with progression. Severe symptoms, respiratory crises and poor drug response. High incidence of thymoma. High mortality rate.

Grade IV: Late severe myasthenia. Symptoms same as grade III, but takes 2 yrs to progress. High mortality rate with life-threatening respiratory impairment.

Q. **What other autoimmune disorders can be associated with myasthenia?**

Ans: I. *Endocranial disorders,* e.g. thyro toxicosis, hypothyroidism, type I DM

II. *Collagen vascular disorders,* e.g. RA, SLE, dermatomyosis, Sjögren's syndrome

III. *Blood disorders,* e.g. pernicious anaemia

IV. *Skin disorder,* e.g. pemphigus

V. *Sarcoidosis*

Q. **What does myasthenic crisis mean? How does it differ from cholinergic crises?**

Ans: Acute exacerbation of myasthenia is called myasthenic crisis. It occurs in about 10% patients with myasthenia.

The precipitating factors include respiratory infection and surgery.

Cholinergic crises means symptoms due to cholinergic stimulation, due to over doses of the drugs (edrophonium, neostigmine).

The difference between the two common crises observed in myasthenia are tabulated (Table 132.2).

Table 132.2: Myasthenic vs cholinergic crisis	
Myasthenic crisis	*Cholinergic crisis*
• It is an acute exacerbation of the disease (disease-induced crisis)	• It is an overstimulation of cholinergic nerves by over-doses of drugs (drug induced crisis)
• It is a life-threatening crisis exacerbated by respiratory infection	• It is due to overdosage of drugs
• Anticholinergic symptoms dominate the crisis	• Cholinergic symptoms, e.g. salivation, confusion, lacrimation mitosis, pallor and collapse dominate
• It needs immediate admission to intensive care unit for respiratory monitoring and support	• It can be treated by tapering the drugs used
• Prognosis is bad	• Prognosis is good

Q.   How does myasthenia gravis differ from myasthenic myopathic syndrome (Eaton-Lambert syndrome)?

Ans: The differences are tabulated (Table 132.3).

Q.   What are the treatment modalities for myasthenia gravis?

Ans: *A. Medical Therapy*

  I. Symptomatic therapy with anticholinesterase drugs, e.g. neostigmine or pyridostigmine or both 4−5 times a day. Avoid overmedication as it may precipitate cholinergic symptoms

  II. Immunosuppressive therapy with drugs such as steroids, azathioprine, cyclosporine, mycophenolate mofetil and rituximab

  III. Immunomodulation therapy with plasmapheresis, immunoglobulin or both.

B. Surgical therapy
  • Thymectomy

Q.   What is the role of thymectomy in myasthenia?

Ans: Thymectomy is the definite mode of treatment in case thymoma is detected. Otherwise thymectomy is indicated in all patients with myasthenia to induce remission or to provide long symptom-free interval (remission).

The role of thymectomy in ocular myasthenia in adults over the age of 55 yrs and in children is debatable.

Table 132.3: Differences between myasthenia gravis and myasthenic-myopathy syndrome

Myasthenia gravis	Myasthenia-myopathic syndrome
• An autoimmune disorder involving AchR, i.e. there is deficiency of acetylcholine receptors	• Presynaptic disorder of neuromuscular junction. AChR are not involved
• More common in females	• Common in males
• Other autoimmune disease may be associated	• No such association
• Deep tendon jerks are preserved	• Tendon jerks are lost
• Muscle weakness is proximal as well as distal	• Muscle weakness is proximal
• Autonomic changes uncommon	• Autonomic changes, e.g. dry mouth, impotence common
• EMG shows decremental response on repetitive nerve stimulation	• Incremental rather decremental response is seen on EMG on repetitive nerve stimulation
• It is caused by antibodies directed against acetylcholine receptors (AChR) which can be assayed	• It is caused by autoantibodies directed against P/Q type calcium channels at the motor nerve terminals. These antibodies can be detected on radioimmunoassay
• Thymoma or thymic hyperplasia is common	• It is associated with malignancy commonly small cell carcinoma of lung

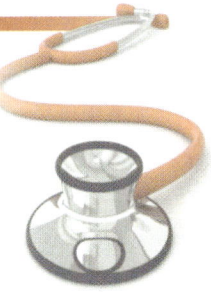

133

Epilepsy

INSTRUCTION

- Ask the relevant history and perform relevant neurological examination

SALIENT FEATURES

- The patient in picture (Fig. 133.1) was brought to hospital by the spouse with history of a fit (seizure) in the morning while doing some work

HISTORY

Ask for the following:

- Take a detailed history regarding description of fit/fits from the attendant (s) or from a person (s) who has/have observed the fit/seizure.

Specific enquiries about fit/fits

- Timing and duration of an attack
- Presence of an aura, its duration and symptoms
- Precipitating event leading to an attack
- Abnormal movements, i.e. jerking of a limb, stiffening or automatism (present)

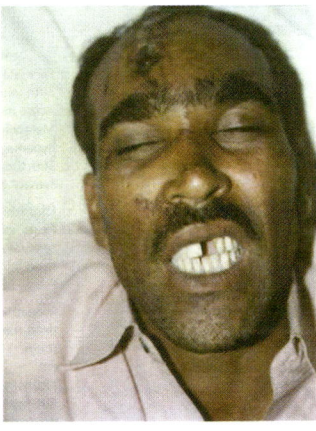

Fig. 133.1: Grand mal epilepsy (tonic-clonic seizures). A patient with grand mal epilepsy sustained injury over forehead and lost a teeth (an incisor) during a fit

- Salivation or frothing at the mouth (present)
- Biting of the tongue (present)
- Incontinence of urine and feces (present)
- Postictal phenomenon, i.e. headache, drowsiness or aches and pain, weakness of a limb or me half of the body (*Todd's paralysis*)
- Cyanosis
- Past history of head injury, diabetes, hypertension, etc.
- Family history of seizure
- Habits, e.g. vegetarian/non-vegetarian (this case)

EXAMINATION

General Physical Examination

- Examination of pulse, BP and heart
- Palpation of carotid arteries and auscultation over them for a bruit or a murmur
- Examination of head for trauma and mouth for tongue injury or loosening or fall of a tooth (Fig. 133.1)
- Skin for epiloia, neurofibromatosis or pigmentation
- Visual fields examination
- Optic fundi examination

Neurological Examination

- Any paralysis of limb/limbs

PROVISIONAL DIAGNOSIS

The patient (a truck driver) has recent onset grand mal seizure (lesion) probably due to intracranial space occupying lesion (aetiology). The patient has to abandon his job as a truck driver as a consequence of this disease (functional status).

QUESTIONS AND ANSWERS

Q. What do you mean by grand mal seizures?
Ans: The grand mal seizure is a generalised complex seizure characterised by following phases:

- *Prodromal Phase:* Patient feels uneasiness or irritability.
- *Aura:* It precedes tonic-clonic phase characterized by hallucinations (e.g. visual, *deja vu phenomenon*), jerking of a limb, GI symptoms.
- *Tonic-clonic phase* characterized by jerking of a limb or one half of the body, frothing from the mouth, biting of tongue, incontinence of sphincters, etc. (present).
- *Unconciousness,* i.e. there is loss of consciousness (present).
- *Postictal phenomenon,* e.g. confusion, headache and automatic behavior

Q. How would you classify epilepsy?

Ans: They are classified into 3 groups:

I. Generalized seizures
- Tonic-clonic seizures (grand mal type)
- Tonic seizure
- Absence seizures
- Akinetic seizures
- Myoclonic seizures

II. Partial seizures
- Simple partial (Jacksonian type)
- Complex partial
- Partial seizures with secondary generalization (tonic-clonic evolution)
- Generalized tonic-clonic seizures with an evidence of focal onset

III. Unclassified seizure

Q. What is the major difference between complex partial and simple partial seizure?

Ans: In simple partial of seizure, awareness is preserved while it is lost in complex partial seizure.

Q. Why is consciousness lost in grand mal seizure?

Ans: The spread of discharge involving both the cerebral hemispheres produces unconscious due to involvement of reticular activating system (RAS) bilaterally.

Q. What is Todd's paralysis?

Ans: Paralysis of a limb or hemiplegia occurring after an epileptic attack is called *Todd's paralysis.* It occurs due to exhaustion of neurons in precentral gyrus. The paralysis is transient and may last few days (1–3 days).

Q. What is Jacksonian epilepsy?

Ans: It is a simple partial seizure of focal onset arising in one portion of the precentral gyrus resulting in a fit involving one part of the body (e.g. thumb) and then spreads to involve that side of the body or the whole body. It suggests usually an intracranial space occupying lesion.

Q. What are the common causes of seizures in an adult?

Ans:
- Idiopathic
- Space occupying lesion (e.g. brain tumor, neurocysticercosis)
- CVA (Cerebrovascular accidents)
- Hypertensive encephalopathy
- Head Injury
- Infections, e.g. meningitis, encephalitis, brain abscess
- Alcohol withdrawal
- Metabolic and electrolyte disturbance, e.g. hepatic failure, renal failure, hypoglycemia, hyponatremia (SIADH), hypocalcemia, etc.
- Alzheimer's disease

Q. What are precipitating factors?

Ans:
- Insomnia
- Physical or mental fatigue
- Drugs
- Flashes of bright light (photosensitivity)
- Loud noise or music
- Stress
- Pyrexia
- Infection
- Alcohol ingestion or withdrawal
- Reading or writing

Q. What are the differences between a psychogenic nonepileptic seizure and an epileptic fit?

Ans: The differences are given below:

Grand mal fits	Psychogenic nonepileptic seizure
• The fits occur in a co-ordinated fashion due to hypersynchronous discharge	• The fits may vary from simple falling to the ground to bizarre attacks
• Stereotyped movements of limbs (tonic and clonic) occur	• There is wild bizarre movements (shaking, twitching) of all the four limbs simultaneously. There is usually no tonic phase
• Attacks can occur during any time of the day	• Attacks occur when patient is being observed or somebody is present
• Patient may injure himself or herself during an attack	• Patient does not hurt himself or herself during an attack
• These are unprovoked fits. There is no purpose behind these fits. These are true seizures	• Attacks occur with some purpose, i.e. to draw the attention of nears and dears or to seek compensation of sympathy. These are pseudoseizures

- There may be biting of tongue during seizure
- There may be urine and faecal incontinence
- The seizures may be precipitated by some known factors
- Pattern of the fits is fixed

- There is no biting of tongue during fit
- There is no urine or faecal incontinence
- There are no known precipitating factors
- Frequent change in the pattern of fits. There may either be an addition or deletion of some symptoms during the fit

- EEG is often abnormal
- Serum prolactin levels 15 – 20 times higher during or after seizure

- EEG is normal
- Serum prolactin level are normal

Q.   What are the metabolic causes of epilepsy?
Ans: Read question on causes of epilepsy.

Q.   How would you investigate such a case?
Ans:
- Complete hemogram
- Blood biochemistry, e.g. urea, creatinine, magnesium, glucose
- Liver function tests
- Serological tests for syphilis and HIV
- X-rays chest and skull
- EEG
- CT scan
- MRI scan

Q.   What does serial seizures mean? How does it differ from status epilepticus?
Ans: *Serial epilepsy* means fits occur in succession, but patient is conscious in between seizures.
  Status epilepticus means seizures follow each others in succession without recovery of consciousness in between seizures.

Q.   How would you treat a patient with epilepsy?
Ans:
- *General advice* regarding Do's and Don'ts in epilepsy.
- *Drug therapy.* The first line drugs in grand mal epilepsy include phenytoin, sodium valproate, carbamazepine, lamotrigine as monotherapy. Several new add-on-drugs have been developed for combination therapy. The main aim of treatment is to control seizure. When seizures are controlled, the drug (s) can be continued for 3 years to produce seizure free period, after which the drug may be withdrawn slowly. If seizure occurs during this period, the drug (s) should be reinstituted and continued throughout life.
- *Advice* about driving.

Q.   What are the do's and don' t sin epilepsy? What precautions should be observed by an epileptic?
Ans:

Do's (to be done)	Don'ts (not to be done)
A. During an epileptic fit	**During an attack of fit**
• Move the patient to a safer place	• Neither put your finger, nor allow any one to put the finger into the mouth
• Loosen the clothes around the neck	• Do not put any thing (liquid) into the mouth
• Make the patient to breath fresh air and comfortable	• **Precautions**
• Try to prevent the tongue biting by putting tighly packed handkerchief or a piece of cloth in the mouth	• Avoid working or recreation near open fires
	• Not to operate dangerous machinery
	• Not to lock bathroom door while taking bath
	• They should take shallow bath in a pond or a canal, that too in the presence of someone
• Remove the artificial denture if any	
B. After the convulsion ceases	• Cycling, swimming, mountaineering should be discouraged until 6 months seizures free interval is achieved.
• Turn the patient to semiprone position	
• Make the air passage clear. Advise the patient to consult a doctor	

Q.   When would you allow this patient to drive a heavy vehicle?
Ans: However, laws differ from state to state and country to country. However, it is responsibility of the physician to apprise the patients about the dangers posed by driving.
  In general, most states allow the patient to drive vehicle after a seizure-free interval of one year (on or off medication).

Q.   What precautions would you advise to an epileptic female using oral contraceptive?
Ans: Patients using drugs such as carbamazepine, phenytoin, phenobarbitone, topiramate, etc. should adopt alternative method of contraception or should modify the anti-epileptic medication because above mentioned drugs antagonise the effects of oral contraceptives.

Q.   How does EEG help in epilepsy?
Ans:
1. Presence of EEG changes (spike and wave activity) helps in the diagnosis, but absence of these changes do not exclude epilepsy.
2. ECG helps in monitoring the drug treatment and its compliance.

134

Neurocysticercosis

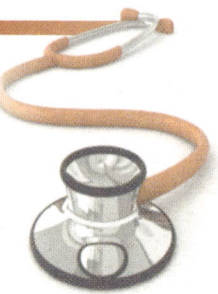

INSTRUCTION

- Take a detailed history and perform relevant neurological examination

SALIENT FEATURES

- The patient, a vegetarian presented with history of grand mal seizures for the last 5 years.

HISTORY

Ask for the following:

- Take the detailed history and ask the relevant points from the patient or spouse or attendant regarding the fits. This has been discussed already in epilepsy.
- Specifically ask about dietary habits. He is a truck driver, takes food from outside (roadside dhabas or restaurants) where food may be contaminated with tapeworm eggs (*T. solium*) from human faces. There may be transmission of infection from the workers of the restaurants who do not keep good hygiene.
- History of psychiatric symptoms
- History of abnormal behaviour and altered cognition
- History of symptoms of raised intracranial tension, e.g. headache, vomiting, photophobia, visual loss and papilledema

EXAMINATION

General Physical Examination

- Look for the physical signs as discussed under epilepsy.
- In addition, palpable the muscles and skin of extremities for subcutaneous or muscular swelling (cysts in the muscles).
- *Eyes:* Examine the eyes including fundus for papilloedema and other intraocular abnormalities.

Neurological Examination

I. *Higher mental function.* There may be altered

mentation due to intracerebral cysticercosis (present). There may be behavioural changes as well

II. *Cranial nerves examination*
   - Examine all the cranial nerves
   - There can be ptosis due to extraocular involvement

III. Motor and sensory system examination for space-occupying lesion or raised ICP

Q. Which investigation would you like to see in this patient?

Ans: CT scan/MRI brain for neurocysticercosis. (Fig. 134.1 – displayed)

PROVISIONAL DIAGNOSIS

The patient has epileptic seizures (lesion) due to neurocysticercosis (aetiology). The patient has still uncontrolled seizures (functional status).

QUESTIONS AND ANSWERS

Q. What do you understand by the term neuro-cysticercosis?

Ans: Involvement of the brain by cysts of *T. solium* is called *neurocysticercosis*.

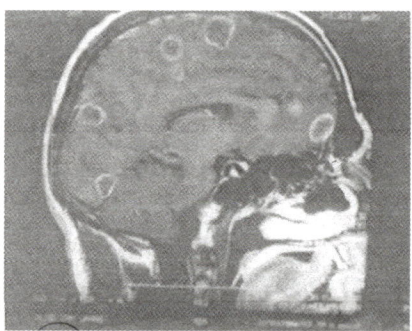

Fig. 134.1: MRI brain showing multiple cysticerci as in the cerebral cortex

Q. How does neurocysticercosis occur in vegetarian humans?

Ans: Though man is a definite host but acts as an intermediate host when humans ingest food contaminated with eggs from human faeces. This is the reason that neurocysticercosis manifests in the vegetarians.

Q. What are the causes of ring enhancing lesions?

Ans: 1. Neurocysticercosis
2. Tuberculoma (Fig. 134.2)
3. Toxoplasmosis
4. Brain abscess

Q. What is a seizure? What do you understand by the term epilepsy?

Ans: A seizure is a transient cerebral dysfunction due to an abnormal paroxysmal neuronal discharge in the brain.

Epilepsy denotes any disorder characterised by recurrent unprovoked seizures, hence, a single seizure may or may not indicate epilepsy.

Q. What is the mode of infection for neurocysticercosis in humans?

Ans: Humans are the definite hosts and pigs are the intermediate hosts for *T. Solium* infection. Intermediate hosts harbour the larval form (cysticercosis) of *T. Solium*. Man will develop cysticercosis if he acts an intermediate host, for example, if humans ingest meat or food contaminated with the eggs of *T. Solium*, then intermediate forms (cysticercosis) hatch out from the eggs and may reach the brain and other tissues.

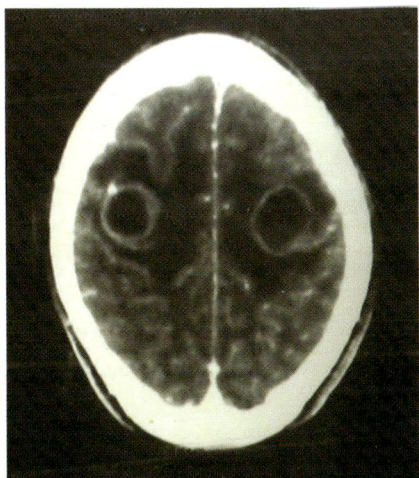

Fig. 134.2: Tuberculoma of brain

Q. What are the various sites of cysticerci?

Ans: Brain, skeletal muscles, subcutaneous tissue and the eyes are the common sites.

Q. What are the clinical manifestations of neurocysticercosis?

Ans: I. *Symptoms and signs due to involvement of brain parenchyma,* e.g. seizures, altered cognition, behaviour disturbance.

II. *Symptoms and signs of hydrocephalus,* e.g. headache, nausea, vomiting, dizziness, changes in vision, ataxia, confusion and papilledema.

III. *Ptosis* due to extraocular muscle paralysis, visual loss can occur due to ocular involvement.

IV. *Symptoms and signs of basal meningitis or arachnoiditis,* e.g. neck rigidity, lower cranial nerve palsy, hydrocephalus or strokes.

Q. How would you diagnose such a case?

Ans: Diagnosis of cysticercosis is difficult. A consensus conference has proposed absolute, major, minor and epidemiological criteria for diagnosis.

I. *Absolute criteria*
- Demonstration of cysticerci in biopsy specimen by histology or microscopy
- Visualisation of the parasite in the eye on fundoscopy
- Demonstration of cystic lesions containing scolex on neuroradiology imaging

II. *Major criteria*
- Neuroradiological lesions suggestive of neurocysticercosis
- Demonstration of antibodies to cysticerci by enzyme-linked immuno-electrotransfer blot
- Resolution of cystic lesions with albendazole or praziquantel alone

III. *Minor criteria*
- Lesions compatible with neurocysticercosis on neuroimaging studies
- Clinical features suggestive of neurocysticercosis
- Demonstration of antibodies to cysticercus antigen in CSF by ELISA
- Evidence of cysticercosis outside CNS (e.g. soft tissue calcification)

IV. *Epidemiological criteria*
- Residence in endemic area of cysticercosis
- Frequent travel to a cysticercosis-endemic area
- Household contact with an individual infected with *T. solium*

Diagnosis is confirmed either with one absolute criteria or a combination of two major, one minor and one epidemiological criteria. A probable diagnosis is considered when (1) one major plus two minor, (2) one major plus one minor plus one epidemiological, or (3) three minor plus one epidemiology criteria are present.

Q.   What are the endemic areas for *T. solium*?

Ans: Parasite is endemic in China, Central and South America, Latin America, Phillipines, South East Asia and Eastern Europe. Cysticercosis is becoming prevalent in industralised nations, largely as a result of immigration of infected person from endemic areas.

Q.   What are the radiological features of neurocysticercosis?

Ans: The radiological findings are:

1. Cystic lesions with or without enhancement (e.g. ring enhancement) (Fig. 134.1)

2. One or more nodular calcified lesions

3. Focal enhancing lesions

Q.   How would you treat neurocysticercosis?

Ans: 1. Seizures can be controlled with antiepileptic treatment. If parenchymal lesions resolve without development of calcification and patients remain free of seizures, antiepileptic therapy can usually be discontinued after 2 yrs.

2. Antiparasitic therapy (albendazole 15 mg/kg/day for 2–4 weeks or praziquantel 50–60 mg/kg/daily in three divided doses for 15 days or 100 mg/kg in 3 doses given over a single day) may be given for faster resolution of the parenchymal lesion. Since both the drugs may exacerbate the inflammatory response around the dying parasite, hence, high dose corticosteroids should be used during treatment to prevent exacerbation of symptoms.

3. For nonobstructive hydrocephalus, ICP should be reduced by drugs. In case of obstructive hydrocephalus, endoscopic removal of the cysticerci is the preferred treatment. An alternative approach is placement of ventriculoperitoneal shunt.

Most authorities recommend prolonged use of antiparasitic treatment and shunting when hydrocephalus is present. For patients with cerebral oedema and raised ICP, steroids with antiparasitic therapy is advised for long-term use.

135

Motor Neuron Disease

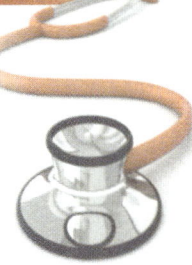

INSTRUCTION

- Examine the nervous system of the patient

SALIENT FEATURES

- Wasting of small muscles of hands

HISTORY

Ask for the following:

- History of muscle twitchings/fasciculations and cramps (these are characteristic features of motor neuron disease)
- Asymmetric muscle weakness involving upper and lower limbs (quadriplegia)
- Difficulty in deglutition (dysphagia) and difficulty in speech (dysarthria)
- Emotional disturbance (uncontrolled episodes of laughing or crying) in case bulbar nuclei are involved

EXAMINATION

General Physical Examination

- It is simlar to case No. 131 (wasting of small muscles of hands)

Neurological Examination

- Examine higher mental functions for emotional lability (common if bulbar nuclei involved)
- Examine cranial nerves (motor cranial nuclei are commonly involved especially lower cranial nerves, e.g. 12th cranial nerve involved (Fig. 135.1)
- Check the tongue for fasciculations (present)
- Examination of Motor System
  - A. Limbs
    - Look for fasciculation (they are visible as flickerings of muscles, if not, can be provoked by tapping the muscle bellies)
    - UMN signs in the upper and lower limbs (spasticity, exaggerated tendon reflexes and plantar extensor response)

- LMN signs, e.g. fasciculations, absent reflexes and wasting of the small muscles of hands (Fig. 135.1 present)
  - B. Neck
    - Check neck muscles, head drop is seen when there is weakness of the thoracic and paraspinal muscles

Note: There can be a combination of above signs.

PROVISIONAL DIAGNOSIS

The patient has LMN signs in upper limbs and a combination of LMN and UMN signs in the lower limbs with atrophy of tongue (lesion) caused by motor neuron disease (aetiology). The patient has marked disability (functional status).

Q.   What are the points in favor of your diagnosis?

Ans: 1. Age (young adults around 40 yrs of age)
2. Speech involvement (dysarthria) and difficulty in swallowing (dysphagia)
3. Generalised fasciculations
4. A combination of LMN paralysis (weakness atrophy, areflexia) in upper limbs and UMN cum LMN paralysis of lower limbs (spasticity exaggerated jerks and plantar extensors).

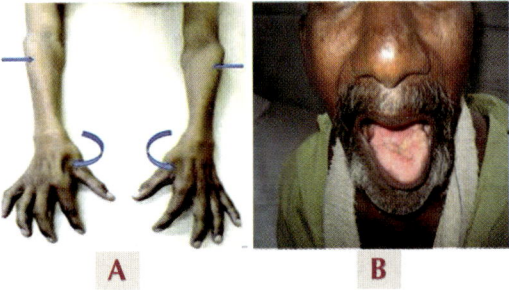

Fig. 135.1: Madras Motor neuron disease. Note the wasting of small muscles of the hands; (A) and tongue (B)

QUESTIONS AND ANSWERS

Q. **What is differential diagnosis?**
Ans: Since the patient has LMN signs (wasting, fasciculation, areflexia) in upper limbs and a combination of UMN signs (spasticity, exaggerated tendon reflexes, bilateral plantar extensors) and LMN in lower limbs, the other condition that can lead to such a clinical picture is cervical cord compression. (Read case discussion on quadriplegia)

Q. **What is motor neuron disease?**
Ans: It is a degenerative disorder involving the anterior horn cells of the spinal cord, the motor cranial nuclei of the lower cranial nerves and the corticospinal and corticobulbar pathways.
The disorder is sporadic, but familial cases may occur and several genetic mutations have been identified.

Q. **What are the various types of motor neuron disease?**
Ans: Five varieties have been recognised on clinical grounds:
1. *Progressive spinal muscular dystrophy* (a LMN paralysis of lower limbs)
2. *Primary lateral sclerosis* (UMN paralysis of the limbs)
3. *Amyotrophic lateral sclerosis* (a mixed UMN and LMN deficit in the limbs)
4. *Progressive bulbar palsy* (involvement of bulbar cranial nerve nuclei)
5. *Pseudobulbar palsy* (bilateral corticobulbar disease, e.g. UMN deficit in addition to bulbar involvement. Emotional disturbance (uncontrolled episodes of laughing or crying) occurs commonly

Q. **What are the characteristic features of MND?**
Ans: 1. Rarely occurs before the age of 40 yrs
2. Presence of UMN and LMN signs involving atleast two limbs or one limb and bulbar muscle nuclei
3. No sensory involvement
4. Ocular muscles are spared
5. Cerebellar and extrapyramidal remain uninvolved
6. Sphincters are involved late
7. Progressive disease with no remission

Q. **What is fasciculation? What are its causes?**
Ans: Read Clinical Methods in Medicine by Prof SN Chugh.

Q. **What is Madras Motor Neuron Disease?**
Ans: It is a disease reported from Southern India (e.g. Madras) which has an early onset (before 30 yrs of age) with asymmetric limb weakness (paralysis), with facial and bulbar involvement along with sensorineural deafness. The course is benign. Fasciculations are marked. It progresses slowly.

Q. **What is pathology of MND?**
Ans: There is degeneration of:
i. Betz cells in cerebral cortex
ii. Pyramidal tracts
iii. Motor cranial nuclei
iv. Anterior horn cells of spinal cord

Q. **Enlist the diagnostic criteria for Amyotrophic Lateral Sclerosis (ALS).**
Ans: Summary of the diagnostic criteria is:
1. *Definite:* LMN and UMN signs in 3 regions.
2. *Probable:* LMN and UMN signs in two regions
3. *Possible:* LMN and UMN signs in one region.
4. *Suspected:* Either LMN signs only or UMN signs only in one or more regions.

Q. **What is the role of genetics in amyotrophic lateral sclerosis (ALS)?**
Ans: Most cases of ALS are sporadic. Only 5–10% cases have familial occurrence due to gene mutations identified in the families. This genetic locus encodes a copper-Zn-binding superoxide dismutase (SOD).

Q. **What is the role of riluzole in MND?**
Ans: Accumulation of toxic levels of glutamate at synapses can cause neuronal death through a calcium-dependent pathway. Riluzoles (50 mg bid), a glutamate antagonist has been shown to be useful in patients with disease of bulbar onset or where one limb is involved.

Q. **What is the role of magnetic cortical stimulation in ALS?**
Ans: It is a technique that allows the detection of degeneration of Betz cells in ALS. The sensitivity of this test is high in patients with ALS with predominant UMN lesion.

Q. **How would you investigate this case?**
Ans: 1. *Serum muscle enzymes* are slightly elevated.
2. *CSF* is normal.
3. *EMG studies* may show changes of chronic partial denervation with abnormal spontaneous activity in the resting muscles. There is also a reduction in the number of motor units under voluntary control. The diagnosis should not be made with confidence unless such changes are found at least in three spinal regions (cervical, thoracic and lumbo

sacral) or two spinal regions and the bulbar musculature.

4. *Motor conduction velocity* is normal or slightly reduced. Sensory conduction studies are normal.

5. *Muscle biopsy shows* changes of denervation.

6. *Genetic analysis* by DNA chips or microassay is used to genotype single nucleotide polymorphism simultaneously. The single nucleotide polymorphism (SNP) is a single nucleotide variation in the DNA sequence that can be used as markers for neighbouring genetic variation. By comparing the prevalence of specific SNP in patients and controls, the chromosomal region represented by the SNP associated with the disease can be determined. This approach has been used by researchers in diagnosis of sporadic ALS.

Q. **What is the role of beta-lactam antibiotics in ALS?**

Ans: Beta-lactam antibiotics (ceftriaxone) have been shown to slow the progression of the disease in experimental mice by enhancing astroglial transport of glutamate.

136

Syringomyelia

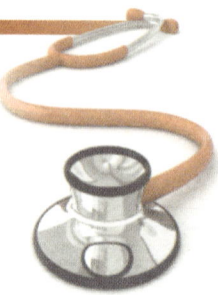

INSTRUCTION

- Examine the nervous system of this patient

SALIENT FEATURES

- Numbness in the upper limbs

HISTORY

Ask for the following:

- Onset of symptoms (slow onset)
- History of numbness in the upper limbs (present)
- History of repeated painless trauma. History of burns with cigarettes (if patient is smoker) or hot water (burn marks present)
- History of chest deformity (scoliosis) since childhood
- History of weakness in upper and/or lower limbs

EXAMINATION

Neurological Examination

1. *Higher mental function*, e.g. emotional lability (It is seen in pseudobulbar palsy variety of MND)

2. *Cranial nerves.* Lower cranial nerve especially 9th to 12th may be involved due to syringobulbia
3. *Motor system*
   A. *Upper limbs*
   - There is wasting of small muscles of the hands and forearm with or without fasciculation (present)
   - Some patients may show hypertrophy in limbs, hands and feet
   - There is hypotonia and areflexia in upper limbs (present)
   - *Dissociated sensory* loss in 'cafe distribution' (present). There is loss of pain and temperature sensations (spinothalamic involvement) with preservation of light touch, vibration sense and joint position sense (intact posterior column)
   - *Charcot joints (senseless joints)* of shoulder and elbow (present)
   - Look for the *Horner's syndrome*
   - Examine the posterior neck for trauma or surgical scar

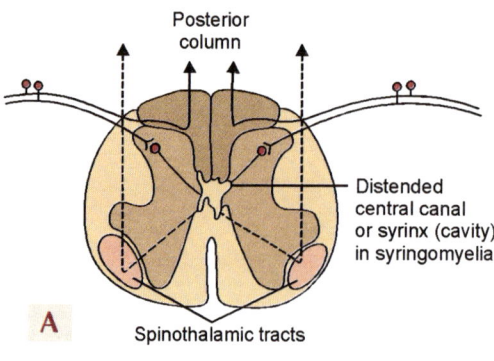

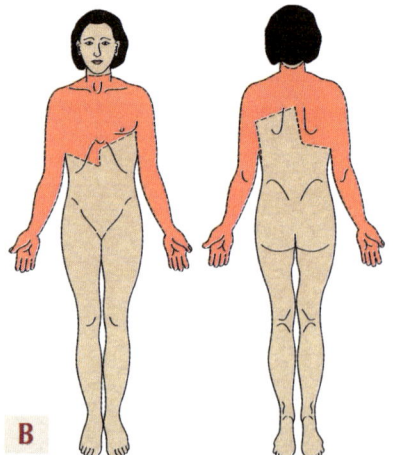

Fig. 136.1: Syringomyelia. (A) Diagram of syrinx (enlarged central canal in lower cervical region; (B) A cape like distribution of sensory loss (e.g. loss of pain and temperature in syringomyelia in the region of lower cervical segments)

B. *Lower limbs*
- Due to enlargement of cavity, there can be spinal cord compression, hence, look for the pyramidal signs is the lower limbs (present)

C. *Face*
- Test the face for loss of pain and temperature sensation due to involvement of V nerve nucleus in syringobulbia
- Look at the eyes for nystagmus and ataxia due to involvement of medial longitudinal fasciculus

PROVISIONAL DIAGNOSIS

The patient has wasting of small muscles of the hands with dissociated sensory loss (lesion) caused by syringomyelia (aetiology). The patient has burn marks of cigarette as well as marks of trauma (functional status).

Q. **Enumerate the points in favor of your diagnosis?**

Ans:
- Slow onset and progressive numbers of hands and upper extremities.
- Presence of burn and trauma marks over hands
- Age between 20 and 40 yrs
- Wasting of small muscles of hands
- Dissociated sensory loss over upper extremities (marked over the hands)
- LMN paralysis of upper extremities
- Charcot shoulder and elbow joints
- Pyramidal signs in the lower limbs

QUESTIONS AND ANSWERS

Q. **What is the differential diagnosis of this case?**

Ans: Following conditions produce clinical picture simulating syringomyelia:
- Intramedullary spinal cord tumor
- Arachnoiditis
- Hematomyelia
- Craniovertebral anomaly
- Spinal cord injury leading to cervical myelopathy

Q. **What investigation would you like to see or advise to confirm the diagnosis?**

Ans: MRI is the standard investigation for diagnosis of syrinx (Fig. 136.2).

Q. **What do you mean by syringomyelia?**

Ans: It means (syrinx-a cavity, myelia-spinal cord) cavitation of the spinal cord adjacent to the central canal as a result of destruction or degeneration of gray and white matter of the cord.

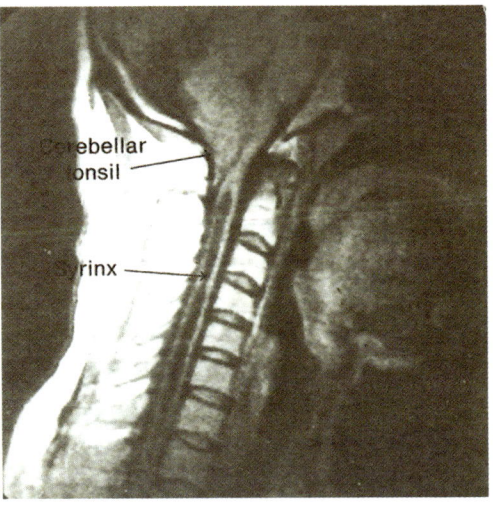

Fig. 136.2: Sagittal MRI scan showing a syrinx extending throughout the length of the cervical cord. There is associated displacement of the cerebellar tonsils (Arnold-Chiari-Type 1) downward

Q. **What is the difference between hydromyelia and syringomyelia?**

Ans: Hydro means fluid and myelia means cord. Collection or accumulation of fluid in a cavity means either hydromyelia or syringomyelia. Both occur due to same pathological process of destruction of the white and gray matter of the cord and accompanying reactive gliosis.

The only difference between the two is that hydromyelia is the expansion of the central canal of the spinal cord in the form of a cavity while syringomyelia is formation of a chest like cavity in the inner substance of the cord with communication with central canal.

Q. **What does syrinx contain?**

Ans: As already discussed, it is a cavity communicating with central canal, hence, it contains CSF with higher protein content.

Q. **What are the clinical characteristics of syringomyelia?**

Ans: I. *Clinical features at the level of cavity (syrinx)*
- There is LMN paralysis due to involvement of anterior horn cells. As cavity is common in cervical cord or medulla, therefore, there will be wasting of the small muscles of hands and forearms with areflexia if cavity is in cervical cord.
- *Dissociated sensory* loss over upper limbs in a *cafe fashion* due to involve-

ment of decussating fibres of the spinothalamic tract with sparing of posterior column.

- Neuropathic upper limb joints (*Charcot's shoulder and elbow joints*). *Trophic changes* in the upper limbs.

II. *Clinical features below the level of syrinx*
- Bilateral pyramidal signs due to involvement of corticospinal tracts.
- Horner's syndrome due to involvement of cervical sympathetic.

Q. **What are the clinical characteristics of syringobulbia?**

Ans: The characteristic features are due to involvement of bulbar nuclei
1. Vertigo and dizziness (cranial nerve 9th and 10th)
2. Wasting of tongue (12th nerve involvement)
3. Dissociated sensory loss over the face in an 'onion-skin' pattern (involvement of 5th cranial nerve)
4. Dyarthria and dysphagia

Q. **What are the treatment modalities available?**

Ans: 1. Syringo-peritoneal shunting in patients with basal meningitis
2. Direct drainage of cavity (syrinx) into subarachnoid space in case of post traumatic syringomyelia

3. In the presence of associated Arnold-Chiari malformation, the pressure is relieved by cervical laminectomy and suboccipital craniectomy to decompress the malformation at the foramen magnum.

Q. **What is *la main succulente*?**

Ans: This is an ugly appearance of hands in syringomyelia due to trophic and vasomotor disturbances leading to cold blue (cyanosed) and swollen hands and fingers.

Q. **What are the causes of dissociated sensory loss?**

Ans: 1. Anterior spinal artery syndrome due to thrombotic occlusion
2. Diabetic small fibre neuropathy
3. Amyloid polyneuropathy
4. Leprosy
5. Malingering (hysterical)

Q. **What is Charcot joint? What are its causes?**

Ans: Read Charcot joint as a separate case discussion in Rheumatology.

Q. **What are associate anomalies in syringomyelia?**

Ans: Arnold-Chiari malformation, spina bifida, platybasia, hydrocephalus and spinal cord tumors.

137

Postpolio Paralysis

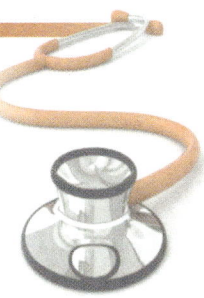

INSTRUCTION

- Examine the motor system of lower limbs of this patient (Fig. 137.1)

SALIENT FEATURES

- Thin lower extremities

HISTORY

Ask for the following:

- Age of onset of weakness (since childhood)
- Weakness whether progressive or stationary (stationary in this patient)?
- History of twitchings or fasciculations (absent in this case)
- History of sensory disturbance (no disturbance)
- Bowel or bladder disturbance (no disturbance)

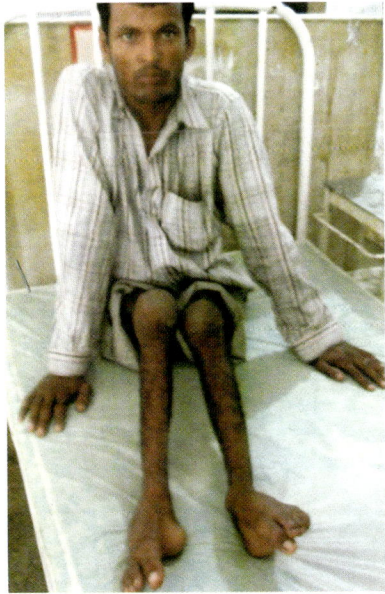

Fig. 137.1: Postpolio paralysis of legs

- Past history of fever in childhood (present)
- Ask about immunisation (not done in this case) for polio during childhood

EXAMINATION

Neurological Examination in this Case

- There is bilateral thinning of the legs due to muscle atrophy (LMN paralysis present)
- Muscular atrophy is asymmetrical
- No fasciculations present
- Muscle power is reduced in the lower limbs in leg muscles
- There is hypotonia of the leg muscles
- Tendon jerks of the lower limbs absent
- No sensory disturbance
- No bowel and bladder involvement

PROVISIONAL DIAGNOSIS

The patient has asymmetric muscular atrophy of both lower legs due to lower motor neuron involvement (lesion) following poliomyelitis (etiology). He finds difficulty in walking (functional status).

QUESTIONS AND ANSWERS

Q. **What are the points in favor of your diagnosis?**

Ans: The points in favor of diagnosis of patient inset in Fig. 137.1 are:

1. History of fever in childhood
2. Weakness since childhood
3. Asymmetric paralysis of lower limbs (Left > Right)
4. Thinning of left lower limb more than right
5. Areflexia of lower limbs with other signs of LMN paralysis
6. No bowel and bladder involvement
7. Weakness is stationary and non progressive

Q. Name the conditions that come into differential diagnosis.

Ans:
- Peripheral neuropathy (read it as a separate case)
- Guillain-Barré syndrome (read it as a separate case)
- Motor neuron disease (discussed as a separate case)
- Cauda equina syndrome (discussed as a separate case)
- Spinal muscular atrophy
- Multiple lumbar disc disease
- Spinal arachnoiditis

Q. What are the causes of unilateral wasted leg?

Ans:
1. Poliomyelitis
2. Lumbar disk prolapse
3. Radiculopathy
4. Wasted leg syndrome, seen in farmers, reported from Punjab, occurs due to compression of sciatic nerve during ploughing of field when farmer keeps one leg over the 'Hal' during ploughing. It is reversible but repeated trauma may result in atrophy
5. Sciatica syndrome

Q. Where is the site of lesion in poliomyelitis?

Ans: In the anterior horn cells of the spinal cord.

Q. Is muscular atrophy in poliomyelitis stationary or progressive?

Ans: Paralytic poliomyelitis usually remains stable after the initial attack. However, in some cases, new muscle weakness and atrophy involving previously affected muscles or even unaffected muscles occur and this deterioration can continue as long as 30 years after first attack called *postpolio syndrome* (the case inset in picture). This progression is slow, but distinct from motor neuron disease. It is not clear why it occurs in some patients not in all. It has been reported to occur in those cases who have widespread paralysis and poor immune status.

Q. What are the characteristics of spinal muscular atrophy?

Ans:
- It is an autosomal recessive neurodegenerative disorders primarily affecting anterior horn cells in spinal cord and bulbar motor nuclei.
- It produces asymmetric weakness and wasting of proximal muscles of limbs in children and adults (type 3), first involves lower limbs and later upper limbs (Fig. 137.2).
- Neck, trunk muscles may be involved. Bulbar nuclei may be affected.

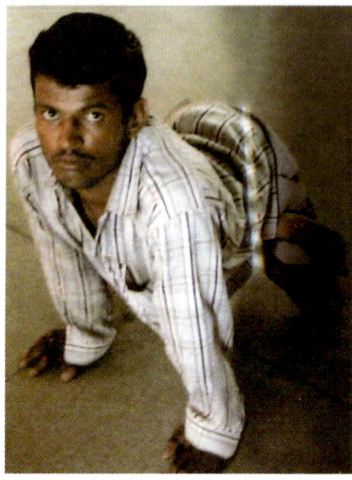

Fig. 137.2: Spinal muscular atrophy

- Lumbar lordosis and calf hypertrophy may be seen in most of cases.
- All the tendon reflexes are diminished, but ankle reflexes are preserved till late.

Q. Which vaccine has been associated with paralytic poliomyelitis?

Ans: Oral polio vaccine particularly in immunodeficient persons has been associated with vaccine associated paralytic polio (VAPP). Such individuals and their household contracts should be given inactivated vaccine.

Q. What do you understand by "provocation poliomyelitis"?

Ans: Provocation poliomyelitis is caused by the administration of intramuscular injection during the incubation period of wild type poliomyelitis or shortly after exposure to oral polio vaccine.

Q. What are the complications of paralytic poliomyelitis?

Ans:
1. Gastric dilatation
2. Intestinal erosions
3. Hypertension
4. Myocarditis
5. Skeletal decalcification

Q. How does polio spread in human?

Ans: By feco-oral route from infected to healthy child.

Q. How does polio virus reach the nervous system?

Ans: Two routes of viral entry have been proposed, i.e. via. bloodstream or via. peripheral nerves. Since viremia precedes the onset of neurologic disease in humans, it has been assumed that virus enters the CNS via. bloodstream. Through the bloodstream, it reaches the muscles where poliovirus receptors are present in the motor end plate region of neuromuscular junction. It travels across the neuromuscular junctions up the axon to the anterior horn cells where it settles down to cause the disease.

Q. **What is bulbar poliomyelitis?**

Ans: Involvement of bulbar nuclei due to polio virus is called *bulbar poliomyelitis*. It is characterised by dysphagia, difficulty in handling secretions or dysphonia, respiratory paralysis and circulatory collapse due to medullary paralysis. Most patients with paralysis recover some functions in weeks to months after infection, about two third of patients have residual disease.

Q. **Which muscles are paralyzed in polio?**

Ans:
- Limb muscles (proximal > distal)
- Thoracic and abdominal muscles
- Bulbar muscles

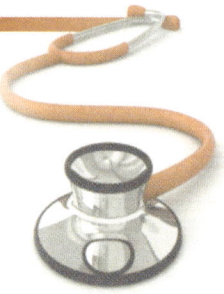

138

Hemiplegia

INSTRUCTION

- Examine the nervous system of the patient

SALIENT FEATURES

- Walking with support due to weakness of one side of the body

HISTORY

Ask and note the following points:

- Note the date and time of onset of stroke
- Mode of onset, e.g. sudden or gradual
- Evaluation of paralysis, i.e. whether it was TIA, stroke-in-evolution or complete stroke
- Any known precipitating factor (s)
- Progress or course of paralysis, e.g. improving, stationary or deteriorating or waxing and waning
- Any associated motor and sensory symptoms
- Any disturbance of consciousness, headache convulsion, visual disturbance, speech disturbance (common in subarachnoid or intracerebral blood)
- Symptoms of raised intracranial tension
- History of similar episodes in the past which recovered completely (TIA)
- History of head injury or epilepsy
- History of HT, diabetes, RHD, meningitis, tuberculosis, migraine, exposure to sexually transmitted disease
- Intake of oral contraceptive
- History of overweight or obesity, smoking, alcoholism
- *Family history* of HT, DM, epilepsy, migraine and similar illness in other family members
- History of functional disturbance, i.e. mobility, pressure sores, visual problem, swallowing or urinary or bowel problem, etc.

EXAMINATION

General Physical Examination

- Is patient conscious or cooperative?
- Posture of the patient

- Neck examination for pulsations, carotid bruits, Horner's syndrome, lymph node, thyroid enlargement
- Vitals, e.g. pulse, BP and temperature
- Edema feet
- Any obvious deformity

Nervous System

(*Read proper nervous system examination*)
- Higher mental functions
- Cranial nerves (UMN or LMN paralysis of 7th nerve), fundus for papilledema,
- Neck rigidity absent or present
- *Position of the limbs* on the paralysed side, arm is held to the side with elbow flexed and the fingers, wrist are also flexed. The leg is extended at both the hip and knee. The foot in inverted and plantar flexed (in this case)
- Signs of UMN (spasticity, exaggerated tendon jerks and planters extensor) are present along with weakness on the paralysed side (in this case)
- Hemiplegic weakness in the upper limbs (shoulder abductor, elbow extensors, wrist and finger extensors, small muscles of hands) and lower limbs (hip and knee flexors and dorsiflexor and evertors of foot) present (Fig. 138.1)
- Cerebellar and autonomic functions are normal (in this case)
- Speech involved if dominant hemisphere is the site of lesion
- Sensory system may show hemianesthesia or hemianopia (homonymous) and sensory inattention
- Gait will be spastic (Fig. 138.1). This patient walks with circumducting gait.

Other Systems

- *CVS* for murmurs (mid diastolic rumble with loud first heart sound in this case), abnormal heart sounds and arrhythmias (AF is present in this case)
- *Respiratory system*
- *GI tract and genitourinary system*
- *Lymphoreticular system*

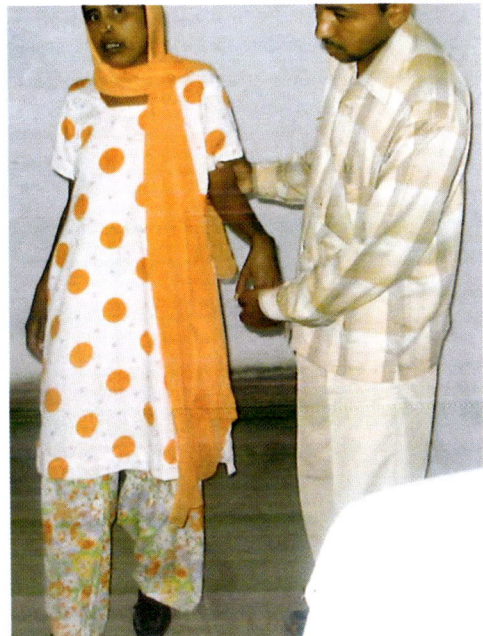

Fig. 138.1: A young female with hemiplegia walking with circumducting gait. She has recovered recently from stroke

PROVISIONAL DIAGNOSIS

This patient is a case of young stroke/CVA (left) with right sided hemiplegia (lesion). The cause of stroke is cerebral embolism (aetiology). She has recovered but still there is difficulty in walking and running (functional status).

QUESTIONS AND ANSWERS

Q. **What are the points in favor of diagnosis?**

Ans: 1. Patient is a case of RHD with MS and AF
2. Sudden onset of hemiplegia without convulsion and speech disturbance
3. 7th supranuclear palsy on right side and hemiplegia on right side (uncrossed hemiplegia) with recovery to some extent
4. UMN signs are still present in right upper and lower limbs
5. Patient is walking with circumducting gait (residual deficit)

Q. **What do you think the cause of hemiplegia in this case and why?**

Ans: Embolic stroke. Points in favour are:
- Catastrophic onset
- Underlying RHD with MS

- Atrial fibrillation is present
- Complete uncrossed hemiplegia
- More or less complete recovery (circumducting gait is a residual deficit)

Q. **What is the site of lesion? What is net neurological involvement in your case?**

Ans: • Site of the lesion is internal capsule
• Neurological deficit is pyramidal tract with 7th supranuclear palsy on the same side

Q. **What are the characteristic features of hemiplegia due to cerebral thrombosis**

Ans: The features are:
1. Onset is sudden, may be slow (stroke-in-evolution)
2. May be transient in TIA
3. Consciousness is preserved or there may be slight confusion
4. Headache is absent but occurs if cerebral edema develops
5. Slowly developing neurological deficit
6. Hypertension, diabetes, dyslipidemia hypothyroidism, hypercoagulable states (pregnancy, puerperium, oral contraceptives), dehydration or shock are precipitating factors
7. Recovery is slow, may be partial or complete

Q. **What is clinical triad of internal capsular lesion?**

Ans: Hemiplegia, hemianesthesia and hemianopia is a triad of capsular lesion.

Q. **Could it be lacunar infarct?**

Ans: Yes, it is a lacunar infarct producing pure motor hemiplegia

Q. **What is lacunar syndrome? What is small vessel infarct?**

Ans: The term lacunar syndrome or infarction implies atherothrombotic or lipohyalinotic occlusion of a small vessel (< 300 μm) in the brain, most of such infarcts being small are not picked up on CT scan. Now, it has been replaced by another term called *small-vessel infarct or stroke* which denotes occlusion of a small penetrating artery and > 50% of these infarcts are picked up on CT scan. Small vessel stroke accounts for > 20% of stroke.

Q. **Name the various lacunar syndromes.**

Ans: 1. *Pure motor hemiparesis* (infarct in posterior limb of internal capsule)
• The face, arm and leg are almost always involved on one side
2. *Pure sensory hemiparesis* (lesion in ventrolateral thalamus)

- Unilateral pure sensory symptoms involving face, arm, legs on one side
3. *Ataxic hemiparesis* (pontine infarct)
   - Ipsilateral cerebellar (ataxia) and corticospinal (hemiparesis) signs
   - There may or may not be dysarthria
   - There is no higher cerebral dysfunction or visual field defect
4. *Dysarthria and clumsy hand or arm syndrome* (infarction in the base of pons or in the genu of internal capsule)
   - There is involvement of one arm
   - Dysathria is present
5. *Aphasic hemiparesis syndrome* (infarction of internal capsule and adjoining corona radiata)
   - There is Broca's (motor) aphasia
   - There is pure motor hemiparesis

Q. **What are the causes of hemiplegia?**
Ans: Read Table 138.1.

Table 138.1: Common causes of hemiplegia

In old age	*In young age*
• CVA (thrombosis, embolism or hemorrhage)	• Demyelination disorder, (multiple-sclerosis)
• Subdural hematoma	• Trauma
• Tumors	• Tumour
• Infections of brain (tuberculosis, syphilis brain abscess, post-encephalitic)	• Embolic stroke
	• Connective tissue disorders
	• Intracranial infection
	• Dural sinus thrombosis

Q. **What do you mean by stroke?**
Ans: A stroke is defined as a neurological deficit occurring as a result of CVA (atherosclerosis, thrombosis, embolism and hemorrhage) and lasting for more than 24 hrs. Stroke in clinical practice is used for hemiplegia, but actually it implies more than that.

Q. **What is TIA and What is RIND? What is completed stroke?**
Ans: 1. *TIA:* It means transient hemiplegia or neurological deficit occurring as a result of ischemia which recovers within 24 hours.
2. *Stroke-in-evolution:* The neurological deficit worsens gradually or in a stepwise pattern over hours or days.
3. *Completed stroke:* Neurological deficit is complete at the onset and persists for days to weeks and often permanently.
4. *Reversible ischemic neurological deficit (RIND):* It means neurological deficit

persisting for more than 24 hours, but recovers totally within a week.

Q. **What are the features of a carotid TIA ?**
Ans: I. *Features of carotid TIAs*
   - Hemiplegia, aphasia or transient loss of vision in one eye only (amaurosis fugax)

Q. **What is crossed or uncrossed hemiplegia?**
Ans: 1. *Crossed hemiplegia:* It refers to ipsilateral LMN paralysis of one of the cranial nerves with contralateral (opposite side) hemiplegia. It signifies the brainstem lesion.
2. *Uncrossed hemiplegia:* It refers to UMN 7th nerve palsy on the side of hemiplegia (i.e. both being opposite to cerebral lesion). For example, if UMN 7th nerve palsy and hemiplegia are on the left side, the cerebral lesion is on the right side.

Q. **What is dense hemiplegia?**
Ans: *Dense hemiplegia:* The complete loss of voluntary functions (weakness) of equal magnitude in both upper and lower limbs on the side of the body involved constitutes dense hemiplegia. This signifies an internal capsular lesion as corticospinal fibers are condensed there.

Q. **What is stuttering hemiplegia?**
Ans: *Stuttering hemiplegia:* Transient speech disturbance (aphasia, dysarthria) with hemiplegia indicates stuttering hemiplegia. It is due to progressive occlusion of internal carotid artery (stroke-in-evolution). It ultimately results in completed stroke.

Q. **What is homolateral hemiplegia?**
Ans: *Homolateral hemiplegia:* It means hemiplegia occurring on the same side of the lesion, is seen in unilateral cervical spinal cord lesion (*Brown-Séquard's syndrome*).

Q. **What is hysterical hemiplegia?**
Ans: Read it in case discussion on abnormal gait.

Q. **What are the risk factors for stroke?**
Ans: • Systemic hypertension, TIA
   - Heart disease, e.g. ischemic, rheumatic with atrial fibrillation, cardiomyopathy
   - Diabetes
   - Hyperlipidemia (familial or non familial), atherosclerosis
   - Homocysteinemia and homocysteinuria
   - Deficiency of proteins C and S
   - Strong family history, smoking
   - Obesity, oral contraceptives

- Hyperviscosity syndrome, e.g. polycy-themia, antiphospholipid syndrome
- Increasing age (old age)

Q. **What are the causes of recurrent CVA/ hemiplegia?**

Ans: Causes are:
- TIA (transient ischemic attack) is common cause
- Post epilepsy — Todd's paralysis
- Hypertensive encephalopathy
- Migrainous hemiplegia (vasospastic hemiplegia)
- Hysterical hemiplegia

Q. **What are the causes of stroke in young?**

Ans: Causes are:
- *Cerebral embolism*
- *Subarachnoid hemorrhage*
- *Hyperviscosity syndrome*, e.g. polycythemia, post-partum state, oral contraceptive
- *Arteritis*
- *Premature or accelerated atherogenesis*
- *Demyelinating disease*, e.g. multiple sclerosis
- *Head injury*
- *Inflammatory disease*, e.g. meningitis, encephalitis, cerebral abscess, tuberculoma, cerebral malaria
- *Migrainous*
- *Intracranial neoplasm*
- *Procoagulant state*, e.g. protein C and S deficiency, homocysteinemia, antithrombin–1 deficiency, antiphospholipid syndrome, puerperium.

Q. **How will you localise the lesion in a case with hemiplegia?**

Ans: The site of lesion can be deduced from associated neurological signs.

1. *Cortical or subcortical (corona radiata) lesion:*

   The characteristic features are:
   i. Contralateral hemiplegia of uncrossed type
   ii. Convulsions (Jacksonian) may occur
   iii. Speech disturbance (aphasia) if dominant hemisphere is involved. The dominant hemisphere is decided from handedness of a person. If a person is right-handed, the left hemisphere is dominant and contains the speech area
   iv. Cortical type of sensory loss (astereognosis, loss of sense of position, tactile localisation and two-point discrimination)
   v. Anosognosia, visual field defect
   vi. Supranuclear 7th nerve palsy

2. *Internal capsular lesions*
   - Contralateral hemiplegia of uncrossed type
   - Contralateral hemianesthesia
   - Dense hemiplegia—complete paralysis of face, upper and lower limbs
   - UMN paralysis of 7th nerve
   - No convulsion, no speech, taste or visual disturbance
   - Pure motor hemiplegia indicates lacunar infarct.

3. *Midbrain lesion*
   - Contralateral hemiplegia of crossed type
   - The 3rd nerve nuclear paralysis with contralateral hemiplegia constitutes *Weber's syndrome*
   - Contralateral hemianesthesia and analgesia

4. *Pontine lesion*
   - Contralateral hemiplegia of crossed type
   - Contralateral hemianesthesia and analgesia
   - Ipsilateral 6th or 7th cranial nerve paralysis (LMN type) with contralateral hemiplegia is called *Millard-Gubler syndrome*
   - Constriction of pupil (*Horner's syndrome*) on the same side of the lesion due to involvement of sympathetic fibers
   - Ataxic hemiplegia with or without dysarthria indicates a lacunar infarct

5. *Medulla oblongata lesion*

   A. Features of medial medullary syndrome
   Ipsilateral
   - Paralysis of half of tongue (XII nerve palsy)
   Contralateral
   - Upper and lower limbs UMN paralysis sparing face.

Q. **How would you classify stroke?**

Ans: Based on Bomford clinical classification, stroke is divided into

1. **Total anterior circulation syndrome**
   i. Hemiplegia (motor deficit of face, arm and leg)
   ii. Homonymous hemianopia
   iii. Higher cortical dysfunction (aphasia, memory, neglect)

2. **Partial anterior circulation syndrome**

Any two of the following may be present:

i. Hemiplegia (motor and/or sensory deficit)

ii. Ipsilateral hemianopia or higher cerebral dysfunction

iii. Higher cerebral dysfunction alone

or

Isolated motor and/or sensory deficit restricted to one limb (monoplegia) or the face.

3. **Posterior circulation syndrome**

One or more of the following features present:

i. Bilateral motor or sensory signs not secondary to brainstem compression by a large supratentorial lesion

ii. Cerebellar signs (ataxic hemiparesis)

iii. Unequivocal diplopia with or without external ocular muscle palsy

iv. Crossed sign, for example, left facial and right limb weakness

v. Hemianopia alone or with any of the 4 features described above.

Q. How would you manage a case of TIA?

Ans: i. Differentiate TIA from stroke by history, examination and CT scan.

ii. Perform duplex ultrasonography of the carotid vessel and/or carotid artery DSA.

iii. Evaluate clinical risk profile and institute life style modifications, ie.
   • Stop smoking and alcohol
   • Dietary management
   • Exercise as advised by the doctor
   • Weight control
   • Maintain the BP and sugar control in diabetes
   • Antiplatelets, e.g. aspirin or aspirin plus clopidogrel or dipyidamole.

iv. *Statins:* Several trials have confirmed that statin drugs reduce the risk of TIA and stroke. Therefore, all patients of TIA must receive one of the statins.

v. Angiotensin-converting enzyme inhibitors or angiotensin-receptor blockers. Lowering of blood pressure to levels below those traditionally defining hypertension with these drugs reduce the risk of stroke.

Q. What is anterior cerebral artery syndrome?

Ans: Occlusion of anterior cerebral artery produces clinical features depending on the site of block as follows:

Symptoms and signs	Area involved
Monoplegia involving a lower limb and paresis of opposite arm to lesser degree (incomplete hemiplegia)	Motor leg area. Arm area of cortex or its descending fibers in corona radita
Loss of cortical sensations over lower limb involved	Sensory leg area
Urinary incontinence	Paracentral lobule (bladder area)
Contralateral primitive reflexes, e.g. grasp, sucking may be present	Supplemental motor area
Akinetic mutism	Cingulate gyrus
Gait apraxia	Frontal cortex near leg area

Q. What is the usual clinical course of hemiplegia?

Ans: A patient of hemiplegia may pass through the following stages:

1. *Stage of neuronal shock:* It is a state when the reflex activity is suppressed, i.e. there is hypotonia. Jerks are absent and plantars are silent. This stage may not be seen in all cases of hemiplegia. This lasts for 2–3 weeks.

2. *Stage of recovery:* After 2–3 weeks the recovery starts. The face recovers first. Power returns in the extensors of lower limb and flexors of the upper limb. Finer movements of the fingers and hands recover last to a variable extent.

3. *Stage of residual paralysis:* The only deficit is little spasticity and a hemiplegic gait.

Q. What are the measures to determine the outcome after an acute stroke?

Ans: The measures used to determine are:

1. *Barthel Index:* It is a measure of the ability to perform activities of daily living, e.g. eating, bathing, walking and using the comode.

2. *Modified Rankin Scale:* It is measure of overall functional ability of the patient in which a score of zero indicates absence of symptoms and a score 5 indicates severe disability.

3. *Glasgow Outcome Scale (global assessment scoring system)*

   Score 1: Good recovery

   Score 2: Moderate recovery

   Score 3: Severe disability

   Score 4: Vegetative existence

   Score 5: Death

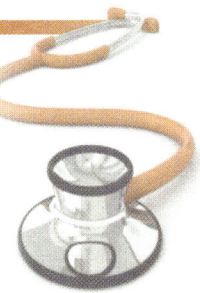

139

Brain Tumor

INSTRUCTION

- Examine the nervous system of the patient

SALIENT FEATURES

- Headache and convulsions

HISTORY

Ask and note the following:

- Age (old age)
- Onset—acute (sudden, catastrophic), subacute or chronic (slow onset suggests brain tumor)
- Disturbance in consciousness: Majority of the patients with brain tumor retain consciousness
- Disturbance of speech (aphasia, dysarthria, dysphonia)
- Convulsions—generalized convulsions preceding the paralysis, Todd's paralysis (postictal) indicate ICSOL (intracranial space occupying lesion). History of Jacksonian fits (present)
- Disturbance of smell, taste, vision (visual field defect, diplopia) suggest frontal lobe tumor
- History of headache before, persistent or mild.

Headache preceding paralysis suggests ICSOL or subdural hematoma
- Symptoms and signs of raised intracranial tension (space occupying lesion)
- Weakness/paralysis of one limb/one half of the body (present)/or of all the four limbs

EXAMINATION

Neurological Examination

- *Higher functions:* They are disturbed in frontal lobe lesions
- *Cranial nerve palsy:* 1st and 2nd cranial of nerves or visual pathway may be involved. There may be supranuclear 7th cranial nerve involvements
- Speech disturbance if dominant hemisphere is involved
- Signs of raised intracranial tension (present in this case)
- Fundus for papilledema (present)
- Lower or upper motor neuron signs involving one limb/one half of the body or UMN signs involving the one side (present) or both side of the body

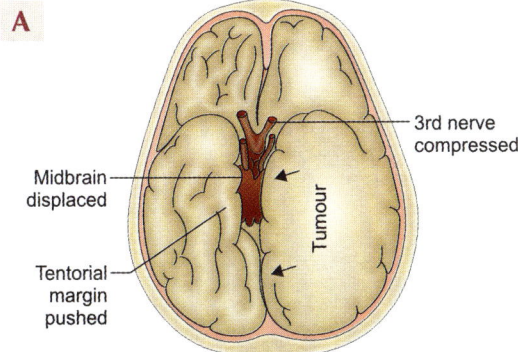

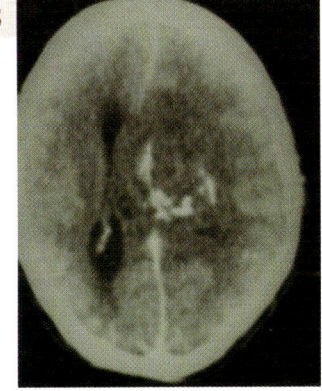

Fig. 139.1: A cerebral tumor producing mass effects. (A) Diagrammatic illustration showing pressure effects; (B) CT scan showing a left-sided tumor with hemorrhage (hyperdense areas) in it causing midline shift to the right

- There may be sensory disturbance if sensory cortex involved (i.e. loss of cortical sensation if sensory cortex involved)

PROVISIONAL DIAGNOSIS

The old person has slow onset hemiplegia with Jacksonian fits (lesion) due to a space occupying lesion (etiology). The patient has disability in walking and is psychological upset (functional status).

Note: Read all the questions regarding hemiplegia in previous case discussion.

QUESTIONS AND ANSWERS

Q. **What are the points in favor of your diagnosis?**
Ans: 1. An old male
2. Slow onset and slow progression of hemiplegia
3. Jacksonian fits
4. Headache vomiting and papilledema (features of raised ICP)
5. False localising signs, e.g. unilateral 6th cranial nerve palsy

Q. **What are the usual features of hemiplegia due to a brain tumor?**
Ans: 1. Slow onset and slow progression
2. *Focal symptoms*—Jacksonian fits (focal epilepsy), aphasia, hemiplegia or monoplegia
3. *Symptoms and signs of raised intracranial tension* (read case discussion on raised ICP or hydrocephalus)
4. *False localising signs*
   - Unilateral 6th nerve palsy (diplopia with lateral deviation of the eye), sometimes it may be bilateral
   - Bilateral plantar extensor response
   - Bilateral grasp reflexes
   - Cerebellar signs
   - Fixed dilated pupils

Q. **What are the features of hemiplegia due to chronic subdural hematoma?**
Ans: The features are:
   i. There may be history of injury or fall. Patient may have underlying liver dis-

ease, bleeding diathesis or may be on anticoagulants
   ii. Slow or chronic onset with fluctuating headache, slow thinking, confusion, drowsiness, personality changes, seizures, etc.
   iii. There may be a lucid interval (weeks, months or more than a year) between the onset of injury and symptoms
   iv. Hemiplegia is uncrossed, due to compression effect on pyramidal tracts.

Q. **What do you understand by true and false localising signs?**
Ans: *True localising signs:* These are the signs due to direct consequence of a lesion or tumor, help in the localisation of the lesion, hence, their name.
False localising signs: They are indirect consequences of a lesion/tumor and have no value in localising of the lesion.

Q. **What are the false localising signs?**
Ans: They have already been enumerated above in clinical features of brain tumour.

Q. **What are the common brain tumors?**
Ans: *Glial tumors* (gliomas) are the most common (50–60%) followed by meningiomas (25%), schwannomas (10%) and rest are other CNS tumors.

Q. **What is the most common malignant tumor of the brain?**
Ans: Medulloblastoma multiforme.

Q. **What are the characteristics of frontal lobe tumor?**
Ans: 1. A left frontal tumour will cause disturbance of personality apathy and impairment of intellectual functions over several months. When speech area is affected (right handed person), an expressive aphasia will result. As the corticospinal pathway becomes involved, a right hemiparesis may follow. Seizures are common.
2. A right parietal glioma involving the optic radiation will cause left homonvmous field defect. Cortical sensory loss and a left hemiparesis may follow. Partial seizures causing episodes of numbness of left limbs may develop.

140

Paraplegia

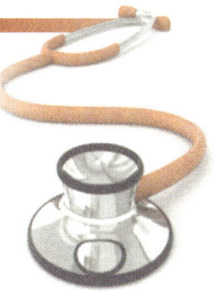

INSTRUCTION

- Examine the nervous system of the patient

SALIENT FEATURES

- Weakness of both lower limbs

HISTORY

Ask for the following:

- Note and ask and the date and time of onset of paralysis
- Mode of onset (sudden or gradual) and course of symptoms
- History of precipitating factors, e.g. spinal trauma, vaccination
- Progress of paralysis, e.g. increasing, stationary, progressive, waxing or waning type
- Motor symptoms including inability or difficulty in walking
- Sensory symptoms, e.g. root pain (radicular pain), history of a constriction band around the waist at the site of lesion
- History of pin and needless sensation (parasthesias), numbness below the level of lesion
- Sphincter disturbance and bladder sensations
- History of urinary infection, pressure sores and venous thrombosis
- Assess functional status by asking the use of wheelchair, walking-aids, orthotic shoes, etc. Has the house been modified for patient's disability?

Past History

- History of fever, tuberculosis, exposure to STD
- History of similar episodes in the past
- History of spinal trauma
- History of diabetes, HT, alcoholism
- Pain in back

Family History

- Diabetes, HT, tuberculosis
- History of paraplegia in other members of the family (hereditary spastic paraplegia)

EXAMINATION

General Physical Examination

- Consciousness or cooperative, posture
- Neck for lymphadenopathy
- Vitals, e.g. pulse, BP and temperature
- Skin, e.g. pigmentation, neurofibroma

Nervous System Examination

- *Higher functions:* Normal/abnormal
- *Neck rigidity:* Absent /present
- *Cranial nerves:* Involved/not involved
- *Cerebellar signs:* Absent/present (cerebellum not involved in this case)
- *Motor system of lower limbs including gait:* There is hypertonia, exaggerated tendon reflexes with bilateral plantar extensors. There is no atrophy (UMN signs present below the lesion)
- *Sensory system of lower limbs:* There is sensory level at the trunk (mid thoracic region, Fig. 140.1). Check for sacral sensation

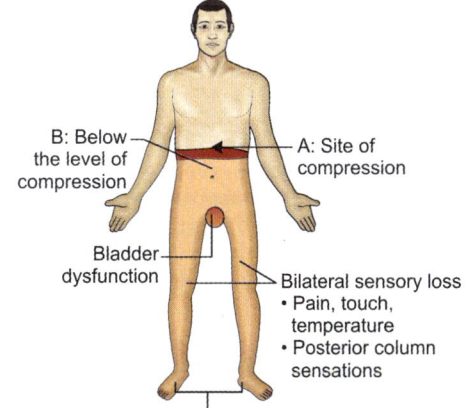

- Bilateral tendon reflexes exaggerated
- Bilateral plantars extensor

Fig. 140.1: Compression paraplegia with transverse thoracic spinal cord lesion with definite level. There are UMN signs below the site of compression. There is bilateral loss of all sensory modalities below the level of compression

Examination of Spine

- Kyphosis, scoliosis, gibbus (present in this case), tenderness (present) and spina bifida (a tuff of hair)

Other Systems

- *Respiratory system examination* for tuberculosis, bronchogenic carcinoma and lymphoma
- *CVS* as discussed in hemiplegia
- *GI tract* for hepatosplenomegaly, ascites
- *Lymphoreticular system* for sternal tenderness, hemorrhagic spots and lymphadenopathy

PROVISIONAL DIAGNOSIS

The patient has compression (spastic) paraplegia (lesion) produced by Pott's disease (aetiology). It is complicated by bladder involvement (functional status).

Q. Why do you say it a compression paraplegia?
Ans: The following points suggest compression:
   i. A level of compression evident
   ii. History of root pain and loss of sensations (radicular) at the level of compression
   iii. UMN paraplegia below the level of compression
   iv. Sensory loss to all modalities below a certain level
   v. Presence of gibbus at midthoracic region
   vi. Presence of sphincter disturbance

QUESTIONS AND ANSWERS

Q. Where is the site of lesion in your case?
Ans: Site of lesion is midthoracic region between $T_4 - T_5$. The points in favor are:
   1. Presence of upper limb reflexes which indicate intactness of all cervical segments and first thoracic.
   2. Loss of abdominal reflexes indicate lesion above T_6.
   3. Weakness of intercostal muscles of T_4, T_5 and a dermatomal sensory loss points the lesion at this site. However, there was no bony deformity of spine at this level.

Q. What is net neurological deficit in your case?
Ans:
- Bilateral pyramidal tract involvement
- Bilateral sensory involvement of all modalities (spinothalamic and posterior column involvement)
- Sphincter involvement (autonomic involvement)

Q. How does tuberculosis cause paraplegia?
Ans: This is as follows:
   1. Compression of the cord by cold abscess (extradural compression)
   2. Tubercular arachnoiditis or pachymeningitis (intradural compression)
   3. Tubercular endarteritis (vascular phenomenon) producing myelomalacia of the cord
   4. Tubercular myelitis, i.e. extension of the lesion from outside to within

Q. What is the type of lesion in your case?
Ans: Extramedullary compression due to Pott's disease. The points in favor are:
   1. Slowly progressive paraplegia, symmetric involvement.
   2. History of root pain and dermatological sensory loss.
   3. Brisk reflexes and sensory loss of all modalities below the level of compression.
   4. Bowel and bladder involvement.
   5. There is no sacral sparing.
   6. Presence of gibbus in mid thoracic region

Q. What are the characteristic signs of compression paraplegia?
Ans:
   1. Signs of LMN paralysis at the site of compression with radicular pain/loss of sensations.
   2. UMN signs below the level of compression.
   3. Sphincter involvement.
   4. Loss of all sensory modalities below the level of compression (sensory level is 3–4 segments below the motor level)

Q. How would you localise site of lesion in case of paraplegia?
Ans: Read Table 140.1.

Table 140.1: Site of localisation in a patient with paraplegia	
Site of lesion	*Symptoms and signs*
Lesion at /above T_6	• Paraplegia with loss of all abdominal reflexes • There is a level of sensory loss over the chest • Deep tendon reflexes below compression are exaggerated and plantars are extensor
Lesion at $T_7 - T_9$	• Paraplegia (UMN) with loss of upper abdominal reflexes
Lesion at $T_9 - T_{10}$	• Umbilicus is turned downwards during rising test (Beever's sign). Upper abdominal reflexes are present
Lesion at $T_{10} - T_{12}$	• Paralysis of both lower limbs (UMN type of paraplegia) • Upper abdominal reflexes are spared but lower abdominal reflexes are lost. Cremasteric being superficial reflexes is also lost

Contd.

Table 140.1: Site of localisation in a patient with paraplegia

Site of lesion	Symptoms and signs
	• Umbilicus is turned upwards during rising test due to paralysis of lower part of rectus abdominis. Beever's sign actually indicates lesions at T_9 and T_{10}
Lesion of L_1	• Paraplegia (UMN) with loss of cremasteric reflex only
	• Superficial sensory loss over sacrum
	• Deep tendon jerks below the level of compression are exaggerated
	• Radicular pain/paresthesia limited to anterior aspect of thigh, groin and testicle
Lesion of $L_2 – L_4$ (cauda equina lesion)	• Paraplegia (LMN) with loss of knee jerks and preservation of ankle jerks
	• Radicular pain/paresthesia over anteromedial aspect of the leg
	• Superficial sensory deficit over anteromedial aspect of leg
Lesion of L_5 and S_1	• Paralysis of movements of foot and ankle, flexion at knee and extension of thigh. There is loss of ankle jerks
	• Radicular pain/paresthesia over dorsum of foot and anterolateral aspect of leg (L_5) or radicular pain/paresthesia over buttock, back of thigh, calf and lateral border of foot

Table 140.2: Distinction between paraplegia-in-extension and paraplegia-in-flexion

Feature	Paraplegia-in-extension	Paraplegia-in-flexion
Posture	Lower limbs adopt an extension posture and extensor muscles are spastic. Extensor spasms occur	Lower limbs adopt flexed posture. Intermittent flexor spasms occur in which there is flexion of both lower limbs
Neurological deficit	Only pyramidal tracts are involved	Both pyramidal and extrapyramidal tracts are involved
Clinical features Positions of limbs	Hip extended and adducted, knee extended and feet plantar-flexed	Thighs and knees are flexed, feet dorsiflexed
Tone	Clasp-knife spasticity in extensor groups of muscles	Rigidity in flexor groups of muscles
Tendon jerks	Exaggerated	Diminished
Plantar response	Extensor	Extensor but evokes flexor spasms
Incontinence of bowel and bladder	Absent	Present
Mass reflex*	Absent	Present

N.B. *Mass reflex* is an area of hyperexcitability of reflex activity. Just stroking the skin of either lower limbs or lower abdominal wall, produces the reflex evacuation of the bladder and bowel with reflex flexor spasms of the lower limbs and lower trunk muscles.

Q. What do you mean by paraplegia-in-flexion and paraplegia-in-extension?

Ans: Paraplegia-in-extension is spastic paraplegia with involvement of pyramidal tract. It indicates partial/incomplete spinal cord compression. On the other hand paraplegia-in-flexion means complete compression of the cord with involvement of pyramidal and extrapyramidal tracts. The differences between the two are summarised in Table 140.2.

Q. Where are the common causes of spastic paraplegia?

Ans: Read Table 140.3.

Q. What are the common causes of noncompressive paraplegia?

Ans: • Motor neurone disease especially amyotrophic lateral sclerosis

Table 140.3: Common cause of spastic paraplegia

I. Compressive

  A. Extramedullary

    i. Intradural

      • Meningioma, neurofibroma, arachnoiditis

    ii. Extradural

      • Pott's disease (caries spine)

      • Vertebral neoplasms, e.g. metastases, myeloma

      • Pachymeningitis

      • Prolapsed intervertebral disc

      • Epidural abscess or hemorrhage

      • Fracture dislocation of vertebra, Paget's disease, osteoporosis

  B. Intramedullary

    • Syringomyelia, hematomyelia

    • Intramedullary tumor, e.g. ependymoma, glioma

    • Spinal cord abscess (e.g. pyogenic, tuberculosis)

- Multiple sclerosis, postvaccinal myelitis
- Acute transverse myelitis
- Subacute combined degeneration (Vit. B$_{12}$ deficiency)
- Lathyrism
- Syringomyelia
- Hereditary spastic paraplegia
- Tropical spastic paraplegia
- Radiation myelopathy

Q. **What is cerebral paraplegia? What are its causes?**

Ans: The lower limbs and bladder (micturition centre) are represented in paracentral lobule (about upper one inch of cerebral cortex), hence, lesion of this area produces paraplegia with bladder disturbance (retention of urine) and cortical type of sensory loss. There may be associated headache, vomiting and convulsions or Jacksonian fits.

The **causes** are:
- Superior sagittal sinus thrombosis
- Parasagittal meningioma
- Thrombosis of unpaired anterior cerebral artery
- Gun shot injury of paracentral lobule
- Internal hydrocephalus

Q. **What are the differences between extra-medullary and intramedullary compression?**

Ans: Read Table 140.4.

Table 140.4: Differentiation between extramedullary and intramedullary spinal cord compression

Extramedullary	Intramedullary
• Root pain common	Rare
• UMN Signs are early and prominent	Late feature and are less prominent
• Segmental sensory loss or absent reflex at the site of compression	Extends to involve few segments with atrophy and fasciculations
• Reflexes brisk, early feature	Less brisk, late feature
• Contralateral loss of pain and temperature with ipsilateral loss of proprioception	Dissociated sensory loss
• Sacral sparing absent	Sacral sparing is a characteristic feature
• Sphincters involvement is late	Early involvement
• Trophic changes are unusual	Common
• Vertebral tenderness may be present	Absent
• 'Froin's syndrome' (CSF change common)	Rare

Q. **How will you distinguish compressive from noncompressive myelopathy?**

Ans: The absolute characteristic of compression of the cord is either motor loss (loss of tendon jerk, muscle wasting, fasciculations) or a sensory sign (hyperesthesia, analgesia) at the site of compression while no such phenomenon is seen in noncompressive myelopathy. The distinction between the two is described in Table 140.5.

Table 140.5: Distinction between compressive and noncompressive myelopathy

Compressive	Noncompressive
• Bone changes, i.e. deformity, tenderness present	No bony change
• Girdle-like pain present (root pain)	No root pain
• Upper level of sensory loss present	No definite level
• Zone of hyperesthesia may be present	Absent
• Usually of gradual onset	Usually of acute onset
• Asymmetrical involvement of limbs	Symmetrical involvement of limbs
• Flexor spasms common	Absent
• Bowel and bladder involvement is early	Late involvement
• Commonest cause is caries spine	Commonest cause is motor neuron disease

Q. **What are the causes of cord compression at multiple sites?**

Ans: Following are the causes:
- Arachnoiditis (tubercular—there is patchy involvement)
- Neurofibromatosis
- Multiple discs prolapse
- Secondary deposits
- Cervical spondylosis

Q. **What are the causes of paraplegia without sensory loss?**

Ans: Causes are:
- Hereditary spastic paraplegia
- Lathyrism
- GB syndrome
- Amyotrophic lateral sclerosis
- Fluorosis

Q. **What are the causes of spastic paraplegia with loss of deep tendon jerks?**

Ans:
- Neuronal shock (spinal shock). All jerks are absent
- Radiculitis—the jerk whose root is involved will be absent
- Associated peripheral neuropathy—bilateral ankle jerk will be absent
- Presence of bedsores or complicating

UTI. The reflex activity in this complication may be suppressed leading to loss of most reflexes

- Hematomyelia (sudden hemorrhage from AV malformation) or myelomalacia causes loss of reflexes
- Hypokalemia

Q.   What is lathyrism?

Ans: It is a slowly evolving epidemic spastic paraplegia due to consumption of *'khesari dal'* (*lathyrus sativus*) for prolonged period. It occurs in areas where drought are commonly seen, e.g. UP, Bihar, Rajasthan and MP where poor people consume often a mixture of wheat, Bengal gram and Khesari dal called *"birri"*. It may invovle many families in a locality. The causative factor is BOAA—a neurotoxin. Initially, patients complain of nocturnal muscle cramps, stiffness of limbs and inability to walk. Ultimately due to increasing spasticity they pass through one-stick stage (scissor type gait), two-stick stage (patient uses two sticks to walk) and crawler stage (patient crawls on hands).

Q.   What are the causes of optic atrophy and paraplegia?

Ans: Optic atrophy may be part and parcel of the disease causing paraplegia.

- Hereditary (Friedreich's) ataxia
- Neuromyelitis optical (Devic's disease—a demyelinating disorder)
- Eale's disease
- Subacute myelo-optic neuropathy, alcohol induced
- Infections like tuberculosis and syphilis
- Deficiency states, e.g. subacute combined degeneration, pellagra

Q.   What is tropical spastic paraplegia (HTLV–I associated myelopathy)?

Ans: It is common in females (3rd, 4th decades) associated with HTLV-1 infection where the patient develops gradual onset of weakness of legs (paraplegia) which *progresses* and patient becomes confined to wheel chair within *10 years*. This is UMN spastic paraplegia without sensory disturbance. Bladder disturbance and constipation are common. This is an example of non-compressive progressive myelopathy. The diagnosis is suggested by seropositivity for HTLV-1.

Q.   How will you investigate the case with paraplegia?

Ans: Investigations are:

1. *Routine blood tests* (TLC, DLC, ESR)
2. *Urine examination*, urine for culture and sensitivity
3. *Blood biochemistry*, e.g. urea, creatinine, electrolytes
4. *Chest X-ray* for tuberculosis or malignancy lung or lymphoma
5. *Lymph node biopsy* if lymph nodes are enlarged
6. *CSF examination*. Features of *Froin's* syndrome will be evident if spinal tumour is the cause of spinal block.
   - Low CSF pressure
   - Xanthochromia
   - Increased protein
   - Normal cellular count
   - Positive Queckensted test
7. *CT myelography* to determine the site and type of compression. Nowadays, it has been replaced by MRI.
   The CT myelography may show:
   i. *Meniscus sign* in intradural compression
   ii. *Brush border sign* in extradural tumors
   iii. *Candle-wax or Candle-guttering appearance* in arachnoiditis
   iv. *Expansion sign* in syringomyelia
8. *MRI to* find out the cause of compression
9. *Other tests* depending on the cause or disease

Q.   What is albumino-cytological dissociation?

Ans: It refers to increased protein content in CSF with no parallel rise in cell count. The causes are:

- GB syndrome
- Froin's syndrome (spinal block due to a spinal tumor)
- Acoustic neurofibroma
- Cauda equina syndrome

Q.   What are the causes of xanthochromia (yellow coloration of CSF)?

Ans:
- Old subarachnoid hemorrhage
- GB syndrome
- Froin's syndrome
- Acoustic neuroma
- Deep jaundice

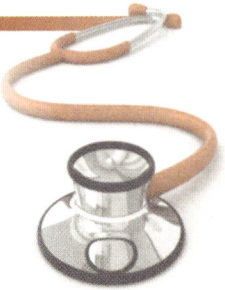

141

Quadriplegia/
Tetraplegia

INSTRUCTION

- Perform neurological examination of this patient

SALIENT FEATURES

- Weakness of all the four limbs

HISTORY

Ask for the following:

- Ask about the onset (acute, subacute, chronic), progression (limb involvement) and course
- Duration of symptoms
- History of neck pain (radicular pain or localised pain)
- History of numbness/paraesthesia involving the upper limbs
- Weakness of all the four limbs, pattern of involvement (gradual, simultaneous or one followed by the other)
- Involvement of bladder and bowel

- History of urinary infections, pressure sores or deep vein thrombosis
- Trauma to neck region
- History of tuberculosis, sepsis and syphilis

EXAMINATION

Neurological Examination

- Higher functions — normal
- Cranial nerves — normal. Look for Horner's syndrome
- Cerebellar functions — could not be tested
- Speech — normal

Motor System

- There is wasting of small muscles of hands (disuse atrophy)
- There is sensory loss of all modalities over the outer arm and forearms and later of aspect of hand (C_5–C_6)
- Hyperreflexia of all the four limbs except biceps jerks which is lost (in this case). There is inversion of biceps jerk.

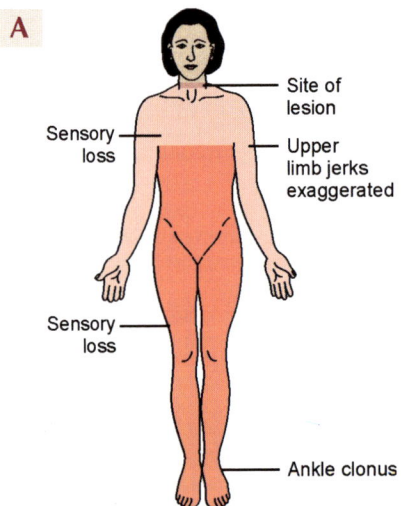

A

Sensory loss

Sensory loss

Site of lesion

Upper limb jerks exaggerated

Ankle clonus

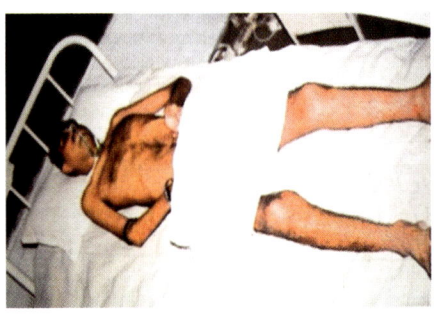

B

Fig. 141.1: Quadriplegia. (A) Site of lesion and clinical features; (B) A patient lying with quadriparesis

- Tone is increased in all the limbs (clasp-knife spasticity present)
- Plantars are bilateral extensors (present)
- No trophic changes or deep vein thrombosis

Sensory System

- Loss of sensory modalities over C_5-C_6 (present)
- Bladder sensations or visceral sensations intact
- Scrotal sensation are intact. Sacral sensations intact

PROVISIONAL DIAGNOSIS

This patient has spastic quadriplegia (lesion) at the level of C_5-C_6 caused by cervical injury (aetiology). Patient is finding difficulty in carrying routine activity due to spasticity (functional status).

QUESTIONS AND ANSWERS

Q. **What are the points in favor of your diagnosis?**
Ans:
- Radicular/neck pain
- Spastic weakness of all the four limbs with bilateral plantars extensor (Fig. 141.1)
- Biceps jerks are lost. There is inversion of biceps jerks
- No bladder and bowel involvement
- Sensory loss over C_5-C_6 dermatomes

Q. **Why do you localise the lesion at C_5-C_6?**
Ans:
1. Radicular neck pain radiating to forearms
2. Biceps jerks are lost with inversion of biceps (it is sine quanon of diagnosis)
3. Sensory loss over C5–C6 dermatomes (outer arm, forearm, thumb and index finger)
4. Spastic quadriparesis

Q. **What are the common causes of hypertonia?**
Ans:
- UMN lesion
- Tetanus
- Strychnine poisoning
- Hysterical
- Voluntary in noncooperative patients
- Extrapyramidal lesion except chorea
- Myotonia
- Catatonia
- Decerebrate rigidity
- The stiff man syndrome

Q. **What is neuronal (spinal) shock?**
Ans: It refers to depression or loss of reflex activity (absent tendon reflexes) in acute lesion of spinal cord. It is transient, may last for few days followed by recovery. This explains the loss of deep tendon reflexes in acute onset UMN lesion of the cord.

Q. **What are the causes of quadriplegia?**
Ans: Quadriplegia means weakness of all the four limbs. It may be spastic (UMN) or flacid (LMN). The causes are:

A. *Spastic quadriparesis* (lesion in the bilateral brainstem or spinal cord up to C_8-T_1)
1. Cerebral palsy
2. Bilateral brainstem lesion
3. High cervical cord compression, e.g. craniovertebral anomaly, high spinal cord injury, etc.
4. Multiple sclerosis
5. Motor neuron disease

B. *Flaccid quadriparesis* (lesion may involve anterior horn cells, peripheral nerves or muscles)
6. Acute anterior poliomyelitis
7. Guillain-Barré syndrome
8. Peripheral neuropathy
9. Myopathy or polymyositis
10. Periodic paralysis (transient quadriplegia)

Q. **How would you localise the lesion in case of quadriplegia?**
Ans: Read Table 141.1.

Table 141.1: Lesions at different sites and their signs

Site of lesion (spinal segment)	Symptoms and signs	
High cervical cord lesion, e.g. at C_1-C_4	• UMN quadriplegia • There may be weakness of respiratory muscles or diaphragmatic palsy • There may be sub-occipital pain radiating to neck and shoulder • Sensory loss over upper part of chest (C_1-C_4)	
Lower cervical cord lesion		
Site	Sensory	Motor
C_5	• Radicular pain/ paresthesia over neck, shoulder, outer arm, forearm	• Muscle weakness of deltoid, supraspinatus brachioradialis
	• Sensory deficit over outer aspect of upper arm	• Jerks affected, e.g. biceps, supinator lost
C_6	• Radicular pain/ paresthesia over neck, shoulder, outer arm, forearm thumb and index finger	• Muscle weakness, e.g. biceps, brachioradialis, extensor carpi radialis longus
	• Sensory loss over thumb and index finger	• Deep tendon jerks affected, e.g. biceps, supinator lost
C_7	• Radicular pain/ paresthesia over neck, shoulder, arm, forearm to index and middle finger	• Muscle weakness of triceps and muscles of forearm

Contd.

Table 141.1: Lesions at different sites and their signs

Site of lesion (spinal segment)	Symptoms and signs
• Superficial sensory loss over middle and index finger	• Loss of tricep jerk
C_8 • Radicular pain/ paraesthesia over neck, shoulder, arm, ring and index fingers	• Muscle weakness of flexors of forearm
• Sensory loss over ring and little fingers	• Finger flexion jerk is lost
T_1 • Radicular pain/ paresthesia over neck, axilla, medial aspects of arm, forearm, little and ring finger	• Muscle weakness of small muscles of hand
• Sensory loss over medial arm and little finger	• Finger flexion jerk is lost

Note: Horner's syndrome may occur at any level of cervical cord compression

Q. What are the causes and clinical features of high cervical cord compression?

Ans: The features of high cervical cord compression are tabulated in Table 141.2.

Q. How will you calculate the level of spinal segments in relation to vertebra in a case with compression paraplegia?

Ans: In case of compression, if vertebra involved is known, then calculation of spinal segment is done as follows:

Vertebra	Spinal segment
• For cervical vertebrae	: Add 1
• For 1 – 6 thoracic vertebrae	: Add 2
• For 7 – 9 thoracic vertebrae	: Add 3
• The T_{10} vertebra overlies	: L_1 and L_2
• The T_{11} vertebra overlies	: L_3 and L_4
• The T_{12} vertebra overlies	: L_5 segment
• The L_1 overlies the sacral and coccygeal segments	

N.B If spinal segment involved is known then vertebral level can also be calculated as detailed above.

Q. What are the classical features of acute transverse myelitis?

Ans: Following are classical features:

• Acute onset of fever with flaccid paralysis. There may be neck or back pain
• Cause is mostly viral
• Bladder involvement is early
• Girdle constriction (constriction band) around the waist is common, indicates mid-thoracic region as the common site of involvement
• Variable degree of sensory loss (complete or incomplete) below the level of the lesion. A zone of hyperesthesia may be present between the area of sensory loss and area of normal sensation
• There is loss of all tendon reflexes (areflexia) due to spinal shock. Abdominal reflexes are absent. Plantar are silent. As the spinal shock passes off, hyperreflexia returns with plantar extensor response.

Q. Is transverse myelitis a compressive or non compressive myelopathy?

Ans: It is non compressive myelopathy but there may be site of lesion due to radicular involvement (radiculomyelopathy).

Q. How would you investigate this case?

Ans: The investigations are same as discussed under paraplegia.

Table 141.2: Features and causes of high cervical cord compression

Causes

1. *Craniovertebral anomalies*, e.g. platybasia, basilar impression, atlantoaxial dislocation, Klippel-Feil anomaly, Arnold-Chiari malformation
2. *High cervical cord (C_1 – C_4) lesion*, e.g. due to craniovertebral anomaly, fracture dislocation, hematomyelia, cervical spondylosis, cord tumours, caries spine.

Features

• A triad of short neck, low hair line and restricted cervical movements
• Spastic quadriparesis of gradual onset, involving one limb followed by the other or
• Spastic paraplegia with:
  Horner's syndrome
  XI nerve palsy
  V nerve palsy (spinal tract of Vth nerve) leading to loss of sensation over face, e.g. 1st and 2nd division of V)
  Vertical nystagmus
• Cerebellar signs may be present
• Mirror image movement, impaired sense of position and vibration

142

Brown-Séquard's Syndrome

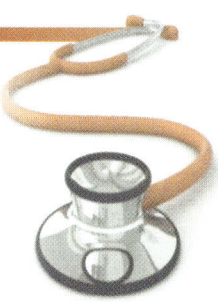

INSTRUCTION

- Examine the neurological system

SALIENT FEATURES

- Numbness over one half of the body or a lower limb

HISTORY

Ask for the following:

- Weakness of one half of the body or a lower limb (present)
- Loss of pain and temperature sensation in the lower limb involved
- History of trauma to thoracic spine (present) or gun shot/stab injury
- History of multiple sclerosis
- History of radicular pain
- History of degenerative spine disease
- History of bladder or bowel involvement

EXAMINATION

Neurological Examination

- Higher function — normal/abnormal
- Cranial nerves — normal/abnormal
- Cerebellar function — normal/abnormal

Motor and Sensory System Examination

A. *Signs below the level of lesion* (Fig. 142.1):

- Ipsilateral monoplegia (right lower limb in this case)/hemiplegia depending on the site of lesion with UMN signs below the level of the lesion
- Ipsilateral loss of posterior column sensations, e.g. sense of position and vibration sense (present)
- Contralateral loss of spinothalamic (pain and temperature) sensation (present). There may be burn marks/injury marks on this side

B. *Signs at the level of lesion*

- Look/elicit the following signs at the level of the lesion, i.e.
  i. Ipsilateral lower motor neuron paralysis, muscle atrophy/loss of tendon jerk

ii. Ispilateral zone of sensory loss or zone of hyperesthesia at the site involved (present)
N.B Always *Look for the signs/symptoms of multiple sclerosis in such a case.*

Other System Examination

- Examination of spine for deformity

PROVISIONAL DIAGNOSIS

The patient has hemisection of spinal cord called *Brown-Séquard's syndrome* at the level $T_6 – T_7$ level (lesion) due to compressive/destructive lesion of the spinal cord (aetiology). This patient is disturbed by weakness of one limb (functional status).

Q. **Enumerate the point in favor of your diagnosis?**

Ans: 1. History of a spinal injury
2. Ipsilateral spastic monoplegia of right lower limb
3. Loss of posterior column sensations on the side involved (ipsilateral loss of position and vibration sense)

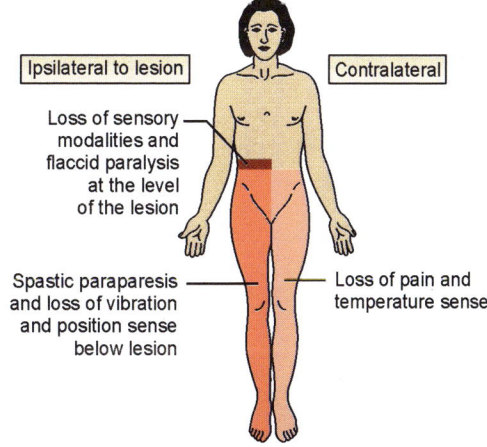

| Ipsilateral to lesion | | Contralateral |

Loss of sensory modalities and flaccid paralysis at the level of the lesion

Spastic paraparesis and loss of vibration and position sense below lesion

Loss of pain and temperature sense

Fig. 142.1: Brown-Séquard's syndrome (hemisection of spinal cord)

4. Contralateral (left side in this case) loss of pain and temperature below the level of the lesion
5. History of unilateral radicular pain with dermatomal sensory loss

Q.   Is there any differential diagnosis?

Ans: Yes, multiple sclerosis with plaques on one side of the cord can simulate this condition, but other features of multiple sclerosis (eye involvement, cerebellar or cerebral involvement) are absent in this case

QUESTIONS AND ANSWERS

Q.   What is hemisection of spinal cord?

Ans: *Brown-Séquard' syndrome*: It is hemisection of spinal cord, commonly due to gun shot injury/trauma to the spin.

It consists of:

- Contralateral loss of pain and temperature with ipsilateral loss of posterior column sensations
- Monoplegia or hemiplegia on the same side of the lesion below the site of involvement

- UMNs signs below the level of lesion, i.e. exaggerated tendon jerks and planttar extensor. Superficial reflexes are lost
- A band of hyperesthesia or a zone of anesthesia at the level of compression
- Segmental signs, i.e. muscle atrophy, radicular pain and loss of a reflex on the side involved

Q.   Why there is contralateral loss of pain and temperature?

Ans: The fibres of pain and temperature cross to the opposite side either immediately of 2–3 segments higher up, hence loss of these sensation occur on the opposite side.

On the other hand the fibres carrying the sensations ascend on the same side upto medulla before crossing, hence there is ipsilateral loss of posterior column sensations.

Q.   What are the causes of Brown-Séquard's syndrome?

Ans:
- Syringomyelia
- Cord tumor
- Bullet or stab injury
- Hematomyelia
- Degenerative disease of spine
- Multiple myeloma

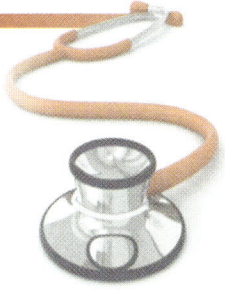

143

Cauda Equina Syndrome

INSTRUCTION

- Perform neurological examination of lower limbs

SALIENT FEATURES

- Numbness of both lower limbs

HISTORY

Ask for the following:

- History of root pain projected to perineum and thighs
- History of trauma
- History of neurogenic claudication (pain or weakness of legs or foot drop while walking which recovers during resting)
- Pain in anterior thigh
- Any trophic change over the lower limbs
- History of leukemia or prostatic carcinoma or bony metastasis
- History of disc prolapse
- Paraplegia without sphincter involvement with sensory loss over the buttocks

EXAMINATION

Neurological Examination

Motor System

- Paraplegia of LMN type
- There is wasting of quadriceps muscles and weakness of inverter of foot
- Nutrition of muscle is normal
- Tone is decreased in the muscles of foot and thigh muscles (present)
- Bilateral foot drop (present)
- Bilateral ankle jerks and knee jerks are absent (in this case)

Neurological Examination

Sensory System

- Saddle distribution of sensory loss (present)
- Sensory loss over the dorsum (Fig. 143.1) and sole of the foot, lateral aspect of the leg and a part of back of the leg

- Plantars are flexors (downgoing)
- Sphincters are not involved (in this case)

PROVISIONAL DIAGNOSIS

The patient has flaccid paraplegia with saddle shaped anaesthesia over the buttocks caused by cauda equina syndrome (lesion) as a result of radicular compression (aetiology).

QUESTIONS AND ANSWERS

Q. How would you justify your diagnosis?
Ans: *The points in favour of the diagnosis are:*
  1. Sudden and symmetrical involvement of both lower limbs
  2. History of root pain, radiating to the distribution of L_3, L_4, L_5, $S_2 - S_3$ segments
  3. Saddle shaped distribution of sensory loss
  4. Flaccid paraparesis with loss of knee and ankle jerks
  5. Bilateral foot drop

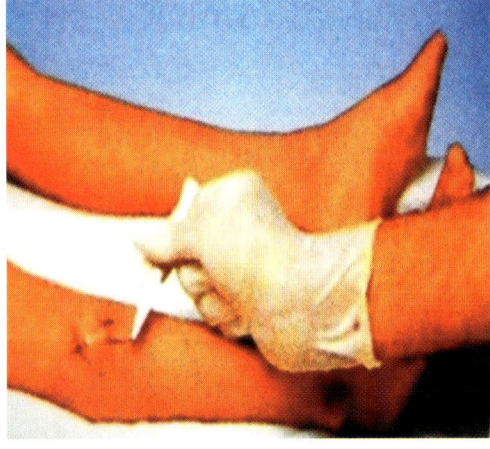

Fig. 143.1: Testing for sensation in cauda equina syndrome

6. Plantars are flexors (downgoing)
7. Bowel and bladder function are spared

Q. What is differential diagnosis?

Ans: All causes of acute onset LMN paraplegia will come into differential diagnosis such as:
1. Guillain-Barré syndrome
2. Diabetes mellitus producing symmetrical neuropathy and amyotrophy
3. Porphyria
4. Paraneoplastic conditions

Q. What is the cause of cauda equina syndrome in your case?

Ans: As there is history of trauma to the spine, therefore, the cause in my case is traumatic compressive lesion involving cauda equina.

Q. What are the causes of cauda equina syndrome?

Ans: Centrally placed lumbosacral disc or spine involvement or spondylolisthesis at the lumbosacral junction can produce cauda equina syndrome. Causes include:
   i. Prolapsed disc due to degeneration, tuberculosis, trauma, etc.
   ii. Leukemic infiltration of the roots of cauds equina
   iii. Tumors of the cauda equina (e.g. ependymoma, neurofibroma)
   iv. Secondaries in the spine causing compression of roots of cauda equina

Q. Which vertebral level is the lesion in the cauda equina syndrome?

Ans: Spinal cord ends at the level of L_1, after that roots of cauda equina emerge. All the lumbar segments (L_2 to L_5) lie opposite to T_{10} to T_{12}. First lumbar vertebra overlies the sacral and coccygeal segments. Therefore, a lesion in the spinal cord at any level below the 10th thoracic vertebra can cause cauda equina syndrome.

Q. What are the various types of cauda equina syndrome in adults?

Ans: I. *Lateral cauda equina syndrome:* It is characterized by:
   • Pain in the anterior thigh
   • Wasting of quadriceps muscle (L_2–L_4)
   • Weakness of foot invertors (L_4)
   • Absent knee jerk (L_2–L_4)
   Cause: e.g. disc prolapse or neurofibroma
   II. *Midline cauda equina syndrome:*
   • Bilateral lumbar (L_2–L_4) and sacral roots (S_1–S_2) lesions leading to (i) wasting of the quadriceps and absent knee jerks, (ii) wasting of the foot

invertors and evertors (L_4–L_5 and S_1) with loss of ankle jerk (L_5–S_1) and (iii) saddle shaped anesthesia over the buttocks

Cause: e.g. disc prolapse, sacral bone tumours (chordomas), secondaries in the bone and leukemic infiltration of the roots.

Q. What are the differences between cauda equina and conus medullaris lesion?

Ans: The conus medullaris is the terminal portion/point at which spinal cord ends and cauda equina (a bunch of roots) starts. Therefore, the main distinctions between the two are the plantars extensor response and symmetrical LMN signs in conus medullaris lesion, while plantars are flexor or not elicitable with asymmetric LMN paralysis in cauda equina syndrome (Table 143.1).

Table 143.1: Differential features between conus medullaris and cauda equina syndrome

Conus medullaris lesion	Cauda equina syndrome
Bilateral symmetrical involvement of both lower limbs	Asymmetric involvement of both lower limbs
No root pain	Severe low back or root pain
No limb weakness	Asymmetric limb weakness
Bilateral saddle anaesthesia	Asymmetric sensory loss
The bulbocavernous (S_2–S_4) and reflexes (S_4–S_5) are absent	Variable areflexia depending on the roots involved
Bladder and bowel disturbance common	They are relatively spared
Plantars are extensor but not always	Plantars are normal or not elicitable

Q. Name the conditions where ankle jerk is absent but knee jerk is preserved.

Ans: • Peripheral neuropathy
   • Tabes dorsails
   • Subacute combined degeneration

Q. Name the conditions where knee jerk is absent but ankle jerk is present. Where is the site of lesion?

Ans: Absent knee jerk indicates LMN involvement of L_2 to L_4. Causes are:
   i. Diabetic amyotrophy
   ii. Proximal myopathy
   iii. Disc prolapse compressing L_2–L_4 due to trauma or bone disease
   iv. Radiculitis invoslving L_2–L_4

Q. What do you know about the term neurogenic claudication?

Ans: It implies that patient develops root pain and leg weakness usually a foot-drop while walking which rapidly recovers on resting.

Q. What is sciatica syndrome?

Ans: It is characterized by low back pain that radiates along the sciatic nerve, occurs due to irritation of roots or nerve anywhere in the spinal canal, intervertebral foramina, in the pelvis or buttocks. Straight leg raising test is positive. There may be sensory or motor deficit with absent or depressed ankle jerk on the side involved. **Causes** include lateral protrusion of the disc, spinal tumours or spondylolisthesis. Spinal canal stenosis can lead to bilateral sciatica with neurogenic claudication.

Q. What is spina bifida occulta?

Ans: It is a failure of closure of one or several vertebral arches posteriorly. The meninges and spinal cord are normal. A dimple or a tuff of hair or lipoma may overlie the defect. Most cases are asymptomatic and discovered incidently on X-rays spines.

Q. What is tethered cord syndrome?

Ans: It presents either as progressive cauda equina syndrome or as myelopathy (cord lesion) or both. The patient is usually young adult who complains of perineal or perianal pain, sometimes following minor trauma. Neuroimaging studies reveal a low lying conus (below L_1–L_2) and a short and thickened filum terminale.

Q. What are trophic changes? Name the trophics changes in skin.

Ans: Trophic changes are neurogenic in origin, involve skin, its appendages and joints (charcot joint), occur due to repeated trauma in the region of anesthesia.

The trophic changes in the skin include:
- Dry and rough skin with lack of sweating
- Pigmentation
- Fall of hairs (hypotrichosis)
- Local cyanosis or edema
- Nails are brittle
- Trophic ulcers, e.g
  On the lateral malleolus, back of heel of the foot/feet, over the sacrum (classical site for bedsore), back of shoulder girdle.

Q. What is flaccid paraplegia?

Ans: Flaccid paralysis means lower motor neuron type of paralysis resulting from the diseases involving anterior horns cells, radicals, peripheral nerves and muscles. Acute onset of UMN type of paralysis may be flaccid instead of spastic if patient is in shock state.

Q. What are the causes of flaccid paraplegia?

Ans: The causes are:
1. Poliomyelitis
2. Radiculitis, polyradiculoneuropathy, tabes dorsalis, cauda equina
3. GB syndrome, peripheral neuropathies
4. Myasthenic gravis, myasthenia-myopathic syndrome (Lambert-Eaton syndrome), periodic paralysis (hypo or hyperkalemic)
5. Myopathy
6. Hysterical

Q. How would you confirm your diagnosis?

Ans: By *CT myelography* and *MRI*

Q. What is the treatment of cauda equina syndrome?

Ans:
1. *To relieve pain*, NSAIDs and paracetamol are effective. Opiates analgesics can be used for short-term if patient is unresponsive to NSAIDs.
2. *Exercise program*: The early resumption of normal physical activity is beneficial. Person should avoid maneuvers which produce stress, e.g. bending, weight lifting, etc.
3. *Traction* can be employed during acute back pain, but is not much effective.
4. Proof is lacking regarding the benefit of accupuncture, transcutaneous electrical nerve stimulation, massage, ultrasound, diathermy or electrical stimulation. Similarly use of ice or heat is not beneficial to relieve pain.
5. Therapeutic nerve root blocks with corticosteroids and local anesthesia is an optimal therapy when conservative measures to relieve acute pain fail.
6. Similarly, a short course of spinal manipulation or physiotherapy for symptomatic relief in uncomplicated cases is an option.
7. Find out the cause and treat it accordingly

144

Peripheral Neuropathy

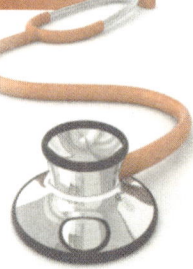

INSTRUCTION

- Perform neurological examination of this patient

SALIENT FEATURES

- Numbness of peripheral parts

HISTORY

Ask for the following:

- Note the duration and onset of symptoms
- Initiation and distribution of sensory disturbance (i.e. glove-stocking anesthesia)
- Evolution of weakness (proximal or distal). Was there any difficulty in holding the things?
- Progression of symptoms, e.g. stationary, progressive, recovering or waxing and waning
- Is there any history of weakness of respiratory muscles or facial muscles? Is there any difficulty in coughing or breathing?
- History of taking drugs (e.g. INH)
- Any precipitating factor or illness
- Bowel and bladder disturbance
- Alcoholism, headache, vomiting, convulsions
- Diplopia, dysphagia, nasal regurgitation

Past History

- Past history of spinal trauma
- History of fever, contact with a patient of tuberculosis, exposure to STD, vaccination
- History of systemic illness, i.e. diabetes (present), renal failure, chronic liver disease, diarrhea or malabsorption, etc.
- History of exposure to solvents, pesticides or heavy metals

Family History

- History of similar illness in other family members.

EXAMINATION

General Physical Examination

- Consciousness and behavior
- Look for anemia, jaundice, edema
- Look for signs of vitamin deficiencies, i.e. tongue, eyes, mucous membranes

- Look for alcoholic stigmata, e.g. gynecomastia, testicular atrophy, muscle wasting, parotid enlargement, palmar erythema or flushing of face.
- Look at the skin for hypopigmented or hyperpigmented patches, scar or burn mark or trophic changes (present)
- Record pulse, BP and temperature

Neurological Examination

- Higher functions — normal/abnormal
- Cranial nerves — normal/abnormal
- Neck rigidity — absent/present

Motor System

- Look for the posture of the limbs (usually decubitus) and foot drop (bilateral foot drop present).
- Note the nutrition, tone, power and coordination of the muscles.
- Elicit the tendon jerks. Bilateral ankle jerks are usually absent in GB syndrome and neuropathy (absent in this case).
- Elicit plantar response (not elicitable)

Sensory System

- Test superficial and deep sensations including cortical sensations. They are lost in the peripheral parts (in this case Fig. 144.1).
- Palpate the various long nerves (ulnar, radial, common peroneal). They may be palpable in diabetes, leprosy, hereditary polyneuropathy.

Other System Examination

1. *CVS* for sounds, bruits and murmurs
2. *Respiratory system* for evidence of tuberculosis, sarcoidosis, malignancy
3. *GI tract* for hepatosplenomegaly
4. *Lymphoreticular system* for lymph node enlargement

PROVISIONAL DIAGNOSIS

This patient has asymmetrical bilateral peripheral neuropathy (lesion) due to diabetes mellitus (aetiology). He is perturbed by loss of sensation (functional status).

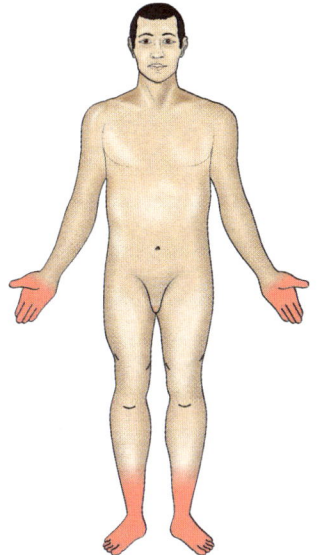

Fig. 144.1: Glove-stocking type of anaesthesia in peripheral neuropathy (diagram)

QUESTIONS AND ANSWERS

Q. **What are the points in favor of your diagnosis?**

Ans: • History of pins and needles in distal parts of all limbs.

• Loss of all types of sensations, i.e. superficial and deep (spinothalamic and posterior column) in peripheral parts of all the four limbs (gloves-stocking fashion)

• Weakness of distal parts of all four limbs with hypotonia, loss of deep tendon jerks and superficial reflexes (plantar response) in the peripheral parts of all limbs.

• Presence of bilateral foot drop.

• Presence of trophic changes.

Q. **What are the causes of peripheral neuropathies with predominant autonomic neuropathy?**

Ans: Most varieties of polyneuropathy affect autonomic functions to a mild extent, but certain neuropathies may have predominant autonomic dysfunctions. The causes are:

• Diabetes mellitus
• Leprosy
• Porphyria
• Amyloidosis
• Alcoholism
• GB syndrome

Q. **What are the causes of palpable thickened peripheral nerves?**

Ans: • Amyloidois, Leprosy

• Guillain-Barré syndrome

• Charcot-Marie-Tooth disease

• Refsum syndrome (retinitis pigmentosa, deafness and cerebellar degeneration)

• Dejerine-Sottas disease (hypertrophic peripheral neuropathy)

• Diabetes

Q. **How would you confirm the diagnosis?**

Ans: **Confirmation of diagnosis** is made by nerve conduction studies. Nerve conduction studies can distinguish demyelinating neuropathy from axonal neuropathy.

• In *demyelinating neuropathy,* there is slowing of conduction velocity, dispersion of evoked compound action potentials, conduction block and marked prolongation of distal latencies.

• In contrast in *axonal type,* there is reduction in amplitude of evoked compound action potentials with preservation of nerve conduction velocity.

Q. **What are the causes of acute, subacute and chronic polyneuropathy?**

Ans: Read Table 144.1.

Table 144.1: Major types of neuropathy (axonal vs demyelinating) and their causes

Oneset	Axonal	Demyelinating
Acute	Porphyria, toxic (As) GB syndrome	All forms of GB syndrome
Subacute	Toxic/metabolic	Relapsing form of CIDP
Chronic	• Toxic or metabolic • Hereditary • Diabetic • Dysproteinemia	• Hereditary • Inflammatory • Autoimmune • Dysproteinemia • Toxic/metabolic

Q. **Which drugs are effective for painful neuropathy in diabetes?**

Ans: • Tricyclic antidepressants

• Antiepileptics, e.g. phenytoin, carbamazepine, valproate, gabapentine/pregabalin

• Topical capsaicin

Q. **What is entrapment neuropathy? What are the common entrapment neuropathies?**

Ans: Entrapment means trapping of the nerve in a tight anatomical compartment leading to compression of the nerve. The common entrapment neuropathies are:

1. *Meralgia paresthetica* (lateral cutaneous nerve trapped)

2. *Carpal tunnel syndrome* (median nerve trapped)
3. *Tarsal tunnel syndrome* (posterior tibial nerve trapped)
4. *Common peroneal nerve entrapment* at head of fibula
5. *Elbow tunnel syndrome* (ulnar nerve trapped)

Q. How would you classify neuropathies? What are their common causes?

Ans: I. *Demyelinating neuropathies*
- Acute inflammatory demyelinating polyradiculoneuropathy (AIDP)
- Diphtheric neuropathy
- Chronic inflammatory demyelinating polyneuropathy (CIDP)
- Charcot-Marie-Tooth disease type I

II. *Axonal neuropathies*
- Acute motor axonal neuropathy (AMA)
- Acute motor and sensory axonal neuropathy (AMSAN)
- Multifocal motor neuropathy
- Neuropathy associated with HIV, diabetes drugs and toxins

III. They can be classified on the basis of diameter of the affected nerves either as small or large fibre neuropathy (demyelinating) (axonal or demyelinating)

Q. Name the types of neuropathy in diabetes.

Ans:
- Large fibre polyneuropathy (symmetric sensory, glove-stocking type)
- Small fibre polyneuropathy (asymmetric polyneuropathy)
- Proximal motor neuropathy (diabetic amyotrophy)
- Acute mononeuropathies (3rd, 6th cranial nerve)
- Mononeuritis multiplex
- Entrapment neuropathies, e.g. median, ulnar, lateral, popliteal, etc.
- Autonomic neuropathy

Q. What are the causes of predominant motor neuropathy?

Ans: Causes are:
- GB syndrome (70%) and CIDP (Chronic inflammatory demyelinating polyradiculoneuropathy)
- Porphyria
- Connective diseases, e.g. SLE, PAN
- Hereditary polyneuropathy
- Acute motor axonal neuropathy
- Delayed neurotoxicity due to organophosphates (TOCP, TCP)

- Diphtheria
- Lead intoxication
- Hypoglycemia
- High doses of dapsone

Q. What are the causes of predominant sensory neuropathy?

Ans: Causes are:
- Hereditary sensory neuropathy
- Paraneoplastic syndrome
- Leprosy
- HIV
- Sjögren's syndrome
- Dysproteinemia
- Vitamin B_1 and B_{12} deficiency

Q. Name few common causes of peripheral neuropathy.

Ans:

Table 144.2: Comon causes of polyneuropathy

Cause	Common conditions
Metabolic/ endocrinal	• Diabetes, chronic renal failure, amyloidosis, hypothyroidism, liver cell failure
Toxic Neuropathy	• Alcohol induced
	• Drug induced, e.g. INH, vincristine, chemical (TOCP)
Inflammatory	• Guillain-Barré syndrome, CIDP
	• Connective tissue diseases
Infective	• Leprosy, diphtheria, typhoid, HIV
Hereditary/ Genetic	• Genetic (Hereditary, sensory, motor neuropathy)
Deficiency states	• Vit B_1, B_6 and B_{12} deficiency
Others	• Paraneoplastic

Q. What do you understand by the term mononeuritis multiplex (multiple mononeuropathy)?

Ans: Mononeuritis multiplex refers to simultaneous or sequential involvement of individual non-contiguous nerve trunks either partially or completely evolving over days to years. Usually there is ischemia of long nerves due to vasculitis involving vasa nervosa which renders the nerves prone to mechanical compression. The causes are:
- Diabetes mellitus
- Leprosy, AIDS
- Collagen vascular disorders, rheumatoid arthritis
- Sarcoidosis, amyloidosis
- Malignancy, neurofibromatosis
- Hypereosinophilic syndrome
- Cryoglobulinemia
- Wegener's granulomatosis

145

Guillain-Barré Syndrome

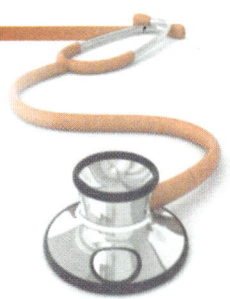

INSTRUCTION

• Perform neurological examination of this case

SALIENT FEATURES

• Bilateral foot drop with thinning of legs

HISTORY

Ask for the following:

• Distal or proximal weakness of lower limbs (difficulty in rising up in sitting position or climbing stairs) followed by upper limbs (difficulty in combing or placing articles on shelf)
• Numbness or paraesthesias in the peripheral parts of the limbs
• Bladder or bowel disturbance
• History of diplopia, drooling of saliva, regurgitation of food due to cranial nerve involvement
• History of fever, myalgia, headache, fatigue (systemic disturbance)
• History of upper respiratory infection, vaccination, inoculation, etc.
• Breathlessness (chest muscle involvement)

EXAMINATION

General Physical Examination

• Measure BP for hyper or hypotension
• Respiration, e.g. rate, rhythm, type/pattern

CNS Examination

• Higher function—normal/abnormal
• Cranial nerves especially 3rd, 7th and 9th cranial nerves involved or not
• Cerebellar function—normal/abnormal
• Gait inability to stand and walk (present)

Motor System

• Lower motor neuron paralysis of lower limbs (thinning of both lower limbs), bilateral foot drop (present in this case)
• Weakness of distal limb muscles more than proximal limb muscles (present Fig. 145.1)

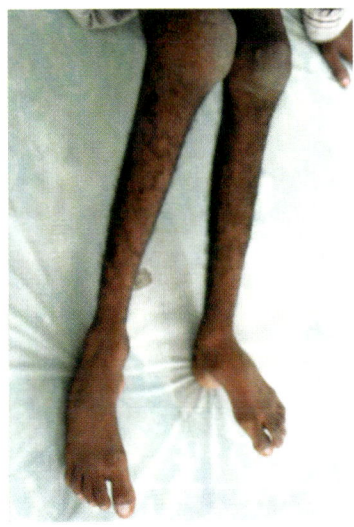

Fig. 145.1: Guillain-Barré syndrome

• Hypotonia and areflexia involving the peripheral parts of the limbs [loss of finger flexion, biceps and supinator jerks in upper limb and ankle jerks in lower limbs (Fig. 145.1)]
• Distal numbness. Plantars are not elicitable due to numbness (in this case)

PROVISIONAL DIAGNOSIS

This patient has Guillain-Barre syndrome (lesion) caused by demyelination following an episode of acute viral respiratory infection (etiology). He is disabled by the weakness of distal muscles (functional status).

QUESTIONS AND ANSWERS

Q. **What are the points in favor of your diagnosis?**

Ans: The points in favor are:

- Short duration and acute onset of symptoms in a young patient
- Progressive weakness of lower limbs
- Areflexia with bilateral footdrop
- Peripheral neuropathy
- Bowel and bladder not involved

Q. What are the characteristic presentation of Guillain-Barre syndrome?

Ans:
- It is an acute, frequently severe and fulminant polyradiculopathy of auto immune origin.
- Peak incidence between 20 and 50 years.
- It manifests as rapidly evolving areflexic motor paralysis (LMN type), with or without sensory disturbance.
- It usually starts from the lower extremities followed by upper extremities or all the four limbs may be involved simultaneously (uncommon). The legs are more affected than arms.
- The lower cranial nerves are also frequently involved, causing bulbar weakness. The VII cranial nerve is frequently involved. Bilateral involvement is common though it can occur unilaterally.
- Deep tendon reflexes are diminished/absent in the limbs.
- Bowel and bladder are rarely involved
- Plantars are either flexor or not elicitable.
- Sensorium is clear throughout the illness.
- The usual variant is *Miller-Fisher syndrome* which comprises a triad of ophthalmoplegia, ataxia and areflexia.

Q. What are the diagnostic criteria for GB syndrome?

Ans: Read Table 145.1

Table 145.1: Diagnostic criteria for Guillain-Barré syndrome

Essential	Supportive
• Progressive weakness of 2 or more limbs due to neuropathy	• Relative symmetric weakness
• Areflexia (loss of reflexes)	• Mild sensory involvement
• Disease course <4 weeks	• Facial and other cranial nerve involvement
• Exclusion of other causes of LMN type of paraplegia or quadriplegia	• Absence of fever
	• Typical CSF changes (acellularity, rise in protein)
	• Electrophysiologic evidence of demyelination

Q. What are the causes of acute onset peripheral neuropathy?

Ans: Causes are:
- GB syndrome
- Diabetes mellitus
- Drugs (TOCP, arsenic, thalidomide, pentamidine sensory neuropathy)
- Cisplatin (antineoplastic)
- Diphtheria
- Porphyria
- Paraneoplastic syndrome
- Alcoholic polyneuropathy

Q. What are the causes of recurrent neuropathy?

Ans: These patients may have several attacks of neuropathy. The common causes are:
- Porphyria
- Chronic inflammatory demyelinating polyneuropathy (CIDP)
- Alcoholic neuropathy
- Occupational toxic neuropathy

Q. What is the differential diagnosis of GB syndrome?

Ans: Read Table 145.2.

Q. What are the characteristics of chronic inflammatory demyelinating neuropathy?

Ans:
- It is a chronic GB syndrome, affects young adults.
- Onset is gradual, sometimes subacute and the initial episode is indistinguishable from that of GB syndrome.
- It is a sensorimotor neuropathy with predominant motor findings, but a small number of patients may present with pure syndrome of sensory ataxia.
- Some patients experience a chronic progressive course, whereas, others have a relapsing and remitting course.
- Some patients may have cranial nerve involvement including external ophthalmoplegia.

The diagnosis is confirmed on typical CSF findings and electrophysiological studies which show findings similar to GB syndrome.

Q. What is Miller-Fisher syndrome?

Ans: It is a variant described under clinical characteristics of GB syndrome

Q. How would you confirm the diagnosis of Guillain-Barré syndrome?

Ans:
- CSF examination for rise of proteins and albuminocytological dissociation
- Immunoelectrophoresis of CSF proteins for rise in immunoglobulins
- Nerve conduction velocities of peripheral nerve
- Sural nerve biopsy and histopathology

Q. **What is pathology of GB syndrome?**

Ans: It is an acute demyelinating polyneuropathy. (Infections (e.g. with *Campylobacter jejuni*) might induce an immune response depends on certain bacterial factors such as specificity of lipooligosaccharide and host factors. Antibodies to lipooligosaccharides can cross react with specific nerve gangliosides and can activate complement leading to immune mediated demyelination.

Genetic polymorphism in the patients might partially determine the severity of GB syndrome.

Q. **What is Landry paralysis?**

Ans: Ascending nature of GB syndrome involving the respiratory muscle is called landry paralysis.

Q. **Which pulmonary function tests are used to assess chest muscle involvement?**

Ans: • Forced vital capacity (FVC)
• Tidal volumes

Q. **How would you treat this case?**

Ans: 1. High-dose immunoglobulin during acute phase
2. Plasma exchange either alone or in combination with IV immunoglobulins
3. Corticosteroids have no role
4. Ventilatory support if respiratory muscles are involved
5. Physiotherapy and occupational therapy

Q. **What is the prognosis of this condition?**

Ans: 1. Due to severe disease, about 3–10% patient die during acute phase

2. About 20% patients still remain unable to walk after 6 months. They can pass on to CIDP.

Q. **What is POEMS syndrome?**

Ans: Read Table 145.2 under the heading of neoplastic neuropathy

Q. **What do you know about diabetic amyotrophy?**

Ans: It is asymmetrical motor polyneuropathy characterised by asymmetric weakness and wasting of the proximal muscles of the lower limbs and sometime upper limbs, diminished or absent knee jerks and sensory loss in the thighs. It is usually accompanied by severe pain in the thighs, often awakening the patient at night. Patient usually recovers, hence, prognosis is good.

Q. **What do you know about diphtheria neuropathy?**

Ans: • Common in children, but now rarely observed due to effective immunization against diphtheria
• Palatal weakness followed by pupillary paralysis and sensorimotor neuropathy
• Cranial nerves 3rd, 6th, 7th, 9th and 10th may be involved
• The condition develops 2–6 weeks after the onset of disease
• Myocarditis may occur in two third of patients with diphtheria. It manifests on ECG as arrhythmias, conduction blocks, ST-T changes and CHF.

Table 145.2: Differential diagnosis of GB syndrome

1. *Prophyric neuropathy*	3. *Neoplastic neuropathy*
• Acute intermittent porphyria produces attacks of paroxysmal neuropathy simulating GB syndrome • This is associated with abdominal colic, confusion, autonomic disturbances and later coma • Alcohol and barbiturates precipitate the attacks 2. *Triorthocresylphosphate (TOCP) neuropathy* It is called *'ginger paralysis'* owing to consumption of fluid extract of ginger which was used in the manufacture of bootleg alcohol and was adulterated with TOCP. It is pure motor neuropathy characterised by bilateral foot and hand drop. It occurs 10–20 days after consumption of adulterated tood (cooking-oil) or drink. *S* stands for skin pigmentation	Polyneuropathy is sometimes seen as a non-metastatic manifestation of a malignancy (paraneoplastic syndrome) which may be motor or sensorimotor. 4. *Multiple myeloma and other dysproteinemias* The polyneuropathy occurs due to demyelination associated with allergic reaction within peripheral nerves. The **POEMS syndrome** is an example of polyneuropathy in multiple myeloma in which, **P** stands for chronic inflammatory demyelinating polyneuropathy **O** stands for organomegaly (hepatomegaly) **E** stands for endocrinopathy (gynaecomastia and atrophic testes) **M** stands for M band on electrophoresis

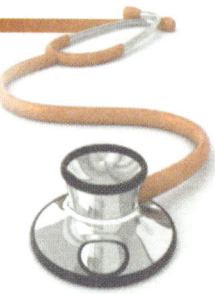

146 Charcot-Marie-Tooth Disease (Peroneal Muscle Dystrophy)

INSTRUCTION

- Examine the nervous system of this patient

SALIENT FEATURES

- Difficulty in walking and doing routine activities

HISTORY

Ask for the following:

- History of thinning of the calves, legs and thighs
- History of deformities such as pes cavus (high-arched foot) or pes planus (flat foot), clawing of toes, shortening of the Achilles tendon
- Difficulty in walking due to bilateral foot drop (wasting of dorsiflexor of feet). High-steppage gait
- History of thinness of palms and clawing of hands (wasting of small muscles of hands)
- History of such disease in the family

EXAMINATION

Neurological Examination

- Higher functions —normal
- *Cranial nerves* —normal
- *Cerebellar functions* —normal
- *Speech* —normal
- *Gait* —high-steppage gait (present)

Motor System

- There is wasting (atrophy) of the muscles of feet, legs especially, calves and lower third of both the thighs giving an inverted champagne bottle appearance (present Fig. 146.1A).
- Pes cavus is present (Fig. 146.1B) with clawing of toes.
- Bilateral foot drop present (Fig. 146.1D) with hammering of toes, clawing of hands and fingers present (Fig. 146.1C).

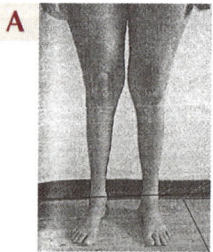

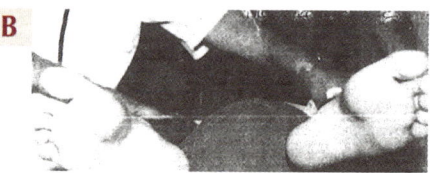

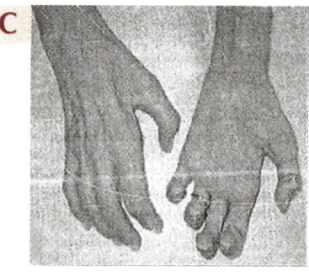

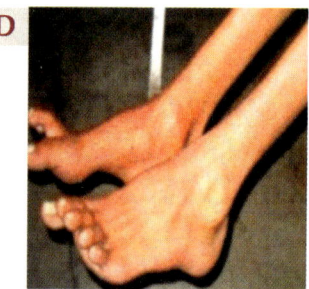

Fig. 146.1: Peroneal muscular dystrophy. (A) Inverted champagne bottle appearance of thighs; (B) Pes cavus; (C) Clawing of hands and fingers; (D) Bilateral foot drop

- Tone is decreased in the dorsiflexors of foot and muscles of the legs (calves present).
- Absent ankle jerks on both sides. Plantars are flexors (in this case) or equivocal.
- Finger flexion jerks are absent (in this case). There is atrophy of muscles of thenar and hypothenar eminence.

Sensory System

- Mild sensory disturbance in glove-stocking fashion (in this case) or no sensory disturbance.
- *Palpation of nerves:* The lateral popliteal and greater auricular or other superficial nerves are not enlarged and not palpable.

Other System Examination

There is no scoliosis.

PROVISIONAL DIAGNOSIS

This patient has hereditary sensory-motor neuropathy or peroneal muscular atrophy called *Charcot-Marrie-Tooth disease* (lesion) which is an heredo familial disorder (aetiology). There is severe feet drop and patient requires calipers (functional status).

QUESTIONS AND ANSWERS

Q. **What are points in favor of your diagnosis?**
Ans: All the features described below in hereditary neuropathy well present.

Q. **What is hereditary neuropathy (Charcot-Marrie-Tooth disease)?**
Ans:
- An autosomal dominant/recessive/X-linked transmission. It occurs in first and second decades of life.
- Sensorimotor neuropathy characterised by distal muscle weakness and atrophy, impaired sensations, absent or hypo-active deep tendon reflexes.
- Pattern of involvement is feet and legs followed by hands and forearm.
- High-steppage gait with frequent falling due to bilateral foot drop.
- Foot deformity (pes cavus, high arch feet) and hand deformity due to atrophy of intrinsic muscles of the hands.

Q. **What are the clinical patterns of this disease?**
Ans: *First:* The muscular atrophy begins in the distal portion of the affected muscles in the lower and upper limbs unlike the global atrophy of the motor neuron disease or muscular dystrophy.
Second: The degree of disability is minimum inspite of marked deformity.

Q. **What are the clinical phenotypes of Charcot-Marrie-Tooth disease?**
Ans: Based on the electrophysiological, clinical and nerve biopsy findings, two phenotypes are recognised.
Type 1: (Demyelinating neuropathy or glial myelonopathy) It is characterised by marked slowing of motor and sensory nerve conduction velocities and absent deep tendon jerks.
Type 2: (Neuronal axonopathy) It is characterised *by little or no slowing of motor and sensory* nerve conduction and normal deep tendon reflexes. Signs of chronic partial denervation are found in the affected muscles on EMG.

Q. **What is distal spinal muscular dystrophy?**
Ans: It is a similar disorder resembling type 2 Charcot-Marie-Tooth disease characterised by no disturbance in motor and sensory loss or nerve conduction velocities. Nerve conduction potentials are normal.

Q. **Name some hereditory neuropathy.**
Ans:
1. Roussy-Levy syndrome
2. Refsum disease (hereditary motor-sensory neuropathy type IV)
3. Dejerine-Sottas-Disease (HMSN type III)
4. Fabry's disease
5. Tangier disease
6. Hereditary amyloidosis
7. Hereditary porphyria

Q. **What is the mode of inheritance in this disease?**
Ans: There is usually an autosomal dominant mode of inheritance, but occasional cases occur on a sporadic, recessive or X-linked basis. The responsible gene is commonly located on the short arm of the chromosome 17 and less often shows linkage to chromosome I or X-chromosome. It is linked to several other chromosomes showing heterogeneity of the disorder.

Q. **What are the causes of pes cavus?**
Ans:
- Congenital
- Friedreich ataxia
- Peroneal muscular atrophy
- Distal spinal muscular atrophy

Q. **What are the uncommon features reported in this disease?**
Ans: Optic atrophy, retinitis pigmentosa and spastic paraparesis have been observed.

Q. **What are the causes of bilateral footdrop?**
Ans: Paralysis of extensors of foot and peronei muscles produce footdrop. The common *causes are:*
- Peripheral neuropathy
- Motor neuron disease (bilateral footdrop)
- Peroneal muscle atrophy (bilateral foot-drop)

147 Subacute Combined Degeneration of the Spinal Cord

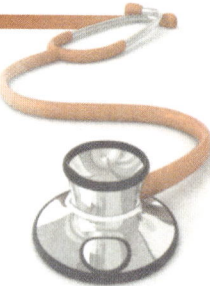

INSTRUCTION

- Perform neurological examination of this patient

SALIENT FEATURES

- Patient complains of weakness of both lower limbs

HISTORY

Ask about the following:

- Mode of onset (acute, subacute or chronic)
- History of prolonged diarrhea or malabsorption
- History of chronic alcoholism (present)
- History of surgery on stomach
- Symptoms of tingling or paraesthesia in peripheral parts of the limbs
- Whether the patient is vegan
- Family history of pernicious anemia

EXAMINATION

General Physical Examination

- Red-fiery tongue (present in this case)
- Patient is anemic (pale mucous membrane)
- Pupils are normal. Fundus—no optic atrophy

CNS Examination

- Higher function—normal (dementia is a feature of SACD)
- Cranial nerve—normal
- Cerebellar function—normal
- Gait—high steppage gait

Motor System

- Tone and power are reduced in the distal muscles of the limbs (present).
- Ankle jerks are absent (due to peripheral neuropathy).
- Knee jerks are brisk as a consequence to absent ankle jerks (present).
- Plantars are extensors due to spinal cord involvement (present).

Sensory System

- There is glove-stocking type of anaesthesia with loss of pain, touch, temperature (present).
- Posterior column sensations, e.g. vibration sense, position sense, deep touch are absent in the periphery of the limbs only (present)
- Ramberg sign is positive due to sensory ataxia (present)

Examination of Abdomen

- Scar marks of gastrectomy
- Toneless flappy abdomen in malabsorption

PROVISIONAL DIAGNOSIS

The patient has red tongue, anemia, peripheral neuropathy and posterior column signs (lesion) due to subacute combined degeneration of spinal cord (aetiology) and paralysis (functional status).

Q. What are the points in favor of your diagnosis?

Ans: 1. Red-fiery tongue (cheilosis), angular stomatitis, anaemia
2. History of chronic diarrhea/malabsorption and alcoholism
3. Symptoms and signs of peripheral neuropathy

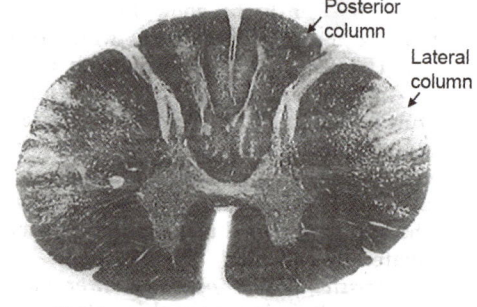

Fig. 147.1: Subacute combined degeneration. Cross section of the spinal cord showing degeneration of posterior and lateral columns (arrows)

4. Loss of posterior column sensations over the periphery of limbs. Romberg sign is positive.

5. Spastic paraplegia with loss of ankle jerks and exaggerated knee jerks. Plantars are extensors.

Q.   What is the cause of vitamin B_{12} deficiency?

Ans: Chronic diarrhea/malabsorption and alcoholism

Q.   What is differential condition in your diagnosis?

Ans: The only other condition which produces similar clinical picture is tabes dorsalis.

QUESTIONS AND ANSWERS

Q.   What do you understand by the term subacute combined degeneration of the cord?

Ans: As the name suggests, the disease is of subacute onset due to deficiency of vit. B_{12} leading to combined degeneration of spinal tracts (posterior column and corticospinal).

Q.   Name the few causes of vit. B_{12} deficiency.

Ans: 1. Vegan diet, inadequate intake, alcoholism
2. Malabsorption
   a. *Intrinsic factor deficiency*
      • Pernicious anemia, gastrectomy, congenital absence
   b. *Intestinal and pancreatic causes*
      • Small bowel resection, ileal disease (Crohn's disease), blind loop syndrome (bacterial colonisation of intestine)
      • Fish tapeworm
   c. *Drugs*
      • PAS (para aminosalicylic acid), colchicine, neomycin

Q.   Name the conditions where ankle jerks are absent and knee jerks preserved.

Ans: • Peripheral neuropathy
• Tabes dorsalis
• Subacute combined degeneration

Q.   What type of anemia do you expect in your case?

Ans: Macrocytic anemia with megaloblastic bone marrow picture.

Q.   What is the pathology of this condition?

Ans: There is degeneration of the ascending tracts of posterior column (sensory), descending pyramidal tracts (corticospinal) of spinal cord and peripheral nerves (neuropathy).

Q.   What is the incidence of gastric carcinoma in such patients?

Ans: There is three-fold rise in incidence of gastric carcinoma in these patients as compared to general public.

Q.   What is the pathogenesis of vitamin B_{12} deficiency in pernicious anemia?

Ans: Intrinsic factor antibodies are seen in 50% cases while other 50% do not have these antibodies. Two types of antibodies, i.e. *type I* (blocking antibody that prevents vitamin B_{12} binding to the intrinsic factor) and *type 2* (binding or precipitating antibody which reacts with intrinsic factor or with vit. B_{12} – intrinsic factor complex) are seen.

Q.   How would you investigate this case?

Ans: • Blood count and complete hemogram for type of anemia
• Bone marrow examination for megaloblastosis
• Vitamin B_{12}, folate and ferritin levels
• Parietal cells and intrinsic factor antibodies
• *Schilling test* (no longer done nowadays)
• MRI (Fig. 147.2) suggests abnormal signal intensity of spinal cord extending from C_1–C_6 (arrows) on T_2-weighted image. There is no enhancement after gadolinium in T_2-weighted image

Q.   What is the role of vit. B_{12} therapy in subacute combined degeneration?

Ans: The neurological response to vit. B_{12} supplementation is variable, i.e. it may improve, deteriorate or remain stationary. Sensory abnormalities improve better than motor. Peripheral neuropathy shows considerable improvement.

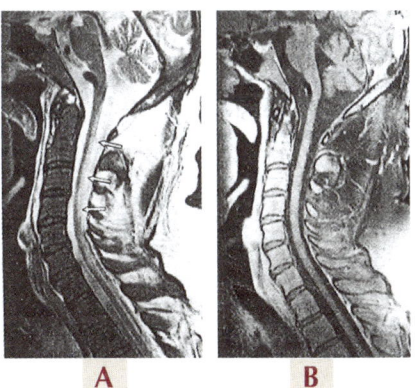

Fig. 147.2: MRI findings in subacute combined degeneration of spinal cord. (A) T_2-Weighted image shows abnormal signal intensity from C_1–C_6 spinal segments (arrows); (B) There is no enhancement after administration of gadolinium in T_2-weighted image

148

Tabes Dorsalis

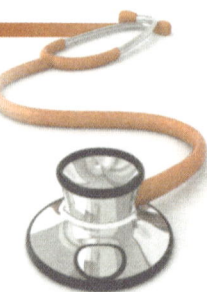

INSTRUCTION

• Examine the nervous system of this patient

SALIENT FEATURES

• Patient feels walking over the cotton-wool

HISTORY

Ask for the following:

• Lightning pains or electrical shock like sensations in the lower limbs, throat and stomach
• Walking as if on the cotton wool (present)
• High steppage gait
• Constipation
• History of incontinence and impotence (in males)

EXAMINATION

General Physical Examination

• Look for stigmata of syphilis, e.g Hutchinson's teeth, A – R pupils (present in this case), saddle-shaped nose
• Fundus for optic atrophy
• Look for trophic changes over the feet and arms
• Look for overflow incontinence

Neurological Examination

• Higher mental function may be normal or abnormal
• Cranial nerves — normal
• Cerebellar functions — normal
• Gait — high steppage gait (present)
• Speech — normal

Motor System

• Ankle jerks are absent (in this case)
• Plantars are normal

Sensory System

• Posterior column sensations are lost over arms and legs (present)
• Loss of pain with normal touch and temperature sensation over the nose, cheeks, inner aspects of arms and legs, a band across the nipple and in the anal area
• Squeeze calf muscles and the Achilles tendon (evokes no pain as deep sensation is lost)
• Visceral sensations are lost. Testicular sensations are also lost (in this case)
• Romberg's sign is positive (sensary ataxia present)

Other System Examination

Joints: Knee and hips may show hypermotility (neuropathic joints)

PROVISIONAL DIAGNOSIS

The patient has small irregular pupils (A – R pupil) with posterior column signs (lesion) caused by tabes dorsalis (aetiology) and has severe ataxia, i.e. positive Romber's sign (functional status).

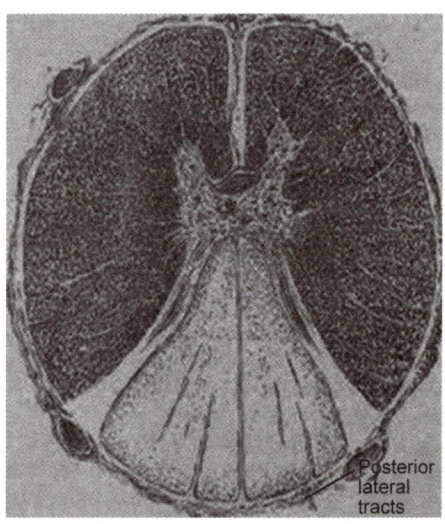

Fig. 148.1: Tabes dorsalis. There is flattening of postero-lateral tracts (diagram)

Q. Name clinical signs in your case which are diagnostic of tabes.

Ans: 1. A–R pupils

2. Loss of posterior column sensations with positive Romberg's sign

3. Loss of visceral sensations, e.g testicular

QUESTIONS AND ANSWERS

Q. What are the various patterns of neuro-syphilis?

Ans: The clinical patterns are:

1. Meningovascular syphilis (occur 3–4 yrs after primary infection)

2. Tabes dorsalis (10–25 yrs after primary infection)

3. General paralysis of insane (GPI) which occurs 10–15 yrs after infection

4. Taboparesis (Tabes combined with GPI)

5. Localised Gummas in the brain

Q. How would you test sensations over testes and eyes?

Ans: 1. Testes are tested for sensations by applying pressure on the testes.

2. Sensation over the eyes are also tested by application of pressure with the closed fist over the eyes.

Q. In which groups of persons in population, syphilis is common?

Ans: Sadhus, saints, sailors and soldiers.

Q. In which groups of patients, syphilis is common?

Ans: In patients with HIV.

Q. What is Argyll Robertson Pupil?

Ans: Read A–R pupil as a separate case discussion.

Q. How would you investigate this case?

Ans: Diagnosis is confirmed on serology.

I. *Nonspecific serological tests*
- Venereal Disease Laboratory Test (VDLT)
- Rapid plasma Reagin (RPR) test

II. *Specific tests*
- *T. Pallidum* Haemagglutination Assay (TPHA)
- Flourescent *T. pallidum* antibody absorption, (FTA – ABS)
- *Treponema pallidum* Immobilisation (TPI)
- Treponemal Elisa test

Q. Name few conditions in which VDRL (Veneral Disease Reference Laboratory) test is positive.

Ans: Rheumatoid arthritis, collagen vascular disorders, chronic active hepatitis, infectious mononucleosis, primary biliary cirrhosis.

Q. What is Jarisch-Herxheimer reaction?

Ans: This is a reaction seen in patients with syphilis treated with penicillins. Toxins from the killed spirochetes cause this reaction which can be fatal.

Q. What are the manifestations of cardio-vascular syphilis?

Ans: 1. Asymptomatic aortitis

2. Aortic dilatation/aortic aneurysm

Q. What is neurogenic bladder?

Ans: Read it as a separate case discussion.

Q. What do you mean by Charcot's joint?

Ans: Read it as a separate case discussion in rheumatology section.

Q. Why do acute abdominal crisis occur in tabes?

Ans: Due to involvement of lower thoracic spinal dorsal roots.

149

Ulnar Nerve Palsy

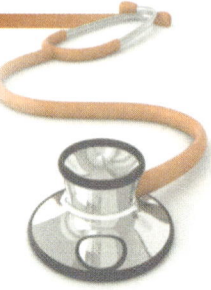

INSTRUCTION

- Perform the neurological examination of upper limbs

SALIENT FEATURES

- Weakness and deformities of the fingers of left hand

HISTORY

Ask for the following:

- History of fracture of the upper arm in childhood (supracondylar fracture of humerus in childhood)
- History of repeated trauma to elbow (over use trauma)
- History of use of elbows by an immobilised patients to shuffle in bed (repeated trauma)

EXAMINATION

Neurological Examination

- There is generalised wasting of the small muscles of the hand on the side involved (left side)
- Clawing of hand (hyperextension at the metacarpophalangeal joints (Fig. 149.1A) and flexion at interphalangeal joints of 4th and 5th fingers
- There is abduction of left little finger while hand is at rest (Fig. 149.1B)
- There is weakness of left movements of the fingers except thumb (i.e. thenar eminence)
- Sensory loss over one and half fingers (little finger and medial side of ring finger (present)
- Inability to flex the distal phalanx of the 4th and 5th digits completely

Examination of Elbow Joint

- Look for the scar and mobility of the joint (osteoarthrosis)
- Look at the carrying angle at the elbow. Large carrying angle due to repeated extension and

flexion in women can result in damage of olecranon and consequently the ulnar nerve

PROVISIONAL DIAGNOSIS

The patient has wasting of the small muscles of left hand, clawing of 4th and 5th fingers and sensory loss over one (little finger) and half medial half of ring finger caused by left ulnar nerve palsy (aetiology). She is unable to perform fine movements (buttoning) with left hand (functional status).

Q. **Enumerate the points in favor of your diagnosis?**

Ans: 1. Weakness and wasting of small muscles of the hand (left in this case)
2. Clawing of 4th and 5th fingers
3. Sensory loss over the little finger and medial half of long finger (one and half finger)
4. History of repeated trauma to elbow (overuse trauma)

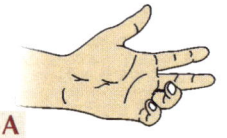

A
Clawing of the fourth and fifth fingers when the fingers and thumbs are held abducted

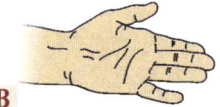

B
Abduction of little finger hand is at rest (Wartenberg sign)

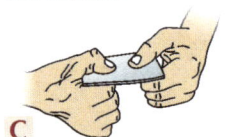

C
Froment's sign to test the adductor pollicis

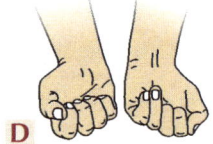

D
Weakness of the flexor digitorum profundus, inability to completely flex the distal phalanx of the 4th and 5th digits of left hand

Fig. 149.1: Left ulnar nerve palsy

QUESTIONS AND ANSWERS

Q. **What is the cause of ulnar nerve palsy in this case?**

Ans: Repeated trauma at elbow.

Q. **What is the root value of ulnar nerve?**

Ans: C_8-T_1

Q. **What are the muscles supplied by ulnar nerve?**

Ans: I. *Muscles in the Forearm*
- Flexor carpi ulnaris
- Medial half of flexor digitorum profundus

II. *In the hand*
- Abductor digiti minimi, flexor digiti minimi and opponens digiti minimi
- Two heads (oblique and transverse) of adductor pollicis
- Dorsal and palmar interossei
- 3rd and 4th lumbricals
- Palmaris brevis
- Inner head of flexor pollicis brevis

Q. **What is the most common cause of ulnar nerve palsy at elbow?**

Ans: It is commonly caused by compression of nerve in the cubital tunnel by fibrous arch of the flexor carpi ulnaris which arises by two heads.

Q. **How can the ulnar nerve be affected at the wrist?**

Ans: The deep motor branch of ulnar nerve is compressed in Guyon's canal at wrist (the canal runs between pisiform and hamate) by a ganglion, neuroma or repeated trauma (in this case).

Q. **What are the causes of claw hand?**

Ans: 1. Rheumatoid arthritis (advanced, deforming), cervical rib, thoracic inlet syndrome
2. Combined lesion of ulnar and median nerves in leprosy
3. Injury to medial cord of brachial plexus
4. Poliomyelitis, amytrophic lateral sclerosis
5. Syringomyelia, intramedullary tumors
6. Peripheral neuropathy
7. Klumpke's paralysis (lower brachial plexus injury)
8. Volkmann's ischemic contracture

Q. **What are the common causes of ulnar nerve palsy?**

Ans: The compression of nerve may occur at elbow or at wrist. The causes are:
I. *At elbow*
- Compression by pressure or trauma at cubital tunnel
- Stretching of nerve due to increase in carrying angle at elbow due to congenital, degenerative and traumatic cause
- Anatomical distortion of cubital tunnel by structures forming the tunnel

II. *At wrist/palm*
- Repeated trauma
- Compression by a ganglion or benign tumors

Q. **How would you differentiate between a lesion above the cubital fossa or a lesion at the wrist?**

Ans: • Flexor carpi ulnaris is supplied by the ulnar nerve in forearm, hence, is involved in lesions above the cubital fossa
• In lesion at the wrist, adductor pollicis is involved

Q. **How would you test flexor carpi ulnaris?**

Ans: Ask the patient to keep the hand flat on the table with palm facing upward towards you. Now ask him/her to perform flexion and ulnar deviation at the wrist agains resistance offered by you.

Q. **How would you test the adductor pollicis?**

Ans: Give a piece of folded paper to the patient and ask him/her to grip it between the thumb and the index finger of each hand so that the thumbs are uppermost (Fig. 149.1C). This causes adductor to contract. When the muscle is paralysed thumb can not be adducted properly, instead gets flexed at the interphalangeal joint due to contraction of flexor pollicis longus (innervated by median nerve). This is called Froment's sign (Fig. 149.1C).

Q. **What is ulnar paradox?**

Ans: Lesion of ulnar nerve at or above the elbow does not produce clawing of 4th and 5th fingers, whereas lesion at the wrist causes ulnar claw hand.

Q. **What do you understand by ulnar claw hand?**

Ans: The ulnar claw hand means the little and ring fingers are flexed at the interphalangeal joints and hyperextended at the metacarpophalangeal joints. The index and middle finger are not affected as first and 2nd lumbricals are supplied by median nerve.

Q. **How would you confirm the diagnosis in this case?**

Ans: The diagnosis is confirmed by electrophysiological studies using nerve stimulation technique.

Q. **What is the treatment in this case?**

Ans: Surgical decompression of the nerve.

150

Carpal Tunnel Syndrome (Median Nerve Palsy)

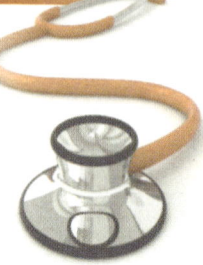

INSTRUCTION

- Perform the neurological examination of patient's upper limb

SALIENT FEATURES

- Nocturnal pain in the hand

HISTORY

Ask for the following:

- Pain in the hand at night (nocturnal pain is common which wakes the patient at night and patient shakes the hand to ameliorate pain called "*wake and shake sign*"
- Pain, paraesthesias (burning, numbness, tingling) on three and half fingers (thumb, index finger, middle finger and radial half of the ring finger) on the palmar aspect of the hand (present)
- History of trauma or injury to the wrist
- History of pregnancy, intake of oral contraceptive
- History of systemic diseases, e.g. rheumatoid arthritis, myxedema, acromegaly, chronic renal failure or sarcoidosis
- History of repeated use of hands (instrument playing, typewriting)
- Family history (abnormal small size of the carpal tunnel runs in the family)

EXAMINATION

General Physical Examination

- *Face:* Edematous (hypothyroidism and chronic renal failure), large face, prognathism (acromegaly)
- *Feet:* Large (acromegaly), fingers short and stubby (acromegaly)
- *Neck:* Lymph nodes (leukemia, sarcoidosis), movements (spondylosis)
- *Joints:* Deforming polyarthritis with deformities of hands (rheumatoid arthritis)
- *Wrist:* Look for the scar of previous surgery
- Look for the fistula for hemodialysis

Neurological Examination

Motor System Examination

- Wasting of the thenar eminence (present)
- Weakness of flexion, abduction and opposition of thumb (present)
- *Flick sign* is positive. This is confirmed by asking the patient "What do you do with your hand when symptoms are worst". If the patient makes flickering movement of the wrist and hand similar to employed in shaking down a clinical thermometer to bring down the mercury, the sign is said to be positive.
- *Tinsel's sign* (Fig. 150.1A): Percuss over the volar surface of the wrist. Patient may experience shock-like pain or tingling. The sensitivity of this test is low (< 50%), but specificity is high (70 – 80%).
- *Phalen's sign* (Fig. 150.1B): Pain or paraesthesia occurs in the distribution of median nerve when the patient flexes both wrists to 90° for 60 seconds.
- *Carpal compression test:* Direct pressure over the carpal tunnel induces numbness and tingling (carpal compression test). It is more sensitive as well as specific than the Tinsel's and Phalen's sign.

PROVISIONAL DIAGNOSIS

The patient has median nerve entrapement neuropathy (lesion) caused by carpal tunnel syndrome, the cause of which has to be found out (aetiology). The patient is disturbed by aching pain at night (functional status).

Q. **What are the points which favor your diagnosis?**

Ans: 1. Pain and tingling at the wrist during night relieved by shaking the hand
2. Radial three and half finger sensory loss
3. Positive Tinsel's Phalen's signs and carpal compression test
4. Wasting of thenar eminence. Weakness of flexion, abduction and opposition of thumb

QUESTIONS AND ANSWERS

Q. What is carpal tunnel syndrome?

Ans: It is painful entrapment neuropathy caused by compression of the median nerve between the carpal ligament and other structures within the carpal tunnel (Fig. 150.1C).

Q. What are the common causes of carpal tunnel syndrome?

Ans: 1. *Local causes,* e.g. tenosynovitis, recent or malhealed fracture, tumours or congenital anomaly.
2. *Systemic causes,* e.g. rheumatoid arthritis, myxedema, acromegaly, hyperthyroidism, chronic renal failure on long-term hemodialysis, sarcoidosis, amyloidosis.
3. Pregnancy and oral contraceptives.

Q. Mention some common entrapment neuropathies?

Ans: 1. *Meralgia paraesthetica* (lateral cutaneous nerve of thigh entrapped)
2. *Elbow tunnel syndrome* (ulnar nerve trapped)
3. *Tarsal tunnel syndrome* (posterior tibial nerve entrapped)
4. *Common peroneal nerve* trapped at fibular head
5. *Morton's metatarsalgia* (trapped medial and lateral plantar nerves)
6. *Radial nerve trapped* in the humeral groove

7. *Anterior interosseous nerve* trapped between the two heads of the pronator

Q. How would you confirm the diagnosis?

Ans: *Nerve conduction velocity* is delayed. Sensory conduction delay is earlier than motor. Increased latency at the wrist on stimulation of the median nerve is diagnostic. Muscles action potential recording from abductor pollicis brevis is also a valuable sign.

Q. Name few diagnostic signs of this syndrome.

Ans: In addition to *Tinel's* and *Phalen's sign,* other diagnostic tests are:
1. *Wrist extension test:* Extension of wrist(s) for 1 minute produces numbness and tingling in the distribution of median nerve.
2. *Tourniquet test:* Raising the BP above systolic pressure by inflating the cuff produces symptoms.
3. *Pressure test:* Direct pressure over the median nerve at the exit of carpal tunnel induces pain.
4. *Durkan's test or carpal compression test:* (already discussed)

Q. How would you treat this condition?

Ans: 1. *Drugs,* e.g. diuretics and NSAIDs
2. Local steroids injection
3. Wrist splinting in neutral position
4. Ultrasound treatment
5. Surgical decompression
6. Treat the underlying cause
7. Alternative therapies, e.g. acupuncture, yoga, chiropractic therapy, etc.

A

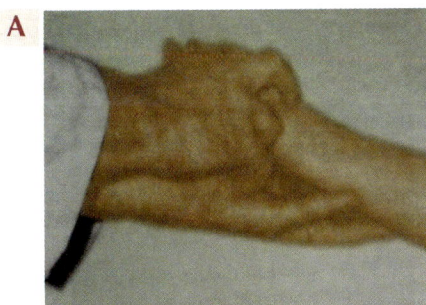

B

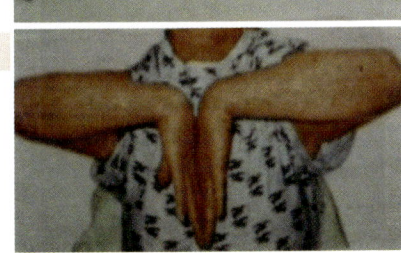

C

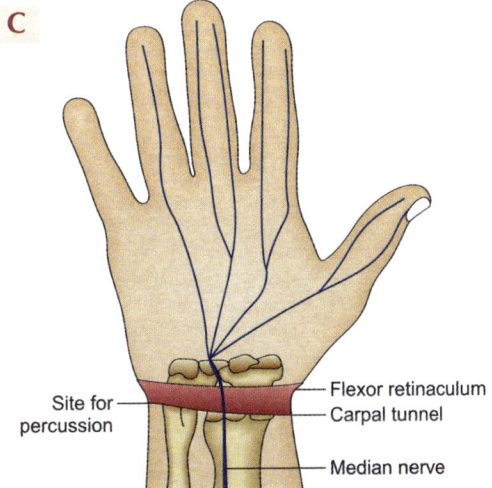

Site for percussion — Flexor retinaculum — Carpal tunnel — Median nerve

Carpal tunnel lying behind the flexor retinaculum contains median nerve (diagram)

Fig. 150.1: Carpal tunnel syndrome; (A) Tinel's sign; (B) Phalen's manoeuvre; (C) Diagram showing anatomy

151

Radial Nerve Palsy

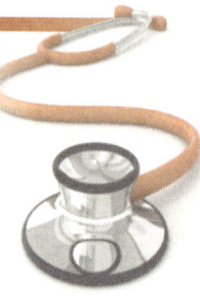

INSTRUCTION

- Perform the neurological examination of the patient

SALIENT FEATURES

- Patient has wrist drop

HISTORY

Ask for the following:

- History of sleeping with the head resting on the upper arm (saturday night palsy in an intoxicated person)
- History of using crutch, shoulder dislocation, fracture of humerus or radius
- History of exposure to lead in lead industry
- History of sitting with arms hanging over the back of chair
- History of deep intramuscular injection over the deltoid area

EXAMINATION

Neurological Examination

- Higher mental functions—normal
- Cranial nerves—normal
- Cerebellar functions—normal
- Gait—normal

Motor System

- There is weakness of extensors of wrist and elbow (flexors are normal). There is right wrist drop in this patient (Fig. 151.1A)
- The patient is unable to straighten the fingers
- Inability to extend the metacarpophalangeal joint, but when the wrist is extended partially, the patient is able to straighten the fingers at the metacarpophalangeal joints (this is due to action of interossei and lumbricals)
- Abductor and adductors of the fingers all are weak on testing in space (present), but this is not present when the hand is kept flat on a table and the fingers are extended
- Weak elbow flexion, i.e. patient is not able to flex the elbow against resistance due to weak brachioradialis
- Test the triceps (extension of elbow normal)

Sensory System

- Check the sensation of pain, touch and temperature over the hand. There is loss of sensation over the dorsum of thumb and index finger extending over the palmar aspect in this patient (Fig. 151.1B)

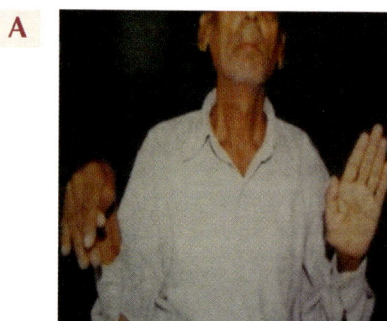

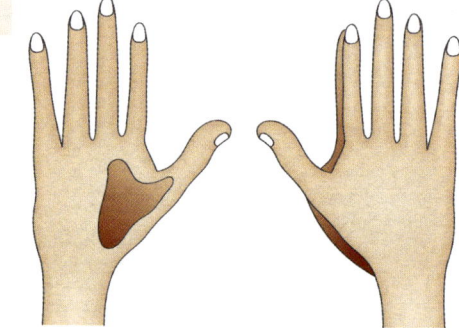

Fig. 151.1: (A) A patient with right radial nerve palsy; (B) Sensory loss (shaded area) in radial nerve palsy

PROVISIONAL DIAGNOSIS

The patient has features suggestive of right radial nerve palsy with sparing of brachioradialis (lesion) caused by recent fracture of humerus (aetiology). He is perturbed by disability (functional status).

Q. **Which characteristic sign in your case suggest radial nerve palsy?**

Ans: Wrist drop.

QUESTION S AND ANSWERS

Q. **Name the radial nerve branches at elbow.**

Ans: • Sensory (superficial radial)
  • Motor (posterior interosseous)

Q. **When does the action of triceps lost in radial nerve palsy?**

Ans: When the injury involves the junction of upper and middle third of the humerus.

Q. **What are the features of high and low radial nerve palsy?**

Ans: Table 151.1 summarises the features of high and low radial palsy.

Q. **What is the cutaneous supply of radial nerve?**

Ans: Only a small area of skin over the first dorsal interosseous is exclusively supplied by radial nerve (Fig. 151.1B)

Q. **What is the root value of radial nerve?**

Ans: C_5–C_8 spinal nerve roots.

Q. **Name the muscles supplied by radial nerve.**

Ans: Brachioradialis, triceps, anconeus, extensor carpi radialis longus, extensor carpi radialis brevis, supinator, extensor digitorum, extensor digiti minimi, extensor ulnaris, extensor indicis and extensors of the thumb.

Q. **What are the physical signs in various brachial plexus injury?**

Ans: Read Table 151.2.

Q. **What are the causes of wrist drop?**

Ans: Paralysis of the extensors of wrist produces wrist drop. The patient is not able to extend the wrist and fingers when asked to do so. In an attempted extension of fingers, there will be flexion of metacarpophalangeal joints and extension of the interphalangeal joints due to unopposed action of lumbricals and interossei.

Table 151.1: High versus low radial nerve palsy

Deficit	High radial palsy	Low radial palsy
Motor	• Accessory forearm flexion and supination • Wrist extension • Digital extension • Radial abduction of thumb	• Finger extension • Thumb extension/abduction
Sensory	• Radial 2/3rd dorsal sensation	• Dorsal radial forearm/hand
Functional disability	• Wrist extension • Digital extension • Radial abduction of thumb	• Digital extension • Radial abduction of thumb

Table 151.2: Physical signs in brachial plexus lesions

Location	Root(s) affected	Weakness of muscles	Sensory loss
1. *Upper plexus (Erb's paralysis)*	C_5 (C_6)	Biceps, deltoid, spinati, rhomboids, brachioradialis, triceps, serratus anterior. Biceps and supinator jerks are lost	Small area over deltoid

Causes: Indirect violence resulting in the nerve being torn by undue separation of head and shoulder, such as birth injury. In adults, it may occur during fall from a motor cycle on one side. Occasionally, it occurs following general anesthesia in patients in whom during the operation the arm has been held abducted and externally rotated.

2. *Lower plexus (Dejerine-Klumpke T_1 (C_8) paralysis)*		All small muscles of hand, claw hand (ulnar/wrist flexors)	Ulnar border of hand/forearm

Causes: Birth injury or may be produced by a fall during which patient tries to save himself by clutching something with the hand.

3. *Thoracic outlet syndrome (cervical rib or a fibrous band)*	C_8/T_1	Small muscles of hands, ulnar/forearm muscles	Ulnar border of hand/forearm (upper arm)

Causes:
- Radial nerve palsy   • Lead neuropathy
- Other peripheral neuropathies

Q. **What are the characteristics of root (radicular) lesion?**

Ans: Following are the characteristics:
- Lesion of the anterior (motor) root(s) produces weakness and atrophy of the muscles innervated by these roots.
- Irritative lesion of posterior (sensory) root produces root pain (increases with coughing), hyperalgesia (calf tender on squeezing) or hyperesthesia related to the segment irritated.
- In compressive lesion (radiculopathy) there is segmental sensory loss as in PIVD or cauda equina syndrome (Saddle-shape anaesthesia).

152

Common Peroneal Nerve Palsy

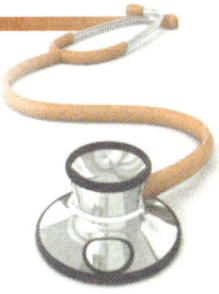

INSTRUCTION

- Perform neurological examination of lower limbs

SALIENT FEATURES

- Thinning of one leg

HISTORY

Ask for the following:

- Trauma to the lateral aspect of the leg (fibular region)
- History of sitting with crossed legs for long periods
- Prolonged bed rest (bed-riddened patients are prone to nerve injury)
- Tight knee plaster (nerve can be compressed because it is superficial)
- History of systemic diseases or any other cause known to produce neuropathy, e.g. diabetes, polyarteritis nodosa, collagen vascular disorders, etc.

EXAMINATION

Neurological Examination

- Higher functions, cranial nerves, cerebellar function and speech are normal

Motor System

- Thinning of the right leg and wasting of the muscles on lateral side of the leg (wasting of peronei and tibialis anterior muscle)
- Weakness of dorsiflexor and evertor of the foot. Foot drop may be present (Fig. 152.1)
- Gait is high steppage (Fig. 152.1)
- Jerks, e.g. ankle jerk is normal

Sensory System

- There is loss of pain, touch and temperature over the lateral aspect of the right leg and dorsum of the foot (Fig. 152.1)

PROVISIONAL DIAGNOSIS

This patient has right common peroneal nerve palsy (lesion) following trauma to upper leg (etiology) and has to wear clippers (functional status).

QUESTIONS AND ANSWERS

Q. What is the root value of common peroneal nerve?

Ans: L_4–L_5 spinal segments

Q. What are the causes of common peroneal nerve palsy?

Ans:
1. Compression of the nerve by tourniquet or plaster of paris cast
2. Direct nerve trauma being superficial
3. Leprosy (commonest cause worldwide)
4. Compression by ganglion arising from the superior tibiofibular joint
5. Compression of the nerve by tendon of peroneus longus

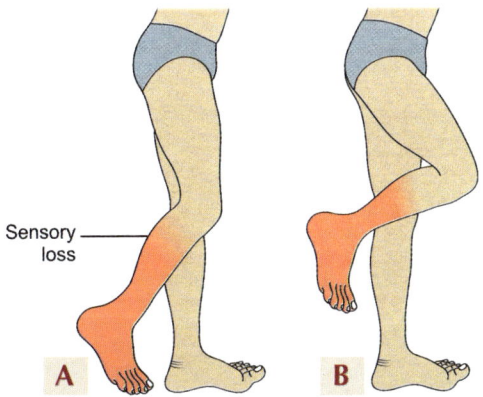

Fig. 152.1: Weakness of ankle dorsiflexors. (A) Foot drop; (B) High-steppage gait (unilateral)

Q.   **What are the various mechanisms of nerve injury?**

Ans: 1. *Neuropraxia* (concussion of the nerve)
2. *Axonotemesis* (the axon is severed)
3. *Neurotemesis* (the nerve is severed)

Q.   **Name few common causes of unilateral foot drop.**

Ans: 1. Peripheral neuropathy
2. L_4–L_5 root lesion
3. Motor neuron disease
4. Sciatic nerve palsy
5. Lumbosacral plexus lesion

Q.   **How would you investigate such a case?**

Ans: By nerve conduction studies which can distinguish between neuropraxia, axontemesis neurotemesis.

Q.   **How would you manage this case?**

Ans: 1. If nerve is severed, surgery is indicated
2. If the nerve is intact but concussed, then 90° splint at night, cliper shoes with 90° stop and galvanic or faradic stimulation to maintain the bulk of muscle is advised.

Q.   **What is meralgia prosthetica? Name the muscle paralysed.**

Ans: Read Table 152.1.

Table 152.1: Syndrome and signs of mononeuropathies of lower limbs

Nerve	Symptoms	Muscle weakness	Sensory loss
1. *Common peroneal*	Footdrop	Dorsiflexors and everter	Nil or dorsum of foot
2. *Lateral cutaneous* (meralgia paresthetica)	Tingling and paresthesia on lateral aspect of thigh	Nil	Lateral border of thigh
3. *Femoral (L_2 – L_4)* (diabetic amyotrophy)	Hip flexion and knee extension difficult	Anterior thigh muscles and loss of knee jerk	Front of thigh and lateral aspect on the back of thigh
4. *Sciatic (L_4 – S_3)* below knee, flail foot and severe disability	Severe leg weakness abductor and all muscles below knee	Hamstring muscles, hip	—
5. *Posterior tibial* (tarsal tunnel syndrome)	Pain and numbness of sole, weak toe flexors	Calf muscles, toe flexors and intrinsic foot muscles	—

153

Lateral Medullary Syndrome

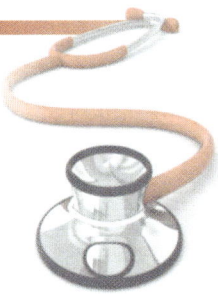

INSTRUCTION

- Examine the nervous system of this patient

SALIENT FEATURES

- Dysphagia and dysphonia

HISTORY

Ask for the following:

- History of anosmia/parosmia (for 1st cranial nerve)
- History of visual disturbance, diplopia (2nd, 3rd, 4th and 6th)
- History of nausea, vomiting, nystagmus/deafness (8th cranial nerve) present in this case
- History of dysphagia, dysphonia, hiccoughs (9th and 10th cranial nerves) is present in this case
- Loss of sensation over the face and neck (5th cranial nerve)

Gait — ataxic gait

Eyes • Nystagmus (present)
- Horner's syndrome (present)

EXAMINATION

Neurological Examination

Examination of Cranial Nerves

- Cranial nerves 1 to 4 are normal
- 5th cranial nerve is involved
- 6th and 7th are normal
- 8th is involved (vestibular division)
- 9th and 10th cranial nerves involved (impaired gag reflex, sluggish palatal movements)

Cerebellar Signs

They are present on the side involved

Sensory System

- Pain and temperature is lost on the opposite side while posterior column sensations are preserved.

Motor System

- Contralateral hemiparesis (present in this case)

PROVISIONAL DIAGNOSIS

The patient has features suggestive of lateral medullary syndrome caused by stroke (aetiology). The patient has dysphagia and dysphonia (functional status).

Q. **What are points in favor of your diagnosis?**
Ans: 1. History of dysphagia, dysphonia and visual disturbance
2. Horner's syndrome, nystagmus (same side) and loss of superficial sensations (contralateral side) with preservation of posterior column sensation
3. Cerebellar features on the side involved
4. Facial anaesthesia on the side involved
5. Contralateral hemiparesis

QUESTIONS AND ANSWERS

Q. **What are the clinical features of lateral medullary syndrome?**
Ans: Read Box 1.

Box 1. Clinical Features of Lateral Medullary Syndrome (Fig. 153.1)

Ipsilateral (same side)
- Facial anaesthesia (V cranial nerve)
- Diplopia, nystagmus, vomiting, ataxia (cerebellar)
- Horner's syndrome (sympathetic)
- IX and X nerve lesions

Contralateral (opposite side)
- Spinothalamic (pain, touch, temperature) sensory loss
- Hemiparesis (mild, unusual)

Q. **Which vessel is involved in this syndrome?**
Ans: Any of the following vessels may be involved:
- Posterior inferior cerebellar artery (common)
- Vertebral artery
- Superior, middle or inferior lateral medullary arteries

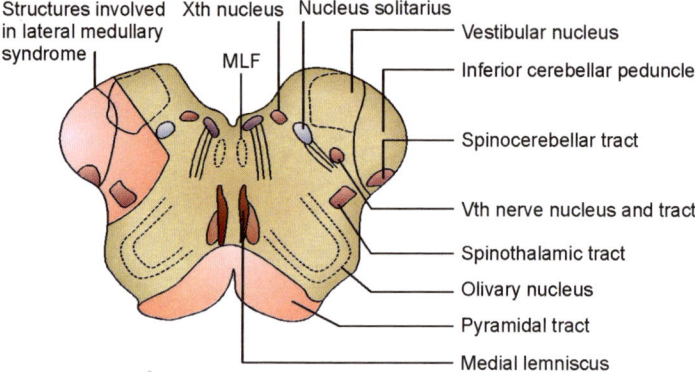

Fig. 153.1: Structure involved in lateral medullary syndrome

Q. What is the site of lesion in this syndrome?

Ans: The site of the lesion is a wedge-shaped area comprising of lateral aspect of the medulla and inferior surface of the cerebellum.

Q. What are the structures involved in this syndrome?

Ans: The structures involved on one side are:
- Nucleus ambiguous, trigeminal nucleus, vestibular nuclei, cerebellar peduncle, spinothalamic tract and autonomic fibres.

Q. What is medial medullary syndrome?

Ans: It is caused by occlusion of the lower basilar artery or vertebral artery. There is wasting and paralysis of the tongue on the side involved with contralateral hemiplegia and loss of vibration and position sense.

Q. Name the various syndromes with crossed hemiplegia.

Ans: Read Table 153.1.

Q. What is Benedikt syndrome? Where is the site of lesion?

Ans: It consists of:
Cerebellar sign on the side opposite to 3rd nerve palsy.
The site of lesion is *midbrain* causing damage to red nucleus interrupting the dentatorubro-thalamic tract from the opposite side.

Table 153.1: Various brainstem syndromes

Syndrome	Site of lesion	Ispilateral	Contralateral
Weber syndrome	Midbrain	LMV 3rd nerve	Hemiplegia (UMN)
Millard gubler syndrome	Pons	LMN 6th cranial nerve	Hemiplegia (UMN)
Foville syndrome	Pons	LMN 6th and 7th with gaze palsy	Hemiplegia (UMN)

154

Cerebellopontine Angle Tumor

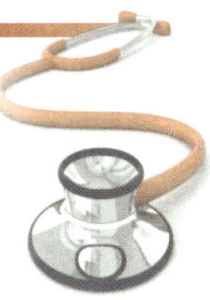

INSTRUCTION

- Examine the nervous system of this patient

SALIENT FEATURES

- History of deafness and ataxia

HISTORY

Ask for the following:

- Onset and progression of the symptoms
- Asymmetry of face
- Deafness and tinnitus, gait abnormality or ataxia
- Taste disturbance
- Nausea, vomiting, papilledema or visual disturbance
- Facial anesthesia

EXAMINATION

General Physical Examination

- *Skin:* Look for neurofibroma
- *Eye:* Fundus for papilledema

CNS Examination

- Higher functions normal
- Cranial nerves, e.g. 7th and 8th are involved. The sensory division of 5th producing facial anesthesia is also involved (in this case)
- Cerebellar signs present on the side involved (in this case)
- Motor and sensory systems are normal

PROVISIONAL DIAGNOSIS

This patient has left cerebellopontine angle tumor (lesion) as a result of acoustic neuroma (aetiology). He is disabled because of hearing loss (functional status).

Q. **Enumerate the points in favor of your diagnosis.**
Ans: 1. History of deafness and involvement of VIIIth cranial nerve on examination on left side

2. Facial anaesthesia (Vth cranial nerve) on left side
3. Cerebellar ataxia (left side)

QUESTIONS AND ANSWERS

Q. **What are the demarcations of cerebellopontine angle?**
Ans: It is a triangular area bounded by cerebellum and pons on the sides and petrous temporal bone as the base.

Q. **What structures traverse this angle?**
Ans: It extends from the 5th nerve above to 9th cranial nerve below, while 6th, 7th and 8th cranial nerves and nervus intermedius traverse the angle to enter internal auditory meatus.

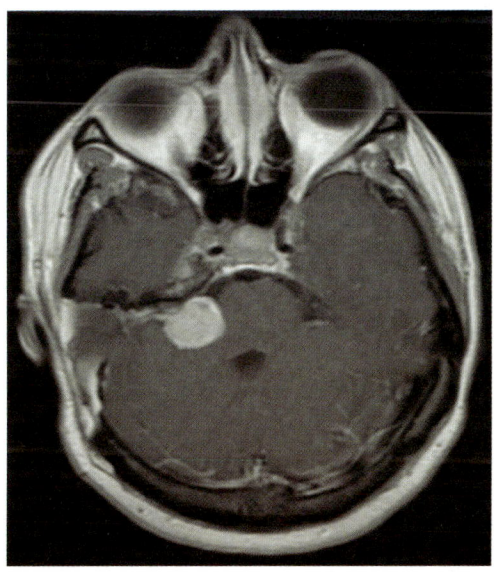

Fig. 154.1: CT scan showing cerebellopontine angle tumor (left)

Q. Name common cerebellopontine angle tumor.

Ans:
1. Acoustic neuroma (commonest 70 – 80%)
2. Pontine glioma
3. Meningioma, cholesteatoma, hemangioblastoma, aneurysm of basilar artery
4. Medulloblastoma
5. Cerebellar tumor
6. Nasopharyngeal carcinoma extending to this angle
7. Syphilitic pachymeningitis

Q. What do you understand by the term acoustic neuroma?

Ans: *Neuromas* also called *schwannomas* are tumors that arise from the schwann cells of the nerve roots most frequently the eighth nerve, hence called *acoustic neuroma* or *vestibular schwannoma*.

Q. What is the other common site for schwannoma?

Ans: Fifth cranial nerve.

Q. How would you investigate this case?

Ans:
1. *Radioimaging* (X-ray skull, tomography of internal auditory meatus) and CT scan
2. *Audiometry/audiography* for hearing loss
3. *Caloric test* for vestibular function
4. *CSF* examination
5. *Serological tests* for syphilis

6. *MRI*
7. *Brain stem auditory evoked potentials*

Q. What is the evolution of acoustic neuroma at CP angle?

Ans: Ipsilateral progressive sensory loss is the initial symptom followed by tinnitis, vertigo, facial weakness or anesthesia and long tract signs.

Q. Name few hereditary syndromes associated with brain tumors.

Ans: Read Table 154.1.

Table 154.1: Hereditary syndromes associated with brain tumor

Hereditary syndrome	Brain tumor
• **Neurofibromatosis** I and II	Schwannoma, glioma, meningioma
• **Tuberous sclerosis** (Bourneville's disease)	Astrocytoma
• **Von-hippel lindau syndrome**	Cerebellar and spinal hemangioblastoma
• **Turcot** (Adenomatous polyposis) **syndrome**	Medulloblastoma
• **MEN type I syndrome**	Pituitary tumors, malignant schwannoma

Q. How would you treat it?

Ans: There are three treatment modalities, i.e.
- Microsurgical resection
- Stereotactic radiosurgery
- Conservative approach

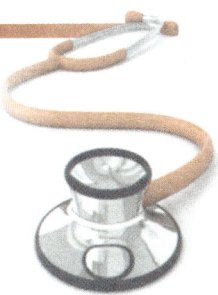

155 Cavernous Sinus Thrombosis

INSTRUCTION

- Examine the cranial nerves of this patient

SALIENT FEATURES

- Fixed eyeballs with chemosis

HISTORY

Ask for the following:

- History of fever or any orbital or sinus infection
- Orbital or facial pain, orbital swelling (present)
- Redness or chemosis of the conjunctiva(e) (present)
- Facial edema, facial neuropathy due to involvement of ophthalmic division of 5th nerve
- Loss of movement of the eyeball, diplopia (present)
- History of diabetes or immunocompromised state
- Progressive dysphagia and dysphonia (nasopharyngeal carcinoma)
- Any granulomatous disorder

EXAMINATION

General Physical Examination

- Look for any evidence of infection on face, around the eye (boil, furunculosis), mucormycosis in diabetic patients. There is chemosis, suffusion of the face and bilateral periorbital edema (Fig. 155.1)
- Examine nose and throat for nasopharyngeal carcinoma
- Elicit tenderness over frontal and maxillary sinus (sinusitis)

Cranial Nerves Examination

- First and second cranial nerves on both sides normal
- 3rd, 4th and 6th cranial nerves on both sides are involved [complete ophthalmoplegia with loss of pupillary reflex, dilated pupils and loss of every movement present (Fig. 155.1)]. Both the eyeballs are immobile

- Sensory loss over the forehead and around the eye (right) due to involvement of ophthalmic division of 5th nerve
- Other cranial nerves are normal
- Auscultate over the orbit for bruit (carotid-cavernous fistula)

PROVISIONAL DIAGNOSIS

The patient has chemosis, suffusion of face, bilateral 3rd, 4th, 6th and first division of 5th cranial nerve involvement (lesion) caused by bilateral cavernous sinus thrombosis following orbital infection. The patient is unable to move the eyes (functional status).

QUESTIONS AND ANSWERS

Q. **Where is the cavernous sinus situated?**
Ans: Lateral aspect of petrous part of temporal bone.

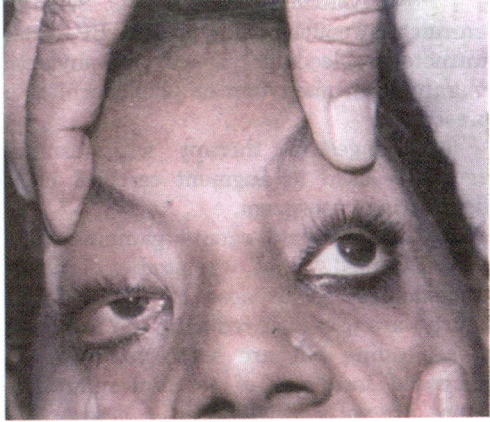

Fig. 155.1: Cavernous sinus thrombosis in a postpartum female. There is chemosis, lid oedema, conjuctional congestion and external ophthalmoplegia of both the eyes immobile eyes due to 3rd, 4th and 6th nerve palsy

Q.   **What structures traverse this sinus?**
Ans: 1. 3rd, 4th, 6th and ophthalmic division of the 5th nerve
     2. Internal carotid artery along with sympathetic plexus
     3. Ophthalmic veins

Q.   **What are the causes of unilateral cavernous sinus thrombosis?**
Ans: 1. Orbital cellulitis or bacterial sinusitis
     2. Aneurysm of carotid artery
     3. Carotid-cavernous fistula
     4. Meningioma, nasopharyngeal carcinoma
     5. Idiopathic granulomatous disorder (Tolosa-Hunt Syndrome)

Q.   **How would you investigate this case?**
Ans: 1. Complete hemogram for leukocytosis
     2. Culture (blood, urine, pus or any other infective material)
     3. Ophthalmic examination by ophthalmologist
     4. Radioimaging (X-rays of paranasal sinuses, CT scan and MRI of orbit)

Q.   **How would you treat it?**
Ans: 1. Find out the underlying cause and treat it such as infection by broad spectrum antibiotics, drainage of any abscess, cavities and identification of the offending organism on culture.
     2. Anticoagulation therapy in cases with primary thrombosis.
     3. Repair or occlusion of the carotid artery in case of fistulas or aneurysms.
     4. Steroids for Tolosa-Hunt Syndrome.

Q.   **What is the cause of pulsating cavernous sinus thrombosis?**
Ans: Carotid-cavernous fistula.

Q.   **What is Tolosa-Hunt Syndrome?**
Ans: Tolosa-Hunt Syndrome is an extension of orbital pseudotumor (an idiopathic inflammatory syndrome of eye muscles called orbital myositis) through the superior orbital fissure into the cavernous sinus leading to compression of its contents.

Q.   **What are the features of superior sagittal sinus thrombosis?**
Ans: Read Fig. 155.2

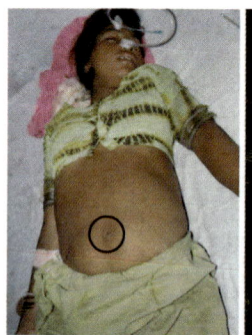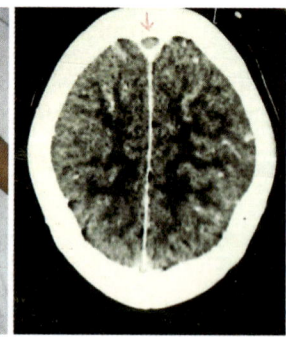

Fig. 155.2: Superior sagittal sinus thrombosis in a postpartum female. The features are:
   i. The patient had bilateral paralysis of UMN type involving lower limbs
   ii. Bladder is distended (encircled)
   iii. There may be symptoms and signs of raised ICP
   iv. CT scan shows an inverse lambda sign (↓)

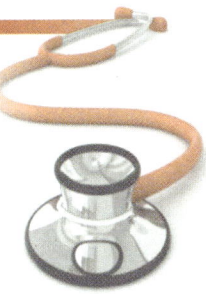

INSTRUCTION

- Examine the nervous system of this case

SALIENT FEATURES

- Paralysis of both lower limbs with visual disturbance

HISTORY

Ask for the following:

- Onset, progression, relapses and remissions of symptoms
- History of fever, infection, inoculation, mental or physical stress
- History of weakness, numbness, tingling or unsteadiness in a limb (incoordination)
- Weakness of both lower limbs (spastic paraplegia present) or all the four limbs (tetraplegia)
- Visual disturbance or loss (present), diplopia, pain during eye movements (retrobulbar neuritis), vertigo, etc.
- Sphincter disturbance (urgency or hesitancy)
- Cognitive dysfunction (impaired attention, memory loss, slow decision-making)
- Ataxia (cerebellar involvement)
- Speech disturbance (dysarthria present), depression, fatigue
- Pregnancy, sexual dysfunction, e.g. impotence, inability to achieve erection or loss of libido
- Family history

EXAMINATION

General Physical Examination

- Patient is unable to stand (ataxic)
- *Eyes:* Test visual acquity, eye movements, visual field and reflexes. Perform fundoscopic examination for retrobulbar neuritis and optic atrophy (present)
- *Face:* Facial weakness

Neurological Examination

- *Higher mental function.* Cognitive dysfunction including memory loss can occur in MS

- *Cranial nerves:* Multiple cranial nerves may be involved
- Speech: Dysarthria (present)
- Gait: Cerebellar ataxia (Romberg's sign negative
- Cerebellar signs (impaired coordination present)

Motor System Examination

- There will be spastic paraplegia (all UMN signs present in this case). Abdominal reflexes are absent
- Impaired coordination both in upper limbs (fingers nose test, etc.) and in lower limbs (heelshin test positive)

Sensory System Examination

- Sensory loss/impairment on the trunk and legs below a horizontal line on the torso (a sensory level) due to spinal cord involvement (present)

PROVISIONAL DIAGNOSIS

The patient has optic atrophy, spastic paraparesis and cerebellar signs (lesion) caused by multiple sclerosis (aetiology). He is disabled and wheelchair bound (functional status).

Q. What are points in favor of your diagnosis?
Ans: 1. History of fever and upper respiratory infection before neurological involvement
2. Retrobulbar neuritis/optic atrophy
3. Cerebellar signs (tested in the upper limbs)
4. Spastic paraplegia
5. Horizontal level of sensory loss
6. Multiplicity of the lesion

Q. What are the sites involved in your case?
Ans: Optic nerve, cerebellum and spinal cord only.

QUESTIONS AND ANSWERS

Q. What do you mean by multiple sclerosis?
Ans: It just means multiple demyelinating plaques

in the brain parenchyma which disseminate in time and space.

Q. What is differential diagnosis of MS?

Ans:
1. Brain tumor with relapsing/remitting or progressive course
2. Acute disseminated encephalomyelitis
3. Some hereditary cerebellar ataxias
4. Functional or somatization disorders

Q. What are the common sites of these plaques?

Ans: Optic nerves, cerebellum, brain stem/cerebrum and the spinal cord are the commonest site.

Q. What is the prevalence of MS?

Ans: The highest known prevalence for MS occurs in Orkney Islands located north of Scotland, throughout Northern Europe, Northern US and Canada.
The prevalence is low (2 per 1,00,000) in UK, parts of Asia and in middle east. Prevalence varies geographically.
Age of onset is between 20–40 years. The females are twice more affected than males.

Q. How does MS present clinically?

Ans:
1. It may present as optic neuritis resulting in diminished visual acquity or decreased colour perception in the field of vision.
2. Weakness of one limb (monoplegia), lower limbs (paraplegia), all the limbs (tetraplegia).
3. Tingling, paraesthesias and loss of posterior coloumn sensations in the extremities.
4. Diplopia, vertigo, nystagmus.
5. Cerebellar ataxia.

Q. What is Lhermitte's sign or Barbar's chair sign?

Ans: It is a tingling or shock-like sensation that radiates to the arms, down the back into the legs on flexion of neck of the patient. It indicates involvement of dorsal column nuclei of the higher cervical cord.

Q. What are the causes of positive Lhermitte's sign?

Ans:
1. Multiple sclerosis
2. Cervical spondylosis/fluorosis
3. Subacute combined degeneration of the cord

Q. What is Uhthoff's phenomenon?

Ans: It is transient exacerbation of symptoms of multiple sclerosis during a hot shower bath or with physical exercise. This phenomenon just indicates heat sensitivity in MS. This is the reason that MS symptoms worsen transiently during febrile illness.

Q. What is disease-course of MS?

Ans: Four clinical disease courses of MS have been described.

1. *Relapsing/Remitting MS (RRMS)*. It is common and accounts for 85% of MS cases which exhibit episodes of acute worsening followed by recovery.
2. *Secondary Progressive MS (SPMS)*. It always begins as RRMS. At some point, however, the RRMS clinical course changes to progressive deterioration in function unassociated with acute attack. About 50% cases with RRMS will develop SPMS after 15 years.
3. *Primary Progressive MS (PPMS)*. There is steady functional decline in symptoms of MS from the onset. It accounts for less than 15% cases.
4. *Progressive/Releasing MS (PRMS)*. There is gradual progressive deterioration of neurological symptoms from the onset with subsequent superimposed relapses.

Q. What is the effect of pregnancy on MS?

Ans: Pregnancy may have mild protective effect but there are increased chances of relapse during perpurium. The overall effect of pregnancy on MS is negligible.

Q. Name some other demyelinating conditions in addition to MS.

Ans:
- Devic's disease (neuromyelitis optica, i.e. myelitis with optic neuritis)
- Leukodystrophies
- Tuberous sclerosis
- Schilder's disease

Q. Which conditions may be considered forme fruste of MS?

Ans:
- Optic neuritis
- Single episode of optic neuritis with myelitis

Q. Name the bad prognostic factors in MS.

Ans:
1. Progressive disease from the onset
2. Frequent relapses during initial 2 yrs
3. Motor and cerebellar signs at presentation
4. Male gender
5. Short interval between first two relapses
6. Poor recovery from relapses
7. Multiple cranial lesions on MRI at presentation

Q. What are the causes of non compressive myelopathy?

Ans: This question has already been answered at many places.

Q.   What are the diagnostic criteria for MS?

Ans: The diagnostic criteria for MS are given in Table 156.1.

Table 156.1: Diagnostic criteria for multiple sclerosis (MS)

1. *Objective abnormalities of the CNS on examination.*

2. *Examination must, reveal CNS white matter involvement* including: (*i*) pyramidal tracts, (*ii*) cerebellum or its connections, (*iii*) medial longitudinal fasciculus, (*iv*) optic nerve and (*v*) posterior column.

3. *Clinical history or examination must reveal involvement of two or more areas of involvement.*
   (*i*) MRI may be used to document second lesion if the examination shows one site of lesion. A MRI (Fig. 156.1) must have either 4 lesions (>3 mm in diameter) involving the white matter or 3 lesions if one is in periventricular area. In patients > 50 years of age, two of the following 3 criteria must also be met, i.e. (*i*) lesion size >5 mm, (*ii*) lesions adjacent to lateral ventricles and (*iii*) lesion in the posterior cranial fossa.
   (*ii*) Evoked potential test may be used to document second lesion not evident on examination.

4. *The clinical pattern must consist of:* (*i*) two or more separate episodes of worsening involving different sites of the CNS, occurring at least one month apart and lasting for at least 24 hours, or (*ii*) gradual or stepwise progression over at least 6 months if accompanied by increased CSF IgG synthesis or two or more oligoclonal bands.

5. *The patient's neurologic condition is best attributed to MS and not to another disease.* Laboratory testing advisable to exclude other conditions include CSF analysis, MRI of brain or spine, serum vit. B_{12} assay, HTLV-I titre, ESR, RA factor and anti-DNA antibodies, serum VDRL, angiotensin-converting enzyme (for sarcoidosis), long chain fatty acids, muscle biopsy and mitochondrial analysis.

Interpretation

1. Definite MS when all five criteria are fulfilled.
2. Probable MS when all five criteria fulfilled except:
   (*i*) Only one objective abnormality despite two symptomatic episodes.
   (*ii*) Only one symptomatic episode despite two or more objective abnormalities.

Q.   What is two-hit model of pathogenesis of MS?

Ans: The two-hit model for cortical demyelination states that two separate pathogenic '*hits*' can (activation hit and a demyelinating hit) trigger the pathologic process in the cortex. An immune-mediated inflammation targets the myelin protein (expressed) which acts on the gray matter endothelial cells to open the blood-brain barrier or alter the endothelial cells to permit the demyelination (antibodies to myelin protein) to produce MS.

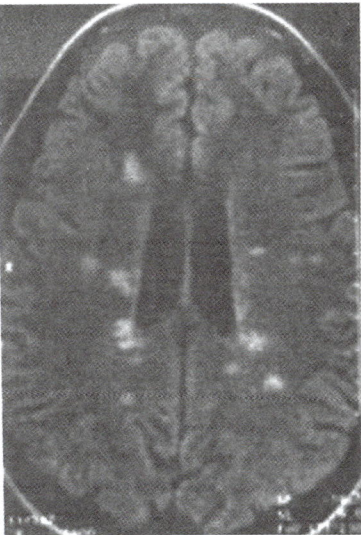

Fig. 156.1: MRI showing periventricular lesions in MS (the dense demyelinated plaques)

Q.   How would you investigate this case?

Ans: • *CSF examination:* There may be mononuclear cell pleocytosis and increased protein concentration especially IgG levels in CSF. Elevated IgG in CSF and discrete bands of IgG (oligoclonal bands) are present in many patients but presence of such bands is not specific.

• *Evoked potentials (EP):* Evoked potential (EP) testing assesses function in afferent (visual, auditory and somatosensory) or efferent (motor) CNS pathways. EPs use computer averaging to measure CNS electric potentials evoked by repetitive stimulation of selected peripheral nerves or of the brain. These tests provide information regarding subclinical involvement of pathways, hence, to confirm or establish the diagnosis of MS, these are necessary.

• *MRI:* MRI can detect about 90% of patients with MS. The T_2-weighted image show hyperintense focal periventricular lesions which are typical of MS, but not pathognomonic of MS.

An increase in vascular permeability of the blood brain barrier is detected by leakage of intravenous gadolinium (Gd) into the parenchyma. Such leakages occur early in MS lesion hence, serve useful markes of inflammation. This is called Gd-enhancement of the lesions.

Q.   What is the management of MS?

Ans: I. *Treatment of acute attack/initial demyelinating episodes*

- Recovery from acute attack can be hastened by IV methylprednisolone 1 g daily for 3 days followed by oral prednisolone 60–80 mg daily for 1 week with tapering doses over a period of 2–3 weeks.
- Plasma exchange (7 exchanges: 54 ml/kg or 1 : 1 plasma volumes per exchange every other day for 14 days) may benefit patients with fulminant attacks who are unresponsive to steroids.

II. *Disease modifying therapies for relapsing forms of MS (RRMS, SPMS with exacerbations)*

- Some agents approved in the US including, (*i*) IFN-βIa, (*ii*) IFN-βIb and (*iii*) glatiramer acetate, have been used in SPMS patients who still experience attacks. They have been shown to reduce the relapse rate in RRMS, delay progression in SPMS, however, SPECTRIMS study showed no significant benefit.

Selective adhesion molecule inhibitor:

Natalizumab (an alpha 4 integrin antagonist) reduces the development of brain lesions and the relapse rate when given IV, once monthly in RR-MS, but is associated with risk of autoimmunity and increased risk of progressive multifocal leukoencephalopathy, hence its use is reserved for non-responders to other modes of treatment.

- *Newer therapies:* Two oral agents, i.e. cladribine and fungolimod have been used in treatment of RRMS to reduce relapse rate.
- *Immunosuppression:* Mitoxantrone– an immunosuppressant has been approved by the US. It reduces rate of clinical relapse and delay the progression of disability in secondary progressive MS.
- *Antimitotic drugs*, e.g. azathioprine, methotrexate, cyclophosphamide have been used as off-label treatment option to delay the disability progression.
- *IV immunoglobulin* (IVIg) have been shown to reduce annual exacerbation rates when used monthly pulses.

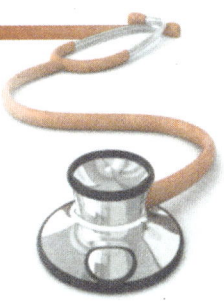

157 Internuclear Ophthalmoplegia

INSTRUCTION

- Examine the patient's eyes

SALIENT FEATURES

- History of squint

HISTORY

Ask for the following:

- Diplopia (double vision)
- History of multiple sclerosis (present)
- History of multiple subcutaneous swellings (neurofibromas)
- Drug history, e.g. phenytoin, carbamazepine

EXAMINATION

Examination of Eyes

- Look for nystagmus (nystagmus is prominent in the abducting eye)
- Divergent squint (present)
- Test the adduction and abduction of the eyes. Abduction in either eye is normal. Adduction is impaired (right eye on attempted lateral gaze to left, Fig. 157.1A). There is dissociation of eye movements on covering the abducting eye (present), the adduction in the other eye becomes normal
- Look for signs of multiple sclerosis, e.g. optic atrophy, cerebellar and pyramidal signs (cerebellar signs and spastic paraplegia are present in this case)

PROVISIONAL DIAGNOSIS

The patient has signs of internuclear ophthalmoplegia (lesion) caused by multiple sclerosis (aetiology)

QUESTIONS AND ANSWERS

Q. Where is the site of lesion?
Ans: Medial longitudinal fasciculus (MLF) is the site of the lesion which ascends from the abducent nucleus in the pons, crosses to opposite side to connect the oculomotor nucleus, thus connects 6th nerve nucleus of one side to 3rd nerve nucleus of opposite side, therefore, called *"internuclear"*.

The eye will not adduct due to 3rd nerve nucleus involvement, therefore, the medial rectus gets disconnected from the lateral gaze centre and 6th nerve nucleus of the opposite side in the pons.

Q. What are the causes of internuclear ophthalmoplegia?
Ans: 1. Multiple sclerosis (commonest)
2. Midbrain vascular lesion or stroke
3. Pontine glioma
4. Brainstem inflammatory lesions
5. Drugs, e.g. phenytoin, carbamazepine

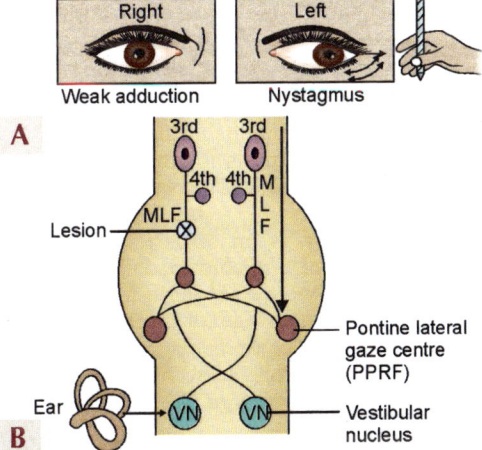

Fig. 157.1: Right internuclear ophthalmoplegia (diagrammatic illustration). (A) On attempted lateral gaze to the left produces weak adduction of right eye and left abducting eye shows nystagmus; (B) The lesion ⊗ lies in right medial longitudinal fasciculus (MLF).

Q.   What is conjugate gaze paralysis?

Ans: Normally the movements of the two eyes are symmetrical, so that visual axes meet at a point of fixation of the eyes. This is called conjugate ocular movements. Supranuclear lesions of 3rd, 4th and 6th cranial nerve leads to paralysis of conjugate movements of the eyes.

Q.   Where is the lesion in lateral gaze palsy?

Ans: Lesion lies in the frontal eye field (FEF) in pons.

Q.   What is one and half syndrome?

Ans: It is a syndrome in which one eye does not move at all while the other eye moves only in abduction (one and a half movements are paralysed). The vertical eye movements and the pupils are normal.

This is due to a lesion involving the PPRF (parapontine reticular formation) and the MLF on the same side. This results in failure of conjugate gaze to the same side, impairment of adduction of the eye and nystagmus on abduction of the other eye.

Q.   What are the causes of one and half syndrome?

Ans: 1. Multiple sclerosis
       2. Brainstem stroke, tumors and AV malformations

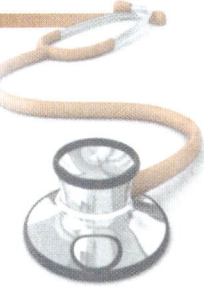

158

Abnormal Gait

INSTRUCTION

- Look at the patient while walking
- Test the patient's gait

SALIENT FEATURES

- Abnormal gait

HISTORY

Ask for the following:

- History of CVA (stroke)
- Paralysis of both lower legs
- Paraesthesias, tingling, foot drop
- Parkinsonism (tremors, rigidity and hypo-kinesia)
- Conversion reaction (hysterical)
- Proximal myopathy, osteoporosis, osteomalacia
- Hereditary ataxia/cerebellar disease

EXAMINATION

Keeping in mind the phases of gait, proceed to examine them as follows:

1. *Heel strike,* i.e. the lateral calcaneus makes contact with the ground and the muscles, tendons and ligaments relax providing adequate energy absorption.
2. *Midbalance,* i.e. the foot is flat and is able to adapt to uneven surfaces to maintain equilibrium and absorbs the shock of touch down in calcaneus below the ankle keeping the front and back of the foot aligned for weight-bearing.
3. *Heal rise:* The ankle (calcaneus) is lifted off the ground, the foot pronates, the muscles, tendons and ligaments tighten and the foot regains its arch.
4. *Toe push off,* i.e. the foot leaves the surface.

Abnormal Gaits

1. *Hemiplegic gait* (Fig. 158.1A):

   It is a circumducting gait in which the patient makes an arc with the leg during walking, i.e moves the leg involved along an arc. It is seen as a residual deficit in a patient recovering or recovered from hemiplegia.

2. *Scissors gait* (Fig. 158.1B):

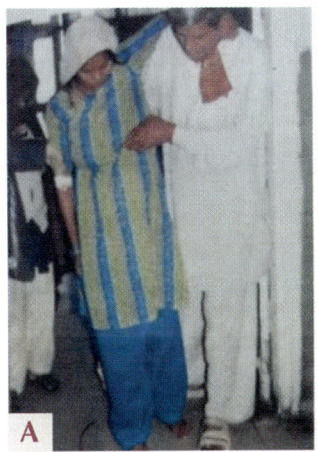 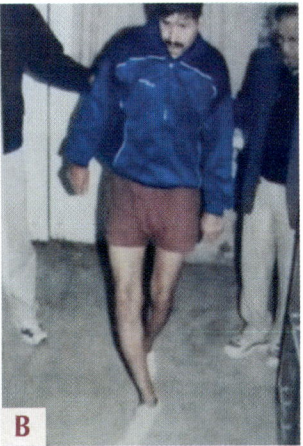

A **B**

Fig. 158.1: (A) Hemiplegic gait. Patient walks with support but circumduction can be seen with spastic leg; (B) Scissor gait. A patient of spastic paraplegia walking with crossing of legs

It is seen in paraplegia/quadriplegia with bilateral spastic lower limbs.

- The limbs are stiff. Each leg is advanced slowly and the legs (thighs) tend to cross forward on each other at each step like a scissor. This is due to spasticity of adductors of hips. The steps are short.

3. *High-steppage or slapping gait* (Fig. 158.1C): It is seen in sensory neuropathy or foot drop (LMN lesion) or dorsal column lesion.

- These patients either drag their feet along the ground or lift them too high to clear the ground and then bring them down with a slap on the floor. They are unable to walk on their heels. The high-steppage gait may be unilateral or bilateral.

4. *Fascinate or short shuffling gait*

It is seen in parkinsonism (Fig. 158.1D) (read parkinsonism as a case discussion).

5. *Cerebellar gait [drunken or reeling gait* (Fig. 158.1E)]

It is seen in patients with a cerebellar or associated tracts involvement.

The gait is ataxic (staggering), unsteady and wide-based with exaggerated difficulty on the turns. These patients cannot stand steadily with feet together, whether their eyes are open or closed.

6. *Rapid tapping gait (magnetic gait)*

It is seen in bilateral corticospinal lesions deep in the cerebral hemisphere (frontal lobe lesion) due to cerebrovascular disease or hydrocephalus. The gait is wide-based, short-stepped like parkinsonism, but rapid tapping *called marche a petits pas* resembling the rapid steps of a ballet dancer on her points. Plantars show extensor response and jaw jerk is exaggerated.

7. *The waddling gait* (Fig. 158.1F)

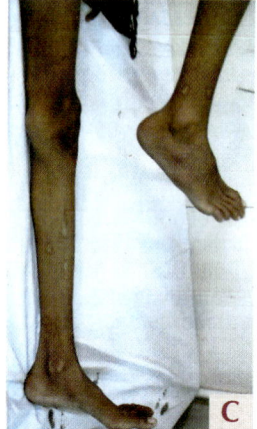

Fig. 158.1C: High-steppage gait

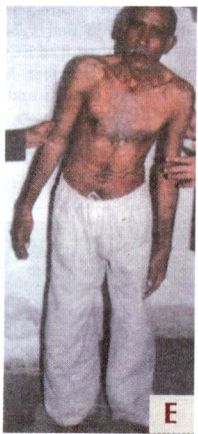

Fig. 158.1E: Cerebellar gait

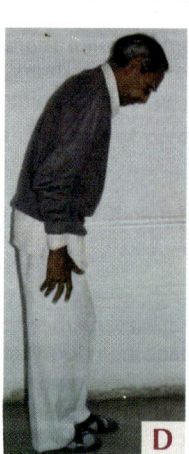

Fig. 158.1D: Fascinate gait

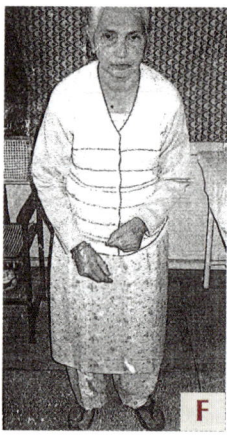

Fig. 158.1F: Waddling gait in osteomalacia

It is seen in proximal myopathy, muscular dystrophy and osteomalacia.

The gait is like the gait of a duck. The body is tilted backwards with increase in lumbar lordosis, the base is wide and the body sways from side to side with each step.

Note: Bilateral hip disease produces a similar gait (*Trendelenburg's sign*)

8. *Hysterical gait* (Fig. 158.2)
   • Bizarre or irregular gait which does not fit into any of the above described patterns. It is seen in hysteria. Miraculously, the patient does not fall. The patient walks with wide base and requires assistance to walk. The feet are put wildly and on each step he/she tends to fall, but does not hurt himself/herself.

QUESTIONS AND ANSWERS

Q. What do you understand by the term Astasia-Abasia?

Ans: This is seen in hysterical patients (conversion reactions) in which patient is unable to stand and walk. The patient deliberately falls to one side on walking (Fig. 158.2), but regains

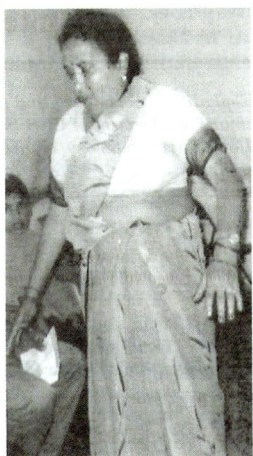

Fig. 158.2: Astasia-Abasia (hysterical gait). Patient is unstable during standing while she can perform all leg movements in bed

balance before hitting the ground. The legs are wide apart and patient knees at each step. The patient has normal coordination of leg movements in bed while lying or sitting, but is unable to stand or walk without assistance. If attention is diverted, stationary balance is sometimes maintained and several steps are taken normally followed by a dramatic demonstration of imbalance and tendency to fall towards examiner's arm or a nearby bed.

Q. What is hysterical hemiplegia?

Ans: The characteristic features are:
1. Hysterical gait
2. Normal tone which increases when you test it by applying fast resistance
3. Tendon reflexes are normal
4. *Plantars are flexor* or down-going
5. Often there is *loss of all forms of sensations* (touch, pain, smell, vision and hearing) on the paralysed side—a group of sensory changes that is never seen in organic brain disease.
6. *Hoover's sign and Babinski's combined leg flexion tests* are helpful in distinguishing hysterical from organic hemiplegia.

"*To elicit Hoover's sign,* the supine patient is asked to raise one leg from the bed against resistance. In a normal individual the back of heel of contralateral leg presses firmly down and the same is true for organic hemiplegia when attempts are made to lift the paralysed leg. The hysterical patient will press down the supposedly paralysed limb more strongly under these circumstances which can be appreciated by placing the hand below the normal heel.

In *Babinski's combined leg flexion test,* the patient with organic hemiplegia is asked to sit up on the bed from lying down position without using his/her arms, in doing this, the paralysed leg flexes (if power is good) at the hip and heel is lifted from the bed, while the heel of the normal leg is pressed into the bed which is appreciated by putting the hand below the heel. This sign is absent in "hysterical hemiplegia".

159

Neurogenic Bladder

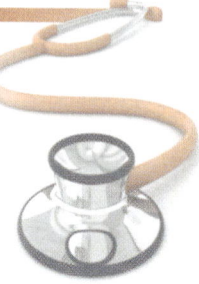

INSTRUCTION

- The patient has paraplegia. He is finding difficulty in passing urine. How would you proceed to examine such a case?

SALIENT FEATURES

- Inability to pass urine

HISTORY

Ask for the following:

- *Bladder sensation* (ask whether patient feels sensation of fullness when bladder is full)
- Urge to pass urine (do you feel to pass urine?)
- Can you stop urine at your own will during mid-micturition?
- Do you have wetting of undergarment?
- Do you suddenly pass large amount of urine?
- Do you feel abdominal discomfort or some mass?
- Do you feel any difficulty in defecation?
- Is there any numbness or anesthesia around the perineal region (do you feel numbness while sitting on chair)?
- History of impotence
- To find out the cause, ask for diseases/conditions that cause paraplegia (history of trauma in this case)

EXAMINATION

Neurological Examination of Lower Limbs

- Examine motor and sensory system of the lower limbs (bladder or sphincture disturbance is part and parcel of cord compression). There will be UMN paralysis and segmental sensory loss and loss of both spinothalamic and posterior column sensation below the compression—present in the case)
- Examine the spine for deformity and cause of compression or cauda equina

PROVISIONAL DIAGNOSIS

The patient has spastic urinary bladder (lesion) due to traumatic spinal cord compression (aetiology).

He requires an indwelling catheter drainage (functional status).

QUESTIONS AND ANSWERS

Q. **What is spastic bladder?**

Ans: It is a small (holds < 250 ml of urine), spastic and hyperreflexive bladder seen in patients with spinal cord lesions at the level of T_5 or higher. A spastic bladder on contrast study appears like *a Christmas tree* with little outpouching of contrast along the lateral margins. There is formation of pseudo-diverticulae due to hypertrophy of the bladder musculature. There is reflex emptying of the bladder as fullness of the bladder is not appreciated. Evacuation of bladder is incomplete hence, has to be emptied by suprapubic compression/catheterisation.

Q. **What are the complications of neurogenic bladder?**

Ans: These patients are prone to urinary infection, calculi and hydronephrosis.

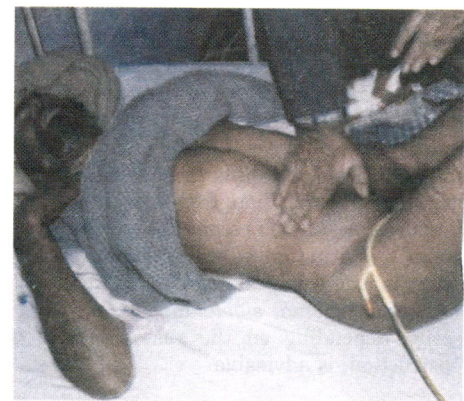

Fig. 159.1: Neurogenic bladder. Patient has traumatic spastic paraplegia with distended bladder. The indwelling catheter is inside the bladder

Q.   What is autonomous bladder?

Ans: This is a senseless (loss of sensation) bladder which is incontinent with continual urine dribbling. Residual urine volume is increased. There is associated loss of perineal sensation and sexual dysfunction.

This type of bladder is seen in lower motor neuron paralysis, i.e. cauda equina syndrome due to any cause. Although these patients have large spacious bladder but, upper collecting system is within normal limits and vesicoureteral reflux is rare.

Q.   What is insensate bladder? What are its causes?

Ans: It is similar to autonomous bladder where there is loss of sensation of bladder fullness. There is also loss of spinal reflex emptying. This results in retention of large volumes of urine, incontinence with dribbling and high volumes of residual urine can be passed by considerable straining.

Causes: It is seen in tabes dorsalis, subacute combined degeneration of the cord and multiple sclerosis.

Q.   What is the type of bladder in paracentral lobule lesion?

Ans: *Uninhibited (uncontrolled) bladder* occurs with lesions affecting the paracentral lobule of frontal cortex (e.g. frontal lobe tumor, parasaggital meningioma, aneurysms of the anterior communicating arteries and dementia) characterised by urgency despite low bladder urine volumes, thus, there is sudden uncontrolled (uninhibited) evacuation. There is no residual urine. If cognitive functions are impaired, patient can pass urine at anytime.

Q.   What is nerve supply of urinary bladder?

Ans: Bladder is supplied by sympathetic system (T_{12} and S_1) and parasympathetic system (S_3).

Q.   What is neurogenic control of the bladder?

Ans: 1. *Central control:* Micturition centre lies in the paracentral lobule of precentral cortex. Ascending afferent inputs from the spinal cord pass through the brain stem to the cortex (micturition centre) where the urgency of micturition is felt.

2. *Sympathetic control:* The sympathetic supply reaches the bladder through hypogastric nerves. As the bladder fills, vesicle afferents get stimulated which in turn stimulate the sympathetic outflow to the bladder to contract the internal sphincter and inhibit detrusor activity. These responses occur through spinal reflex pathways that promote continence.

3. *Parasympathetic control:* As the bladder becomes full, afferent fire more intensely and reach the central micturition centre from where the efferents reach the para sympathetic system to initiate micturition. Micturition follows through activation of parasympathetic system which contracts the detrusor muscle and inhibits the external uretheral sphincter so as to pass urine.

Q.   How would you investigate such a case?

Ans: The investigations include cystometry, ultrasound, sphincter electromyography, dynamic uroflowmetry, uretheral pressure measurements and electrophysiological studies for bladder innervation.

Q.   What are the various types of urinary incontinence?

Ans: 1. *Total incontinence* (patient passes urine at all times and in all positions).

2. *Stress incontinence.* It occurs due to rise in intra-abdominal pressure on coughing, sneezing, straining, etc. It occurs in multiparous women.

3. *Urge incontinence.* A strong urge forces the patient to void urine. It occurs in cystitis or neurogenic bladder.

4. *Overflow incontinence.* It occurs when the bladder is full due to retention of a large amount of urine, thus urine spills from distended bladder during sitting or walking, etc.

5. *Enuresis* (nocturnal involuntary incontinence) usually seen in children.

160

Argyll-Robertson Pupil

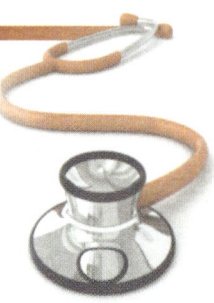

INSTRUCTION

- Examine the patient's eye

SALIENT FEATURES

- Abnormal pupil

HISTORY

Ask for the following:

- Lancinating pains
- History of syphilis, sarcoidosis, multiple sclerosis
- Difficulty in walking or history of walking just as on the wool

EXAMINATION

Examination of Eyes

- **Pupils:** They are small, irregular and unequal (Fig. 160.1)

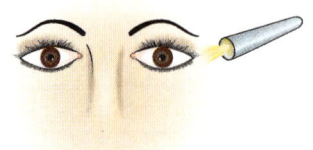

Light reflex absent (in this case)

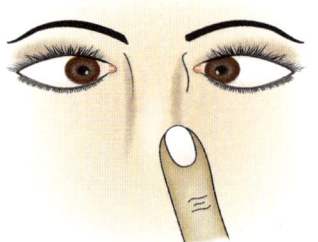

Accommodation reflex present (in this case)

Fig. 160.1: Argyll-Robertson pupil (small, irregular, unequal)

- Light reflex is absent
- Accommodation reflex is present (Fig. 160.1)
- No depigmentation of iris
- Bilateral ptosis and over compensation by frontalis muscles

Relevant Neurological Examination

- Examine posterior column sensations, e.g. sense of position and sense of vibration
- Look for Romberg's sign (positive in tabes dorsalis)
- Elicit deep tendon jerks (diminished in this case)

PROVISIONAL DIAGNOSIS

The patient has Argyll-Robertson pupils (lesion), the aetiology of which has to be found out.

QUESTIONS AND ANSWERS

Q. What is A-R Pupil?
Ans: • The involved pupil is small and irregular
  • Light reflex on the side involved is absent
  • Accomodation reflex is retained

Q. What are the common causes of A-R pupil?
Ans: • Tabes dorsalis (neurosyphilis)
  • Brainstem encephalitis
  • Sarcoidosis
  • Lyme disease
  • Pinealoma, tumor of 3rd ventricle
  • Multiple sclerosis
  • Autonomic neuropathy due to any cause (e.g. diabetes)
  • Syringobulbia

Q. What is neurological pathway of light reflex?
Ans: • The afferent pathway is through optic nerve
  • The efferent pathway is oculomotor nerve (Edinger-Westphal nucleus)

Q. **Where is the lesion in A-R pupil?**
Ans: Pretectal region of the midbrain from where fibres relay to Edinger-Westphal nucleus of 3rd nerve.

Q. **Name the muscle of accommodation.**
Ans: Ciliary muscle.

Q. **What is 'Reversed' Argyll-Robertson Pupil?**
Ans: This means pupils react to light, but not to accommodation. This is seen in encephalitis lethargica causing parkinsonism.

Q. **What is anisocoria? What are its causes?**
Ans: Anisocoria means unequal pupils. The causes are:

1. 3rd nerve palsy
2. Iritis/iridocyclitis
3. One eyed person
4. CVA or severe head injury
5. Hemianopia caused by optic nerve involvement
6. Horner's syndrome
7. Normal individual (20% cases)

Q. **Mention few causes of small pupil.**
Ans: • Senile pupil
• Use of pilocarpine in glaucoma

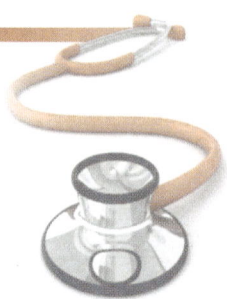

161 Holmes-Adie Syndrome (Tonic Pupil)

INSTRUCTION

• Examine the patient's eyes

SALIENT FEATURES

• Abnormal pupil

HISTORY

Ask for the following:

• Onset (it is acute)
• Age and sex (common in young female)
• History of impaired sweating

EXAMINATION

• The pupil is large (right pupil in this case), oval/circular, regular/irregular
• The pupil (right) reacts sluggishly to light (Fig. 161.1)
• *Myotonic pupil,* i.e. normally, pupil is sluggish, reacts to light slowly, but when a strong and persistent stimulus is applied, it can contract strongly to a very small size and when the stimulus is removed, then it slowly returns to its original size, hence, called *tonic pupil* (present).
• *Test near vision:* Pupil constricts slowly and redilate late after near vision.
• *Test accommodation:* It is impaired.
• There is segmental spontaneous movement of the iris.
• *Tendon jerks:* The ankle jerks are absent (in this case).

PROVISIONAL DIAGNOSIS

The woman has large sluggishly reacting right pupil, i.e. tonic pupil with absent ankle jerk (lesion) caused by Holmes-Adie syndrome (aetiology). This is a benign condition of no consequence (functional status).

QUESTION AND ANSWERS

Q. What is the significance of this syndrome?
Ans: It is benign, hence, carries no significance.

Q. What is the importance of this syndrome?
Ans: It is important clinically because it has to be differentiated from A-R pupil.

Q. What are the causes of large (dilated) pupil?
Ans: • Mydiatric eye drops (these dilate the pupil)
• Oculomotor nerve palsy
• Holmes-Adie pupil
• Ciliary ganglion lesion (herpes infection, trauma)
• Irectomy, lens implant
• Post-traumatic iridoplegia (blunt trauma)
• Anticholinergic/parasympatholytic poisoning, e.g. atropine, belladona
• Drug overdoses, e.g. amphetamines, sympathomimetics, cocaine
• Deep coma
• Death

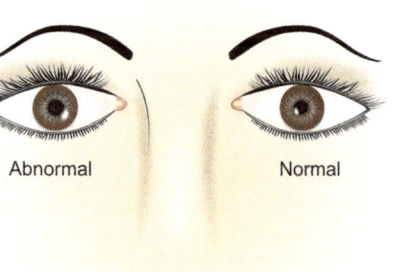

Abnormal   Normal

Fig. 161.1: Ciliary ganglion lesion (Adie's myotonic pupil)
· Light reaction absent on side affected
· Accommodation reaction is slow and sustained

Q. What are the causes of a small pupil (miosis)?

Ans: A small, constricted pupil occurs in:
- Senility, old age
- Pilocarpine eye drops (miotic agent)
- Horner's syndrome
- A-R pupil
- Lateral medullary syndrome
- Pontine lesion (hemorrhage, tumor)
- Narcotics, e.g. morphine poisoning, heroin, OP poisoning

Q. Where is the lesion in Adie's tonic pupil?

Ans: There is involvement of parasympathetic fibres within or outside ciliary ganglion.

Q. What is the difference between Adie's tonic pupil and Holmes-Adie syndrome?

Ans: Adie's tonic pupil with absent deep tendon jerks is called Holmes-Adie syndrome.

Q. Name the conditions associated with this syndrome.

Ans:
- *Ross syndrome* (occurrence of Adie's syndrome with segmental loss of sweating)
- Cardiac arrhythmias

Q. Is Adie's pupil sensitive to parasympathomimetics?

Ans: Yes, there is supersensitivity of Adie's pupil to acetylcholine secondary to parasympathetic denervation in this syndrome.

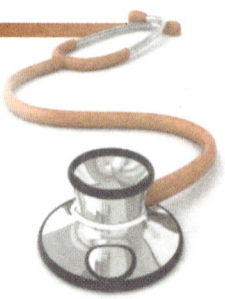

162

Bitemporal Hemianopia

INSTRUCTION

- Examine the patient's eyes and visual fields

SALIENT FEATURES

- Defective vision

HISTORY

Ask for the following:

- Onset of symptoms (insidious onset due to compression of optic chiasma)

- History of pituitary hypogonadism, e.g. impotence in males and amenorrhea in females
- Headache (expanding mass lesion)
- Diabetes insipidus (craniopharyngioma as the cause)
- Tall stature (acromegaly/gigantism)

EXAMINATION

- Test the visual fields
- There is bitemporal field loss of vision (Fig. 162.1)

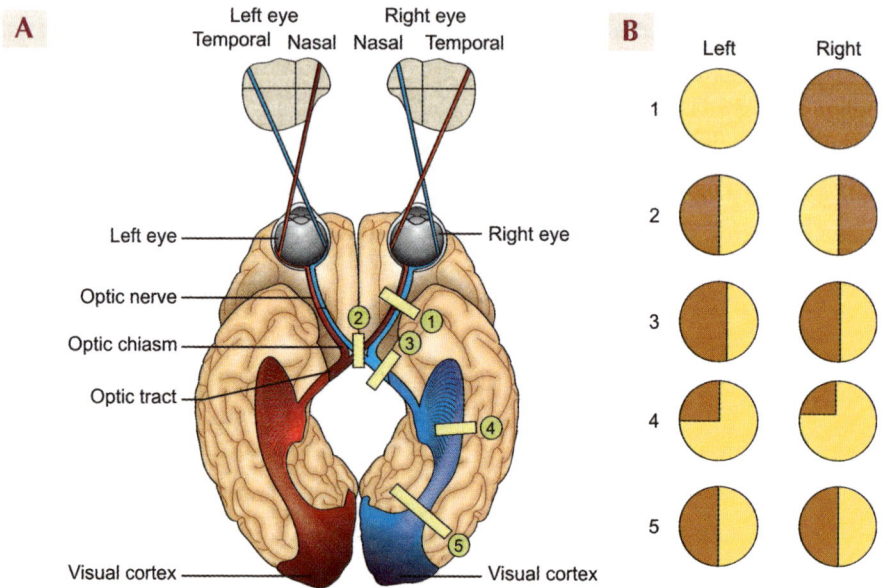

Visual pathways from the retina to the visual cortex   Visual defects

Fig. 162.1: The visual pathways with sites of the lesions denoted by bars in (A) and consequent visual defects are depicted in (B)

Site 1. Blind right eye (right optic nerve lesion). There is loss of direct light reflex
2. Bitemporal hemianopia (optic chiasmal lesion)
3. Left homonymous hemianopia (right optic tract lesion)
4. Homonymous left upper or quadrantic defect (right optic radiation lesion-partial)
5. Left homonymous hemianopia (right optic radiation)

- Look for face and hands for acromegaly (GH secreting tumor)
- Look for the signs of hypogonadism and hypo-pituitarism (read case discussion)

PROVISIONAL DIAGNOSIS

The patient has bitemporal hemianopia (lesion) due to compression of optic chiasma, the cause of which has to be found out.

QUESTIONS AND ANSWERS

Q. **What are the causes of bitemporal hemi-anopia?**

Ans: The causes are:

1. Pituitary tumor
2. Craniopharyngioma
3. Suprasellar meningioma
4. Metastatic tumors
5. Glioma
6. Aneurysm

Q. **How would you investigate?**

Ans: 1. *X-ray skull* for size and shape of pituitary fossa, destruction of clinoid processes and calcification.
2. Serum prolactin and other pituitary hormones.
3. CT scan/MRI of head for confirmation of mass lesion.

Homonymous Hemianopia

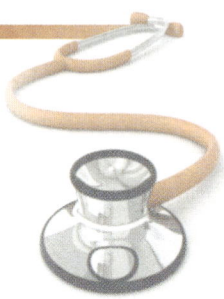

INSTRUCTION

- Examine the patient's visual field

SALIENT FEATURES

- Defective vision, difficulty in reading the news paper

HISTORY

Ask for the following:

- History of fall or bumping into the things on one side
- History of accidents of the vehicle/car on one side. The vehicle may be damaged on one side without the knowledge of the patient
- Patient may complain of having one bad eye
- Difficulty in reading the news paper/books (present)
- Determine whether patient is aware of the defect (if patient is not aware of the defect, then defect is macular sparing or inattention hemianopia, if aware of defect then defect splits the macula and bisects the central vision)

EXAMINATION

Examination of Eyes

- Test for homonymous hemianopia (read the Clinical Methods in Medicine by Prof SN Chugh). Sit at a distance from the patient. Ask the patient to see at your forehead. Bring moving fingers of both the hands from both the sides and instruct the client to point it as soon as he/she is able to see and determine the attention field defect.
- Test the whole field of vision of each eye using a white hat pin or any other object.

- Revaluation of the field in each eye for macular sparing or macular splitting using a hat pin.
- Lastly, formal field testing if necessary by using tangent screen or using a perimeter.
- Check the visual acquity.
- Examine the fundus.
- Perform relevant neurological examination. It should be done to find out the cause. Ask the examiner, that you would like to examine the neurological system to find out the cause.

PROVISIONAL DIAGNOSIS

The patient has left homonymous hemianopia (lesion) the cause of which has to be determined (aetiology).

QUESTIONS AND ANSWERS

Q. **What is the site of the lesion in homonymous hemianopia?**

Ans: Homonymous hemianopia with intact visual field indicate retro-chiasmal lesion. The Fig. 163.1 shows the site of the lesion and the visual field defect.

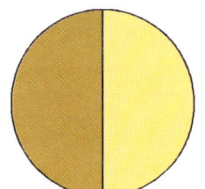 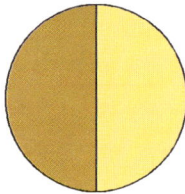

Fig. 163.1: Left homonymous hemianopia due to right optic radiation involvement

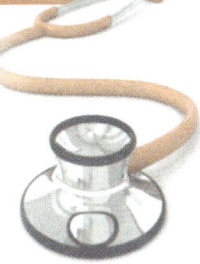

INSTRUCTION

- Examine the nervous system of this patient

SALIENT FEATURES

- Limb muscle pains, aches and weakness

HISTORY

Ask for the following:

- Age of onset and duration of symptoms, course
- Difficulty in getting up from a low chair, climbing stairs, lifting and running (present)
- Inability to raise the head, difficulty in raising arm above the head, difficult kneeling (present)
- Dysphagia, dysphonia
- Limb muscle pains and aches (present)
- Weakness and fatigue
- Episodic discoloration of fingers (Raynand's phenomenon)
- Rash or photosensitivity on sun exposure
- Any endocranial disorder, i.e. Cushing's syndrome, thyrotoxicosis (to exclude proximal myopathy)
- Heart problems, e.g. swollen ankles, shortness of breath, regular heart rate
- Drug history (e.g. steroids, triamcinolone, clofi-brate, penicillamine, chloroquin, colchicine, statins)
- Diabetes (to exclude amyotrophy)
- Myasthenia (to exclude myasthetic myopathic syndrome)
- History of fever, inoculation, upper respiratory infection (to exclude Guillain-Barré syndrome)
- Cough, fever, dyspnea, hemoptysis (lung malignancy or interstitial lung disease)
- Postmenopause/early menopause, oral contraceptive use
- Alcoholism

EXAMINATION

General Physical Examination

Face

- Look for dusky red (violaceous) rash with malar distribution. Depressive look

- Periorbital edema and purplish suffusion over the eyelids (heliotrope rash present)
- Erythema over other areas, i.e. neck, shoulders, upper chest and back (*shawl sign*)
- *Gottron sign,* i.e. scary patches over the dorsum of the hands and fingers
- Periungal erythema and dilatation of nail bed capillaries

Joints

- Look for inflammatory polyarthritis

Hands

- Look for hyperkeratosis of radial and palmar aspects of finger with irregular dirty horizontal lines (*mechanic's hands*)

Neurological Examination

- Higher functions, cranial nerves, cerebellum are normal
- Gait—waddling gait

Motor System

- Tone and power is decreased more in the proximal than distal muscles of the limbs (present). Neck muscles are weak
- Muscle bulk is normal. Muscles are tender to touch (present Fig. 164.1)
- The jerks are preserved/normal (in this case)
- Superficial reflexes are normal

Sensory System

- All sensory modalities are normal

Examination of Other System

- *Respiratory system* should be examined for interstitial lung disease

PROVISIONAL DIAGNOSIS

The patient has dermatomyositis/polymyositis (lesion) due to collagen vascular disease (aetiology)

Q. What are the points in favor of your diagnosis?

Ans: • A young female
- History of muscle pains, aches, arthralgia
- Heliotropic skin rash
- Proximal muscle weakness more than distal weakness. Muscles of thigh and legs swollen and tender (Fig. 164.1)
- Tendon jerks are preserved despite weakness

Q. What are the causes polymyositis?

Ans: 1. Viral infection (HTLVI)
2. Autoimmune, idiopathic
3. Inherited, i.e. an abnormal inherited gene involved
4. Collagen vascular disorder
5. Malignancy
6. Drug induced

QUESTIONS AND ANSWERS

Q. What is dermatomyositis?

Ans: As the name suggests myopathy associated with rash is called *dermatomyositis*.

Q. What do you understand by the term polymyositis?

Ans: It is subacute inflammatory myopathy affecting adults and rarely children who do not have any other cause to explain it. It is diagnosis of exclusion, i.e. exclusion of myopathy due to drugs, toxins, endocrinopathy, neurogenic disease, muscular dystrophy and biochemical muscle disorders.

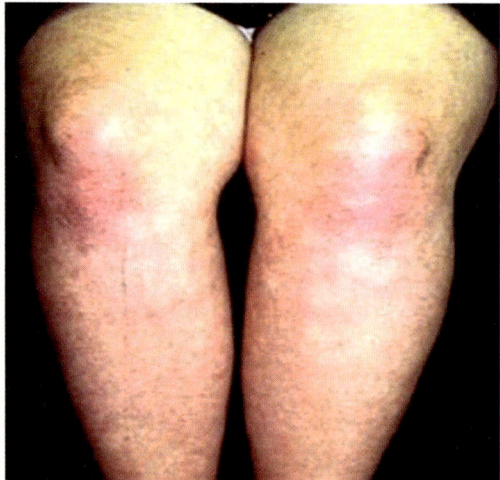

Fig. 164.1: Polymyositis. The thighs and legs and swollen, tender and muscles are weak

Q. What are the causes of proximal muscle weakness?

Ans: This question has already been answered in case discussion on proximal myopathy.

Q. Which groups of muscles are spared in dermatomyositis/polymyositis?

Ans: Facial and ocular muscles.

Q. What is the type of dysphagia in dermatomyositis/polymyositis?

Ans: As dermatomyositis/polymyositis involves the striated muscles, therefore, dysphagia is motor where initiation of swallowing is difficult.

Q. Name the proximal muscle weakness where serum creatinine levels are normal?

Ans: Steroid induced myositis.

Q. Name the conditions where serum muscle enzymes are raised with myositis (proximal weakness).

Ans: • Drugs such as statins, colchicine, lovastatin clofibrate, penicellamine, chloroquine, etc.
- Patients on hemodialysis
- Vaccine injury

Q. How would you classify dermatomyositis/polymyositis?

Ans: Aetiological classification of dermatomyositis/polymyositis into 5 groups is as follows:
I. Primary idiopathic polymyositis
II. Primary idiopathic dermatomyositis
III. Dermatomyositis/polymyositis associated with malignancy
IV. Childhood dermatomyositis or polymyositis associated with vasculitis
V. Polymyositis/dermatomyositis associated with collagen vascular disease

Q. What are the systemic manifestations in polymyositis?

Ans: • *Systemic symptoms*, e.g. fever, arthralgia, Raynaud's phenomenon, etc.
- *Joint manifestations*, e.g. arthritis, contractures
- *GI symptoms*, e.g. dysphagia, GERD, retrosternal discomfort
- *Cardiac manifestations*, e.g. myocarditis, arrhythmias, conduction disturbance, CHF
- *Pulmonary manifestations*, e.g. interstitial lung disease
- *Skeletal muscles*, e.g. proximal myopathy with tender muscles and preserved jerks

Q. What is the difference between polymyositis and myasthenia myopathic syndrome?

Ans: Read case discussion 'myasthenia gravis'.

Q. **What are the differences between polymyositis and inclusion body myositis?**

Ans: Read Table 164.1.

Q. **What do you understand by the term overlap syndrome?**

Ans: Overlap syndrome means the association of polymyositis with other connective tissue diseases. Dermatomyositis can overlap with systemic sclerosis and mixed connective tissue disorder. Patients with overlap syndrome of dermatomyositis and systemic sclerosis may have specific antinuclear antibodies, anti PM/SCL directed against a nucleolar protein complex.

Q. **How would you investigate your case?**

Ans: 1. Estimation of CPK or aldolase, ESR, C-reactive protein.
2. Antinuclear antibodies and anti-Jo-I.
3. *EMG.* It may show myopathic changes (spontaneous fibrillation potentials, short duration of polyphasic potentials of low amplitude and high action potentials).
4. *Muscle biopsy.* It may show muscle degeneration/necrosis with interstitial and perivascular infiltration of lymphocytes/mononuclear cells.
5. *MRI and MR Spectroscopy* may show abnormal signals from the involved striated muscles and abnormalities in muscle metabolism.
6. A search for cancer is recommended in all adult patients with polymyositis.

Q. **How would you treat such a patient?**

Ans: 1. *Corticosteroids.* Most cases respond to them.
2. Resistant cases of dermatomyositis/polymyositis may be treated with methotrexate, azathioprine and IV immunoglobulin.
3. Dermatomyositis/polymyositis associated with tumor, resolves after removal of the tumor.

Table 164.1: Differences between polymyositis and inclusion body myositis

Feature	Polymyositis	Inclusion body myositis
• Age	Occurs usually <50 years of age	>50 years of age
• Familial association	No	Yes
• Weakness of muscles	Proximal group is involved more then distal	Distal muscles are involved early and more than proximal groups.
• Pattern of muscle involvement	Symmetric involvement	Asymmetric muscle involvement
• Disease onset and progression	Insidious	Slow onset and slow progression than polymyositis
• CPK and other muscle enzymes	They are highly raised and useful in diagnosis	Creatinine kinase and other muscle enzymes are mildly raised or normal (in 25% cases)
• Muscle biopsy	The characteristic finding is endomysial lymphocytic infiltration	Light microscopy shows intracellular vacuoles. Electron microscopy shows filamentous or tubular inclusions in the nucleus or cytoplasm
• EMG	Shows only myopathic changes	EMG shows both myopathic and neuropathic changes
• Response to treatment	Good	It is treatment resistant polymyositis

165

Episodic (Hypokalemic) Periodic Paralysis

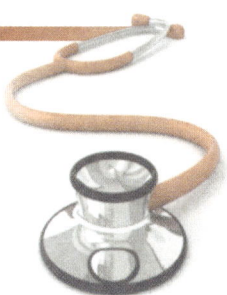

INSTRUCTION

- Examine the motor system of the patient

SALIENT FEATURES

- Intermittent muscle weakness

HISTORY

Ask for the following:

- Age of the patient (adolescent <20 yrs), onset of weakness (acute)
- History of repeated episodes of such weakness followed by recovery (present)
- Precipitation by heavy meal or high carbohydrate diet (present)
- Intake of a diuretic (thiazide, loop)
- Worsening of weakness or occurrence of weakness after vigorous exercise (present)
- Symptoms of thyrotoxicosis, i.e. sweating, palpitation, diarrhea, exophthalmos, etc.

EXAMINATION

General Physical Examination

- Look at the neck for goitre and signs of thyrotoxicosis

Neurological Examination

Motor System Examination

- Patient may be completely normal if an attack has been treated or aborted
- Immediately after acute attack, the examination reveals weakness of proximal muscles than distal. There is LMN paralysis of all the four limbs. Planters are flexor (present)
- There is no involvement of ocular, bulbar and respiratory muscles at this moment

Sensory System

- Normal

Other System Examination

Tell the examiner that you would like to look into other features of hypokalemia, i.e. distension of abdomen, absent/diminished bowel sound and cardiac arrhythmias as.

PROVISIONAL DIAGNOSIS

The patient had acute episodic paralysis of all the four limbs following exertion (lesion) caused by hypokalemic periodic paralysis (aetiology) and he has now recovered (functional status).

Q. Enumerate the points in favor of your diagnosis

Ans: 1. A young age
2. Acute onset of muscle weakness involving all the limbs. Proximal muscles are involved more than distal
3. Weakness has been precipitated by exertion/exercise
4. History of similar episodes in the past

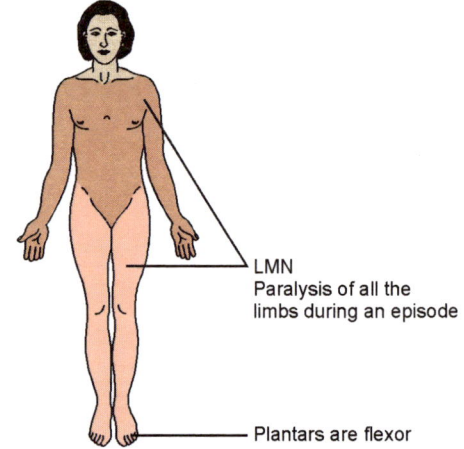

LMN
Paralysis of all the limbs during an episode

Plantars are flexor

Fig. 165.1: Hypokalemic (serum K$^+$ <2.5 mEq) periodic paralysis

5. Recovery of weakness
6. LMN paralysis of all the limbs. Plantars are flexors

QUESTIONS AND ANSWERS

Q. **What do you mean by hypokalemic periodic paralysis?**

Ans: It is an autosomal dominant disorder of calcium channel characterised by acute episodic muscle weakness with hypokalemia (serum $k^+ < 3.0$ m Eq/L). The acute paralysis improves after administration of potassium.

Q. **What are precipitants for hypokalemic periodic paralysis?**

Ans: Exercise, heavy meal or large carbohydrate meal, a diuretic, high salt diet are common precipitants.

Q. **What are the common causes of periodic paralysis?**

Ans: • Hypokalemia and hyperkalemia
• Thyrotoxic periodic paralysis
• Paramyotonia
• Idiopathic syndrome (channelopathy)
• Anderson's syndrome (channelopathy)

Q. **Where is the genetic defect in hypokalemic periodic paralysis?**

Ans: It is caused by mutations in the CACNLIA 3, SCN4A or KCNE3 gene.

Q. **What is hyperkalemic periodic paralysis?**

Ans: Hyperkalemia like hypokalemia can lead to episodic paralysis, which is acute in onset, brief, precipitated by rest following exercise or fasting; and proximal muscles are involved sparing the facial and bulbar muscles. It is associated with mutations in the SCN4A gene.

Q. **What is normokalemic periodic paralysis?**

Ans: It is similar to hyperkalemic paralysis but k^+ levels are normal in this condition.

Q. **What is Anderson's syndrome?**

Ans: It is potassium-channel disorder, characterised by episodic weakness, cardiac arrhythmias and dysmorphic changes (short stature, scoliosis, clinodactyly, hypertelorism, low set ears, micrognathia and broad forehead).

Q. **How would you investigate your case?**

Ans: 1. Serum potassium levels
2. ECG
3. EMG
4. Thyroid function tests to rule out thyrotoxic periodic paralysis

Q. **How would you treat this condition?**

Ans: 1. Administration of potassium chloride will improve the attack. Potassium chloride should be given either orally or parenterally in mannitol not in glucose or saline (this will precipitate hypokalemia)
2. Low carbohydrate and low salt should be given for few days.
3. Some patients improve on treatment with spironolactone or triamterene. Prophylactically, acetazolamide may be used to abolish the attack.

166

Multisystem Atrophy

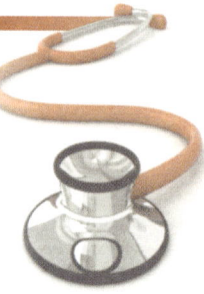

INSTRUCTION

• Examine the patient

SALIENT FEATURES

• Tremors, abnormal gait, rigidity, giddiness

HISTORY

Ask for the following:

• Dizziness, vertigo, blackout before eyes (postural hypotension)
• Dysphagia, dysphonia
• Difficulty in walking, frequent falls, ataxia
• Ask for symptoms of Parkinson's disease (rigidity, bradykinesia)
• Impotence, bladder disturbance (urinary incontinence)
• Loss of sweating

EXAMINATION

General Physical Examination

• *Skin*, dry (anhidrosis)
• *Face*—Mask-like face, rigidity, tremors. Glabellar sign positive
• *Gait* —Cerebellar ataxia (Romberg's sign negative)
• *Blood pressure* (sitting and standing for postural drop)
• *Eyes*: Look for signs of autonomic dysfunction, e.g. pupillary asymmetry, Horner's syndrome

Neurological Examination

1. Look for signs of parkinsonism
2. Look for signs of cerebellar involvement

PROVISIONAL DIAGNOSIS

The patient has cerebellar signs, parkinsonism and autonomic disturbance (lesion) caused by multiple system atrophy—a degenerative disorder (aetiology). He has marked disability (functional status).

QUESTIONS AND ANSWERS

Q. **What are the points in favor of multiple system atrophy?**
Ans: 1. Parkinsonism (extrapyramidal system degeneration)
2. Cerebellar ataxia (cerebellar degeneration)
3. Autonomic disturbance, e.g. anhydrosis, urinary incontinence, postural hypotension (autonomic system involvement)

Q. **What is Shy-Drager syndrome?**
Ans: It is parkinsonism plus syndrome due to degeneration or loss of brain stem neuron ganglia and autonomic nerves in spinal cord characterised by parkinsonism plus dysautonomia.

Q. **What do you understand by multiple system atrophy?**
Ans: It is a neurodegenerative syndrome representing a sporadic group of disorders characterised by varying degrees of extrapyramidal

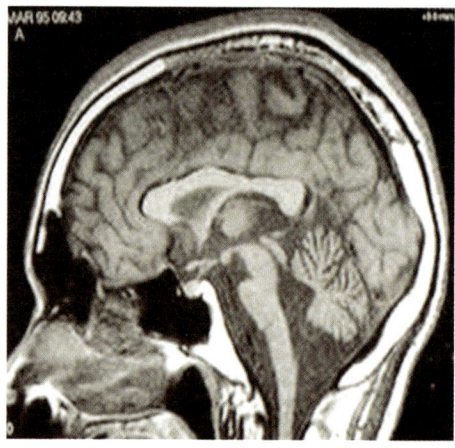

Fig. 166.1: Multisystem atrophy. MRI shows degeneration of basal ganglia, brainstem, cerebellar atrophy in a patient with multisystem atrophy

parkinsonism, cerebellar, corticospinal and autonomic dysfunction. There is normal pressure hydrocephalus.

Q. **What is the hallmark of multiple system atrophy?**

Ans: Multiple system atrophy is progressive degenerative disorder of parkinsonism associated with abnormal metabolism of α-synuclein, hence α-synuclein-positive inclusions are present in the various brain regions.

Q. **What is olivoponto cerebellar atrophy?**

Ans: Olivoponto cerebellar atrophy is also a multisystem atrophy involving the olives (located in the medulla), the pons and the cerebellum of posterior cranial fossa.

Q. **What is the mechanism of normal pressure hydrocephalus in multisystem atrophy?**

Ans: There is an increase in CSF volume in the cisterns which get distributed in the cisterns due to associated atrophy of brainstem and cerebellum, with the result the pressure of CSF does not increase inspite of hydrocephalus, hence, called normal pressure hydrocephalus.

Q. **What is the mechanism of autonomic dysfunction in multisystem atrophy?**

Ans: The increase in CSF volume in the cistern causes dysautonomia.

167 Acute Glomerulonephritis (Acute Nephritic Syndrome)

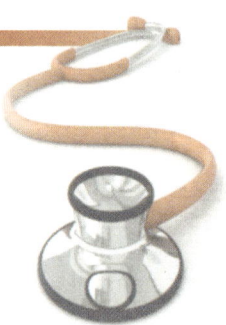

INSTRUCTION

- Look at the patient. Perform relevant examination
- What is the functional renal status?

SALIENT FEATURES

- Puffiness of face and low urine output

HISTORY

Ask for the following:

- *Age:* The patient is usually a child or adolescent
- History of fever, sore throat (present), tonsillitis, pharyngitis, otitis media or cellulitis
- History of collagen vascular disorder or a hematological disorder
- History of vaccination (DPT)
- History of oliguria, puffiness of face, change in color of urine (present)
- History of drug, rash, jaundice, breathlessness, headache and edema feet
- History of disturbance in consciousness, lazziness, lethargy, nausea, vomiting, pruritus, palpitation (features of uremia present)

EXAMINATION

General Physical Examination

- *Face* [periorbital edema, puffiness present (Fig. 167.1A)]
- *Pulse* and *BP* (BP is high)
- *JVP.* It is raised (in this case)
- *Edema* feet, sacral edema (present)
- Note the change in color of urine (red, brown or smoky present)

Systemic Examination

I. Examination of CVS: Look for the signs of cardiomegaly. Auscultate the heart for any murmur or rub or abnormal sound (3rd heart sound)

II. Examination of Lungs: Auscultate the lungs for crackles or rales for fluid overload or noncardiogenic pulmonary edema due to LVF

III. Abdominal Examination:

- Inspect the abdomen for distension or ascites
- Elicit the signs for presence of ascites or edema of abdominal wall
- Palpate the abdomen for any organ enlargement

IV. Examination of CNS

- Features of hypertensive encephalopathy
- Fundoscopy for hemorrhage/exudate and papilledema

PROVISIONAL DIAGNOSIS

The young female patient has acute nephritic syndrome also called acute glomerulonephritis (lesion) probably due to post-streptococcal infection (aetiology). Patient has acute renal failure (functional status).

QUESTIONS AND ANSWERS

Q. What are the points in favour of your diagnosis?

Ans:
1. A young patient
2. History of sore throat, fever and flank pain
3. Puffiness of face, pedal edema, abdominal distension (no ascites)
4. Hypertension
5. Oliguria. Urine is smoky
6. Features of uraemia (acute renal failure)

Q. How do you define acute nephritic syndrome?

Ans: *Acute nephritic syndrome* is characterized by an acute transient inflammatory process involving mainly the glomeruli and to lesser extent the tubules, manifests clinically with oliguria, hypertension, hematuria, (smoky urine Fig. 167.1B) edema and acute renal failure. Acute glomerulonephritis (AGN) is interchangeably used with acute nephritic syndrome. The clinical features of AGN are depicted in Fig. 167.1C.

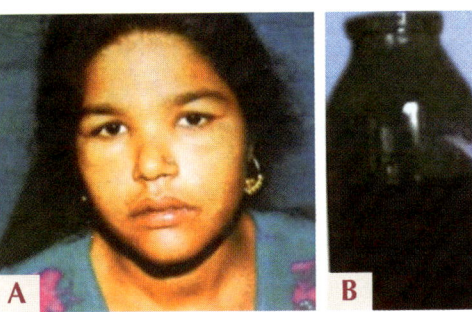

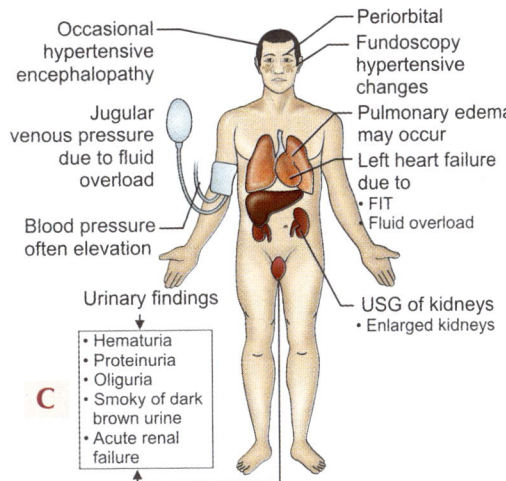

Fig. 167.1: Acute glomerulonephritis (acute nephritic syndrome). (A) A young female patient having puffiness of face; (B) 24 hour urine of the patient which is small in amount, smoky and shows RBCs and proteinuria; (C) Clinical manifestations of acute nephritic syndrome

Q. What is rapidly proliferative glomerulonephritis?

Ans: The term *rapidly proliferative glomerulonephritis* (RPGN) is used for those patients of AGN who do not go into remissions after acute nephritis, spontaneously develop acute renal failure over a period of weeks to months. These patients belong to either a primary glomerular disease or a complicating multisystem disease (secondary glomerular disease).

Q. What is its etiopathogenesis?

Ans: It is an immune complex glomerulonephritis characterised by production of antibodies against glomerular antigen, deposition of immune complexes in the walls of glomerular capillaries which modify the immune system leading to inflammation of the glomeruli. The stepwise pathogenesis is

1. *Binding of antibodies* directed against glomerular basement membrane antigen.
2. *Trapping* of soluble immune complexes in the glomerular capillary wall (subepithelial or subendothelial).
3. *In situ immune complex formation* between circulating antibody and fixed antigen or antigen planted either in the mesangium and/or in capillary wall.
4. *Action of circulating primed T cells* with macrophages.

Q. What are the causes of acute nephritic syndrome?

Ans: Causes are:

I. Infectious diseases
   a. Post-streptococcal glomerulonephritis
   b. Non-streptococcal glomerulonephritis
      i. *Bacterial:* Infective endocarditis, staphylococcal and pneumococcal infection, typhoid, syphilis and meningococcemia
      ii. *Viral:* Hepatitis B, infectious mononucleosis, mumps, measles, coxsackie and echoviruses
      iii. *Parasitic:* Malaria

II. Systemic disorders
   Systemic lupus erythematosus (SLE), vaculitis, Henoch-Schönlein purpura, Goodpasture's syndrome

III. Primary glomerular disease
   Mesangiocapillary glomerulonephritis, mesangioproliferative glomerulonephritis

IV. Miscellaneous
   Guillain-Barré syndrome, serum sickness, DPT vaccination, IgA nephropathy

Q. What conditions can lead to RPGN?

Ans: Following are the conditions that can progress of RPGN:

I. Infectious diseases
   a. Poststreptococcal glomerulonephritis
   b. Infective endocarditis

II. **Multisystem diseases**
   a. Systemic lupus erythematosus (SLE)
   b. Goodpasture's syndrome
   c. Vasculitis
   d. Henoch-Schonlein purpura
III. **Primary glomerular disease**
   a. Idiopathic
   b. Mesangiocapillary glomerulonephritis
   c. Membranous glomerulonephritis (anti glomerular basement membrane antibodies nephritis)

Q. When would you suspect RPGN?

Ans: It is suspected on clinical grounds due to following manifestations.

1. **Signs and symptoms of azotemia**
   Nausea, vomiting, weakness. The azotemia develops early and progresses faster.
2. **Signs and symptoms of acute glomerulonephritis**
   It includes oliguria, abdominal flank pain due to large kidneys, hematuria, hypertension and proteinuria.

Q. How would you investigate such a case?

Ans: The investigations to be done are given in Table 167.1.

Q. What are the common complications of acute nephritic syndrome (AGN)?

Ans: Complications are:
- Fluid overload
- Hypertensive encephalopathy
- Acute left heart failure
- Noncardiogenic pulmonary edema (ARDS)
- Rapidly progressive glomerulonephritis (RPGN)
- Uremia
- Massive hemoptysis

Q. How would you treat such a patient?

Ans: The condition is usually self-limiting, hence treatment is symptomatic as well as specific to the cause.
   i. *Relief of edema* by salt restriction, rest and diuretics.
   ii. *Control of Hypertension*, i.e. salt restriction, diuretics, ACE inhibitors
   iii. *Treatment of oliguria.* Fluid and electrolyte balance is to be maintained. Diuretics may help.
   iv. Depending on the nature and severity of AGN, high dose steroids and cytotoxic agents (cyclophosphamide) can be used. *Plasmapheresis* is useful in Goodpasture syndrome and immune complex nephritis.

Table 167.1: Investigations for acute nephritic syndrome

Investigation	Positive finding
1. Urine microscopy	1. RBCs and red cell casts
2. Urine complete	2. High specific gravity, proteinuria present
3. Blood urea and serum creatinine	3. May be elevated
4. Culture (throat swab, discharge from ear, swap from infected skin)	4. Nephrogenic streptococci may be isolated but not always
5. ASO titre	5. Elevated in post-streptococcal nephritis
6. C3 level	6. Reduced
7. Antinuclear antibody (ANA)	7. Present in significant titres in lupus (SLE) nephritis
8. X-ray chest	8. Cardiomegaly, pulmonary edema—not always
9. Renal imaging (Ultrasound)	9. Usually normal or large kidneys
10. Renal biopsy	10. Glomerulonephritis

168

Nephrotic Syndrome

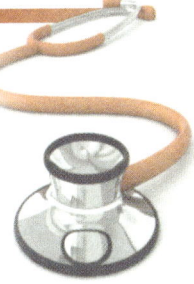

INSTRUCTION

- Examine the patient

SALIENT FEATURES

- Swollen legs and feet

HISTORY

Ask for the following:

- Symptoms, their duration, progression, relapse or remission, aggravating and relieving factors, diurnal variation
- History of streptococcal throat or skin infection, hepatitis (blood transfusions)
- History of jaundice, diabetes (present in this case), hypertension, neck swelling (lymphoma)
- Past history of infections (malaria, toxoplasmosis, schistosomiasis, leprosy) collagen vascular disorder (SLE), skin rashes, neoplasms (lymphoma, solid tumors)
- Drug history (NSAIDs, ACE inhibitors, heroin, gold, penicillamine, chlorpropamide, tolbutamide, rifampicin)
- Family history suggestive of Alport's syndrome

EXAMINATION

General Physical Examination

- *General appearance* — moon facies or puffiness of face, periorbital edema (present Fig. 168.1), xanthelasma
- *Nutritional status* (poor nutrition)
- Look for *jaundice, anemia* (pallor), *cyanosis*
- *Neck veins* for JVP
- *Lymph nodes* for leukemia, lymphomas
- *Pulse* and *BP*
- *Skin* for alopecia, rash, xanthomas
- *Feet* for pitting edema (Fig. 168.1)
- *External genitalia* for edema and hydrocele
- An evidence of *infection* (these patients are more prone to infection, Fig. 168.1)

Systemic Examination

1. *Abdomen:* Distended, presence of ascites (present), edema of abdominal wall, shiny skin, nontender renal angle, scrotal (or vulval) edema, presence of hydrocele.
2. *Respiratory system:* Thoracoabdominal respiration, edema chest wall and legs, pleural effusions. Sometimes evidence of infection may be present.
3. *CVS examination:* No cardiomegaly, no murmur and no abnormal sound.

PROVISIONAL DIAGNOSIS

The patient has nephrotic syndrome (lesion) caused by diabetic nephropathy (lesion). Patients has gross edema of legs (functional status).

QUESTIONS AND ANSWERS

Q. **What are the points in favor of your diagnosis?**
Ans: • Gross pedal, leg edema and ascites

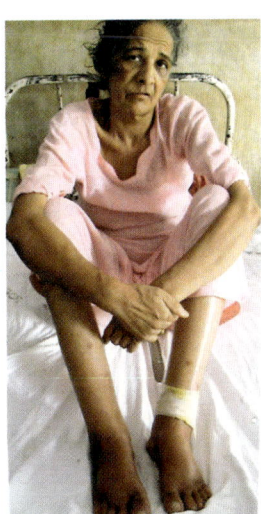

Fig. 168.1: Nephrotic syndrome

- Evidence of infection (wound is bandaged)
- Presence of diabetes for many years

Q. What bedside test would you like to perform to confirm the diagnosis?

Ans: The urine examination for protein and sugar.

Q. What are the components of nephrotic syndrome?

Ans: 1. Massive proteinuria > 3.5 g/day or protein creatinine ratio of > 400 mg/mmol
2. Hypoalbuminemia/hypoproteinemia
3. Pitting pedal edema
4. Hyperlipidemia and lipiduria
5. Hypercoagulopathy

Q. What are the other conditions which can produce this picture?

Ans: The following conditions which can lead to generalised anasarca come into one's mind:
1. Congestive heart failure
2. Cirrhosis of the liver
3. Constrictive pericarditis
4. Hypoproteinemia (malabsorption syndrome)

Q. What are the causes of nephrotic syndrome?

Ans: Read Table 168.1.

Table 168.1: Common causes of nephrotic syndrome

I. Primary glomerular diseases

- Minimal change disease
- Glomerulonephritis (mesangioproliferative, membranous and membranoproliferative)
- Focal glomerulosclerosis

II. Secondary glomerular diseases

A. Infections
- a. Post-streptococcal glomerulonephritis
- b. Post-streptococcal endocarditis
- c. Secondary syphilis
- d. Malaria (vivax and malariae infection)
- e. Lepromatous leprosy
- f. Hepatitis B and C

B. Drugs and toxins
  Gold, mercury, penicillamine, captopril, NSAIDs antitoxins, antivenoms and contrast media

C. Heredo-Familial
- Congenital and Alport's syndrome

D. Miscellaneous
- a. Toxemia of pregnancy
- b. Renovascular hypertension
- Renal tumors, leukemia, lymphoma

Q. What is etiopathogenesis of nephrotic syndrome?

Ans: I. *Immunological* (deposition of immune complexes in the glomeruli leading to glomerular injury.

II. *Non immunological injury,* i.e. drugs, toxins, diseases (diabetes) can cause glomerulopathy.

Q. What is selective and nonselective proteinuria?

Ans: *Selective proteinuria* means filtration of low molecular weight proteins especially the albumin through the glomeruli. It is seen in minimal change glomerulonephritis and early phase of other glomerulonephritis. These cases respond well to steroids.

Nonselective proteinuria means filtration of albumin along with high molecular weight proteins, e.g. globulins, antithrombin III, transferrin, immunoglobulins, thyroxine-binding globulins, calciferol-binding globulin, etc. This occurs in advanced glomerular disease and does not respond to steroids.

Q. What is orthostatic proteinuria?

Ans: It occurs on standing and disappears on lying down. It is due to compression of inferior vena cava by liver during standing. The prognosis is good. Proteinuria is absent in the morning on rising from the bed.

Q. What is glomerular proteinuria? How does it differ from tubular proteinuria (Tamm-Horsetall protein)

Ans: 1. Glomerular proteinuria is >1 g/day and is associated with cells and casts.
2. Tubular proteinuria is <1 g/day and may contain only epithelial or granular casts.

Q. What are the causes of hypertension in nephrotic syndrome?

Ans: Hypertension is not a component of nephrotic syndrome, but may be seen in:
- Diabetic nephropathy
- SLE (lupus nephritis) and polyarteritis nodosa
- Nephrotic syndrome complicated by CRF
- Focal glomerulosclerosis

Q. What is the indication of renal biopsy in nephrotic syndrome?

Ans: The renal biopsy is done in adults
- To confirm the diagnosis
- To know the underlying pathological lesion

Q. What are the complications of nephrotic syndrome?

Ans: Common complications are as follows:
1. **Vascular**
   - Accelerated atherogenesis
   - Hyperlipidemia

- Peripheral arterial or venous thrombosis, renal vein thrombosis and pulmonary embolism due to hyper-coagulable state.
2. **Metabolic**
   - Protein malnutrition
   - Iron-resistant microcytic hypochromic anemia
   - Hypocalcemia and secondary hyperparathyroidism
3. **Infections**
   - Pneumococcal and staphylococcal infections (respiratory and peritoneum)
4. **Chronic renal failure**

Q. **Which glomerulonephritis responds favorably to treatment?**

Ans: Minimal change glomerular disease. It carries good prognosis.

Q. **What are the characteristics of minimal change disease?**

Ans: The characteristic features are:
   i. Most common cause of nephrotic syndrome in children (70–80%) and more common in males than females.
   ii. It is named so because light microscopy of renal biopsy specimen does not reveal any abnormality of glomeruli. Electron microscopy reveals effacement of the foot processes of epithelial cells.
   iii. Proteinuria is highly selective.
   iv. Hematuria is uncommon.
   v. Spontaneous relapses and remissions are common.
   vi. Majority of the patients respond promptly to steroids. The disease may disappear after steroid therapy.
   vii. Progression to acute renal failure is rare.

Q. **How will you investigate such a patient?**

Ans: Investigations to be done are as follows:
   1. *Urine examination* for proteinuria and lipiduria (fatty casts). Hematuria is uncommon.
   2. *24 hours urine* for excretion of albumin or proteins >3.5 g daily or protein/creatinine ratio >400 mg/mmol. In early disease or in patients receiving treatment, the proteinuria may be less.
   3. *Full blood count, ESR and C-reactive protein.*
   4. *Serum lipids:* Low density lipoproteins and cholesterol are increased in majority of the patients (dyslipidemia).
   5. *Serum proteins or albumin:* Total serum proteins may be normal or low. Serum albumin is usually low <3 g/dl (an important diagnostic criteria).
   6. *Other renal function tests,* are normal.
   7. *DNA antibody, antinuclear antibody (ANA), complement level.*
   8. *Chest X-ray* may show hydrothorax.
   9. *Ultrasound of kidneys:* The kidneys may be normal, small or large depending on the cause. Amyloid and diabetic kidneys are large, while kidneys in glomerulonephritis are small.
   10. *Renal biopsy:* It is done in adult nephrotic syndrome to diagnose the nature of underlying disease, to predict the prognosis and response to treatment.

Q. **What is the treatment of patients with nephrotic syndrome?**

Ans:
   1. *Diuretics* (loop diuretics, thiazide and potassium-sparing) to relieve edema and ascites.
   2. *ACE inhibitors* to reduce proteinuria. They are renoprotective agents.
   3. *Steroids and cytotoxic drugs* (8 week course) for minimal change and other glomerulonephritis.
   4. *Prevention of venous thrombosis* and thromboembolism by elastic stocking and anticoagulants (heparin, warfarin).
   5. *Albumin infusion* in severe symptomatic hypoproteinemic patients resistant to other treatment.
   6. *Plasma ultrafiltration* in severe cases.
   7. *Pneumococcal vaccination.*
   8. Interferone-alpha for hepatitis-associated nephrotic syndrome.
   9. Lipid lowering agents if there is severe dyslipidemia.

169

Polycystic Kidneys

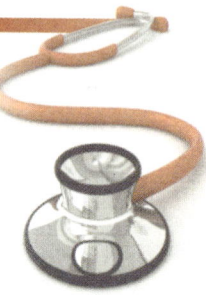

INSTRUCTION

• Examine the abdomen of the patient

SALIENT FEATURES

• Flank pain with red colored urine

HISTORY

Ask about the following:

• Acute flank/loin pain, red coloured urine (gross hematuria present)
• Abdominal or loin discomfort due to large kidneys present (history of dragging pain in polycystic kidneys)
• Family history of polycystic disease of kidneys (present)
• Symptoms and signs of hypertension
• History of stroke (as a result of rupture of berry aneurysm)
• Family history of brain aneurysm (hemorrhage in young age)

EXAMINATION

General Physical Examination

• Look for anemia (CRF) or polycythemia (increased erythropoietin)
• Measure BP (hypertension present)
• Edema feet
• Arteriovenous fistula in the arm (present) or subclavian dialysis catheter

Systemic Examination

Abdominal Examination in this case

• No scar marks
• Renal angles on the back are full (in this case)

Palpation

• There are two masses, one each in the lumbar region
• Each mass is small, nontender having irregular

surface, moves slightly with respiration. Mass is bimanually palpable and ballotable. Fingers can be insinuated between the mass and costal margins
• *Renal angles* on the back are nontender

Percussion

• There is resonant note over the masses

Auscultation

• There is no bruit, rub or hum

PROVISIONAL DIAGNOSIS

The patient has bilateral renal masses with hypertension and hematuria (lesion) due to polycystic kidney disease (aetiology) and is currently on dialysis (functional status).

QUESTIONS AND ANSWERS

Q. **What are the points in favor of your diagnosis?**

Ans: The points in favour of the diagnosis are:
  1. History of flank pain with dysuria and haematuria
  2. Positive family history
  3. Presence of hypertension
  4. Bilateral palpable kidneys
  5. An arteriovenous fistula in the arm for dialysis

Q. **What is your differential diagnosis?**

Ans: • Bilateral hydronephrosis
  • Bilateral pyonephrosis
  • Bilateral masses can be confused with hepatosplenomegaly, i.e. liver enlargement with right kidney and enlarged spleen with left kidney. For differentiation read clinical methods by Prof SN Chugh
  • Para-aortic and mesenteric lymphadenopathy. These masses are irregular, firm, nontender, nonmobile neither bimanually palpable nor ballotable

Q. What is adult polycystic kidneys disease (ADPKD)?

Ans: Adult polycystic kidney disease is a heredo-familial (autosomal dominant and autosomal recessive) disorder in which cysts are present in kidneys making it palpable and enlarged. These cysts cause compression of the intervening renal tissue and progressive loss of excretory function.

Q. How does polycystic kidney disease manifest?

Ans: It usually manifests in 3rd and 4th decade with:

- Pain in the lumbar region (s) hematuria, hypertension
- Urinary tract infection, urinary tract obstruction, symptoms of uremia
- Subarachnoid hemorrhage due to rupture of associated berry aneurysm

Q. What is genetic defect in ADPKD?

Ans: Three forms of autosomal dominant genes have been recognized:

1. *ADPKD1 gene* accounts for 90% of cases and localized to short arm of chromosome 16.
2. *ADPKD2 gene* is less common (10%) and is localised to short arm of chromosome 4. These patients develop symptoms of renal failure later than ADPKD1.
3. *ADPKD3 gene* not mapped to any specific chromosome.

Both ADPKD1 and ADPKD2 encode for the polycystic protein 1 and 2, the mutation of which leads to the disease.

Q. What are the causes of pain abdomen in ADPKD?

Ans: 1. Urinary tract obstruction by clot or stone
2. UTI
3. Sudden hemorrhage into a cyst

Q. What is the cause of hypertension in ADPKD?

Ans: Hypertension is secondary to intrarenal ischemia leading to stimulation of renin-angiotensin-aldosterone system.

Q. What are the extrarenal manifestations of ADPKD?

Ans: These are as follows:

1. **Cysts in the other organs,** i.e. liver (50–70%) spleen pancreas and ovaries.
2. **Intracranial aneurysms (berry aneurysms)** can occur in 5–10% cases.
3. **Diverticulosis** of the colon may occur and patients are more vulnerable to perforation than general population.
4. **Mitral valve prolapse (25% cases).** Mitral, aortic and tricuspid regurgitation can occur.

Q. What are the causes of palpable kidney or kidneys?

Ans: Read the Clinical Methods in Medicine by Prof. SN Chugh.

Q. What are the causes of mass in lumber region?

Ans: Read the "Clinical Methods in Medicine" by Prof SN Chugh.

Q. What are the causes of death in ADPKD?

Ans: 1. *End-stage renal disease* and *progressive renal failure*
2. *Hypertension* and its related complications, i.e. CHF, cerebral hemorrhages
3. Rarely due to *unrelated causes*

Q. What are the renal consequences of ADPKD?

Ans: 1. Cysts formation and their further enlargement causes tubular dysfunction
2. Loss of renal concentrating ability
3. Increased secretion of renin resulting in hypertension and increased secretion of erythropoietin results in polycythemia

Q. What are the complications of ADPKD?

Ans:
- *Recurrent urinary tract infection* including infection of the cyst (pyocyst)
- *Urinary tract obstruction*
- *Nephrolithiasis* (calcium oxalate and uric acid stones) is common
- *End-stage renal disease* (ESRD) due to progressive decline of renal function is a late complication
- *Renal failure*

Q. How will you investigate a case of ADPKD?

Ans:
- *Ultrasound* is the preferred technique for diagnosis of symptomatic patients and for screening of asymptomatic family member. It has replaced intravenous pyelography (IVP) used to be done previously for diagnosis.

At least 3–5 cysts in each kidney is standard diagnostic criteria for ADPKD (Fig. 169.1)

- *IVP:* It has been superceded by USG. It detects cysts and distortion of pelvicalyceal system and gives typical "Spidery leg appearance". It gives an idea of renal excretory function.
- *CT Scan:* It is more sensitive than USG.
- *Genetic linkage analysis:* Genetic probes are available for analysis. The genetic analysis is reserved for cases where radiographic imaging is negative and there is need to confirm the diagnosis, for example, screening of family members for potential kidney donation.

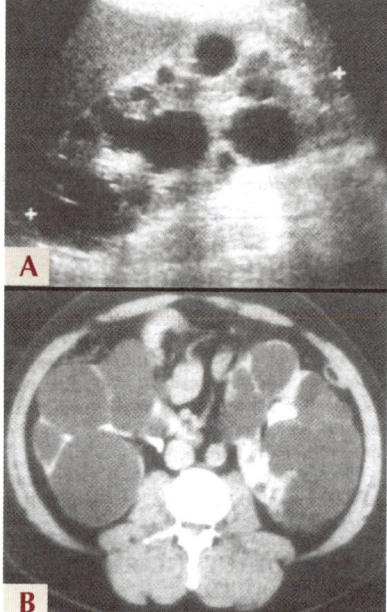

Fig. 169.1: Adult polycystic kidney disease. (A) Ultrasound shows multiple cysts (>3) in the kidney; (B) CT scan confirms the diagnosis showing bilateral cystic disease of kidneys (>3 cysts are seen in each kidney)

Q.   How will you treat ADPKD?

Ans: As it is genetically related disorder, hence, there is no definite treatment. The aim of treatment is to retard the progress of the disease and preserve renal function as long as possible by:

- *Control of hypertension* by antihypertensives especially ACE inhibitors
- *Treatment of urinary tract infection* by appropriate antibodies
- *Relief of chronic pain* by an analgesic. If no relief, cyst may be punctured and sclerosed with ethanol
- *Dialysis* and *kidney transplantation* when renal failure occurs

Q.   What are the causes of renal cysts on USG?

Ans: The causes are:

1. ADPKD (autosomal dominant)
2. ADPKD (autosomal recessive)
3. *Tuberous sclerosis* (adenoma sebaceum, shagreen patch, benign tumors of CNS, renal angiomyo lipomas and renal cysts may occur)
4. *Von Hippel-Lindau disease* (e.g. hemangioblastoma of retina and CNS, bilateral renal cysts may occur)
5. Medullary spongy kidney
6. Medullary cystic disease

170

Unilateral Palpable Kidney

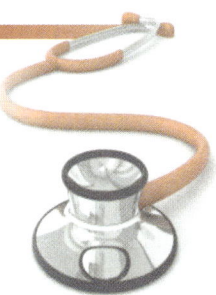

INSTRUCTION

- Examine the patient's abdomen

SALIENT FEATURES

- Heaviness and dragging pain in right lumbar region

HISTORY

Ask for the following:

- Age of the patient
- Flank pain or dragging pain due to abdominal mass, hematuria (red colored urine)
- Paraneoplastic manifestations, e.g. fever, flushed face (polycythemia), hypercalcaemia, cushing facies (Cushing's syndrome)
- Congenital absence of one kidney
- Nephrectomy (one kidney has been donated)
- Features of renal failure
- Look for an arteriovenous fistula in the arm or an subclavian catheter for hemodialysis

EXAMINATION

General Physical Examination

- Visible swelling in one of the lumbar region
- Anemia or polycythemia
- Signs of uremia, e.g. bone pain, alterations in mentation, pruritus, bruishing, etc.
- Features of paraneoplastic syndrome

Abdominal Examination

- Right kidney is bimanually palpable, ballottable and moves slightly with respiration (Fig. 170.1). Renal angle is full. On percussion, there is a band of colonic resonance in front of the mass. Fingers can be insinuated between the mass and costal margins. The mass is right renal mass.

PROVISIONAL DIAGNOSIS

A old person presenting with a triad of abdominal pain, gross hematuria and a palpable renal mass (lesion), the provisional diagnosis is renal cell carcinoma (aetiology). There is no evidence of renal failure or an arteriovenous fistula for dialysis (functional status).

QUESTIONS AND ANSWERS

Q. What are the causes of unilateral palpable kidney?

Ans:
1. Polycystic kidney disease in which one kidney is involved or multiple cysts in one kidney (renal cysts)
2. Renal cell carcinoma or oncocytomas (benign renal tumor)
3. Hydronephrosis
4. Perinephric abscess
5. Hypertrophy of solitary functioning kidney following nephrectomy or after kidney donation

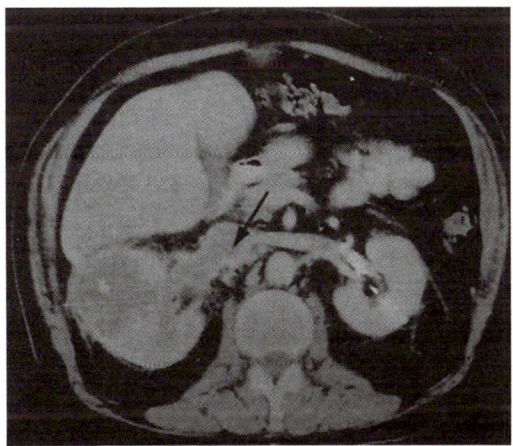

Fig. 170.1: Unilateral enlarged kidney due to renal cell carcinoma. The CT scan shows enlarged right kidney which is filled with a low-density tumor which fails to take up contrast material. Tumor is extending into the renal vein and inferior vena cava

Q. What are paraneoplastic syndromes associated with renal cell carcinoma?

Ans:
- Hypercalcemia
- Cushing's syndrome
- Polycythaemia or erythrocytosis
- Fever

Q. What are the risk factors for renal cell carcinoma?

Ans:
1. Cigarette smoking
2. Familial predisposition for renal cell carcinoma have been identified (Von Hippel-Lindau disease) as well as an association with dialysis related acquired cystic disease and genetic aberrations.

Q. How would you investigate this case?

Ans:
- *Complete hemogram* for polycythemia or erythrocytosis.
- *Urine* for hematuria and cells and casts.
- *Serum calcium* levels may be high.
- *USG* will confirm the renal mass. Duplex Doppler USG will be useful to defect tumor thrombus within renal vein.
- *CT Scan* is done to confirm the mass and further stage the lesion with respect to regional lymph node, renal vein or hepatic involvement. CT scan also provides valuable information regarding the anatomy and function of contralateral kidney.
- *Chest X-ray* for pulmonary metastases.
- *Bone scans* should be performed for large tumors and in patients with bone pain.
- *MRI* is excellent tool to detect tumor thrombus within renal vein or superior vena cava.

Q. What changes can occur in a kidney when other has been removed?

Ans: In patients having solitary kidney (one kidney removed), the renal function remains stable for a long time with reduction in renal mass. However, these patients are at increased risk of developing changes of hyperdynamic circulation through the kidney. These changes are:

i. Proteinuria

ii. Hyperdynamic glomerulopathy

iii. Progressive renal failure

Hence, patients with solitary kidneys must be monitored for renal function.

On the other hand, most kidney donors (one kidney donated) had preserved GFR, normal albumin excretion and enjoy a good quality of life. Renal failure has gradually developed in small number of cases and according to the United Network for organ sharing, a few of kidney donors have ultimately been registered for kidney transplantation. Some donors may develop

i. Hypertension

ii. Microalbuminuria (occasional)

Hence, it is worth considering to use renoprotective therapy to prevent these complications.

Q. What are the risks of donation?

Ans:
1. Risk of bleeding during and after the procedure.
2. Risk of infection.
3. Post-operative problems.
4. Loss of time. About 4–5 weeks are lost from work/job.
5. Rare death can occur.

171

Transplanted Kidney

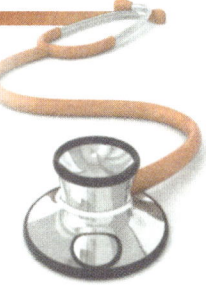

INSTRUCTION

• Examine the patient's abdomen

SALIENT FEATURES

• Kidney has been implanted

HISTORY

• Ascertain history of chronic kidney disease, duration, type and cause
• History of hemodialysis (frequency and duration)
• History of arteriovenous fistula
• History of transplantation

EXAMINATION

General Physical Examination

• Look for the signs of uremia, e.g. coated tongue, uremic breath, pruritus, anemia, bleeding, urine output
• Look for laparotomy scar over the abdomen (to confirm transplantation)
• Ascertain presence of arteriovenous fistula in the arms
• History of diabetes (present), hypertension, glomerulonephritis (chronic), pyelonephritis

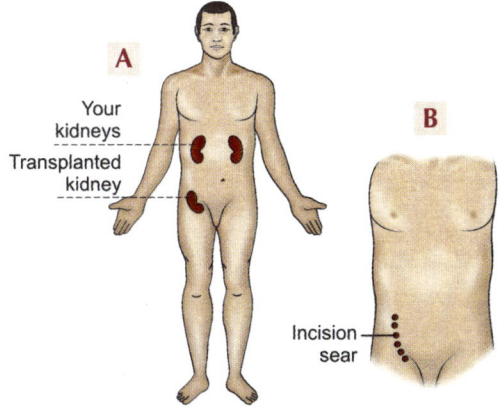

Fig. 171.1: Transplanted kidney. (A) Diagram; (B) Implanted kidney in a patient

Abdominal Examination

• There will be a scar over the abdomen (present).
• There is a mass in the right iliac fossa which is ballotable and bimanual palpable. This is kidney mass (present).

PROVISIONAL DIAGNOSIS

The patient has a transplanted kidney on right side (lesion) probably required for diabetic nephropathy (patient is diabetic). The kidney functions are preserved (functional status).

QUESTIONS AND ANSWERS

Q. What are the causes of mass in right iliac fossa?

Ans: Read the case discussion on masses in the abdomen.

Q. Tell few indications for renal transplantation?

Ans: The sole indication of renal transplantation is end-stage renal disease (ESRD) due to any cause such as:
  • Diabetic nephropathy with ESRD
  • Hypertension with ESRD
  • Chronic glomerulonephritis/interstitial nephritis with ESRD
  • Cystic kidney diseases

Q. What do you mean by the term End Stage Renal Disease (ESRD)?

Ans: End stage renal disease is defined as stage 5 chronic kidney disease characterised by GFR ≤ 15 ml/min/1.73 m^2 on dialysis and these patients are candidates for renal replacement therapy.

Q. What are the contraindications of renal transplantation?

Ans: A positive cross-match by cytotoxicity testing between recipient serum and donor cells is a contraindication.

Q. What are the complications of renal transplant?

Ans: The complications are related to procedure and toxicity to drugs:
1. Opportunistic infections, e.g. pneumomycosis, CMV
2. Premature CAD (coronary artery disease)
3. Hypertension
4. Lymphomas and other cancers
5. *De novo* glomerulonephritis in transplanted kidney
6. Steroid-induced complications

Q. Would you refer the patient for transplantation before instituting dialysis?

Ans: Yes, it is acceptable and infact preferable to refer the patient to renal transplant before dialysis with judicious planning between renal physician and transplant surgical team.

Q. What is the survival rate following kidney transplant?

Ans: The 1 and 3 years kidney graft survival for living donor transplant is 89% and 78% respectively, whereas in cadaveric donor transplantation, it is about 70%.

Q. What immunosuppressive regimen is used to prevent graft rejection?

Ans: A combination of corticosteroid, an antimetabolite (azathioprine, mycofenolate mofetil) and a calcineurin inhibitor (tacrolimus or cyclosporin) or mTor inhibitor (sirolimus).

Q. What are the advantages of renal transplantation over long term dialysis?

Ans: The advantages are:
1. Better quality of life
2. Reduction in long-term risk of death
3. Reduction in medical expenses

Q. What are the signs and symptoms of rejection of the graft?

Ans: Rejection can be acute or chronic. It should be suspected when:
1. The graft becomes tender
2. Urine output falls
3. Creatinine clearance starts rising

Q. How would you evaluate for suspected graft rejection?

Ans: Graft biopsy is done if rejection is suspected on clinical grounds. It is subjected to histopathology.

Acute rejection is characterised by lymphocytic interstitial infiltration with destruction of epithelial cells. *Chronic rejection* is characterised by interstitial fibrosis, tubular atrophy and proliferation of vascular intima.

Q. What are the factors that determine outcome of transplantation?

Ans:
1. *Antigenic disparity* (ABO blood group and histocompatibility or HLA) between donor and recipient
2. *Type of immunological response* by the host
3. *Immunosuppressive regimen* used to prevent graft rejection
4. *Nonimmunological factors*, i.e. age and race of recipient, donor age, length of time on dialysis and coexisting hyperlipidemia, hypertension or CMV infection

Q. Is HLA-matching advantageous for transplantation?

Ans: Yes. There is recent evidence that HLA-matched kidneys (HLA-DR, HLA-B and HLA-A antigens) are associated with long term survival of the patient. Complete matching of HLA-DR, HLA-B and HLA-A is associated with better chances of survival respectively.

Q. Should repeated blood transfusions be avoided in a patient ready for renal transplant?

Ans: Yes. Patients with CRF can tolerate anemia without blood transfusions per se. However, blood transfusion should be avoided in patients waiting for transplant because of risk of HLA sensitization.

Q. What are the other factors known to cause HLA sensitization?

Ans:
1. Previously failed transplant
2. Pregnancy

Q. What is the role of pancreas-kidney transplantation in patients with diabetic nephropathy and ESRD?

Ans: Simultaneous renal and pancreas transplantation in type I DM with end-stage renal disease prolongs survival because pancreas transplantation can reverse the lesions of diabetic nephropathy.

172

Uremia

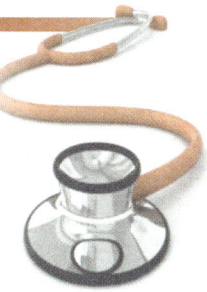

INSTRUCTION

- Perform general physical examination and ask relevant questions

SALIENT FEATURES

- Nausea, vomiting, anaemia, high BP urinous breath

HISTORY

Ask about the following (Fig. 172.1):

- Headache, visual disturbance, confusion, disorientation
- Nausea, vomiting (present), anorexia, hiccups, GI bleed (hematemesis)
- Fatigue, lethargy, malaise (present)
- Polyuria, nocturia
- Swelling of face, feet
- Breathlessness (present), cough, orthopnea, PND
- Pruritus
- Restless legs
- Paraesthesias (hypocalcemia or peripheral neuropathy)
- Bone pain (renal osteodystrophy, osteomalacia)
- Proximal myopathy
- History of diabetes, HT (present) and recurrent UTI (fever)

- Family history of polycystic kidney disease or other renal disease
- History of impotence in males, amenorrhea in females

EXAMINATION

General Physical Examination

1. Look for *signs of anemia*, e.g. pallor, sallow look, rapid pulse (present)
2. *Mouth* for urinous breath (uremic breath present)
3. Neck for JVP (fluid overload)
4. *Stature* of the patient (renal rickets)
5. *Pulse and BP* (hypertension present or hypotension)
6. *Nails*, e.g. 'half and half' nails [proximal half portion is white while distal portion is brownish (Fig. 172.2)]
7. *Skin*, e.g. scratch marks, lemon tingue of the skin, pallor. Look for uremic frost, skin pigmentation
8. *Arms:* Asterixis (flapping tremors), hemodialysis fistula (arteriovenous fistula)
9. *Breathing*, e.g. Kussmaul (acidotic) breathing or hyperventilation (rapid breathing)
10. *Feet:* Pitting edema

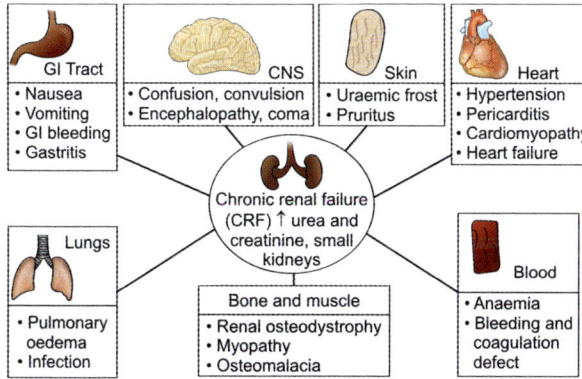

Fig. 172.1: Clinical manifestations of uremia

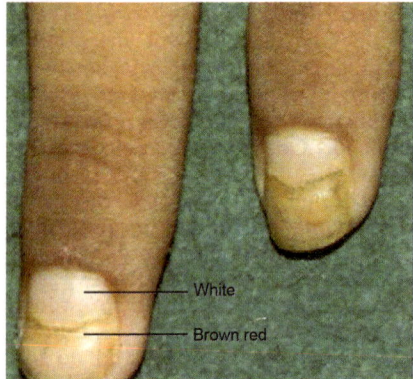

White

Brown red

Fig. 172.2: Half and half nail (proximal part of nail plate is white and distal part brown) in a patient with chronic renal failure

Relevant System Examination

Abdominal examination kidney mass/palpable kidneys, i.e. polycystic kidneys, hydronephrosis, pyonephrosis
- Palpate the bladder and elicit signs for ascites

Cardiovascular system for cardic enlargement, left ventricular failure, pericardial rub

Respiratory System Examination for crackles and rales (LVF, fluid overload)

Nervous system for disturbance in sensorium (uremic encephalopathy) and peripheral neuropathy, proximal myopathy

Fundus examination for diabetes, hypertension

Rectal and vaginal examination for urinary obstruction (palpable bladder)

PROVISIONAL DIAGNOSIS

The patient has features of uremia (chronic renal failure) due to diabetic nephropathy (aetiology) and is currently undergoing dialysis (functional status).

QUESTIONS AND ANSWERS

Q. What are the points in favor of your diagnosis?

Ans: Symptoms of uremia, e.g. nausea, vomiting, uremic breath, shallow look, lethargy, fatigue, etc.
- Presence of anaemia, oedema, hypertension
- History of chronic kidney disease (diabetic nephropathy for the last many years (>6 month)
- Presence of pericardial rub
- Presence of AV fistula for dialysis

Q. What is chronic kidney disease (CKD) and kidney damage?

Ans: *Chronic kidney disease* (CKD) is defined as either kidney damage or GFR <60 ml/min/ 1.73 m² for 3 or more months.
Kidney damage is defined as presence of pathologic abnormalities or markers of damage including abnormalities in blood or urine tests or imaging studies.

Q. How would you classify CKD?

Ans: CKD is classified based on the clinical parameters and GFR (Table 172.1).

Stage	Decription	GFR (ml/min/1.73 m²)
	Table 172.1: Classification of CKD	
1.	Kidney damage with normal or increased GFR	≥ 90
2.	Kidney damage with mild reduction in GFR	60 – 89
3.	Moderate reduction in GFR	30 – 59
4.	Severe reduction in GFR	
5.	Kidney failure (ESRD)	<15 or dialysis

Q. What do you understand by the term uremia and azotemia?

Ans: *Uremia:* It implies a deterioration of renal function associated with symptoms (GFR < 20% of normal). *Chronic renal failure* is defined as serum creatinine >3 mg%.
Azotemia: It implies a raised level of nitrogenous products (urea, creatinine) without symptoms (GFR about 20 – 35 % of normal).

Q. What are the common causes of CRF?

Ans: 1. Glomerulonephritis (primary or secondary)
2. Diabetes mellitus (diabetic nephropathy)
3. Chronic pyelonephritis/interstitial nephritis
4. Hypertensive kidney disease (nephropathy)
5. Cystic kidney diseases (polycystic kidney diseases)
6. Analgesic nephropathy
7. Obstructive nephropathies

Q. What are the reversible causes of chronic kidney disease (CKD)?

Ans: 1. Infection
2. Obstruction
3. Fluid volume overload
4. Hypertension
5. Nephrotoxic agents
6. Electrolyte disturbance
7. Left ventricular failure

Q. What are the consequence of CRF?

Ans: Read the clinical consequences in Fig. 172.1.

Q. Name the drugs to be avoided in CRF.

Ans: Nephrotoxic drugs to be avoided are:
- Aminoglycosides, tetracycline, angiotensin receptors blockers, cephalosporins, potassium sparing diuretics.

Q. What is renal osteodystrophy?

Ans: Bone changes in CRF are renal osteodystrophy which is characterised by:
  i. Osteomalacia (renal rickets)
  ii. Osteitis fibrosa cystica (secondary hyperparathyroidism)
  iii. Osteosclerosis (increased bone density producing rugger-jersey spine)

Q. How ACE inhibitors are renoprotective?

Ans: The renoprotective effects of ACE inhibitors are due to:
  1. Control of hypertension by antagonising the renin-angiotensin mechanism, hence prevent the progression of chronic kidney disease.
  2. Anti proteinuric effect of these drugs
  3. ACE inhibitors can help reduce hyperfiltration injury and thus slows the progression of CKD.

Q. What is the basis of secondary hyperparathyroidism in CRF?

Ans: There is failure of phosphorous excretion early in CKD leading to rise in its level. To normalise the levels of phosphorous and calcium, parathyroid hormone is released (secondary hyperparathyroidism) which leads to bone disease (osteitis fibrosa cystica). This is called *Bricker's trade off hypothesis.*

Q. How would you investigate this patient?

Ans: 1. *Complete urine examination,* i.e. specific gravity, sugar, protein, microscopy, GRF (creatinine clearance), 24 hours urinary proteins, electrophoresis.
  2. *Blood counts* and *ESR.*
  3. *Serum biochemistry,* e.g. urea, creatinine electrolytes (Na^+, K^+), calcium and phosphorous, proteins, uric acid, etc.
  4. *Ultrasonography* for kidneys (usually small contracted kidneys) and bladder.
  5. *Special investigations,* e.g.
     - Pyelograms (nephrograms)
     - Protein electrophoresis
     - Complement levels
     - Autoantibody screening
     - Serum cryoglobulins
  6. *Kidney biopsy.*

Q. What is the management of CRF?

Ans: 1. Restriction of dietary proteins to 0.8 to 1 g/kg/day (No benefit of protein restriction claimed by randomised studies).
  2. Avoidance of smoking.
  3. Control of hypertension by ARBs or ACE inhibitors, dose adjusted to bring down the BP to ≤ 130/80 mm H_2.
  4. *Diuretics:* A thiazide or a loop diuretic added to control salt retention and control of BP. A beta blocker/calcium channel blocker may be added if target BP is not achieved.
  5. *Treatment of hyperlipidemia* with a statin if present.
  6. Treatment of anemia with diet, iron and folate supplements and recombinant erythropoietin to achieve the target harmogobin of 10–11 g/L.
  7. Phosphate binder (antacids) may be added to the therapeutic regimen to bring down phosphate levels.
  8. Calcitriol (vit D active analogue) to combat hypocalcaemia and secondary hyperparathyroidism.
  9. Acidosis if severe may be treated with bicarbonate.
  10. Dialysis.

Q. What are the indications of dialysis?

Ans: 1. Hyperkalemia.
  2. Severe acidosis.
  3. Raised blood urea (>100 mg%) with uremic symptoms and serum creatinine >3 mg%.
  4. Fluid overload unresponsive to diuretics.
  5. According to the Kidney Disease Outcomes Quality Initiative (KDOQI) guidelines, dialysis initiation should be considered when GFR is 10 ml/min or serum creatinine is 8 mg/dl in nondiabetic patients or GFR <15 ml/min or serum creatinine is 6 mg/dl in diabetic patients.
  6. Uremic pericarditis.

Q. What is renal replacement therapy?

Ans: I. *Temporary:* Dialysis (hemodialysis, peritoneal dialysis, hemofiltration).
  II. *Permanent:* Renal transplantation.

Q. What are the complications of hemodialysis?

Ans:
  - Hypotension, if excess fluid has been removed
  - Anaphylactic reactions to ethylene oxide which is used to sterilise the dialyser
  - Bleeding
  - Hard-water syndrome
  - Hemolytic reactions, muscle cramps
  - Air-embolism
  - Dialysis disequilibrium syndrome
  - Transmission of infection

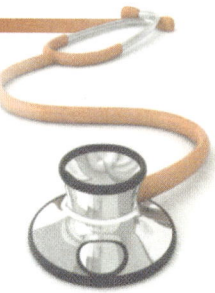

173

Anemia

INSTRUCTION

- Perform general physical examination

SALIENT FEATURES

- Generalised pallor, dyspnoea on exertion

HISTORY

Ask about the following:

- History of blood loss from any source, e.g. hematemesis, malena, hemoptysis, injury, bleeding piles or per recum
- Menstrual history of excessive blood loss
- Postpartum blood loss
- Surgery (gastrectomy)
- Loose motions malabsorption, parasitic infestation
- Nutritional history, e.g. poor diet, alcoholics, elderly patients
- Drug history, e.g. NSAIDs, phenytoin, chloramphenicol
- Associated symptoms, e.g. fatigue, dyspnea on exertion, generalised pallor, weakness and weight loss
- Family history (hemolytic anemia)
- History of hematuria (adult polycystic kidney disease)

EXAMINATION

General Physical Examination

- The patient has generalised pallor (Fig. 173.1B). Conjunctiva and tongue are pale (present)
- Look for koilonychia (present) or platynychia (iron deficiency), clubbing of the fingers (bacterial endocarditis)
- See the tongue for glossitis (magenta colored tongue) baldness [iron deficiency and angular stomatitis (vitamin B complex deficiency). Tongue is pale in anemia
- Examine mouth for ulcers, bleeding gums and angular stomatitis (malnutrition)

- Look for lymphadenopathy at different sites, e.g. neck, axillae, groin, etc.
- Skin for purpura, bruising (aplastic anemia)
- Look for jaundice (hemolytic anemia)
- Legs for ulcers in hemoglobinopathies

Relevant Systemic Examination

- *Examine the abdomen* for hepatomegaly and splenomegaly or any other mass
- *CVS* for murmurs, cardiomegaly, CHF, bacterial endocarditis

PROVISIONAL DIAGNOSIS

Patient has generalised pallor with koilonychia indicating anemia (lesion) due to iron deficiency (aetiology). Patient is symptomatic due to low hemoglobin (functional status).

QUESTIONS AND ANSWERS

Q. What do you understand by the term anemia?
Ans: A haemoglobin of ≤ 11.0 g% in an adult female and < 12.0 g% in an adult male is called anemia.

Q. What are the common causes of anemia?
Ans: 1. *Nutritional* (poor intake with increased demands or nutrient loss)
- Poor diet
- Chronic diarrhea
- Pregnancy, lactation
- Hook worm infestation
2. *Bleeding from different sites*, e.g.
- Hematemesis (peptic ulcer, gastritis, gastric cancer, cirrhosis)
- Piles or bleeding per rectum
- Bleeding from gums (thrombocytopenia, leukemia)
- Hematuria (glomerulonephritis, adult polycystic kidneys)

3. *Excessive blood destruction (hemolysis)*
   - Malaria
   - Drug induced in G6PD deficiency
4. *Anemia of bone marrow suppression*
   - Aplastic anemia
5. *Anemia of chronic illness and malignancy*
   - Rheumatoid arthritis, SLE, tuberculosis, uremia, endocranial diseases
   - Malignancies, leukemia, lymphoma

Q.   What are the sites where anemia should be seen?

Ans: Sites to be looked for anemia:
   - Conjunctiva
   - Oral mucosa and tongue (under surface)
   - Soft palate
   - Nails
   - Creases of the palm
   - Inner aspect of lips
   - Skin

Q.   How would you classify anemia?

Ans: Based on red cell size, haemoglobin content and red cell indices, anemias are classified into 4 types:
   1. *Microcytic hypochromic:* MCV, MCH, MCHC all are reduced. Examples include iron deficiency anemia, sideroblastic anemia, thalassemia, etc.
   2. *Normocytic normochromic:* MCV, MCH, MCHC are normal. Examples include anemia of blood loss, hemolytic anemia, aplastic anemia, etc.

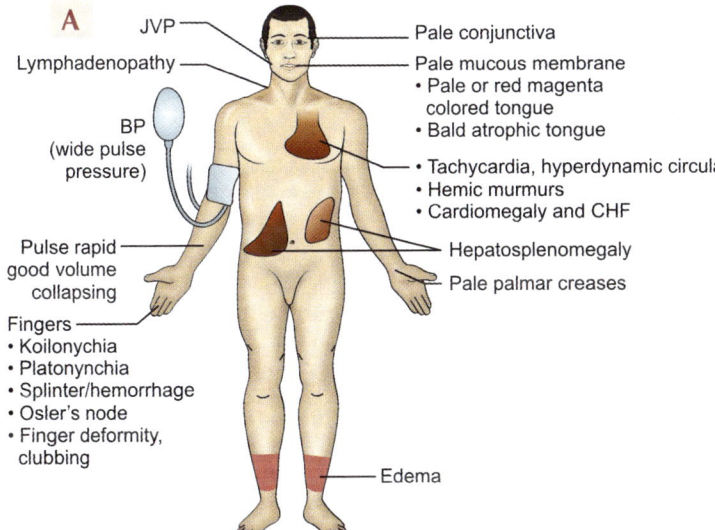

A
JVP — Pale conjunctiva
Lymphadenopathy — Pale mucous membrane
• Pale or red magenta colored tongue
• Bald atrophic tongue
BP (wide pulse pressure)
• Tachycardia, hyperdynamic circulation
• Hemic murmurs
• Cardiomegaly and CHF
Pulse rapid good volume collapsing
Hepatosplenomegaly
Pale palmar creases
Fingers
• Koilonychia
• Platonynchia
• Splinter/hemorrhage
• Osler's node
• Finger deformity, clubbing
Edema

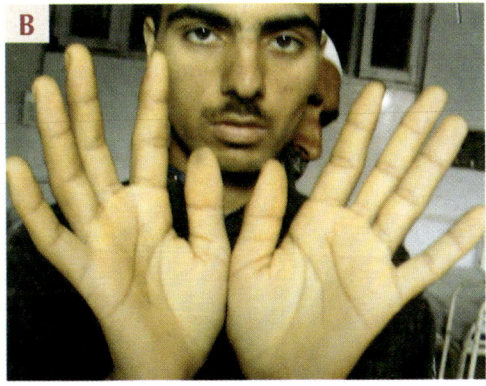

B

Fig. 173.1: Anemia. (A) Clinical manifestations; (B) Pallor of hands, palmar creases, lips and even face in a patient with anemia

3. *Macrocytic:* MCV is raised. Examples include macrocytic and megaloblastic anemia (folate, vitamin B_{12} deficiency), myelodysplasia, hypothyroidism, liver disease, etc.

4. *Dimorphic:* When two populations of red cells (microcytes as well as macrocytes) are seen on peripheral blood examination, anemia is said to be dimorphic due to combined deficiency of iron as well as folic acid/vit B_{12}.

Q. What are the symptoms and signs of anemia?

Ans: Read Fig. 173.1A.

Q. How would you classify anemia physiologically?

Ans: Physiological basis of evaluation of anemia is depicted in Fig. 173.2.

Q. What is reticulocyte production index? How is it calculated? What is its significance?

Ans: Reticulocyte production index indicates bone marrow response to anemia.

Reticulocyte production index is calculated in two steps:

a. First reticulocyte count is corrected for degree of anemia. For example, if Hb is 7.5 g of the patient against 15 g of normal, and reticuloyte count is 9%, then corrected reticulocyte count will be

$$= 9 \times 7.5 \div 15 = 4.5$$

b. Now corrected reticulocyte count is corrected for maturation time depending on hematocrit. Thus for hematocrit correction, the factor of 1 to 3 is applied (generally factor 2 is applied). Thus reticulocyte production index of above patient will be; corrected reticulocyte divided by PCV of the patient against normal (or factor of 2). Suppose PCV is 23% against 45% then divide corrected reticulocyte count by 2, hence index will be

$$4.5 \div 2 = 2.25$$

Clinical significance of this classification is that it separates hemolytic/hemorrhagic group (reticulocyte production index ≥ 2.5) from hypoproliferative/maturation defect group (reticulocyte production count ≤ 2.5).

Q. What are the signs of iron deficiency anemia?

Ans: • Pallor
• Glossitis (bald atrophic tongue)
• Angular stomatitis

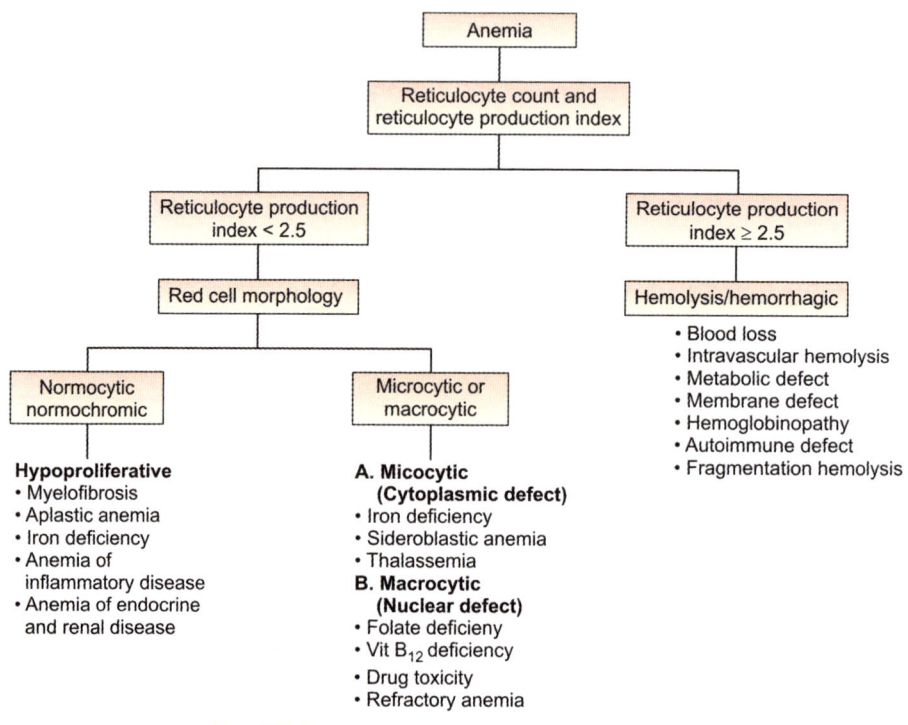

Fig. 173.2: The physiologic classification of anemia

- Cheilosis
- Koilonychia
- Mild splenomegaly
- History of pica (eating of strange items, earth, coal)
- Dysphagia (Plummer-Vinson syndrome)

Q. What is Plummer-Vinson (Paterson-Kelly) syndrome?

Ans: It consists of koilonychia (spoon shaped depressed nails), iron deficiency anemia (bald atrophic tongue) and dysphagia due to oesophageal webs. This is seen in middle aged females and considered as a premalignant condition.

Q. What are the diagnostic clues to hookworm anemia?

Ans: 1. Occupation (common in farmers, gardeners, etc.)
2. History of walking with bare feet
3. Ground itch in interdigital areas
4. Pain abdomen and diarrhea
5. Prevalence of hookworm disease in that area

Q. How does hookworm cause anemia?

Ans: 1. By consuming the nutrients
2. By bleeding from the intestines
3. By diarrhea or malabsorption

Q. How would you investigate a case of anemia?

Ans: Investigations done are:
1. Hemoglobin and RBC count.
2. Stool examination for hookworm ova.
3. Peripheral blood film for type of anemia, shape of RBCs, malarial parasite and any other abnormal cells. Reticulocyte count and reticulocyte production index can be calculated.
4. Bone marrow examination. It provides cellularity, stages of developing RBCs, assessment of iron stores, presence of marrow infiltration by parasites, fungi and secondary carcinoma.
5. Specific tests depending on the type of anemia.

Q. How would you investigate microcytic anemia?

Ans: • Peripheral blood film
- Serum iron is low (normal 50–150 mg/dl)
- Iron binding capacity is raised (normal 300–360 mg/dl)
- Serum ferritin low (normal about 100 µg/dl in males and about 30 µg/dl in females)
- Transferrin saturation low (normal 25 – 50%)
- Stool for occult blood
- Upper GI endoscopy
- Colonoscopy, barium studies
- Prothrombin time and INR
- Hemoglobin for electrophoresis
- Bone marrow for iron stores and reticulocyte index (low)

Q. How would you investigate macrocytic anemia?

Ans: • Peripheral blood smear
- Plasma LDH markedly elevated
- Serum iron elevated
- Serum ferritin elevated
- Serum bilirubin—unconjugated hyperbilirubinemia
- Antiparietal cell antibodies and an abnormal vit. B_{12} absorption studies (Schilling test) may be done in vit B_{12} deficiency anemia or pernicious anemia
- Serum folate levels/Red cell folate levels may be low
- Upper GI endoscopy
- Bone marrow examination

Q. How would you investigate hemolytic anemia?

Ans: • PBF for morphology of the RBCs (spherocytes, ovalocytes, elliptocytes, sickle cells) and for malarial parasite
- Hemoglobin electrophoresis for thalassemia (HbF > 2%)
- Coombs' test (direct and indirect)—may be abnormal
- Osmotic fragility test may be positive
- Serum bilirubin shows unconjugated hyperbilirubinemia
- Red cell survival studies may reveal decreased survival
- Sickling test is positive in sickle cell anemia

Q. What are the causes of refractory anemia?

Ans: The anemia that does not respond to appropriate treatment given for optimal period is called *refractory anemia*. The causes are:
- Aplastic anemia
- Thalassemia
- Sideroblastic anemia (pyridoxine responsive)
- Refractory anemia due to myelodysplastic syndrome
- Anemia due to leukemia, e.g. erythroleukemia or aleukemic leukemia

174

Sickle Cell Anemia

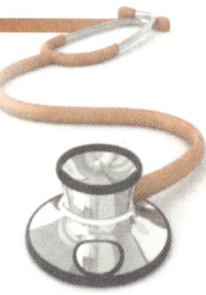

INSTRUCTION

- Perform general physical and relevant systemic examination

SALIENT FEATURES

- Recurrent abdominal and chest pain and anemia

HISTORY

Ask for the following:

- History of recurrent painful crises involving connective tissue and muscles (e.g. chest pain (present), back pain, bone pain) and viscera (hematuria)
- History of recurrent abdominal pain (present in this case)
- Priaprism (painful erection of penis)
- Provocation of vaso-occlusive (microinfarct) episodes by dehydration, infection, cold, acidosis and hypoxia
- History of repeated infections, e.g. pneumonia
- Past history of stroke
- Family history of such episodes
- Painful infarcts of digits and dactylitis

EXAMINATION

General Physical Examination

- Look for anaemia
- Fundus for hemorrhage, retinal detachment and neovascularisation
- Look at the digits for microinfarcts (present) and tender pulp of fingers and toes (Hand-foot syndrome)
- Examine the legs for chronic leg ulcers
- Priapism (due to penile infarction)

Systemic examination

- *Abdominal-examination* for tenderness and splenomegaly (present in this case).
- *Examine CVS* for cardiomegaly and hyperdynamic circulation
- *Examine chest* for pulmonary hypertension and cor pulmonale

PROVISIONAL DIAGNOSIS

Patient has old digital infarcts (lesion) due to sickle cell anemia (aetiology). Patient has severe difficulty in using the hands in performing routine daily activities (functional status).

QUESTIONS AND ANSWERS

Q. **What are the points in favor of your diagnosis?**

Ans: 1. History of intermittent pain episodes precipitated by the infection, dehydration, cold, etc.
2. Anemia (hemolytic)
3. Splenomegaly, hepatomegaly (due to hemolytic anemia)
4. Retinopathy (neovascularisation, retinal detachment)
5. Recurrent chest pain (pulmonary infarcts)

Q. **What is abnormality of hemoglobin in this patient?**

Ans: This patient has hemoglobinopathy in which there is structural abnormality of hemoglobin chain, i.e. HbS is present.

Q. **What are the characteristics of HbS?**

Ans: The HbS being abnormal, polymerises on deoxygenation leading to sickling shapes of RBCs results in short span of RBCs hemolysis and obstruction to microcirculation leading to small vessels infarct.

Q. **Is splenomegaly a feature of sickle cell anemia?**

Ans: The splenomegaly is seen in children and adolescents with sickle cell anemia due to hemolytic anemia. Later on these patients have hyposplenia (autosplenectomy) due to repeated splenic infarcts.

Q. **What is genetic basis of this disease?**

Ans: The sickle cell anemia occurs in homozygous state when both genes (both parents) are abnormal (HbSS).

The sickle cell trait occurs in heterozygous state where only one gene (parent) is abnormal (HbAS).

Q. **What are the complications of this condition?**

Ans: 1. Priaprism
2. Chronic leg ulcers
3. Pigmentary gall stones due to repeated hemolytic episodes
4. Renal failure (repeated renal infarction)
5. Aseptic necrosis of the hip (femoral heads)
6. Repeated pulmonary infections, e.g. pneumonia, acute chest syndrome
7. Pulmonary infarcts, pulmonary hypertension and chronic cor pulmonale

Q. **What is sickle cell trait?**

Ans: It occurs when an individual inherits one gene from a parent. It is a mild disease and person leads a normal life.

However, problem may arise when they undergo surgery or go to high altitudes; sickling may occur under these conditions and pain crises or infarction can be precipitated.

Q. **Is sickle cell trait protective against malaria?**

Ans: Yes, HbAS protects against Falciparum malaria.

Q. **What are the effects of sickling of RBCs?**

Ans: 1. Sickling increases blood viscosity.
2. Sickled cells tend to adhere to or entangle each other and obstruct the blood flow completely or incompletely.
3. Sickling predisposes to thrombosis and infarction resulting in pain crises.
4. Sickling reduces the life span of RBCs and predisposes them to hemolysis.

Q. **What happens to the level of hemoglobin during sickle cell crisis?**

Ans: The hemoglobin during sickle cell crisis remains in steady state and stable. It does not fall unless or until there is bone marrow aplasia produced by *parvovirus infection* or *hemolysis* induced by drugs or there is mass scale sequestration of RBCs in liver and spleen.

Q. **How would you investigate this patient?**

Ans: 1. Complete hemogram, blood counts and reticulocyte count.
2. Peripheral blood film for sickle cell (Fig. 174.1), Howell-Jolly bodies, target cells (hyposplenemia).

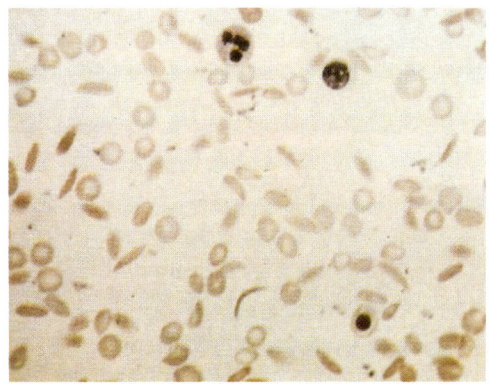

Fig. 174.1: Sickle cell anemia (blood film): Sickle cells and target cells with nucleated red cells are present indicating homozygous state (HbSS)

3. *Sickling test:* Sickling of RBCs can be produced by a reducing substance (sodium metabisulphite) in sickle cell anemia (HbSS), but not in sickle cell train (HbAS).
4. Hemoglobin electrophoresis shows no HbA, 80–95% HbSS and 2–20% HbF.
5. Family study to differentiate whether patient is homozygous or heterozygous for sickle cell disease.

Q. **How would you manage it?**

Ans: Management of sickle cell anemia includes:
1. *Anemia* is treated by folic acid supplementation.
2. *Treatment and prevention of precipitating factors*, e.g. infection by antibiotics, dehydration (fluid therapy). Chilling should be avoided.
3. Treatment of *pain crisis by analgesics*.
4. *Blood transfusions:* Most of these patients being in steady state do not require blood transfusions. It is indicated only when the anemia is severe or frequent episodes of crisis are occurring particularly during pregnancy.
5. *Exchange transfusion* is used for intractable pain crisis, priapism and stroke.
6. *Hydroxyurea and erythropoietin* are given to increase the synthesis of HbF which reduces sickling and pain crisis.
7. *Bone marrow transplantation*.
8. *Counseling* regarding psychosocial problems, drug therapy and birth control.

Pregnant woman with sickle cell trait should have their partner tested as there is risk of severe hemoglobin defect if both the parents are affected.

175

Hemophilia

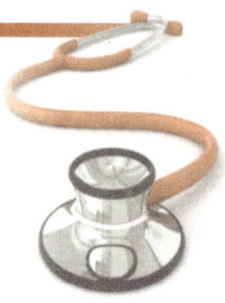

INSTRUCTION

• Examine the patient musculoskeletal system

SALIENT FEATURES

• Swollen right knee following mild trauma

HISTORY

Ask for the following:

• History of bleeding into the joints, bruising and purpura, bleeding from mucous membranes
• Family history of bleeding disorder (X-linked recessive) present in this case
• History of swelling (hematoma) after intra-muscular injection or minor trauma (present)
• Hematuria
• History of recurrent pain abdomen
• History of continuous bleeding after trauma (present)/or dental procedure
• History of headache, TIAs (intracranial bleed)
• No history of spontaneous bleeding

EXAMINATION

Examination of Musculoskeletal System

• A male patient
• There is swelling of right knee with fixed equinus deformity of right leg (Fig. 175.1)
• There is no muscular hematoma or bruishing
• There is no compression of femoral nerve

PROVISIONAL DIAGNOSIS

The young adolescent male has swollen right knee with fixed deformity of the right leg [lesion Fig. 175.1)] caused by hemophilia A (aetiology). The patient is handicapped due to deformity.

QUESTIONS AND ANSWERS

Q. What do you mean by the term hemophilia A?
Ans: It is an inherited disorder of factor VIII deficiency. It is inherited as X-linked recessive trait, manifests clinically as coagulation disorder in males, while females act as carriers.

Q. What is the inheritance of hemophilia A?
Ans: It is a sex-linked disorder. All daughters of hemophilic males are carriers and sons are normal. If the female carrier has a son, he has 50% chances of having hemophilia and a daughter will have 50% chances of being carrier. Hemophilia breeds true within a family, i.e. all the members will have same abnormality of the gene and severity of the disease.

Q. What is basic defect in hemophilia? How does hemophilia manifest clinically?
Ans: It is a disorder of coagulation due to defici-ency of factor VIII. It manifests clinically depending on the concentration of factor, i.e.

1. *Severe deficiency* (factor VIII < 1%) mani-fests spontaneous bleeding into the joints and muscles.

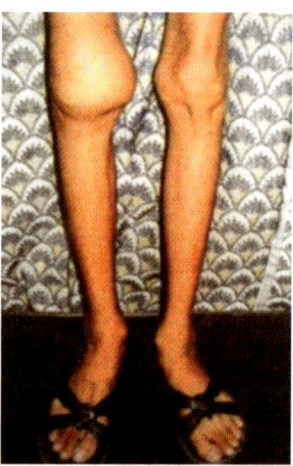

Fig. 175.1: Hemophilia (there is hemarthrosis of right knee joint)

2. *Moderate deficiency* (factor VIII 1–5%) manifests clinically as episodes of bleeding following minor trauma or surgery.
3. Mild deficiency (factor VIII 5–50%) manifests as bleeding episode after severe trauma or major surgery.

Q. What are the differences between bleeding and coagulation disorder?

Ans: Read Table 175.1.

Table 175.1: Distinguishing features between bleeding and coagulation disorder

Feature	Bleeding disorder (Thrombocytopenia)	Coagulation disorder (Hemophilia A)
1. Petechiae and ecchymosis	Characteristic	Rare
2. Deep dissecting muscle hematoma	Rare	Characteristic
3. Superficial ecchymo, sis, bruising	Small, multiple	Large solitary
4. Site of bleeding	Into skin, mucous membrane, nose	Joints, muscles and retroperitoneal space
5. Hemarthrosis	Rare	Characteristic
6. Onset of bleeding	Immediate	Delayed
7. Bleeding from superficial cuts and scratches	Profuse	Minimal
8. Sex of the patient	Mostly males	Mostly females
9. Positive family history	Rare	Common
10. Measure to stop bleeding	Local measures	Systemic therapy

Q. How would you treat an episode of bleeding?

Ans: 1. If bleeding is minor or follow dental extraction/procedure, factor VIII concentrate may be given to raise its concentration 20–30% of normal.
2. *For severe bleeding*, factor VIII should be raised to 50% of normal.
3. *For major surgery*, or life threatening bleeding factor VIII should be raised to 100% for 1–2 weeks then maintained at least 50% of the normal until wound healing.
4. Desmopressin can also raise factor VIII level when given I.V. It is useful for minor bleeding depending on the initial factor VIII level.

Q. What are the complications of hemophilia?

Ans: 1. Recurrent hemarthrosis leads to crippling deformity.
2. Severe intracranial bleed.
3. Sudden death due to internal hemorrhage and shock.

Q. What are the complications of factor VIII therapy?

Ans: Factor VIII infusion is associated with transfusion associated diseases such as:
1. Hepatitis B, C and delta infection.
2. AIDS and its related diseases and syndromes.
3. Development of factor VIII inhibitors (antibodies) which neutralise factor VIII activity and prevent effect of therapy.

Q. What are the potential risks of blood transfusions?

Ans: 1. Transmission of infections, e.g. HIV, hepatitis B, C and malaria
2. Transfusion iron overload (hemosiderosis)
3. Transfusion related complications, e.g. hemolytic reactions, thrombocytopenia, etc.

176

Leukemia

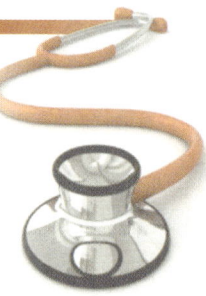

INSTRUCTION

- Examine the abdomen of this patient

SALIENT FEATURES

- A mass abdomen

HISTORY

Ask about the following:

- Age of the patient
- History of a lump or a mass (present)
- History of dragging pain (present)
- History of bleeding/bruising
- Breathlessness on exertion, palpitation, headache, weakness due to anemia (present)
- Generalised pallor (present)
- Fever, night sweat, weight loss (present)

EXAMINATION

General Physical Examination

- Age of the patient (CML is common). Men in age groups of 20–40 yrs
- Anemia is present
- Skin for ecchymosis/bruises
- No bleeding from the gums

Abdominal Examination

- Hepatosplenomegaly present
- Sternal tenderness may/may not be present (present in this case)
- No lymphadenopathy

PROVISIONAL DIAGNOSIS

The middle aged male has slow onset of anemia with hepatosplenomegaly (lesion) due to chronic myeloid leukemia (etiology). He is incapacitated by severe anemia (functional status).

QUESTIONS AND ANSWERS

Q. What are the points in favor of your diagnosis?

Ans: 1. Middle age male
2. Slow onset of anemia

3. History of fever, night sweats, weight loss, lassitude
4. Bone pains/sternal tenderness
5. Massive splenomegaly (> 8 cm) and mild to moderate hepatomegaly

Q. **What is Philadelphia chromosome (Ph[1] chromosome)? What is its significance?**

Ans: Philadelphia chromosome (Fig. 176.2) is an chromosomal abnormality that occurs in CML. Philadelphia chromosome is a reciprocal translocation between the long arm of chromosome 9 and 22. A large portion of 22 q is translocated to 9 q and a smaller portion of 9 q moves to 22 q. The portion of 9 q that is translocated contains abl, a protooncogene that is cellular homolog of Abelson murine leukemia virus. This abl gene is received at specific site on chromosome 22 called *bcr region* (*break point cluster region*). The fusion gene *bcr/abl* gene possesses tyrosine kinase activity, hence, is pathogenic to cause the disease.

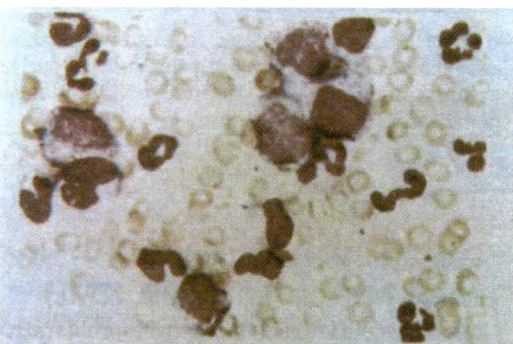

Fig. 176.1: Chronic Myeloid Leukemia (CML). Chronic myeloid (granulocytic) leukemia. Note the increased number of granulocytes and their precursors in the peripheral blood. The majority of granulocytes are segmented or present in band forms. Myelocytes, promyelocytes and myeloblasts are not seen in this plate

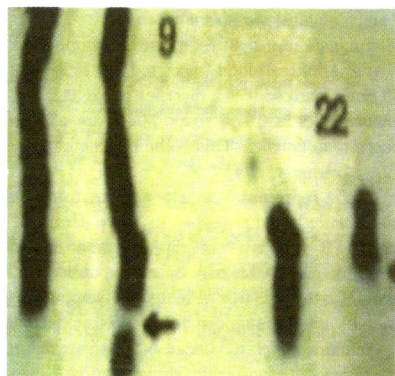

Fig. 176.2: Philadelphia chromosome (Ph[1] chromosome). This chromosome is positive in 90% cases of CML

The patients with Philadelphia chromosome respond better to treatment and have good median survival.

Q.   What is the cause of anemia in CML?

Ans: The enchroachment of erythropoietic tissue by the proliferative myeloid tissue in the bone marrow leads to anemia.

Q.   What is the cause of hepatosplenomegaly in CML?

Ans: Myeloid mtaplasia is the cause.

Q.   What is myeloid metaplasia and myelofibrosis?

Ans: *Myeloid metaplasia* means the hematopoiesis occurring outside the bone marrow due to loss of bone marrow activity. It may be of unknown origin called *agnogenic meyloid metaplasia* or may be secondary to myelofibrosis.

   Myelofibrosis means loss of marrow elements due to fibrosis which may be primary or secondary.

Q.   What are the complications of CML?

Ans: 1. Myelofibrosis with pancytopenia
2. Acute blastic transformation (acute blastic crisis)

3. Hyperuricemia
4. Rupture of massive spleen
5. Repeated infections and fatal septicemia
6. Priaprism

Q.   How would you investigate this patient?

Ans: 1. Mean hemoglobin (low in CML)
2. WBC count will be high (in lacs)
3. Mean platelet count initially will be high, but falls to low levels (thrombocytopenia) as the disease progresses
4. Blood film (Fig. 176.1) may shows more than 30% immature cells (myelocytes, promyelocytes, myeloblasts, metamyelocytes). Myeloblasts are less than 10.5%
5. Bone marrow is hypercellular. Myeloblasts constitute <5%.
   Cytogenetic studies show presence of Ph[1] in 90% cases. DNA probe can confirm the presence of *abelson BCR* gene
6. PCR can detect *bcr/abl gene* in peripheral blood film

Other investigations

- Neutrophil alkaline phosphatase is raised
- Vitamin B_{12} levels are high
- Blood LDH levels are elevated

Q.   How would you treat CML?

Ans: The drug of choice is imatinib mesylate, a tyrosine kinase inhibitor of bcr/abl fusion gene. It is well tolerated and results in universal (98%) hematological control of chronic phase of CML. The standard dose is 400 mg/day. **Side effects** include, edema, rash and myalgia. The drug is given to achieve hematologic as well as cytogenetic remission (i.e. 3 log reduction in bcr/abl gene on PCR). Those patients who have good cytogenetic response have good prognosis.

   Allogeneic bone marrow transplantation was the only curative therapy before imatinib, but now it is reserved for those who either do not respond to it or who fail to respond after initial response or who have an accelerated phase of the disease (acute blastic crisis).

177

Purpura

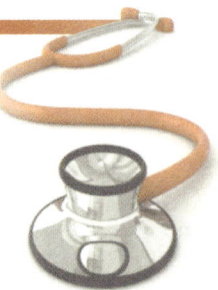

INSTRUCTION

- Perform general physical and relevant systemic examination

SALIENT FEATURES

- Bleeding spots over both legs and the body

HISTORY

Ask for the following:

- Age for senile purpura and allergic purpura (young age)
- Drugs, e.g. steroids, anticoagulants, phenyl-butazone, carbimazole, chloramphenicol, gold salts, etc. for drug-induced purpura
- History of chronic liver and renal disease
- History of joint pains, abdominal pains, etc. for Henoch-Schönlein purpura (present)
- History of mouth ulcers or necrotising mouth lesions, etc. for neutropenia or pancytopenia

EXAMINATION

General Physical Examination:

- *Mouth* examination for ulceration and infection (for pancytopenia)
- Signs or stigmata of *chronic liver disease* or *chronic renal failure*
- *Anemia* for marrow aplasia, leukemia and marrow infiltration
- *Signs/deformities of rheumatoid arthritis* and drugs-induced purpura
- *Symptoms/signs of scurvy*, e.g. bleeding gums, corkscrew hair, perifollicular hemorrhage
- *Cutis laxa* and *hyperextensibility* of the *joints* (Ehlers-Danlos syndrome)
- *Bleeding from punctured sites, e.g. for DIC*
- Examine the neck for lymph nodes

Abdominal Examination

- For spleen and liver enlargement

PROVISIONAL DIAGNOSIS

There are purpuric spots (Fig. 177.1), bruishes and echymoses (lesion) caused by a bleeding disorder (aetiology). Patient is upset with fresh episode of bleeding.

Q. Which bleeding disorder do you expect in this case and why?

Ans: Henoch-Schönlein purpura—an allergic purpura due to following reasons:
1. An adolescent male
2. Purpura occurring after an episode of sore throat
3. Well-circumscribed purpuric spots over the legs
4. History of polyarthritis and abdominal pain

Q. Which bed-side test would help you in the diagnosis?

Ans: Normal bleeding and clotting time.

Q. What are the other differential conditions?

Ans: 1. Thrombasthenia
2. von Willebrand's disease
3. Thrombocytopenia

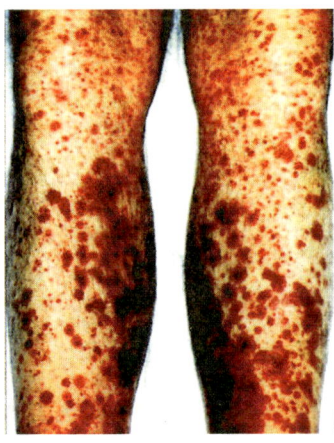

Fig. 177.1: Purpura (Anaphylactoid)

4. Spotted fever
5. Meningococcemia
6. Vasculitis

QUESTIONS AND ANSWERS

Q. **What is Henoch-Schönlein purpura (ana-phylactoid purpura)?**

Ans: It is self-limiting type of vasculitis, occurs in children and young adults, characterized by purpuric spots or urticarial rash on the extensor surfaces of the arms and legs, polyarthralgia or arthritis, abdominal colic and hematuria (focal glomerulonephritis). The syndrome follows an episode of URI or *Streptococcus pharyngitis*. All the coagulation tests are normal despite purpura. Bleeding time is normal.

Q. **What is purpura? How does it differ from petechiae and ecchymosis? What is its characteristic feature?**

Ans: *Purpura* is defined as hemorrhagic spots of pin-head size, occurs due to extravasation of blood (RBCs) into the dermis.

Petechiae are smaller hemorrhagic spots (≤ 2 mm) while purpuric spots are larger (≥3 mm). The *echymosis or bruises* are still larger purpuric spots/lesions.

The *characteristic feature* of purpuric spots is that they do not blanch with pressure by a pin head or glass slide. This feature differentiates it from vasculitis produced by vasodilatation that blanches with pressure. The *telangiectasia, mosquito bite marks, spider nevi* blanch on pressure, hence, can easily be differentiated.

Q. **What are the common causes of purpura?**

Ans: • Thrombocytopenia due to any cause
• Vascular purpura, e.g. scurvy, connective tissue diseases, amyloidosis
• DIC, thrombotic thrombocytopenic purpura
• Anticoagulants
• Steroids (Cushing's syndrome, steroid induced purpura)
• Renal and liver disease

Q. **What are the causes of palpable purpura?**

Ans: i. *Vasculitis*
• Allergic purpura (Henoch-Schönlein)
• PAN (polyarteritis nodosa)
ii. *Infections/emboli*
• Meningococcemia
• Disseminated gonococcal infection
• Rocky Mountain spotted fever
• Ecthyma gangrenosum

Q. **What are the causes of non-thrombocyto-penic purpura?**

Ans: Causes are as follows:
• *Infections*, e.g. meningococcal, gonococcal, rickettsial and viral
• Allergic purpura (*Henoch-Schönlein*)
• Hereditary telangiectasia
• Drug-induced (thiazides sulphonamides, phenylbutazone, sulphonylureas, barbiturates, steroids)
• Senile purpura, Vasculitis, Uremia
• Purpura simplex (Devil's pinches)
• Steroid-induced (Cushing's syndrome)
• Paraproteinemia

Q. **How will you investigate a case with purpura?**

Ans: The **investigations** are as follows:
• *Hemoglobin* — may be low
• *Urine* for hematuria, proteinuria
• *Platelet count* — low in thrombocytopenic purpura, normal in non-thrombocytopenic purpura
• *Bleeding time* is prolonged. Clotting time is normal *PTTK and PT* (prothrombin time) are normal
• *Antiplatelets antibodies.* They are present in immune thrombocytopenic purpura
• *Serological tests for hepatitis*, cytomegalovirus, Epstein-Barr virus and HIV
• *Bone marrow examination.* It should be done when platelet count is >50,000/μl and there is no bleeding
• *Antinuclear antibodies* (ANAs) for SLE
• *Radiolabelled platelets* and their destruction in the spleen will confirm hypersplenism

Q. **What are the causes of splenomegaly with purpura?**

Ans: Following are the causes:
1. *Lymphoreticular malignancy*, e.g. leukemia and lymphoma, acute blastic crisis of CML and CLL
2. *Infections*, e.g. subacute infective endocarditis septicemia
3. *Connective tissue disorders*, e.g. SLE
4. *Myelofibrosis*
5. *Hypersplenism*

Q. **What is thrombotic thrombocytopenic purpura (Moschcowitz's syndrome)?**

Ans: Thrombotic thrombocytopenic purpura is an acute disorder characterized by thrombocytopenic purpura, microangiopathic hemolytic anemia, transient or fluctuating neurological features, fever and renal involvement (read Emergency Medicine by Prof SN Chugh).

178

Thrombocytopenia

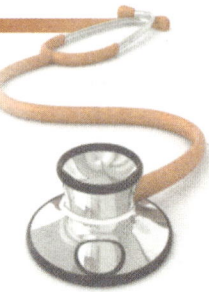

INSTRUCTION

- Perform general physical examination

SALIENT FEATURES

- Bleeding spots over the legs

HISTORY

Ask the following:

- Age and sex (adult females in child bearing age involved)
- History of viral infection or fever or upper respiratory infection
- History of epistaxis, menorrhagia (present)
- History of other autoimmune diseases, e.g. SLE, Hashimoto's thyroiditis, autoimmune hemolytic anemia, etc.
- History of relapses and remissions (present in this case)

EXAMINATION

General Physical Examination

- Pin-head sized purpuric spots in front of both the legs (Fig. 178.1)
- There is a large ecchymotic patch in front of the left leg (present, Fig. 178.1)
- There may be nasal bleeding (epistaxis present)
- No joint bleeding or hematoma

PROVISIONAL DIAGNOSIS

The young female has bleeding into the skin and from nose (lesion) caused by idiopathic thrombocytopenic purpura (aetiology). Patient is distressed by repeated episodes.

QUESTIONS AND ANSWERS

Q. **What are the points in favor of your diagnosis?**

Ans: • A young female (24 years)

- Pin-head sized purpuric spots and an ecchymotic patch over the leg (s)
- Replapses and remissions
- Spleen is not palpable

Q. **What will be your differential diagnosis?**

Ans: All the conditions causing thrombocytopenia listed below will constitute the differential diagnosis.

Q. **What are the common causes of thrombocytopenia?**

Ans: • ITP (Idiopathic thrombocytopenic purpura)
- SLE
- Hypoplasia of marrow/myelofibrosis
- Drug-induced
- Thrombotic thrombocytopenic purpura
- DIC
- Infections, e.g. dengue hemorrhagic fever

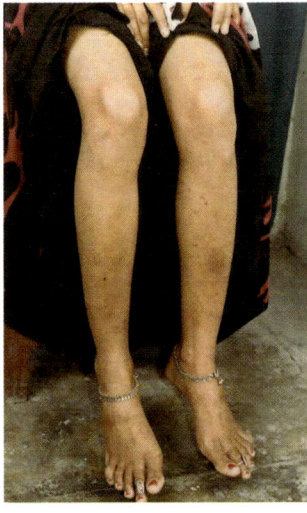

Fig. 178.1: Thrombocytopenia. There are bleeding spots and ecchymotic patches in front of legs in a patient with thrombocytopenia

Q. What is critical platelet count?

Ans: Critical platelet count means the lowest platelet count at which spontaneous bleeding into the skin, brain or internal organs may occur and may be fatal. The critical count is <20,000/µl. The count between 20,000/µl and 50,000/µl leads to bleeding only after minor trauma or stress.

Q. Name the drugs producing thrombocytopenic purpura.

Ans: I. *Drugs causing suppression of platelets production*
- Myelosuppressive drugs, e.g. cytosine arabinoside, daunorubicin, cyclophosphamide, busulfan, methotrexate, 6-MP, Vinca alkaloids
- Thiazide diuretics
- Ethanol (binge drinker)
- Estrogen

II. *Drugs and toxins producing immunological destruction of platelets*
- Antibiotics, e.g. sulphonamide, tetracyclines, novobiocin, PAS, rifampicin, chloramphenicol
- Cinchona alkaloids, e.g. quinine, quinidine
- Sedatives, hypnotic and anticonvulsants (carbamazepine)
- Digoxin, Alpha-methyldopa
- Anti-inflammatory, e.g. aspirin, phenylbutazone
- Chloroquine, gold salts, arsenicals
- Insecticides

Q. What is pathogenesis of ITP (Idiopathic thrombocytonic purpura)?

Ans: It is an autoimmune disorder of platelets. Autoantibodies are formed against the membrane glycoproteins IIb, IIIa leading to accelerated destruction and removal of platelets by mono-macrophage system with normal or increased megakaryocytes in the bone marrow.

Q. What are the clinical characteristics of ITP?

Ans: The three clinical characteristics are:

1. Bleeding is the characteristic feature of ITP which occurs at the following sites:
   - Skin, e.g. petechiae, purpura, ecchymosis
   - Mucous membrane and gum bleeding
   - Nasal bleeding (epistaxis)
   - Genitourinary tract bleeding (hematuria, menorrhagia)
   - Intracranial and intra-abdominal bleeding
2. Reduced platelet count
3. Hypercellular marrow with megakaryocytosis

Q. What is the treatment of ITP?

Ans: This is as follows:
- Specific therapy (platelet infusion) is not necessary unless platelet count is <20,000/ml. Analgesic (codeine and paracetamol) may be used for pain or fever.
- *Corticosteroids* are used to control bleeding in acute ITP. Oral prednisolone is given in dose of 40–60 mg/day for few weeks followed by tapering of the dose to maintenance dose of 5–10 mg/day.
- *IV immunoglobulin (IVIG)* is reserved for patients with severe thrombocytopenia and clinical bleeding who fail to respond to steroids and other measures.
- *Plasmapheresis means removal of immune complexes, is as useful as I.V immunoglobulin in ITP.*
- *Blood transfusions/platelets transfusion.*
- *Splenectomy:* It is indicated in patients with ITP who are resistant to other measures.
- *Immunosuppressive therapy:* Patients who remain thrombocytopenic after steroid therapy or splenectomy or who relapse within months to years after initial therapy are candidates for immunosuppression with azathioprine, cyclophosphamide or vincristine/vinblastine.

Q. What is dengue hemorrhagic fever? What is Hess capillary test?

Ans: Dengue hemorrhagic fever is characterised by all manifestations of classic dengue fever, thrombocytopenia (platelet count <1 lac/cumm), vascular instability and increased permeability and local hemorrhage (spontaneous petechiae and/or purpura) with positive tourniquet test called *Hess capillary test*. The hemorrhage in dengue is due to combined effect of vascular damage and thrombocytopenia.

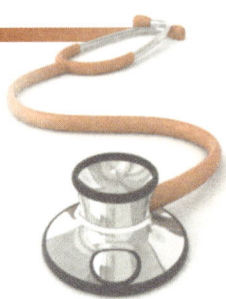

179 Disseminated Intravascular Coagulation (DIC)

INSTRUCTION

- Perform general physical examination

SALIENT FEATURES

- Sheets of bleeding over trunk and arms, and gum bleeding

HISTORY

Ask about the following:

- History of bleeding from nose, gums, urine, mucous membrane and into the skin
- History of bleeding from surgical incisions, venepuncture, catheter sites, etc.
- History of thrombosis or gangrenous toes/fingers
- History of fever (gram-negative septicemia, meningococcemia, malaria, viral)
- History of snake bite (present in this case)
- History of abruptio placentae, missed abortions/miscarriages, pre-eclampsia, pregnancy
- Trauma or surgery
- Malignancies
- Burns
- Puffiness of face, hypertension, oliguria (AGN or hemolytic uremia syndrome)

EXAMINATION

General Physical Examination

- There are fang marks of snake bite present (Fig. 179.1). Patient passed dark red urine
- There is bleeding from the gums
- There is sheets of hemorrhages into the skin over the limbs and trunk (Fig. 179.1)
- Pulse is fast. BP is normal

PROVISIONAL DIAGNOSIS

The patient had bleeding from more than two sites (gums, skin, urine) following snake bite (lesion), could be due to Disseminated Intravascular Coagulation (etiology). The patient is not in shock (functional status).

QUESTIONS AND ANSWERS

Q. What do you understand by the term Disseminated Intravascular Coagulation (DIC)?

Ans: It is an acquired bleeding disorder with thrombohemorrhagic manifestations. It is also called *defibrination syndrome* or *consumption coagulopathy*.

Q. What is its pathogenesis?

Ans: Endothelial damage due to any cause, for example, endotoxins produced in gram negative septicaemia activate platelets, leucocytes and factor XII leading to initiation and promotion of intravascular coagulation.

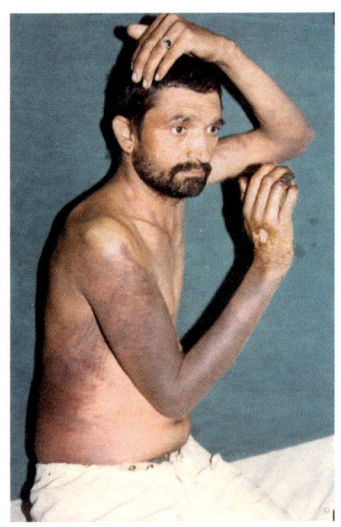

Fig. 179.1: DIC. A patient bitten by snake shows thrombotic (gangrene of right ring and little fingers) and the hemorrhagic manifestations (sheets of hemorrhage are seen over upper limb and trunk)

Similarly, thromboplastin released from the damaged tissues, placenta, fat embolus or trauma may activate the coagulation system. Once coagulation system is activated, it gets self propagated with consumption of platelets factor V, factor VIII and fibrinogen leading to their low levels resulting in defective hemostatic mechanism and hemorrhagic manifestations as a result of excess fibrin formation. As a protective mechanism, fibrinolytic system gets activated and causes breakdown of fibrin and formation of fibrinogen degradation products (FDP) which further promote bleeding by inhibiting fibrin polymerisation.

Q. **What are the common causes of DIC?**

Ans: 1. *Infections*
- Gram negative septicemia
- Meningococcal septicemia
- Certain viral infection
- Malaria (falciparum)
- Snake bites

2. *Liberation of tissue factor (thromboplastin)*
- Abruptio placentae
- Retained dead fetus
- Amniotic fluid embolism
- Pre-eclampsia
- Massive trauma, surgery
- Malignancies

3. *Widespread endothelial damage*
- Aortic aneurysm
- Hemolytic uremic syndrome
- Severe burns
- Acute glomerulonephritis

Q. **How do the patients with DIC present?**

Ans: The clinical presentation varies with the stage and severity of the disease. The patient is often acutely ill and is in shock. Majority of patients have skin (Fig. 179.1) and mucous membrane bleeding and hemorrhage from multiple sites, i.e. surgical incisions, venepuncture, catheter sites. Bleeding from more than two sites suggests DIC. Less often patients may have thrombosis and pregangrenous changes in digits, genitalia and nose. Thrombosis may involve any organ.

Q. **What are the laboratory parameters for DIC?**

Ans:
- Platelet count is low
- Blood film shows schistocytes and fragmented red cells
- Prothrombin time (PT)—prolonged
- Thrombin time—prolonged
- Activated Partial thromboplastin time (aPTT)—prolonged
- Plasma fibrinogen levels—low
- Fibrinogen degradation products (FDP)—raised. D-dimers are present

Q. **How does DIC differ from coagulation disorder?**

Ans:
- In DIC, there is consumption of the platelets leading to thrombocytopenia, hence, it is basically a bleeding disorder. In coagulation disorders, platelets are normal.
- In DIC, both thrombotic and hemorrhagic manifestations occur where there are no thrombotic manifestations in coagulation disorder.
- In DIC, bleeding occurs from the multiple site simultaneously which is not must for coagulation disorder.

Q. **How would you treat DIC?**

Ans: Treatment is aimed at treating the underlying cause for DIC and taking measures to control the major symptoms either bleeding or thrombosis. Aggressive antibiotic therapy is recommended for infection. Exacerbating factors such as acidosis, dehydration, hypoxia and renal failure should be corrected. Patients with bleeding should receive (i) fresh frozen plasma, red cell concentrate and cryoprecipitate to replace depleted clotting factors and (ii) platelet concentrates to correct thrombocytopenia.

The use of heparin is controversial. It is used in those patients who have thrombosis or those rare patients who continue to bleed despite vigorous treatment with plasma and platelets. Antithrombin and/or activated protein C concentrates have been found useful in selected cases. Antifibrinolytics (e.g. tranexamic acid) are contraindicated.

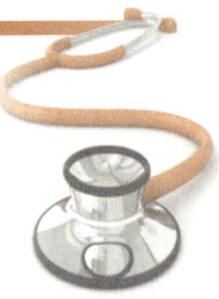

INSTRUCTION

- Examine abdomen of this patient

SALIENT FEATURES

- Recurrent jaundice with dark urine

HISTORY

Ask about the following:

- Age of the patient and onset of symptoms (childhood or young age)
- History of growth failure or delayed milestones
- History of recurrent jaundice with dark colored stool and urine (present)
- Bony deformities (frontal bossing present)
- History of repeated blood transfusions (present)
- History of congestive heart failure (dyspnea, orthopnea, PND, cardiomegaly)
- Positive family history
- Symptoms and signs of chronic anemia, headache, fatigue, malaise, palpitation, dyspnea on exertion

EXAMINATION

General Physical Examination

- Patient has frontal bossing and malor prominence (Fig. 180.1)
- Mild jaundice (present)
- Anemia (present)
- JVP is normal

Abdominal examination

- The liver is enlarged, nontender, soft (in this case)
- Spleen is also enlarged, soft, nontender, 5 cm below the costal margin (in this case)
- No other mass palpable

PROVISIONAL DIAGNOSIS

An adolescent female has anemia, jaundice and hepatosplenomegaly (lesion) caused by hemolytic jaundice due to thalassemia (etiology). The patient requires repeated blood transfusions (functional status).

QUESTIONS AND ANSWERS

Q. **What are the points in favor of your diagnosis?**
Ans:
- Onset of symptoms in young age
- Bony deformities, e.g. frontal bossing and malar prominences (Fig. 180.1B)
- Chronic severe anemia
- Repeated mild jaundice with dark colored urine and stool
- Moderate hepatosplenomegaly
- Positive family history
- Past history of blood transfusions

Q. **What is the type of anemia in beta-thalassemia?**
Ans: Microcytic hypochronic anemia.

Q. **What do you mean by thalassemia?**
Ans: The thalassemias are hereditary disorders characterised by reduction in the synthesis of globin chains (α and β) of hemoglobin. Reduced globin synthesis causes reduced hemoglobin synthesis and eventually produces hypochromic microcytic anemia because of defective hemoglobinisation of RBCs.

Q. **What are the various hemoglobins and their constituents?**
Ans:
1. Normal adult hemoglobin (98%) is HbA formed from tetramer of two α chains and two β chains ($\alpha_2 \beta_2$)
2. Hemoglobin A$_2$ (1–2% of adult hemoglobin) comprises of $\alpha_2 \delta_2$
3. Hemoglobin F (fetal hemoglobin) which comprises <1% of adult hemoglobin is formed by tetramer of $\alpha_2 \gamma_2$.

Q. **What are the various types of thalassemia?**
Ans: Two common types of thalassemias are:

I. The α-*thalassemia* seen commonly in persons from southeast Asia and China and less common in blacks. They have 4 copies of α-globin chain. When three alpha globin genes are present, patient is normal (silent carrier), when two α-globulin genes are present, patient is called α-thalassaemia trait (thalassemia minor). When one α-globin gene is present, the patient has hemoglobin H disease (chronic hemolytic anemia of variable severity between minor and intermedia). These patients are hematologically normal, do not require blood transfusions except during stresses or infection.

II. The *β-thalassemia* affects Italians, Greek, Asians and Blacks. Patient homozygous for β-thalassaemia have severe disease called *thalassemia major*, requires blood transfusions. They have growth failure, bony deformities, hemolytic jaundice and hepatosplenomegaly. Patients homozygous for β-thalassaemia can have intermediate disease, i.e. only chronic hemolytic anemia and do not require blood transfusions except during period of stress. They survive adult life with hepatosplenomegaly with bony deformities. Patients heterozygous for the disease have thalassaemia minor and have clinically insignificant microcytic anemia.

Q. What are the common causes of microcytic hypochromic anemia?

Ans: • Iron deficiency anemia

• Hookworm disease

• Thalassemias

• Sideroblastic anemias

• Anemia of chronic infection

Q. How would you investigate this case?

Ans: 1. Hemoglobin is low

2. Peripheral blood film shows marked poikilocytosis, hypochromia, microcytosis (Fig. 180.1A), target cells, basophil stippling and nucleated RBCs

3. Hemoglobin electrophoresis shows little or no HbA, variable amount of HbA$_2$ and major hemoglobin present is HbF in thalassemia major. In thalassemia minor, there is elevation of HbA$_2$ to 4–8% (normal 1–3%) and HbF to 1–5% (normal <1%)

4. Serum unconjugated bilirubin is raised

5. Red cell survival studies show decreased survival

6. Prenatal diagnosis can be made

Q. How would you treat it?

Ans: 1. Patients with mild disease do not require treatment.

2. Patient with hemoglobin H disease requires folic acid supplementation and avoidance of iron and oxidative drugs, e.g. sulphonamides.

3. Patients with severe thalassemias require repeated blood transfusions and folic acid supplementation.

4. Splenectomy is performed if hypersplenism is present.

5. Patients on regular blood transfusions therapy require iron chelation by subcutaneous deferroxamine or oral deferasirox.

6. Allogeneic bone marrow transplantation is the treatment of choice for thalassemia major.

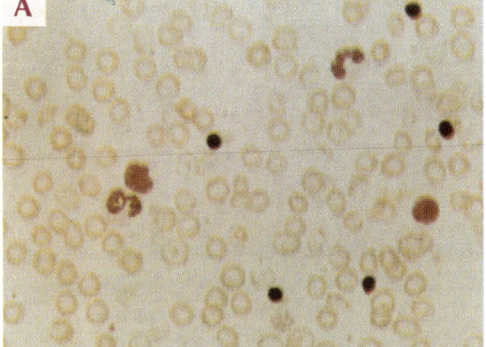
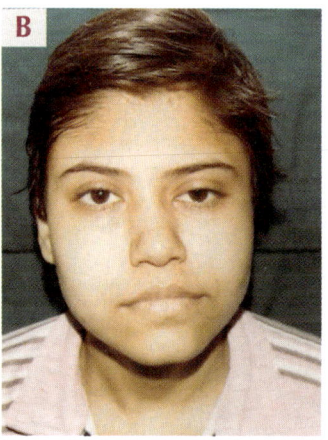

Fig. 180.1: (A) Thalassemia minor (peripheral blood film). There is microcytic hypochromic anemia with target cells, nucleated red blood cells; (B) A patient with thalassemia minor showing pallor due to chronic moderate anemia

181

Rheumatoid Arthritis (RA)

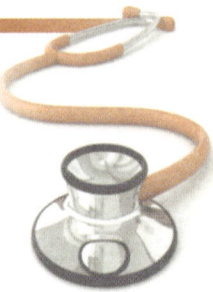

INSTRUCTION

Examine the musculoskeletal of system

SALIENT FEATURES

- Small joints polyarthritis and deformities of hands

HISTORY

Ask for the following:

- Note the age and sex of the patient
- Ask for symptoms of joint disease, e.g. pain, swelling, restricted movements
- Morning stiffness
- Number of joints involved
- History of palpitation, dyspnea
- History of extra-articular manifestations
- History of joint deformities (present)

EXAMINATION

Musculoskeletal System Examination

Examine the hands as follows:

1. Pain, swelling, tenderness of joints present (Fig. 181.1)
2. Number of joints involved (polyarthritis)
3. Pattern of joint involvement, i.e. symmetrical (in this case) or asymmetrical

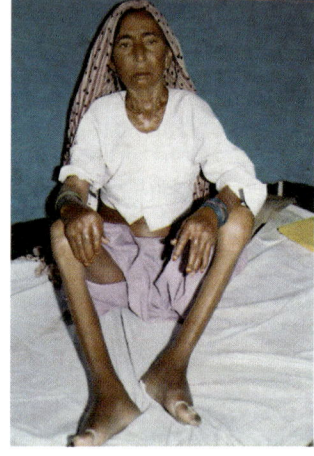

Fig. 181.1: Rheumatoid arthritis—a deforming poly-arthritis in a female. Note the deformities of the hands. There is edema of feet due to renal involvement (amyloidosis of the kidneys)

4. Types of joints involved, i.e. small joints (in this case) or big joints
5. Look for the following deformities:
   - Ulnar deviation of hands (Fig. 181.2A)
   - Swan-neck deformity (Fig. 181.2C)
   - Boutonniere deformity (Fig. 181.2B)

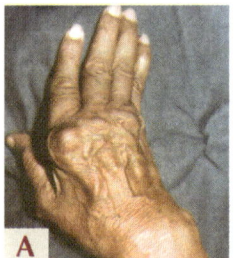
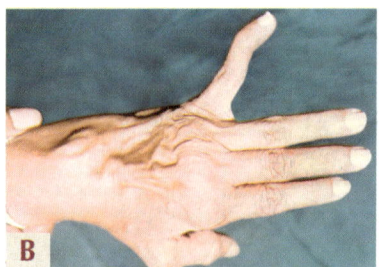
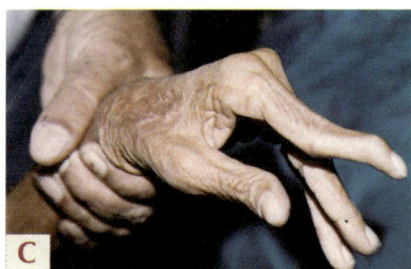

Fig. 181.2: Hand deformities in rheumatoid arthritis. (A) Ulnar deviation; (B) Boutonniere deformity; (C) Swan-neck deformity

- Z deformity of the thumb
- Square hands
- Subluxation at metacarpophalangeal joints
- Dorsal subluxation of ulna at carpal joint

6. *Look at hands for:*
   - Palmar erythema
   - Wasting of first dorsal interossei and other small muscles of hand (present)

7. *Examine the fingers*
   - Nail fold infarct or skin lesions

8. *Examine elbow*
   - Rheumatoid nodules

9. Look for features of carpal tunnel syndrome, i.e.
   - Test for weakness of abductor *Pollicis brevis* and interossei. Test sensations over index and little finger (one and a half finger involved if median nerve is compressed)
   - Test the hand grip strength
   - Ask the patients to perform simple tasks, e.g. fasten shirt buttons, writing, combing hair etc.
   - Examine other joints
   - Examine for extra-articular manifestations, e.g. eye involvement, lung involvement, heart involvement
   - Look for other associated autoimmune diseases
   - Look for felty syndrome (RA, splenomegaly, thrombocytopenia or pancytopenia)

PROVISIONAL DIAGNOSIS

The patient has symmetric bilateral polyarthritis of small joints with deformities (lesion) caused by rheumatoid arthritis (aetiology). Patient is incapacitated due to deformities of the hands.

QUESTIONS AND ANSWERS

Q. Which joints are involved in RA?

Ans:
- Small joints of hands and feet, i.e. proximal inter-phalangeal joints, metacarpophalangeal joints of the hands and metatarsophalangeal joint (toes)
- Wrist joints
- Temporomandibular joint, atlantoaxial joint
- Uncommonly knee joints

Q. What is a rheumatoid nodule? What is its significance? Where are they found?

Ans: These are hard nodules found over the flexor and extensor tendons of hands, achilles tendon, sacrum, lungs and myocardium (read Clinical Methods in Medicine by Prof SN Chugh).

The presence of nodules indicate active disease and seropositive arthritis.

Q. Name the extra-articular manifestations of RA.

Ans:
I. *Ocular manifestations*
   - Scleritis, episcleritis, iridocyclitis
   - Keratoconjunctivitis sicca or Sjögren syndrome

II. *Lung manifestations*
   - Fibrosing alveolitis
   - Caplan syndrome
   - Pleuritis and pleural effusion
   - Rheumatoid nodules
   - Small airway disease

III. *Neurological manifestations*
   - Peripheral neuropathy
   - Mononeuritis multiplex
   - Carpal tunnel syndrome
   - Entrapment neuropathy
   - Atalanto-axial dislocation with cervical myelopathy

IV. *Cardiovascular manifestations*
   - Pericarditis, pericardial effusion
   - Mitral or aortic regurgitation
   - Myocarditis

V. *Soft tissue manifestations*
   - Rheumatoid nodules
   - Bursitis, tenosynovitis
   - Muscle wasting

Q. What is Felty syndrome?

Ans: It occurs in children, consists of:
1. Rheumatoid arthritis
2. Splenomegaly
3. Anemia, thrombocytopenia, leukopenia (Pancytopenia) due to hypersplenism
4. Leg ulcers

Q. What are the skin manifestations of RA?

Ans:
- Palmar erythema
- Nail fold infarcts
- Vasculitis

Q. What are the causes of anemia in RA?

Ans: The anemia could be due to
- Chronic disease itself (anemia of chronic illness)
- Folate deficiency
- Felty syndrome (hypersplenism)
- Drug induced. Drugs causing iron deficiency or bone marrow suppression

Q. What is pathogenesis of anemia in RA?

Ans: Anemia in RA is similar to anemia in other chronic illness. The mechanisms of pathogenesis are:
1. Decreased production of RBCs due to substrate deficiency

2. Ineffective erythropoiesis
3. Abnormal development of erythroid progenitor cells
4. Increased destruction of RBCs (decreased RBCs survival)

Q. What is palindromic RA?

Ans: It is a variant of RA. It is characterised by recurrent episodes of arthritis in individual joints lasting for only a few hours or days. The rheumatoid factor is positive in 50% cases and one third cases develop chronic RA.

Q. What precaution would you take in RA before upper GI endoscopy or general anaesthesia?

Ans: Cervical spine X-ray must be taken to rule out the atlanto-axial dislocation or subluxation.

Q. How would you diagnose RA?

Ans:

Table 181.1: The 2010 ACR/EULAR classification criteria for rheumatoid arthritis

Domain: Joint involvement	Domain: Duration of synovitis
• 1 large joint (0 points)	• Less than 6 weeks (0 points)
• 2–10 large joints (1 point)	• 6 weeks or longer (1 point)
• 1–3 small joints (2 points)	
• 4–10 small joints (3 points)	
• >10 joints [at least 1 small joint] (5 points)	
• RF/CCP negative (0 points)	• Normal ESR/CRP (0 points)
• RF or CCP positive at low titer <3 times ULN (2 point)	• Abnormal ESR/CRP (1 point)
• RF or CCP positive at high titer, defined as >3 times ULN (3 points)	

ULN = upper limit of normal

Joint involvement refers to any swollen or tender joint on examination which may be confirmed by imaging evidence of synovitis. Distal interphalangeal joints, first carpometacarpal joints, and first metatarsophalangeal joints are excluded from assessment.

"Large joints" refers to shoulders, elbows, hips, knees, and ankles.

"Small joints" refers to the metacarpophalangeal joints, proximal interphalangeal joints, second through fifth metatarsophalangeal joints, thumb, interphalageal joints, and wrists.

Q. How does RA lead to nephrotic syndrome?

Ans: Nephrotic syndrome in RA is either due to development of amyloidosis of kidneys or may be drug induced (gold and penicilla-mine).

Q. How would you treat RA?

Ans: 1. *NSAIDs* to relieve pain and inflammation. They are used to control arthritis and induce remission.

2. *DMARDs* (Disease modifying anti-rheu-matic drugs) are used when NSAIDs fail to induce remission. Hydroxychloro-quine, sulfasalazine and penicillamine are used to modify the course and progre-ssion of the disease. Low dose metho-trexate and gold salts are used to prevent disease progression.

Biological DMARDs that inhibit the action of TNF-α, e.g. infiximab, etanercept and adalimumab and one that inhibit the action of interleukin-I (anakinra) produce significant improvement in the severity of arthritis.

Alternative agents include lefunomide, an TNF or interlukin blocker, rituximab, an anti CD-20 monoclonal antibody and abatacept which blocks selective costimu-lation of T cells.

Q. What is pathogenesis of ulnar deviation of hand in RA?

Ans: Normally during a grip, the fingers move to the ulnar side of the hand due to weakening of the radial side of the joint capsule and radial insertion of the interosseous ligaments.

This phenomen is exacerbated in RA due to following reasons:

i. The volar support of the flexor tendon sheath are weakened by inflammation in RA; allowing the tendon to move in the direction of ulna during gripping.

ii. Ulnar deviation of extensor tendons make them slip if the dorsal metacarpopha-langeal joint is rigid and this potentiates the development of ulnar deviation.

iii. Joint capsules of metacarpophalangeal joints are weaker on radial sides than on ulnar sides.

182

Ankylosing Spondylitis (AS)

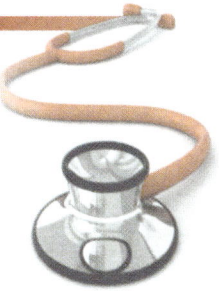

INSTRUCTION

Examine the musculoskeletal system

SALIENT FEATURES

- Difficulty in bending

HISTORY

Ask about the following:

- Age of the patient. Onset of symptoms and their progression
- Back pain and stiffness worst in the morning, improves on activity and worsens on rest
- Joints involved, i.e. shoulder, knee, axial.
- Nocturnal exacerbation of pain
- Extra-articular manifestations, e.g. conjunctivitis (red eyes), cough, dyspnea (pulmonary fibrosis), palpitations (aortic regurgitation), diarrhea (GI manifestations)

EXAMINATION

Musculoskeletal System Examination

- Typical 'Question mark' posture due to loss of lumbar lordosis and increased kyphosis (present)
- Loss of spinal mobility with limitation of anterior and lateral flexion and extension of lumbar spine (present)
- Limited chest expansion
- Protuberant abdomen
- Tenderness over sacroiliac joint on direct pressure (present)
- Tenderness and spasm of paraspinal muscles (present)

Manoeuvres to be done

- Ask the patient to look to either side. The patient's whole body turns to that side when he tries to do so
- Ask the patient to stand with heel and back against the wall. The head does not make contact due to limitation of thoracic and cervical spine (present). Measure the occiput to wall distance.
- Perform Schober's test. It is positive (Fig. 182.1)

The schober test is useful measure of flexion of lumbar spine. The patient stands erect with heels together. Two cross marks are drawn directly over the spine 5 cm below and 10 cm above the lumbo-sacral junction (identified by a horizontal line between posterospinal iliac spines called dimple of Venus). The patient then bends forward maximally and the distance between the two marks increases 5 cm or more in case of normal mobility and <4 cm in the case of decreased mobility (spinal stiffness). Chest expansion on maximal forced inspiration is decreased in AS (normal expansion is ≥5 cm or more).

- Examine for extra-articular manifestations, e.g.
  1. *Eyes* for iridocyclitis
  2. *CVS* for aortic regurgitation (occurs in 4% patients with disease >15 yrs duration) and conduction defects
  3. *Lungs* for fibrosing alveolitis and hypoventilation syndrome due to rigid spine
  4. *CNS* for quadriplegia
  5. *Foot* for Achilles tendinitis and plantar fascitis

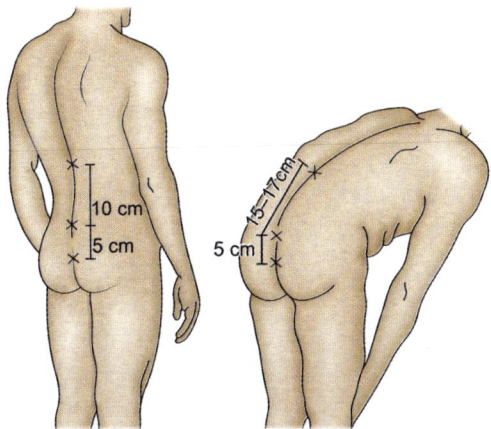

Fig. 182.1: Ankylosing spondylitis: Schober's test. Measuring forward flexion of the spine

PROVISIONAL DIAGNOSIS

The patient has rigid spinal column, fixed kyphoscoliosis of thoracic spine with loss of lumbar lordosis (lesion) caused by ankylosing spondylitis (aetiology). He is incapacitated with rigid spinal column (functional status).

QUESTIONS AND ANSWERS

Q. **What are the points in favor of your diagnosis?**

Ans:
- Male patient
- Symptoms of back pain and stiffness of spinal column
- Pain of inflammatory origin, i.e. aggravated at rest, exacerbated during activity. Pain radiates to both legs
- Restriction of spinal movements with positive Schober's test
- Presence of extra-articular mainifestation
- Limited chest expansion
- Asymmetric distal joints arthritis. Joints of hands and feet spared

Q. **What are the complications of AS?**

Ans:
1. *Spinal fracture* with minor trauma.
2. *Cauda equina syndrome*.
3. *Pulmonary fibrosis*.
4. *Aortic insufficiency* leading to congestive heart failure and complete AV block can occur with prolonged disease.
5. *Amyloidosis* is rare association.

Q. **Name the seronegative HLA B$_{27}$ spondyloarthropathies.**

Ans:
1. Ankylosing spondylitis
2. Psoriatic arthritis
3. Reiter's syndrome
4. Enteropathic synovitis
5. Reactive arthritis

Q. **What are the common characteristic features of HLA B$_{27}$ arthropathy?**

Ans:
1. Low back pain
2. Asymmetric distal joints involvement
3. Familial aggregation
4. HLA B$_{27}$ positivity
5. Anterior uveitis or other extra-articular features
6. Seronegativity (rheumatoid factor absent)
7. Sacroiliitis on X-ray

Q. **How would you investigate this patient?**

Ans: Following investigations are done;
1. *ESR* is raised and *C-reactive protein* raised.

2. A mild normocytic normochronic anemia may be present.
3. *Rheumatoid factor* and anti-nuclear antibodies are absent in blood.
4. Elevated serum IgA levels are common.
5. *X-ray of lumbar spines and pelvis*
   - In the early stages, sacroiliac joint is eroded with blurred margins, and there is sclerosis of the adjacent bone.
   - As the disease progresses, the sacroiliac joint may fuse (fibrous or bony ankylosis).
   - The spines show syndesmophytes, that grow between the margins of vertebrae.
   - There is calcification and ossification of interspinal ligaments so that with syndesmophytes, the X-ray (PA view) shows three continuous lines connecting vertebral bodies anteriorly and laterally giving the so called "tramline appearance" or "bamboo spine". (Fig. 182.2)
   - In addition there is squaring of vertebrae with straightening and sclerosis.
6. **HLA B$_{27}$** (measured in blood lymphocytes) is useful supporting evidence in a difficult case, but one must remember that many normal people carry the gene. HLA B$_{27}$ is present in 90% cases of AS.

Q. **What are the diagnostic criteria for AS?**

Ans: Modified New York 1984 criteria for AS define AS is present if the radiological criteria is associated with at least one clinical criteria.

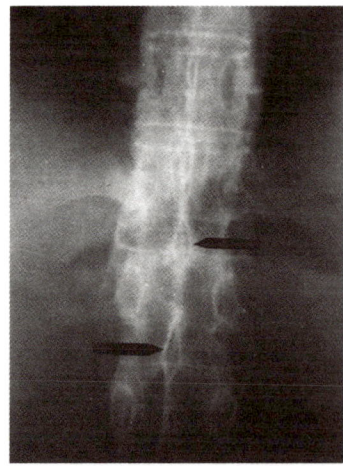

Fig. 182.2: X-rays spines showing calcification of interspinous ligaments producing "bamboo-spine"

Clinical criteria:

i. Low back pain and stiffness for more than 3 months that improve with exercise, but is not relieved by rest.

ii. Limitation of motion of the lumbar spine in the sagittal (sideways) and frontal (forward and backward) planes.

iii. Limitation of chest expansion relative to normal values correlated for age and sex.

Radiological criterion:

– Sacroiliitis grade 2 bilaterally or grade 3–4 unilaterally or bilaterally.

Q.   How do you grade sacroiliitis?

Ans: Sacroiliitis grades are:

- **Grade 0:** Normal
- **Grade 1:** Some blurring of the joint margins-suspicious
- **Grade 2:** Minimal sclerosis with some erosions (mild sacroiliitis)
- **Grade 3:** Severe erosions with widening of joint space + \ – some ankylosis (moderate sacroiliitis)
- **Grade 4:** Complete ankylosis

Q.   What is the earliest radiological features of AS?

Ans: 1. Earliest radiographic change is bilateral symmetric sacroilitis of joints which is picked up by MRI.

Q.   What is the risk of "bamboo spine"?

Ans: The risk of bamboo spine is increased whiplash injury and restricted lateral vision during driving. Accidents are common.

Q.   What is the treatment of AS?

Ans: 1. NSAIDs to relieve pain

2. Physical exercise to preserve back extension

3. Methotrexate and sulphasalazine

4. Tumor necrosis factor blockers decrease pain and stiffness and improves overall functioning and decrease disease activity (reduce ESR, CRP, increase chest expansion).

183

Osteoarthritis

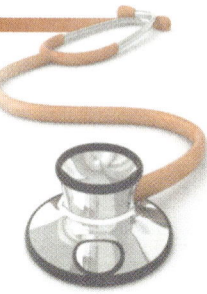

INSTRUCTION

Examine the musculoskeletal system

SALIENT FEATURES

- Pain in both knees and difficulty in walking

HISTORY

Ask about the following:

- Age of the patient (middle or old age)
- Pain in the joints (mention the joints involved). Morning stiffness usually lasts > 30 min (Fig. 183.1A)
- Stiffness of joints after a period of inactivity
- Gait abnormality
- Difficulty in climbing stairs, getting out of the chair and walking long distances
- Nocturnal hip pain is common

EXAMINATION

Musculoskeletal Examination

- Patient appears to have vacant look or appear depressed.
- Look for Herberden's nodes and Bouchard's nodes at terminal and proximal inter-phalangeal joints respectively (present, Fig. 183.1B).
- Examine the knee for crepitus (present). The joints may be red, swollen if inflamed or disorganised with bulging due to effusion.
- Examine the hip and elicit tenderness by direct pressure. Perform range-of-motions. Pain in the hip is exacerbated during internal and external rotation when knee is in full extension. The movements at hip are restricted (present).

PROVISIONAL DIAGNOSIS

The old men has involvement of big joints, i.e. knee, hip, with Heberden's nodes at the distal inter-

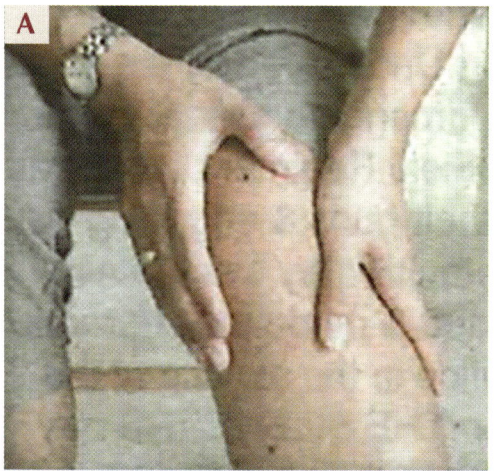

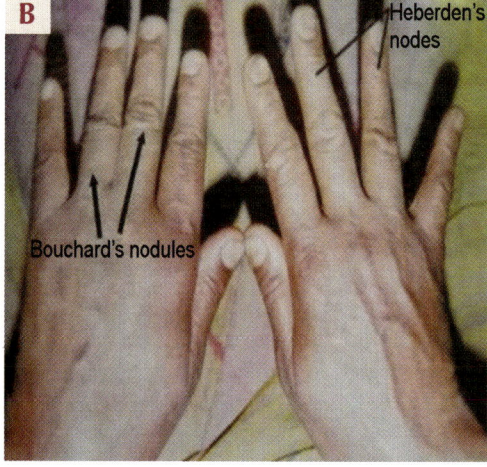

Fig. 183.1: (A) Knee joint pain in OA. (B) Nodular osteoarthritis. Note the prominent involvement of distal interphalangeal joint with Heberden's nodes and proximal interphalangeal joints with Bouchard's nodes indicated by arrows in a patient with nodular osteoarthritis

phalangeal joints and Bouchard's nodes at proximal interphalangeal joints (lesion) caused by osteoarthritis—a degenerative disorder (aetiology). He is unable to perform normal activities of daily life (functional status).

QUESTIONS AND ANSWERS

Q. Which joints are commonly involved in OA?

Ans: The knees, hands, hip, feet, ankle and lumbar and cervical spines are involved.

Q. What is pthogenesis of OA?

Ans: Osteoarthritis is a degenerative disease of cartilage which is composed of a matrix of collagen II fibres stuffed with proteoglycan molecules. The degenerative process is initiated by a variety of stimuli which cause degradation of matrix of cartilage. This process is limited or inhibited by inhibitors of matrix degrading enzymes. Therefore, the imbalance between the two processes (Fig. 183.2) predispose to cartilage destruction.

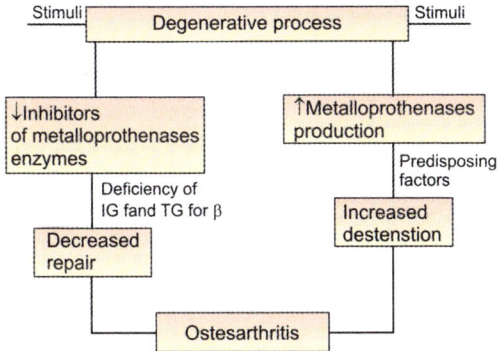

Fig. 183.2: Pathogenesis of osteoarthritis

Q. What are Bouchard's and Heberden's nodes?

Ans: Bouchard's nodes are bony swellings seen over the proximal interphalangeal joints in OA while *Heberden's nodes* are seen over distal interphalangeal joints.

Q. What are the causes of OA?

Ans: The osteoarthritis may be primary and secondary.

Primary OA commonly affects some or all of the following, i.e. DIP and proximal interphalangeal joints (PIP), joint of fingers, carpometacarpal joint of thumb, the hip, the knee and metatarsophalangeal joints (MTPs) of big toe and the cervical and lumbar spines. Secondary OA on the there hand, can occur in any joints as a sequela to articular injury

resulting from RA or any other causes. The cause are given in Table 183.1.

Table 183.1: Aetiology of OA
I. Primary (cause unknown)
II. Secondary

i. *Congenital abnormalities*, e.g. hypermobility and congenital dysplasia.

ii. *Structural disorder*, e.g. Perthes disease

iii. *Trauma* and *mechanical factors* (this affects athletes and mechanics)

iv. *Inflammatory arthropathies*, e.g. RA, septic arthritis, gout

v. *Neuropathic joint* (Charcot joint), e.g. diabetes, syringomyelia, tabes dorsalis

vi. *Endocranial*, e.g. hyperparathyroidism, acromegaly, hypothyroidism

vii. *Metabolic*, e.g. hemochromatosis, chondrocalcinosis (pseudogout)

Q. What are the risk factors for OA?

Ans: All the secondary causes of OA as discussed above are actually risk factors or predisposing conditions. In addition obesity, old age, hypermobility of the joints, osteoporosis, trauma and occupation and sports injury also contribute to it.

Q. What are the radiological hallmarks of OA?

Ans: Joint space reduction, subchondral bone sclerosis, subchondral cysts formation, osteophytosis and osteochondral (loose) bodies in joints.

Q. What does synovial fluid examination show in OA?

Ans: The fluid is clear with < 3000 WBCs/litre.

Q. What do you understand by the term nodular osteoarthritis?

Ans: Nodular osteoarthritis is a primary generalised osteoarthritis with following characteristics:

1. Peak incidence in middle age women
2. Strong genetic predisposition (autosomal dominant)
3. Polyarticular finger interphalangeal joints OA
4. Heberden's nodes and Bouchard's nodes
5. Arthritis may be acute. The deformities are marked (square hand deformity). Functional disability is little
   - Later on the hips, knee, joints of thumb and apophyseal joints may be involved

Q. What is the role of aggrecan in pathogenesis of OA?

Ans: It has been shown in experimental studies that loss of aggrecan is the primary event that can lead destruction of cartilage in OA. Therefore, three enzymes that can degrade aggrecans have been identified (ADAMTS I, ADAMTS4 and ADAMTS5) which can play a role in treatment of OA in near future.

Q. **How would you manage this condition?**

Ans: Life style modifications such as cessation of smoking, alcohol, reduction of weight and physical exercise may help to improve OA. Physical exercise that strengthen muscles and exercise program of water aerobics or with physiotherapist at a frequency of twice a week will be most helpful.

- *Relief of pain:* The applications of heat to joint may reduce pain and stiffness
- *Drug therapy:* There is no specific drug to control the disease. NSAIDs are used to reduce pain and inflammation. NSAIDs, rubifacients and cox 2-inhibitors are used for acute flare up. Capsaicin cream can be used locally to reduce pain.

Intra-articular corticosteroid injection (triamcinolone 20–40 mg) may obviate the need for NSAIDs, are used for acute flare-ups and patients unfit for surgery. Intra-articular injection of hyaluronidase is used to the reduce symptoms of OA knee.

- *Surgery*
    i. Arthroscopic removal of loose bodies and radioisotope synovectomy for persistent arthritis.
    ii. Joint replacement is the final answer for hip and knee OA.

184

Gout

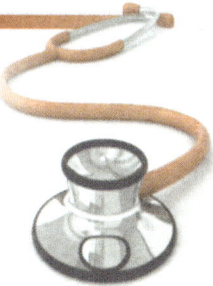

INSTRUCTION

Examine the musculoskeletal system

SALIENT FEATURES

- Pain in joints of foot and swelling of a big toe

HISTORY

Ask about the following:

- History of acute attack of pain involving the joints of foot especially big toe (present)
- Nocturnal attacks of pain (present)
- Alcohol and fasting state precipitate the attacks
- *Drug-history:* Certain drugs (diuretics) may precipitate the attack
- Note the number of joints involved
- History of fever, malaise
- Presence of tophi (present, Fig. 184.1A)
- Renal colic (gouty nephropathy)

EXAMINATION

Musculoskeletal Examination

- There are chronic gouty tophi in the interphalangeal joint and joints of foot (Fig. 184.1A). They are tender and mobile.
- There is an ulcerated tophus over the lateral malleolus (Fig. 184.1B).
- There is swelling of first metatarsophalangeal joint (podagra).

  Now look for tophi at the following sites:
  - Ear lobules
  - Achilles tendons
  - Elbow and olecranon bursae
  - Forearm

PROVISIONAL DIAGNOSIS

The patient is an alcoholic who has swellings of intertarsal joints and an ulcerated tophus over the

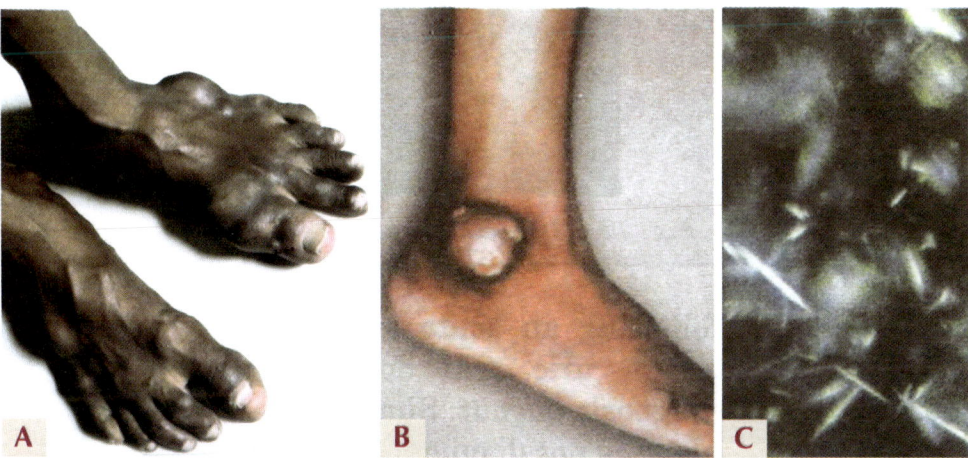

Fig. 184.1: Podagra; (A) Acute gouty arthritis of first metacarpophalangeal joint if feet. (Note the swelling of the joints and tophi which were painful and tender); (B) Tophus (ulcerated ulcer over lateral malleolus). Urate crystals can be demonstrated from this lesion; (C) Needle shaped crystals in synovial fluid under polarised light

ankle (lesion) caused by chronic tophaceous gout (aetiology). He is unable to walk because of pain over ulcer (functional status).

QUESTIONS AND ANSWERS

Q. **What is gout?**

Ans: Gout is a disorder of purine metabolism, characterised by hyperuricemia caused by either overproduction or under excretion of uric acid leading to deposition of monosodium urate crystals in joints, soft tissue and kidneys.

Q. **What are the clinical manifestations of gout?**

Ans: 1. Asymptomatic hyperuricemia
2. Acute gouty arthritis
3. Chronic erosive and deforming arthritis
4. Chronic tophaceous gout
5. Gout nephropathy, hypertension and renal stones

Q. **What are the precipitants of acute gouty arthritis?**

Ans: Alcohol intake, fasting state, dehydration, surgery, food rich in purine (sweet breads, liver, kidney and sardines) and drugs (thiazides) are major precipitants of acute gout.

Q. **When would you treat hyperuricemia in gout?**

Ans: 1. Hyperuricemia associated with repeated acute arthritis
2. Hyperuricemia associated with gouty nephropathy

Q. **How would you treat acute attack of gout?**

Ans: Acute attack of gout is treated by
  i. *NSAIDs*. Nonsteroidal anti-inflammatory drugs (indomethacin ibuprofen, diclofenac, etc.) give an excellent response.
  ii. *Colchicine* is given during, acute attack or during interictal period within first 24 hrs to prevent recurrent attacks of severe gout.
  iii. *Corticosteroids* give dramatic symptomatic relief. They are useful in patients with contraindications to NSAIDs. They can be used orally (prednisolone) or IV (methyprednisolone)
  iv. *Anakina*: This drug being an interleukin-I receptor antagonist has efficacy for treatment of acute attack.

Q. **Name the drugs that lower serum uric acid.**

Ans: Two classes of drugs may be used to lower the serum uric acid, but none of them is useful for acute attack.

1. *Uricosuric agents:* These drugs lower the serum urate levels via increased excretion through kidneys if kidneys functions are preserved. Therefore, these drugs (probenecid) are useful where there is undersecretion of uric acid, i.e. a value of 24 hr urine uric acid is <800 mg/day.
2. Xanthine oxidase inhibitors (e.g. allopurinol, febuxostat). They inhibit the synthesis of uric acid, hence, are used when uric acid production is high, i.e. 24 hr urine uric acid excretion is >800 mg/day.

Q. **What are the diagnostic criteria of acute gout?**

Ans: American Rheumatism Diagnostic criteria 1977 for acute gout includes the presence of seven or more of the following:
1. More than one attack of gout
2. Involvement of single joint (monoarthritis)
3. Maximum inflammation occurs within 1 hr of an attack
4. Redness over the other joints
5. First metatarsophalangeal joint red and swollen (podagra)
6. Unilateral attack of first metatarsophalangeal joint
7. Unilateral attack of tarsal joint
8. Tophus (suspected or proven)
9. Hyperuricaemia
10. Asymmetric swelling within a joint on radiology
11. Monosodium urate crystals in joint glued during attack
12. Culture of joint fluid negative for organism during an attack

Q. **How would you decide whether the patient is over producer or underexcretor of uric acid?**

Ans: It has already been answered that patients with 24 hr urinary excretion of uric acid less than 800 mg/day are presumed to be underexcretor and less producer. An overproducer is one who excretes > 800 mg on 24 hr urine sample.

Q. **What is pseudogout?**

Ans: Pseudogout is an acute arthritis due to deposition of calcium pyrophosphate dehydrate (CPPD) crystals in articular cartilage and periarticular tissue. It is associated with hyperparathyroidism, haemochromatosis, hypothyroidism, Wilson's disease and true gout.

185

Charcot's Joint

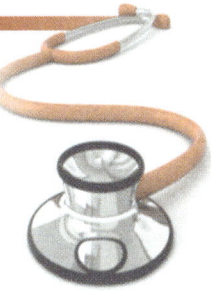

INSTRUCTION

- Examine the musculoskeletal system. Perform other relevant system examination

SALIENT FEATURES

- Painless joint swelling

HISTORY

Ask about the following:

- History of painless joint swelling (present)
- History of diabetes (present), tabes dorsalis (lancinating pains) and syringomyelia
- Abnormal gait
- Atrophy of muscles around the joint (present)

EXAMINATION

Musculoskeletal System Examination

- Painless swollen affected joint (left ankle) as compared to other side (Fig. 185.1)
- Hypermobile and instability of the joint (present)

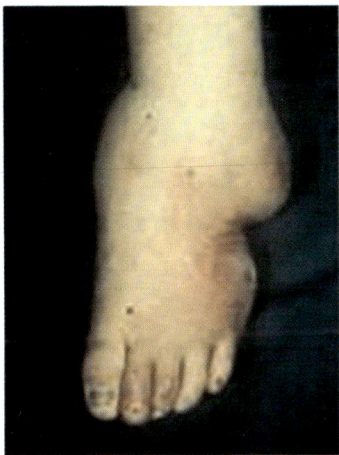

Fig. 185.1: Charcot's joint (left ankle)

- On palpation of the joint, crepitus may be felt (present in this case)
- Collapse of the longitudinal arch resulting in rocker-bottom deformity
- Look for Argyll-Robertson pupil (tabes dorsalis)
- Look for hypopigmented macules (leprosy)

Neurological Examination

- There is atrophy of muscles around the joint involved
- There is hypotonia and decreased muscle power
- Loss of sensations of pain, touch and temperature as well as loss of sense of position and vibration sense in the affected limb (both legs in this case) having the affected joint/joints (left ankle)
- Check the limb for dissociated sensory loss (syringomyelia)
- Check for peripheral neuropathy (present) or amyotrophy (diabetes)
- Palpate the peripheral nerves (leprosy)

PROVISIONAL DIAGNOSIS

The patient has Charcot's joint (lesion) caused by neuropathy due to diabetes mellitus (aetiology). There is marked deformity of the joint (functional status).

Q. What are the points in favor of your diagnosis?

Ans: 1. The affected joint (ankle) is swollen and painless
2. Joint is disorganised and mobility is increased
3. Presence of diabetic peripheral neuropathy
3. Presence of atrophy of small muscles of foot

QUESTIONS AND ANSWERS

Q. How do you say the hypermobile ankle joint?

Ans: Hyperextensibility of the ankle beyond 90° indicates hypermobility.

Q.   What do you understand by the term Charcot's joint?

Ans: It is a progressive degenerative arthropathy as a result of sensory loss (neuropathic arthropathy). It occurs as a result of various disorders affecting the sensory system of CNS. It results in gross deformity, osteoarthrosis and new bone formation due to repeated trauma.

Q.   What are the causes of Charcot's joint?

Ans: 1. *Diabetes mellitus* affecting the tarsal joints (diabetic foot)
2. *Tabes dorsalis* affecting the knees and the ankles
3. *Syringomyelia* affecting the shoulder and elbow joints
4. *Subacute combined* degeneration affecting knees and ankles
5. *Ehlers-Danlos syndrome*
6. *Miscellaneous disorders*
   - Leprosy
   - Peripheral neuropathies
   - Peripheral nerve injury

Q.   What are the clinical characteristics of Charcot's joint?

Ans: It is a neuropathic joint characterized by:
- Painless joint swelling (e.g. knee, hip, shoulder joint)
- Hypermobile joint
- Disorganized and destroyed joint
- Loose bodies or osteophytes in the joint cavity
- Palpable crepitus

Q.   How do you classify Charcot's foot?

Ans: The Rogers and Bevilacqua classified charcot foot based on the clinical examination, radiology and anatomy of the foot into 4 stages:

Stage A : Acute deformity
Stage B : With deformity progression
Stage C : With deformity and ulceration
Stage D : With osteomyelitis

With the progression of the stage, the risk of amputation increases, therefore patient at stage A is at the lowest risk and at stage D, he/she is at a highest risk.

Q.   What is the significance of measuring skin temperature in Charcot's foot?

Ans: The average temperature difference measured by contact or noncontact thermometer between the acute Charcot's foot and unaffected foot of 9°F (5°C) is considered significant and diagnostic of Charcot's joint.

Q.   What is the pathogenesis of Charcot's foot in diabetes?

Ans: Read diabetic foot as a case report.

Q.   How would you treat it?

Ans: • Treat the underlying cause
- Stabilise the joint by braces and splints

186

Acute Monoarthritis (Acute Septic Arthritis)

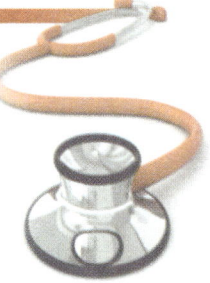

INSTRUCTION

- Examine the musculoskeletal system

SALIENT FEATURES

- Painful swollen elbow

HISTORY

Ask about the following:

- Painful knee/ankle/shoulder/any other joint
- Swelling of the joint (elbow joint in this case)
- Restricted movements (present)
- History of fever and trauma (present)
- History of RA, gout, hemophilia, tuberculosis, gonorrhea, syphilis, otitis media, osteomyelitis, skin infection
- History of intra-articular injection
- History of surgery over the joint

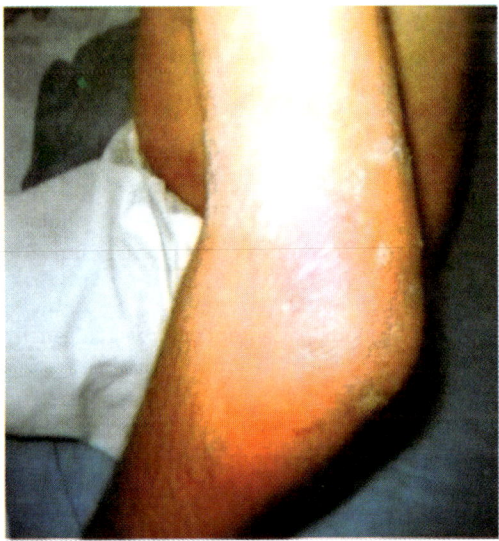

Fig. 186.1: Acute septic arthritis elbow

EXAMINATION

Musculoskeletal System Examination

- The involved joint may be red, painful and swollen (elbow in this case). Temperature over the joint may be raised (acute inflamed joint)
- Both active and passive movements over the joints are restricted (in this case)
- There is disuse atrophy of the humeral muscles on the left side (present)
- No other joint is involved

PROVISIONAL DIAGNOSIS

The patient has painful left elbow with restricted movements and disuse atrophy of humeral muscles (lesion) caused by septic arthritis following trauma (aetiology). The patient finds difficulty in using left upper limb (functional status).

QUESTIONS AND ANSWERS

Q. **What are the causes of painful elbow joint?**
Ans: 1. Trauma to the elbow
2. Acute arthritis, e.g. septic, viral, etc.
3. Acute rheumatoid arthritis
4. Acute osteoarthritis
5. Acute gout and pseudogout
6. Hemarthrosis (hemophilia)

Q. **What are the causes of acute monoarticular arthritis?**
Ans: The causes are:
1. *Bacterial arthritis* (septic arthritis) due to *Staph. aureus, Gonococcus, Meningococcus, Streptococcus*
2. Reactive arthritis
3. Sarcoidosis
4. Hemarthrosis (hemophilia)
5. Traumatic arthritis
6. Gout and pseudogout
7. Rheumatoid arthritis

Q.   What are the causes of acute polyarthritis?

Ans: 1. Infective endocarditis
2. Acute hepatitis B infection
3. Serum sickness
4. Acute rheumatic fever
5. Rheumatoid arthritis
6. Collagen vascular disorder, e.g. SLE
7. HIV and parvovirus infection
8. Acute osteoarthritis of knee

Q.   What are the predisposing factors for septic arthritis?

Ans: 1. Immunocompromised individuals, i.e. patients with diabetes or cancer patients on immunosuppressive therapy
2. History of surgery on the joint
3. Trauma
4. Neuropathic joint
5. Patients of rheumatoid arthritis or osteoarthritis

Q.   How would you confirm your diagnosis?

Ans: The supportive diagnostic investigations are:
1. Blood test for leucocytosis
2. Blood culture may be sometimes positive
3. Aspiration of synovial fluid is diagnostic if it is purulent and typically contains 1,00,000 WBCs/μL predominantly neutrophils
4. CT/MRI is useful in detecting joint effusion, bony erosions and osteomyelitis

187

Ehlers-Danlos Syndrome

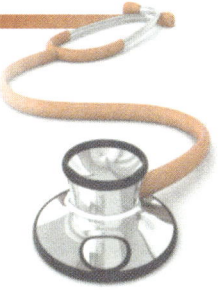

INSTRUCTION

- Examine the musculoskeletal system. Perform other relevant system examination

SALIENT FEATURES

- Hyperelastic skin and hypermobile joints

HISTORY

Ask the following:

- History of loose fragile skin (present)
- History of bleeding diathesis
- History of the disease running in families
- Hypermobile joints (present)
- History of dyspnea, palpitations (mitral and aortic regurgitation)
- History of gaping wounds, rectal prolapse
- History of polyuria (renal tubular defect)

EXAMINATION

Musculoskeletal System Examination

- The skin over the neck, cheeks, axillae and groin is smooth and elastic (Fig. 187.1)
- It can be stretched like a rubber (Fig. 187.1) and

when released it returns back to normal. The skin can become loose and wrinkled later on
- Look for bruising over the bony prominences
- Look for hematomas and gaping wounds. Wound may heal with thin-paper "cigarette paper" scars
- Look and palpate the joints for hypermobility (present) and hemarthrosis
- Kyphoscoliosis
- Look at the hernial sites for any hernia
- Examine the eyes for myopia or retinal detachment

Other System Examination

- Examine the heart for aortic or mitral regurgitation
- Examine the lungs for pneumothorax

PROVISIONAL DIAGNOSIS

The patient has fragile skin and hypermobile joints (lesion) caused by Ehlers-Danlos syndrome (aetiology). He is at risk of trauma (functional status).

Q. **What is the type of EDS in your case?**
Ans: Type II (mitis variety) due to presence of hyperelastic skin and hypermobile joint (read Table 187.1).

A   **B**

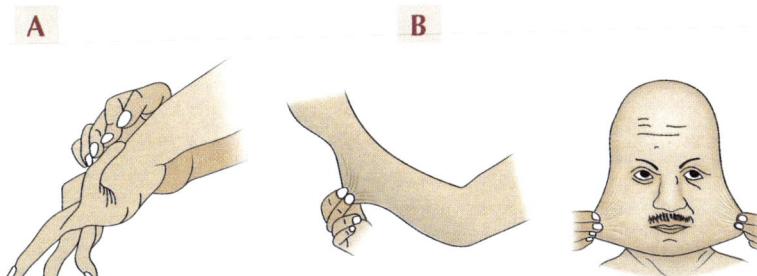

Fig. 187.1: Ehlers-Danlos syndrome (diagram). (A) Demonstration of joint hypermobility; (B) Demonstration of hyperextensibility (cutis laxa)

Table 187.1: Clinical types, mode of inheritance and clinical features of EDS

Type	Mode of inheritance	Clinical features
i. Gravis	Autosomal dominant	Skin manifestations, hypermobile joints, varicose veins, prematurity
ii. Mitis	–do–	Similar to type I but less severe
iii. Familial hypermobility	–do–	Soft skin, no scaring, hypermobility
iv. Ecchymotic (vascular type)	–do–	Thin skin with visible veins, easy bruisability, arterial, bowel and uterine rupture. Skin and joints have normal extensiblity
v. X-linked	X-linked recessive	Similar to type II, but occurs in male only
vi. Lysyl hydroxylase enzyme deficiency (kyphoscoliotic type)	Autosomal recessive	Hyperextensibility, soft skin, joint hypermobility, ocular fragility and keratoconus
vii. Arthrochalasis multiplex congenita	Both autosomal dominant and recessive	Marked joint hypermobility, soft skin with normal scarring
viii. Periodontal	Autosomal dominant	Generalised periodontitis, skin similar to type II (mitis)
ix. Cutis laxa occipital horn syndrome	Not known (abnormal copper metabolism). Menkes's syndrome is X-linked	Occipital horn, bony exostosis, widened and bowed bones
	Autosomal recessive	This has platelet aggregation defect, correctable with fibronectin, hypermobility and hyperextensibility also present

QUESTIONS AND ANSWERS

Q. What is the basic defect in Ehlers-Danlos syndrome?

Ans: Ehlers-Danlos syndrome comprises of heterogenous disorders in which there is defect in collagen synthesis which vary genetically and clinically from one another.

Q. What are the gastrointestinal manifestations of this syndrome?

Ans:
1. Tendency to herniation (inguinal and diaphragmatic)
2. Achalasia cardia
3. Eventration of diaphragm
4. Megacolon
5. Rectal prolapse
6. Internal piles

Q. What are the cardiac manifestations of this syndrome?

Ans:
- Aortic root dilatation, aortic regurgitation
- Mitral valve prolapse and mitral regurgitation
- Intracranial aneurysm
- Raynaud's phenomenon

Q. What precautions a surgeon should take while managing skin wounds?

Ans: As skin wound tends to gap, therefore, surgeon must keep this thing in mind while closing the wound. The wound should be approximated properly with care, removable sutures used should be left in place for double the time than usual time.

Q. Name another disorder of defect in collagen metabolism.

Ans: Osteogenesis imperfecta.

Q. What are the criteria for joint hypermobility?

Ans: Nine points scoring system is used by *Beighton* for hypermobility of the joint. Two points are assigned for each of the following four paired (8 points) manoeuvres.

1. Hyperextension of the fifth metacarpophalangeal joint to 90°
2. Apposition of the thump to the volar aspect of forearm
3. Hyperextension of elbow to beyond 10°
4. Hyperextension of the knee to beyond 10°
5. The ninth point is assigned for the ability to place the palms of the hands on the floor with knees extended

In addition, there is laxity of small joints while the large joints are less lax.

Q. What are the clinical types of Ehlers-Danlos syndrome? What are their clinical features?

Ans: Read Table 187.1.

Q. **What is the effect of pregnancy in a patient with EDS?**

Ans: There are chances of:
- Severe postpartum hemorrhage
- Uterine prolapse
- Abdominal hernias
- Increased incidence of premature births

Q. **What profession is most suitable to patients with EDS?**

Ans: The patients with Ehlers-Danlos syndrome can become good flute players and string players because of laxity of fingers and wrist joints.

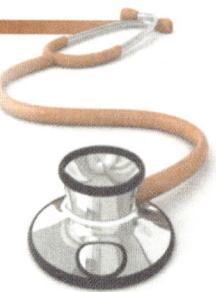

188

Alopecia Areata

INSTRUCTION

Perform general physical examination

SALIENT FEATURES

- Hair loss

HISTORY

Ask for the following:

- Age of the patient (75% are below the age of 40 years)
- Sex of the patient
- History of drugs
- History of atopy
- Family history of loss of hair (25% patients have positive history)
- History of local skin disease, pruritus
- History of wearing wigs
- History of other autoimmune disorder

EXAMINATION

General Physical Examination

Scalp: There are well defined, discrete patches of hair loss over the scalp and eyebrows (Fig. 188.1)
Nails: There is nail pitting with transverse lines, dystrophy, fragmentation and ridging. Nails are brittle with rough nail surface (present).
Look for evidence of vitiligo.

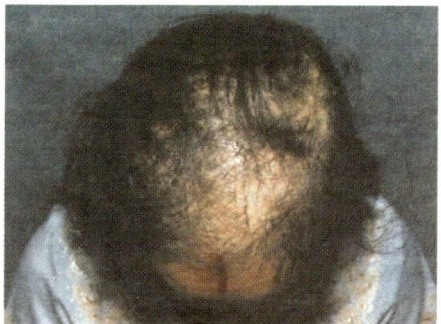

Fig. 188.1: Alopecia areata, e.g. patchy loss of scalp hair in a young female

PROVISIONAL DIAGNOSIS

The patient has alopecia areata (lesion) which is presumed to be autoimmune (aetiology) causing disfiguring of head and face (functional status).

QUESTIONS AND ANSWERS

Q. What is alopecia areata?

Ans: It is probable an autoimmune disorder involving, skin, hair and nails causing patchy nonscarring alopecia with pitting, ridging and furrowing of nails. It is nonscarring alopecia.

Q. What is differential diagnosis of alopecia areata?

Ans:
- Androgenic alopecia (common male baldness)
- Telogen effluvium
- Taenia capitis
- Traumatic alopecia
- Drug-induced (anti cancer drugs)
- Thyroid disorders

Q. What are the causes of nonscarring alopecia?

Ans: Read Table 188.1. The causes of nonscarring alopecia are:

Table 188.1
A. *Primary cutaneous disorders*
• Telogen effluvium
• Androgenic alopecia
• Alopecia areata
• Taenia capitis
• Traumatic alopecia
B. *Drugs,* e.g. Thallium, heparin, antimetabolites, antithyroid, hypervitaminosis, retinoids, oral contraceptives.
C. *Systemic diseases*
• SLE
• Secondary syphilis
• Hypo- and hyperthyroidism
• Deficiency of proteins, biotin and Zn
• HIV infection

Q. **What are the causes of scarring alopecia?**

Ans: The causes are:

A. *Primary cutaneous disorders*
- Cutaneous discoid lupus
- Lichen planus
- Folliculitis decalvans
- Linear scleroderma (morphea)

B. *Systemic diseases*
- SLE
- Sarcoidosis
- Cutaneous metastases

Q. **What are the sites of alopecia areata?**

Ans: The sites are:
1. Scalp
2. Beard, eyebrows and eyelashes
3. Moustache

Q. **What is pathognomonic sign of alopecia areata?**

Ans: The presence of *"exclamation mark hair"* at the periphery of lesion is the pathognomonic sign of disease activity. These hair are short that taper and become depigmented as the scalp is approached. Plucking reveals that the hair are in telogen phase.

Q. **Which systemic disorders are associated with alopecia areata?**

Ans: Alopecia areata being an immune-mediated non-inflammatory disorder is associated with other autoimmune disorders such as
- Autoimmune thyroid disorders, Addison's disease
- Vitiligo
- Down syndrome
- Pernicious anemia
- Atopy
- Hypogammaglobulinemia

Q. **Name the drugs causing alopecia.**

Ans: Read Table 188.1.

Q. **What is the commonest cause of alopecia?**

Ans: Alopecia areata.

Q. **Name the commonest systemic disorder producing alopecia.**

Ans: SLE

Q. **What is the treatment of alopecia areata?**

Ans:
- Steroids (topical and systemic)
- PUVA therapy but alopecia returns after stoppage of therapy
- Dithranol is left on the scalp for 20–30 minutes
- Topical minoxidil

Q. **What is alopecia totalis and alopecia universalis?**

Ans: If all the hair on the scalp are lost, it is called *alopecia totalis*, and if there is complete loss of body hair from all sites, it is called *alopecia universalis*.

Q. **What is trichotillomania?**

Ans: It is mechanical pulling of hair leading to broken hair. Hair loss is irregular and there is always hair growing as they are not long enough to be pulled out. The patch of hair loss is unilateral and occurs on the same side as the patient's dominant hand. The patient may be unaware of this habit.

Q. **What is telogen effluvium?**

Ans: It is transitory dying of the hair causing sudden diffuse shedding off normal hairs. The hair loss occurs due to major stresses, e.g. pregnancy, postpartum, acute psychiatric illness, emotional and physical trauma, surgery, oral contraceptives. It reverses without treatment.

Q. **What do you understand by male pattern baldness (androgenic alopecia)?**

Ans: In some men who are predisposed to this pattern of baldness, androgens cause a switch from terminal to vellus or vellus like follicles on the scalp hair of men and a reduction in the duration of an anagen phase. These individuals have increased androgens receptors and 5α-reductase activities (converts testosterone to 5-dehydrotestosterone) in frontal hair follicle is greater than in occipital follicles. This is an explanation of frontal baldness in men. Based on this concept, finasteride-5α-reductase inhibitor is useful for treatment as it causes regrowth of hair in 70% men after 2 years of continuous use.

Q. **How much hair loss occurs daily in normal person?**

Ans: About 70–100 hairs/day.

Q. **What do you understand by the term trichorrhexis nodosa?**

Ans: It is the fracture of hair shaft and is common in black patients who straighten their hair. If healthy care practices are followed, then hairs regrow healthily.

189

Erythema Nodosum

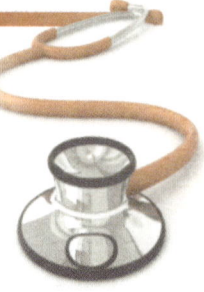

INSTRUCTION

Perform general physical examination

SALIENT FEATURES

- Skin lesion over the leg

HISTORY

Ask for the following:

- Ask history of fever preceding lesion.
- History of arthralgias
- Sore throat (β-hemolyticus streptococcal infection)
- Drugs (oral contraceptives, penicillins, sulphona-mides)
- Gastrointestinal symptoms (*Yersinia entero-colitica infection*)
- Infections, e.g. tuberculosis, leprosy, cocci-dioidomycosis, histoplasmosis
- Sarcoidosis

EXAMINATION

General Physical Examination

- The skin lesions are multiple, red erythematous nodules which are non-itchy, but painful and tender (Fig. 189.1)

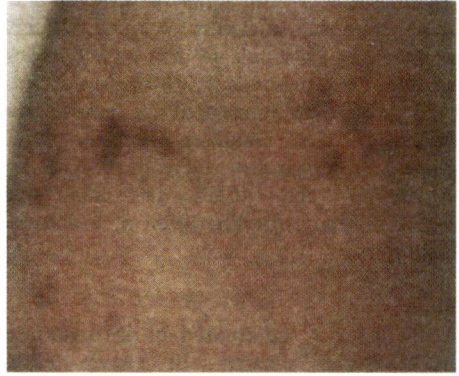

Fig. 189.1: Erythema nodosum

- They are bilateral and symmetrical (only one side is shown)
- They are present on the shin (in this case)

PROVISIONAL DIAGNOSIS

The patient has tender subcutaneous nodules due to erythema nodosum (lesion) on the legs caused by some drug (aetiology).

QUESTIONS AND ANSWERS

Q. What is erythema nodosum? What is com-mon site of this lesion?

Ans: *Erythema nodosum* is a panniculitis (inflam-mation of fat) characterized by painful, tender, subcutaneous, red (erythematous) nodules. The lesions are present on the extensor surfaces, e.g. anterior portion of leg (over the shin), thigh, upper arm or forearm. The lesions appear in crops, therefore, les-ions in different stages of evolution may be seen. Shin is the commonest site.

Q. What are the common causes of erythema nodosum?

Ans: Common *causes* are:
- Primary pulmonary tuberculosis
- Infections, e.g. β-*hemolyticus streptococci, yersinia, salmonella and chlamydia*
- Lepromatous leprosy
- Inflammatory bowel disease, e.g. ulcera-tive colitis or Crohn's disease
- Sarcoidosis
- Drug hypersensitivity, e.g. sulphona-mides, penicillins, oral contraceptives and barbiturates
- Fungal infections, e.g. *histoplasmosis or coccidioidomycosis*
- Behset's syndrome
- Brucellosis
- Rarely in rheumatic fever

Q. What is the basic pathology of the lesion?

Ans: This is type III (immune complex) hypersensitivity reaction, involves the fat (panniculitis) and the blood vessels (vasculitis).

The shin is the most common site of involvement because foreign proteins and bacteria are slowly removed from the "front of the legs" due to poor lymphatic drainage.

Q. How would you confirm the diagnosis?

Ans: By a *deep wedge biopsy* of the tissue which shows inflammatory reaction in the subcutaneous fat, i.e. edema, widening of connective tissue septae, fibrin, exudation and neutrophils infiltration followed by infiltration of lymphocytes, histiocytes and giant cells in later stages.

Q. What are the other common skin lesions over the shin?

Ans: In addition to erythema nodosum, other lesions are:
- *Pretibial myxedema* (a feature of Graves' dermopathy)
- *Necrobiosis lipoidica diabeticorum* (seen in diabetes)
- *Lichen amyloidosis*

Q. What is erythema nodosum leprosum?

Ans: Read the question on lepra reactions in leprosy (Case No 192).

Q. What are the causes of red (erythematous), subcutaneous nodules?

Ans: *Causes* are:
1. Inflamed epidermal inclusion cysts, acne cysts and furuncles
2. Panniculitis due to any cause
3. Cutaneous/systemic vasculitis, e.g.
   - Polyarteritis nodosa
   - Allergic granulomatosis
   - Wegener's granulomatosis
4. Cutaneous metastases

Q. How would you treat such a patient?

Ans: *Local:* Hot and cold compresses

Systemic: NSAIDs, salicylates, steroids or potassium iodide.

Q. What is panniculitis? What are its causes?

Ans: It is inflammation of subcutaneous fat, characterized by tender nodules either singly or in multiple crops.

Causes
- Collagen vascular disorders
- Factitious
- Lymphoma
- Weber-Christian disease
- Pancreatitis
- α_1 antitrypsin deficiency

N.B Erythema nodosum is a common examples of panniculitis.

190

Erythema Multiforme and Stevens-Johnson Syndrome

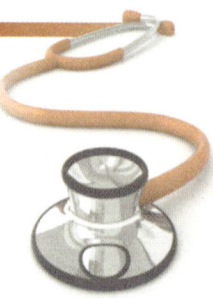

INSTRUCTION

Perform general physical examination

SALIENT FEATURES

- Fever with skin lesions

HISTORY

Ask for the following:

- History of previous sore throat, URC or cold
- Fever, joint pain
- Drug history (history of intake of NSAIDs present)
- History of mouth, lips and tongue ulceration (oral cavity involvement), nasal mucosa and conjunctival involvement
- Recurrent episodes

EXAMINATION

General Physical Examination

- Target-shaped lesions (Fig. 190.1) usually over the palms, soles and the skin (present). A target

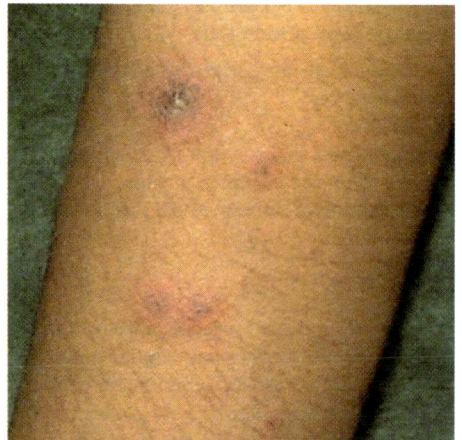

Fig. 190.1: Erythema multiforme caused by sulphonamides

lesion consists of a central dark purple area or blister surround by a pale edematous round zone which is further surrounded by a peripheral rim of erythema, hence, has pleomorphic appearance

- Eruptions of varying shapes and sizes, i.e. macules, papules and bullae/blisters
- *Mouth*: Look the buccal mucosa, gums, lips and tongue for mucosal lesions (present in Stevens-Johnson syndrome)
- *Genitalia*: Examine the genitalia for ulcers.

PROVISIONAL DIAGNOSIS

The patient has typical skin eruptions called erythema multiforme (lesion) caused by a drug (NSAIDs) which usually resolves on discontinuance of the drug (functional status).

QUESTIONS AND ANSWERS

Q. **What is erythema multiforme? What are its causes?**

Ans: Erythema multiforme is an abnormal cutaneous vascular cell-mediated hypersensitivity reaction to a number of stimuli.

The *causes* are:

1. Herpes simplex viral infection
2. Bacterial (streptococcus, mycoplasma) infection
3. Fungal infection, e.g. histoplasmosis
4. Parasitic infestations
5. *Drugs*, e.g. sulphonamides, barbiturates, penicillins, antimalarials
6. *Systemic diseases*, e.g. SLE, lymphoreticular malignancies (lymphomas), multiple myeloma
7. Pregnancy
8. Idiopathic. In 50% cases, no cause is found out.

Q.   What is Stevens-Johnson syndrome?

Ans: Stevens-Johnson syndrome (Fig. 190.2) is severe or major form of erythema multiforme characterized by erosions of skin and mucous membrane with hemorrhagic crusting, may lead to shock or hypotension creating an emergency situation in dermatology.

Q.   What is erythema marginatum?

Ans: It is an erythematous lesion (rash) seen in patients with acute rheumatic fever. It is a type of erythema multiforme, characterized by red/pink macules with pallor centre and irregular, red spreading margins. It is a migratory lesion, i.e. appears and disappears before the examiner's eyes.

It is nowadays rare lesion and usually not appreciated in the dark-complexion patients.

Q.   What is the histology of erythema marginatum?

Ans: There are three types of histological lesions:

I.   *Early lesions:* There is degeneration and necrosis of keratinocytes with superficial perivascular lymphocytic infiltration.

II. *Late lesions:* There is upward migration of lymphocytes from dermo-epidermal junction into epidermis, epidermal necro-sis resulting in blisters formation and subsequently sloughing and erosion of epidermis.

III. *Target lesions:* Central necrosis with perivenular inflammation.

Q.   How would you investigate such a case?

Ans: • Viral serology for herpes simplex type-I
 • Complement test for mycoplasma
 • ASO titres (antistreptolysin titre)
 • Urine for Bence-Jones protein
 • Protein electrophoresis

Q.   How would you manage erythema multiforme?

Ans: It is a self-limiting condition, may be treated as follows:

 • Symptomatic treatment with antibiotics, antipyretics and I.V. fluids
 • Systemic corticosteroids
 • *Other immunosuppressive drugs* used include levamisole, azathioprine, dapsone, thalidomide and high dose I.V immuno-globulin for recurrent erythema multiforme
 • *Aciclovir* is recommended on empirical basis in severe, recurrent disease even when there is no history of preceding herpes infection
 • *Local treatment,* e.g. antibiotic cream, ointments, sterile dressing, special beds containing beads, amnion dressing on denuded skin
 • *For eye care,* artificial tears and topical vit A is recommended.

Q.   What is the treatment of Stevens-Johnson syndrome?

Ans: Read Emergency Medicine by Prof SN Chugh.

Q.   What is Behçet's syndrome?

Ans: It is a syndrome of recurrent orogenital mucocutaneous ulceration of unknown etiology. Systemic manifestations involving the eyes, joints, brain may also occur. The mucocutaneous lesions are treated by colchicine or thalidomide while systemic manifestations require steroids or anti-mitotic drugs.

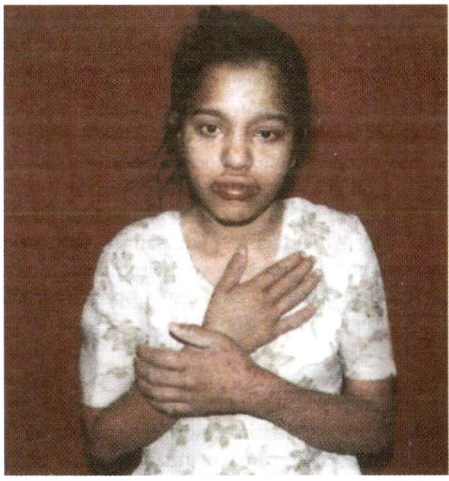

Fig. 190.2: Stevens-Johnson syndrome

191

Erythema Ab Igne

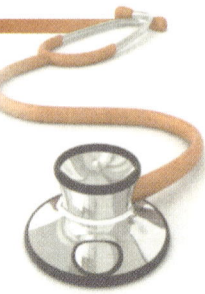

INSTRUCTION

Perform general physical examination

SALIENT FEATURES

- Readness over the back of abdomen

HISTORY

Ask about the following:

- History of loss of weight and loss of appetite, anemia, asthenia (internal malignancy)
- History of heat exposure to legs or abdomen (hot water bottle in this case), etc.
- History of severe abdominal pain (pancreatitis, renal/ biliary/ intestinal colic)

EXAMINATION

General Physical Examination

- Pulse and BP for hypothyroidism
- There is erythematous rash over the back of the abdomen (Fig. 191.1)

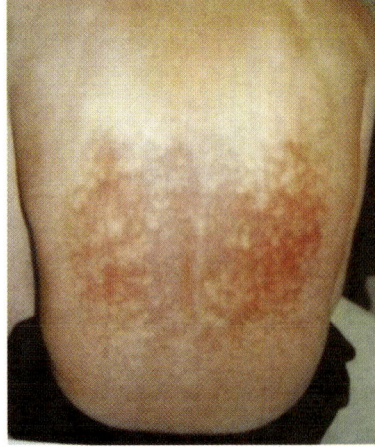

Fig. 191.1: Erythema ab igne produced by hot water bottle

- Look for the features of hypothyroidism (thick dry road like skin) and non pitting edema.
- Elicit the ankle jerks.

PROVISIONAL DIAGNOSIS

The patient has reticulated erythematous rash over the abdomen (lesion) caused by exposure to heat by using hot water bottle repeatedly (aetiology).

QUESTIONS AND ANSWERS

Q. What is erythema ab igne?

Ans: It is dusky discoloration of the skin due to repeated exposure to heat. The heat (<45°C) which is not painful and does not burn the skin, but produces reticulated net-like pigmentation over the exposed part (front of the legs in old person who sit in front of open fire places or abdomen or back of patients who use hot water bottles or heating pads for relief of pain in chronic painful conditions).

Q. What are the causes of erythematous rash over the abdomen?

Ans: • *Erythema ab igne* due to use of hot water bottle or heating pads
 • *Chronic hemorrhagic pancreatitis* (rash is present over the front of abdomen or lumbar region—Cullen's sign)
 • *Intra-abdominal malignancy*

Q. What is the complication of erythema ab igne?

Ans: Epithelioma

Q. What are the causes of reticulated rashes?

Ans: • Erythema ab igne
 • Livedo reticularis caused by PAW, SLE, occult malignancy, microembolisation in the skin.

Q. Name the heat related disorders.

Ans: • Heat stroke
 • Heat exhaustion
 • Heat hyperpyrexia
 • Heat cramps

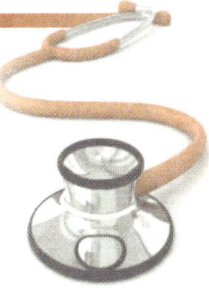

192

Leprosy

INSTRUCTION

Perform general physical examination

SALIENT FEATURES

- Hypopigmented lesion of forearm (Fig. 192.1)

HISTORY

Ask for the following:

- History of skin contact or with nasal secretions of a leprosy patient
- History of fever and pigmentation (kala azar)
- History of self-mutilation of fingers/toes
- History of cough, lever, arthralgia, lymphadenopathy, hepatosplenomegaly (sarcoidosis)
- History of tuberculosis
- Features suggestive of discoid lupus (SLE)

EXAMINATION

General Physical Examination

- The patient has a large well defined hypopigmented macular lesion which is anesthetic on testing. There is loss of hair over this patch (Fig. 192.1)
- Superficial nerves, e.g. superficial temporal, ulnar are palpable (in this case)
- No organomegaly

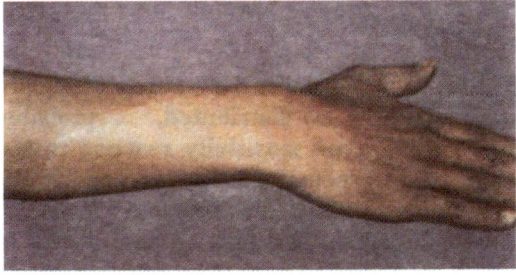

Fig. 192.1: Tuberculoid leprosy. A large well defined hypopigmented and hypoaesthetic macular lesion

PROVISIONAL DIAGNOSIS

The patient has a hypopigmented anesthetic macular lesion with palpable nerves (lesion) caused by tuberculoid leprosy (aetiology). He is depressed due to psychosocial stigma (functional status).

QUESTIONS AND ANSWERS

Q. What are the points in favor of your diagnosis?

Ans:
- A hypopigmented macule over the back of forearm
- The lesion is anesthetic on testing
- There is loss of hair over this patch
- The ulnar nerve is palpable
- Superficial temporal nerve is also palpable

Q. What is differential diagnosis of leprosy?

Ans: *Differential diagnosis of leprosy*

SLE: An early diffuse maculopapular lesion or circular lesion (discoid lupus) with erythematous rim may be seen over the face with depigmentation and follicular plugging.

Lupus Vulgaris: Well defined annular/arcuate plaques with erythermatous periphery is characteristic. Centre is depigmented and atrophic hence resembles leprosy. Sensations over the lesion are normal. Nerves are not palpable. The site of lesion is face and buttocks.

Sarcoidosis: Maculopapular rash with pruritus is common cutaneous lesion in sarcoidosis. Lupus pernio is common in black patients. Other features of the disease such as cough, fever, arthralgia lymphadenopathy, hepatosplenomegaly, ocular and cardiac features may be present.

Yaws: It is a chronic relapsing, nonveneral treponematosis characterised by early maculopapular lesions which can be confused with leprosy. These lesions are not anesthetic. Rheumatic like pains and palmar and plantar hyperkeratosis usually accompany these lesions. In late yaws, bones, cartilage, CNS, eyes, aorta or other organs are involved.

Post kala-azar dermal leishmaniasis: Even after successful treatment about 10% patients in India develop post kala-azar dermal leishmaniasis characterized by depigmented macules or pinkish papules and nodules. These macules are not anesthetic and LD bodies can be demonstrated in >60% cases in macules and >90% cases with nodules/papules.

Q. How is leprosy caused? What is the mode of transmission?

Ans: It is caused by *Mycobacterium leprae*—a gram-positive acid-fast and alcohol-fast bacillus called *Hansen's bacillus.*

Mode of Transmission: Man is only reservior of infection, hence, untreated patients with extensive disease (smear positive) are potential source of transmission to healthy persons. The routes of transmission are, nasal (aerosol) and oral while skin contact may also be a mode if lesion is ulcerated. Foamites and vectors do not play any role in its transmission.

Q. How do you classify leprosy? What are its different clinical types?

Ans: Depending on the cell-mediated immunity (CMI), the leprosy is classified into two polar forms and a borderline form (Fig. 192.2).

Note: *Lepromatous leprosy* means multibacillary (highly bacillated), low resistance with systemic disease, while *tuberculoid leprosy* means paucibacillary, high resistance with localized disease

Q. What are the causes of thickened peripheral nerves?

Ans: Causes are:
- Leprosy
- Sarcoidosis
- Diabetic neuropathy
- Charcot-Marie-Tooth disease
- Idiopathic hypertrophic neuropathy
- Neurofibromatosis
- Post-Guillain-Barré syndrome
- Dejerine-Sottas type neuropathy or Refsum's disease
- Amyloidosis
- Acromegaly

Q. What are the systemic manifestations of leprosy?

Ans:
1. Hepatosplenomegaly/lymphadenopathy
2. Nephrotic syndrome
3. Symmetric peripheral neuropathy with gloves and stocking type of anesthesia
4. Granulomatous uveitis and keratitis
5. *Leonine facies*
6. Testicular atrophy/Gynecomastia
7. Anemia (hemolytic, megaloblastic or iron deficiency)

These systemic manifestations occur in lepromatous leprosy.

Q. What is leonine facies?

Ans: Leonine facies (Fig. 192.3) includes:
- Lines on the forehead become deeper as well as upper central incisor teeth loosen or may fall. There is hoarseness voice
- Loss of hair on lateral thirds of eyebrows and thickened eyebrows
- Saddle deformity of nose
- Perforation of nasal septum
- Thickened skin of face due to massive infiltration especially earlobes

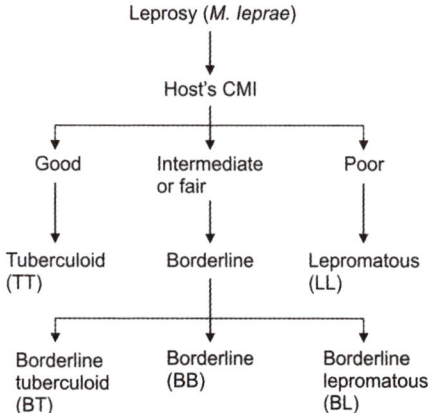

Fig. 192.2: Clinical types of leprosy depending on host immune status/CMI

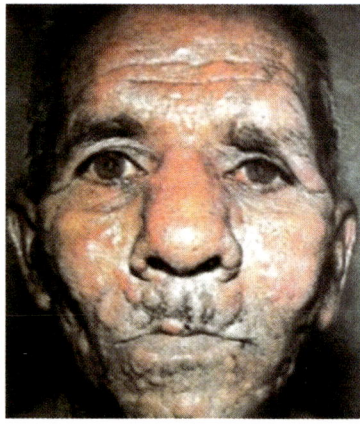

Fig. 192.3: Lepromatous leprosy. Note the typical leonine face in this type of leprosy

Q. What are the causes of leonine facies?

Ans:
- Albright disease
- Carcinoid syndrome
- Amyloidosis
- Cleidocranical dysostosis
- Primary hypertrophic osteoarthropathy
- B-cell lymphoma

Q. What are the complications of leprosy?

Ans: Complications are:
- Crippling deformities, e.g. claw hand
- Blindness
- Tuberculosis
- Secondary amyloidosis
- Social stigma

Q. What is lepromin test? What is its significance?

Ans: Lepromin is suspension of autoclaved *M. leprae* obtained from human or armadillos. 0.1 ml is injected intradermally and test result is read after 48–72 hours (*Fernandez reaction*) and 4 weeks (*Mitsuda reaction*). Fernandez reaction represents the delayed hypersensitivity while *Mitsuda reaction* represents cell-mediated immunity (CMI).

The test is strongly positive in tuberculoid leprosy, just positive in borderline tuberculoid and negative in lepromatous. In borderline it is weakly positive and negative in borderline lepromatous.

Q. What are the various reactions in leprosy?

Ans: 1. *Type I lepra reaction (reversal reaction* Fig. 192.4*):* It can complicate all the three borderline (BB, BT, BL) types, existing skin lesions develop erythema and swelling, new lesions may appear and the nerves become tender. It is managed by aspirin, corticosteroid and chloroquin.

2. *Type II Lepra reaction or erythema nodosum leprosum (ENL):* It occurs in lepromatous (LL) or borderline lepromatous (BL) patients. It occurs in patients in their second year of treatment. Tender, inflamed

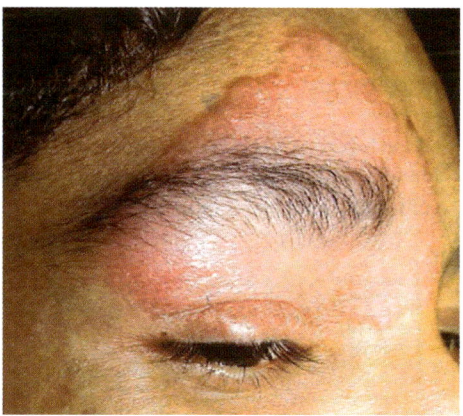

Fig. 192.4: Type I reaction in borderline tuberculoid leprosy erythematous plaque

subcutaneous nodules develop in crops with pain in the nerves. Fever, arthritis, lymphadenopathy may accompany severe ENL. Each nodule lasts for a week or two, but new crops may continue to appear.

It is treated by analgesics, antipyretics, thalidomide (contraindicated in pregnancy) or steroid and increasing the dose of clofazimine.

ENL develops due to immune-mediated (immune complex) reaction.

3. *Lucio phenomenon*: It is characterized by arteritis, is limited to patients with diffuse infiltrative non-nodular lepromatous leprosy. The patients develop angular ulcers. It is a complication rather than reaction.

Q. What are the disabilities/deformities in leprosy?

Ans: Exposure keratitis, claw hand, deformities of the fingers, contractures of toes and fingers, trophic changes as well as joint deformities can cause disabilities.

Q. How would you grade disabilities in leprosy?

Ans: Read Table 192.1.

Grade	Hands and feet	Eye
	Table 192.1: WHO grading of deformities/disabilities in leprosy	
Grade 0	No anesthesia. No visible deformity or damage	No eye problem due to leprosy. No Visual impairment
Grade 1	Anesthesia present. No visible deformity or damage	Eye problems due to leprosy are present Vision 6/60 or better, the patient can count fingers at 6 meters
Grade 2	Visible deformity or damage present	Severe visual impairment (vision less. than 6/60), the patient is unable to count fingers at 6 meters

Q. What is claw hand? What are its causes?

Ans: (Read case discussion 149 on ulnar nerve palsy)

Q. How do you diagnose leprosy?

Ans: Diagnosis is based on

1. *Slit skin smear stained with modified Ziehl-Neelsen* concentration (>104/g of tissue). Two indices are calculated. *Bacteriological index* (number of bacilli living or dead) is calculated on 6 points logarithmic scale. Bacteriological index in LL is 5 – 6 Bacteriological index in TT is 0
The morphological index (MI) of smear (% of all bacilli that stain solidly indicating living bacilli) is also calculated. This confirms the diagnosis.
2. *Skin biopsy*: It is done where diagnosis is in doubt and to classify the disease accurately.
3. *Nerve biopsy*: It is done in pure neuritic leprosy.
4. *Lepromin test* (positive in LL).
5. *Sweat function test* by pilocarpine or acetylcholine. Loss of sweat indicates leprosy.
6. *Fluorescent leprosy antibody absorption* (FLA-ABS) test to detect *M. leprae* specific antibody.
7. *ELISA* for antibody.
8. *Polymerase chain reaction* (PCR).

Q. How do you treat leprosy?

Ans: The WHO and NLEP regimens for treatment of paucibacillary (tuberculoid, borderline tuberculoid and indeterminate classes) and multibacillary (borderline lepromatous, lepromatous leprosy and indeterminate classes) leprosy are tabulated (Table 192.2).

Side Effects of Anti-leprosy Drug:

1. Clofazimine—red coloration of skin, urine and body secretions, abdominal pain, anorexia, nausea, vomiting, pruritus.
2. Dapsone—exfoliative dermatitis, hemolytic anemia, agranulocytosis, hepatitis, psychosis and hypoproteinemia.

Q. What is the possibility of vaccine in leprosy?

Ans: *Vaccine*: Attempts have been made to achieve quicker control of leprosy after the drugs have killed the lepra bacilli. For this various agents like BCG and mycobacterial vaccine (BCG + killed *M. leprae*, killed ICRC vaccine and killed M.W.) are being tried.

Table 192.2: WHO and NLEP regimens for leprosy				
Group	*Drugs*	*Adult dose (mg)*	*Regimen*	*Duration*
1. Paucibacillary (PB), i.e. BT, BB and TT	• Rifampicin • DDS	600 100	Once monthly supervised Daily self-administered	6 monthly pulses to maximum of 9 month
2. Multibacillary (MB), i.e. BL, LL	• Rifampicin • Clofazimine • Dapsone • Clofazimine	600 300 100 50	Once monthly supervised Daily self-administered	12 monthly pulses to maximum of 18 months

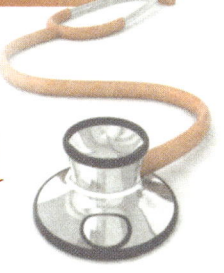

193 Systemic Lupus Erythematosus and Discoid Lupus

INSTRUCTION

Perform general physical examination

SALIENT FEATURES

- Joints pain with rash

HISTORY

Ask about the following:

- Tiredness and fatiguability
- Polyarthritis (Small joints involvement present)
- Digital gangrene (vasculitis)
- Skin rash, alopecia, Raynaud's phenomenon
- Mouth ulcer
- Puffiness of face, edema
- Fever and lymphadenopathy
- Bleeding from gums, nose or menstrual bleeding
- History of seizures
- History of relapses and remission
- Drug history

EXAMINATION

General Physical Examination

- *Face* for butterfly rash (present), edema and cushingoid features
- *Conjunctiva* for anemia
- *Mouth* for oral ulcers (present)
- *Scalp* for alopecia (patchy alopecia present)
- *Blood pressure* (may be raised in SLE)
- *Neck* for JVP and lymphadenopathy
- Look for subcutaneous nodules and vasculitic rash over sun exposed areas
- *Nails* for splinter hemorrhages, finger infarcts and digital gangrene
- *Hands* for palmar erythema, Raynaud's phenomenon, vasculitis
- *Joints* for arthritis (present)
- *Feet* for pitting edema (nephrotic syndrome present)

- *Urine* for proteinuria (present)
- *Abdomen* for hepatosplenomegaly

PROVISIONAL DIAGNOSIS

The patient has malar rash over the face with telangiectasia (lesion) caused by SLE (aetiology). Patient has nephrotic syndrome (lupus nephritis) as evidenced by massive edema legs and proteinuria (functional status).

QUESTIONS AND ANSWERS

Q. **What do you understand by the term lupus face?**

Ans: This patient has typical lupus face consisting of:

- Classical photosensitive 'butterfly' rash over the nose extending over the malar areas (Fig. 193.1)
- Patchy alopecia
- Lupus hairs—short broken hair seen above the forehead
- Oral ulcers seen on opening the mouth

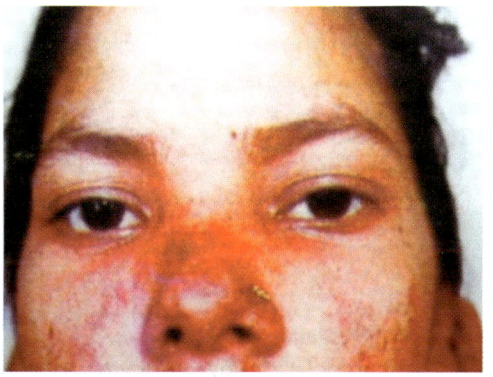

Fig. 193.1: Butterfly rash—malar rash of systemic lupus erythematosus

Q. **What are the skin manifestations of SLE?**

Ans: The cutaneous manifestations of SLE can be divided into acute, subacute and chronic (i.e. discoid LE). In addition to 'butterfly rash', the other lesions are:

- Ill-defined, discrete erythematous papules (papulosquamous form) on the back, chest, shoulders and extensor surfaces of arms and hands. There is associated scaling.
- Sometimes annular lesions resembling erythema multiforme may appear as an oral or circular erythematous papules
- Purpura
- Bullous lesion
- Panniculitis
- Digital infarcts
- Livedo reticularis
- Raynaud's phenomenon
- Angioneurotic edema
- Pigmentation and patchy alopecia

Q. **What is discoid lupus?**

Ans: Discoid lupus is a chronic skin lesion seen in 20% patients with SLE characterized by:

- Circular lesions with an erythematous rim over the face, scalp or external ears
- Follicular plugging (thick scales oclude the hair follicles). When scales are removed, its underside will show small excrescences that correlate with the openings of hair follicles and is termed as "*carpet track appearance*". This finding is specific for DLE
- Long-standing lesions develop scarring and atrophy
- Hypopigmentation
- Telangiectasia

Q. **What are the causes of SLE?**

Ans: Etiological factors incriminated in SLE are:

1. *Genetic*
   HLA B8, DR3, DR2
   Inherited complement deficiencies, C4 null allele
2. *Environmental*
   - UV light
   - Physical and emotional stress
   - Infection
   - Female sex hormones
   - Drugs, e.g. procainamide, quinidine, hydralazine, methyldopa, isoniazid, chlorpromazine

Q. **What are the hematological manifestations of SLE?**

Ans: • Anemia, leukopenia, thrombocytopenia

- Lupus anticoagulant (anti-phospholipid syndrome)
- Splenomegaly and lymphadenopathy

Q. **What are the neurological manifestations of SLE?**

Ans: • Headache, migraine
- Cognitive dysfunction
- Organic brain syndromes (e.g. psychosis, seizures)
- Cranial nerve involvement, hemiplegia
- Transverse myelitis
- Peripheral neuropathy
- Extrapyramidal disorders (chorea) and cerebellar dysfunction

Q. **What are the cardiopulmonary manifestations of SLE?**

Ans: • Pleurisy, pneumonia, pleural effusion, ARDS
- Pericarditis/myocarditis
- Endocarditis (Libman-Sachs)
- Interstitial fibrosis/fibrosing alveolitis
- Heart blocks and arrhythmias

Q. **What are the renal manifestations of SLE?**

Ans: • Proteinuria, hematuria
- Renal failure
- Nephrotic/nephritic syndrome
- Urinary tract infection

Q. **What are ocular manifestations of SLE?**

Ans: • Conjunctivitis/episcleritis
- Sicca syndrome
- Retinal vasculitis

Q. **How would you classify SLE?**

Ans: Read Table 193.1.

Q. **Name the autoantibodies in SLE.**

Ans: The autoantibodies in SLE are:

1. *Antinuclear antibodies* against multiple nuclear antigens. These are sensitive but not specific autoantibodies.
2. *Anti-ds DNA* is more specific than anti-s DNA.
3. *Anti-Sm* (specific for SLE).
4. *Anti-RNP*–present in mixed connective tissue disease.
5. *Anti-RO (SS-A)* is associated with ANA negative lupus.
6. *Anti-LA (SS-B)* occurs in neonatal lupus, in elderly Sjögren's syndrome.
7. *Anti-histone,* e.g. drug-induced lupus.
8. *Antiphospholipid antibodies* (e.g. three types are recognized such as lupus anticoagulant, anti-cardiolipin and anit-β_2 glycoprotein-I
9. *Anti-erythrocytes* antibodies.

Table 193.1: SLICC⁺ Classification criteria for systemic lupus erythematosus

I. CLINICAL CRITERIA

1. **Acute/Subacute Cutaneous Lesion**
   - **Acute cutaneous lupus:** lupus malar rash (do not count if malar discoid), bullous lupus, toxic epidermal necrolysis—variant of SLE, maculopapular lupus rash, photosensitive lupus rash (in the absence of dermatomyositis)
   - **Subacute cutaneous lupus:** nonindurated psoriaform and/or annular polycyclic lesions that resolve without scarring, although occasionally with postinflammatory dyspigmentation or telangiectasias

2. **Chronic Cutaneous Lupus**
   - Classic discoid rash localized (above the neck) or generalized (above and below the neck), hypertrophic (verrucous) lupus, lupus panniculitis (profundus), mucosal lupus, lupus erythematosus tumidus, chilblains lupus, discoid lupus/lichen planus overlap.

3. **Oral Ulcers Or Nasal Ulcers**
   - Oral: palate, buccal, tongue, nasal ulcers in the absence of other causes, such as vasculitis, Behcet's disease infection (herpes virus), inflammatory bowel disease, reactive arthritis and acidic foods.

4. **Nanscarring Alopecia**
   - Diffuse thinning or hair fragility with visible broken hairs in the absence of other causes such as alopecia areata, drugs, iron deficiency and androgenic alopecia.

5. **Synovitis Involving 2 or More Joints**
   - Characterized by swelling or effusion **OR**
   - Tenderness in 2 or more joints and at least 30 minutes of morning stiffness.

6. **Serositis**
   - Typical pleurisy for more than 1 day **OR** pleural effusions **OR** pleural rub
   - Typical pericardial pain (pain with recumbency improved by sitting forward) for more than 1 day **OR** pericardial effusion **OR** pericardial rub **OR** pericardins by electrocardiography
   - This should be in the absence of other causes, such as infection, uremia and Dressler's pericarditis.

7. **Renal**
   - Urine protein-to-creatinine ratio (or 24-hour urine protein) representing 500 mg protein/24 hours OR red blood cell casts.

8. **Neurologic**
   - Seizures, psychosis, mononeuritis multiplex (in the absence of other known causes such as primary vasculitis), myelitis, peripheral or cranial neuropathy (in the absence of other known causes such as primary vasculitis, infection and diabetes mellitus), acute confusional state (in the absence of other causes, including toxic, metabolic, uremia, drugs)

9. **Hemolytic Anemia**

10. **Leukopenia ($<4000/mm^3$) OR Lymphopenia ($<1500/mm^3$)**
    - Leucopenia at least once in the absence of other known causes such as Felty syndrome, drugs and portal hypertension.
    - Lymphopenia at least once in the absence of other known causes such as corticosteroids, drugs and infection.

11. **Thrombocytopenia ($<100,000/mm^3$)**
    - At least once in the absence of other known causes such as drugs portal hypertension and thrombotic thrombocytopenic purpura.

II. IMMUNOLOGIC CRITERIA

1. *ANA level* above laboratory reference range
2. *Anti-dsDNA antibody* level above laboratory reference range (or 2-fold the reference range tested by ELISA)
3. *Anti-Sm:* presence of antibody to Sm nuclear antigen
4. *Antiphospholipid antibody positivity,* as determined by
   - Positive test for lupus anticoagulant
   - False-positive test result for rapid plasma reagin
   - Medium or high-titre anticardiolipin antibody level (IgA, IgG or IgM)
   - Positive test result for anti-β_2-glycoprotein I (IgA, IgG or IgM)
5. *Low complement* (C3, C4 or CH50)
6. *Direct Coombs test* (in the absence of hemolytic anemia)

Diagnostic criteria (at least 4 clinical and 1 laboratory criteria)
OR biopsy-proven lupus nephritis with positive ANA or anti-DNA

10. *Anti-platelet*, anti-lymphocyte antibodies.
11. *Anti-neuronal*, e.g. in diffuse CNS lupus.
12. *Anti-ribosomal* P, e.g. in psychosis, CNS lupus.

Q. How will you investigate a case of SLE?

Ans: The investigations done are:

- *Hemaglobin* for anemia. ESR will be raised
- *Total and differential leukocyte count* for leukopenia, lymphopenia and thrombocytopenia
- *Urine* for hematuria, proteinuria and casts
- *Serological tests for syphilis* may be positive
- *Autoantibodies detections.* The ANA, anti-Sm, anti-DNA and antiphospholipids antibodies are done commonly
- *Coombs' test*—Direct test may be positive
- *Serum complement* may be low
- *Other tests* depending on the organ/system involvement.

Q. What is the treatment of SLE?

Ans: Treatment according to severity is as follows:

I. *Therapy for mild to moderate disease*
  - Bed rest
  - NSAIDs and Cox-2 inhibitors
  - Antimalarials, e.g. hydroxychloroquin, chloroquin for treating lupus rashes and arthritis that do not respond to NSAIDs. Chloroquin 200 mg/day is given. Patient is advised eye checkup after every 6 months.

II. *Therapy for SLE with life-threatening manifestations*

- Topical steroids are used for skin lesions.
- Systemic steroids in immunosuppressive dosage are used in SLE with life-threatening manifestations such as glomerulonephritis, hemolytic anemia, myopericarditis, CNS involvement and thrombotic thrombocytopenic purpura.
- Methylprednisolone can also be used in the dose of 1 g daily for 3 days followed 0.5 to 1 mg/kg/day of oral prednisolone.
- Lupus nephritis needs renal biopsy for confirmation. Focal renal lesions respond to steroids. However, diffuse proliterative of membranoproliferative forms of nephritis (WHO grades III, IV, V) need cyclophosphamide or azathioprine along with steroids. Dialysis is indicated in renal failure.
- Antiphospholipid syndrome is treated with aspirin and anticoagulation.
- Infection is treated with appropriate antibiotics.
- *Pregnancy with lupus*: SLE is controlled with the lowest dose of prednisolone for the shortest period. Pregnancy with recurrent fetal loss and antiphospholipid antibodies is treated with aspirin and low molecular heparin.
- SLE with thrombotic thrombocytopenic purpura or hemolytic uremic syndrome is treated by plasmapheresis.

194

Antiphospholipid Syndrome

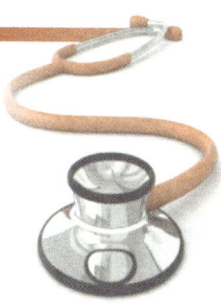

INSTRUCTION

- Take the detailed history
- Perform general physical examination

SALIENT FEATURES

- Repeated abortions

HISTORY

Ask for the following:

- History of recurrent thromboembolism, DVT
- History of repeated abortions (Fig. 194.1)
- History of bleeding
- History of gangrene
- Stroke
- Fever
- Chest pain or coronary artery disease
- Visual disturbances or blindness

EXAMINATION

General Physical Examination

- Look for features of SLE (read it as a case report 193)
- Look for valvular heart disease

PROVISIONAL DIAGNOSIS

The female has history of recurrent fetal loss (lesion) due to antiphospholipid syndrome (aetiology), the cause of which is still unknown. The lady is mentally disturbed (functional status).

QUESTIONS AND ANSWERS

Q. **What is an autoantibody? Which antibody is more sensitive and which one is more specific for SLE?**

Ans: Autoantibody means antibody produced against own (self) antigen. Antinuclear antibodies (ANAs) mean antibodies produced against nuclear components of a cell. Antinuclear antibodies are the best screening test as they are more sensitive. A positive ANA test is not specific for SLE. Anti-Sm is specific for SLE.

Q. **What are the causes of ANA?**

Ans:
- Normal individual (low titer)
- Other autoimmune diseases
- Viral infections
- Chronic inflammatory diseases
- Several drugs-induced ANA

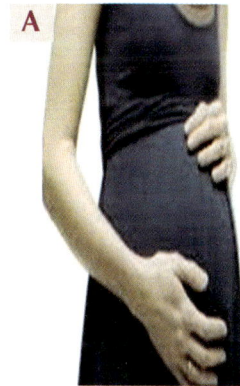

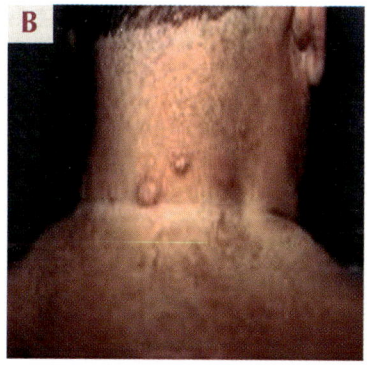

Fig. 194.1: Antiphospholipid syndrome. (A) Pregnant woman at risk of abortion; (B) Sweet's syndrome

Q. **What are antiphospholipid antibodies and what is their significance?**

Ans: A syndrome resulting from the production of antiphospholipid antibodies (e.g. lupus anticoagulant, anticardiolipin, anti-β_2 glycoprotein-I and false-positive VDRL) is called *antiphospholipid syndrome*, commonly seen in SLE and other autoimmune disorders.

The presence of these antibodies is associated with:
- Increased coagulopathy (arterial, venous thrombosis)
- Fetal loss
- Thrombocytopenia
- Valvular heart disease

Q. **Can woman with antiphospholipid syndrome (APS) have successful pregnancy?**

Ans: Yes, if woman has one antiphospholipid antibody test positive. If all the three antibodies tests, i.e. lupus anticoagulant, anticardiolipin antibodies and antibodies to beta-2 glycoprotein-I are positive, the woman is at highest risk.

Q. **What is antiphospholipid antibody syndrome (APS)?**

Ans: The antiphospholipid antibody syndrome (APS) is said to be present if the patient has persistently elevated (twice at least 3 months apart) levels of antiphospholipid antibody and/or positive lupus anticoagulant test and the presence of one of the following, i.e. arterial or venous thrombosis, fetal loss, thrombocytopenia.

Q. **What are the causes of APS?**

Ans: 1. *Primary*—no definite cause is known
2. *Secondary*
   - SLE
   - Infections
   - Drug-induced lupus
   - Malignancy

Q. **What are the clinical features of APS?**

Ans: • Recurrent thromboembolism
- Recurrent fetal loss (2 or more)
- Livedo reticularis
- Nonstroke neurological manifestations
- Valvular heart disease
- Thrombocytopenia
- Catastrophic vascular occlusion

Q. **How do you classify APS?**

Ans: *Classification of APS is as follows:*
Type 1 : DVT with pulmonary embolism
Type 2 : Coronary and peripheral artery thrombosis
Type 3 : Cerebrovascular or retinal artery thrombosis
Type 4 : Mixed type

Q. **How would you treat APS?**

Ans: • Anticoagulants, e.g. heparin including low molecular weight (LMWH)
- Antiplatelets, e.g. aspirin
- Intravenous immunoglobulins (IgG)
- Immunosuppressants and steroids

Q. **What is Sweet's syndrome?**

Ans: Sweet's syndrome (Fig. 194.1B) also referred to as acute febrile neutrophilic dermatosis, is characterised by a constellation of symptoms and findings, i.e. fever, neutrophilia, erythematous painful skin lesions (pseudovesicular nodules/plaques) and prompt improvement of symptoms and lesions after treatment with systemic steroids. It is seen in patients with systemic diseases, internal malignancy, antiphospholipid syndrome and may be drug-induced.

195

Hyperpigmentation

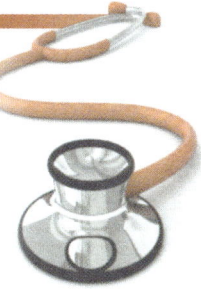

INSTRUCTION

Perform general physical examination

SALIENT FEATURES

• Excessive pigmentation

HISTORY

Ask for the following:

• History of fever (kala-azar)
• Pain in abdomen or distension of abdomen
• GI hemorrhage or rectal bleeding
• Family history of such disease
• History of diabetes (hemochromatosis)
• Drug history

EXAMINATION

General Physical Examination

• BP for Addison's disease
• Look for pigmentation over the creases of palms
• Circumoral pigmentation (Peutz-Jeghers syndrome)

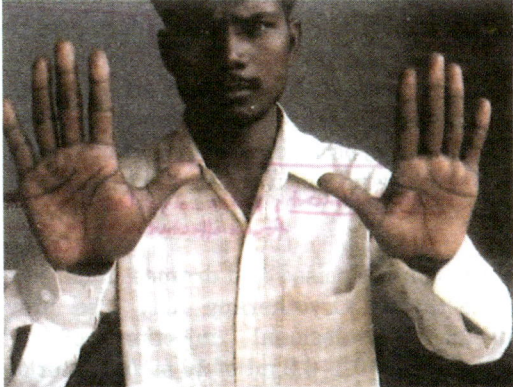

Fig. 195.1: Idiopathic pigmentation of face and hands in a young adult

• Look for pigmentation of buccal mucosa (Addison's disease, malabsorption, Peutz-Jeghers syndrome)
• Pigmentation over the face (melasma or chloasma)
• Pigmentation over face, forehead, mouth (kala-azar)

Systemic Examination

• Hepatosplenomegaly for kala-azar

PROVISIONAL DIAGNOSIS

The patient has hyperpigmentation of face, mouth, lips and hands (lesion). The cause of which has to be found out, could be familial (aetiology).

QUESTIONS AND ANSWERS

Q. **What is hyperpigmentation? What are its causes?**

Ans: Abnormal increased pigmentation is called *hyperpigmentation* which may be localized (due to skin disorders) or generalized (due to systemic disorders).

The causes of hyperpigmentation are:

I. Localised pigmentation

• *Acanthosis nigricans*
• Lentigo, ephelids (freckles)
• Peutz-Jeghers syndrome
• LEOPARD, LAMB, NAME syndrome
• Café au lait spots

II. Generalised pigmentation

• Addison's disease
• Porphyria
• Hemochromatosis
• Pellagra
• Biliary cirrhosis
• POEM syndrome
• Drugs

Q. Name the drugs causing pigmentation.

Ans: • Minocycline, cancer chemotherapy, clofazimine, psoralens, bleomycin.

Q. What is kala-azar? What is the type and site of pigmentation?

Ans: Kala-azar (Hindi version of "black fever") is caused by Leishmania, hence called *leishmaniasis*.

The skin lesions including hyperpigmentation develop in some patients during or within a few months of therapy (e.g. in East Africa) or years after therapy (e.g. in India). The lesions are pigmented macules, papules, nodules or patches typically seen over the face around the mouth, on the temple and forehead.

Q. What are the sites of pigmentation in Addison's disease?

Ans: Sites are:
1. Pressure points (elbow)
2. Normally pigmented areas (areola, genitalia, knuckles, palmar creases and scars)
3. Mucous membranes (mouth)

Q. What is the site and type of pigmentation in hemochromatosis?

Ans: Skin pigmentation is called *bronze pigmentation*, occurs due to excessive deposition of melanin and iron, gives a metallic or slate gray hue to the skin. The pigmentation is diffuse and generalized, but may be more pronounced on the face, neck, extensor surfaces of lower forearms, dorsum of the head, lower legs, genitalia and in scars.

Q. What is Peutz-Jeghers syndrome?

Ans: It is a heritable (autosomal dominant) disorder characterized by polyposis of small intestine and colon with mucocutaneous (circumoral) pigmentation and tumors of the ovary, breast, pancreas and endometrium. The chances of malignant transformation of polyposis are rare.

Q. What is chloasma or melasma?

Ans: This is symmetrical hyperpigmentation seen on malar prominences and bridge of the nose mostly in young females (very rare in males) precipitated by pregnancy (chloasma gravidarum) or following prolonged use of oral contraceptives—called *mask of pregnancy*.

Q. What is malar flush?

Ans: • Read malar flush in mitral stenosis (mitral facies).

Q. Name the syndromes associated with localized hyperpigmentation (lentigines).

Ans: 1. *LEOPARD syndrome*
- **L** stands for lentigines (localized multiple hyperpigmentation)
- **E** stands for ECG abnormalities (conduction defects)
- **O** for ocular hypertelorism
- **P** stands for pulmonary stenosis and aortic stenosis
- **A** stands for abnormal genitalia (cryptorchidism, hypospadias)
- **R** stands for retardation of growth
- **D** stands for deafness—sensorineural

2. *NAME and LAMB syndromes*

Localized pigmentation, e.g. lentigines are associated with atrial myxomas in two syndromes, i.e. NAME (Nevus, Atrial myxoma, Myxoid neurofibroma and Ephelides) and LAMB (Lentigines, Atrial myxoma, Mucocutaneous myxomas and Blue nevi). These patients can have endocrinopathies in the form of Cushing's syndrome, acromegaly or sexual precocity.

Q. What is lentigines? How do they differ from freckles?

Ans: Lentigines are light brown or dark brown macules of varying sizes (1–10 mm), discrete and present on any part of the body. The differences between freckles and lentigines are given in Table 195.1.

Table 195.1: Freckles vs Lentigines

Freckles	Lentigines
• Individuals are fair skined	Any skin color
• Located to photoexposed areas	Any part of the skin and even mucosa
• Variable in color, e.g. light to dark	Each lesion is of uniform color
• Darken on exposure to sunlight	No change in color

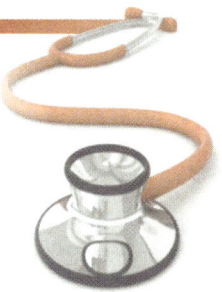

196

Raynaud's Phenomenon

INSTRUCTION

Perform general physical examination

SALIENT FEATURES

- Colour change of the fingers

HISTORY

Ask for the following:

- Whether the condition is precipitated by cold, emotion and relieved by heat (yes, in this case)?
- Whether episodes of skin change is painful or not?
- It there any sensory disturbance in hands (e.g. numbness), stiffness, aching pain?
- What is occupation of the patient? (polishing tools, vibrating tools)
- Is there any dysphagia (ask for CREST syndrome)?
- History of use of electrically heated gloves.
- History of SLE or other collagen vascular disease (butterfly rash, arthralgia, dry mouth, etc.)

EXAMINATION

General Physical Examination

- Examine the face for signs of scleroderma, i.e. mask-like face, thickening and tightening of skin over face and mouth, inability to open the mouth, telangiectasia of face, lip, tongue, etc.
- Look for butterfly rash, polyarthritis.
- Examine the hands. The hands and fingers are painful, tender, cyanosed and cold (Fig. 196.1) or may be warm or red or blue. The thumbs are rarely affected.
- Examine upper limb pulses.
- Blood pressure in both the upper limbs for cervical rib.

PROVISIONAL DIAGNOSIS

The patient has cold blue (cyanosed) hands (lesion) caused by a vasospastic phenomenon called

Raynaud's phenomenon (aetiology). The episodes are painful (functional status).

QUESTIONS AND ANSWERS

Q. What is Raynaud's phenomenon?

Ans: Raynaud's phenomenon is characterized by episodic vasospasms of digital arteries leading to sequential development of tricolor response (digital blanching, cyanosis and rubor) of the fingers or toes following cold exposure and subsequent return on rewarming. In this phenomenon, patient experiences pallor or whiteness of fingers or toes when exposed to cold environment or touching a cold object. Emotional stress precipitates this phenomenon.

Q. What is differential diagnosis of Raynaud's phenomenon?

Ans: The differential diagnosis lies within the causes of Raynaud's phenomenon, i.e.
   1. Raynaud's disease
   2. Scleroderma (systemic sclerosis)
   3. Vasculitis (connective tissue disease)
   4. Thoracic outlet syndrome or cervical rib

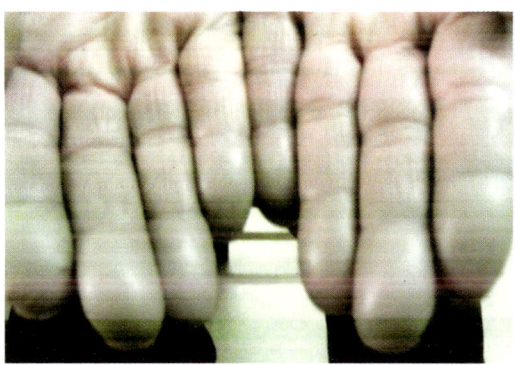

Fig. 196.1: Raynaud's phenomenon

Q. What is pathophysiology of Raynaud's phenomenon?

Ans: Raynaud's phenomenon is cold-induced episodic digital ischemia secondary to reflex sympathetic vasoconstriction or an enhanced vascular response to cold or normal sympathetic stimuli.

Q. How do you classify Raynaud's phenomenon?

Ans: It is divided into two categories:
1. *Raynaud's disease:* It is idiopathic.
2. *Secondary Raynaud's phenomenon:* It is secondary to some identifiable cause.

Q. Can Raynaud's phenomenon lead to gangrene?

Ans: Yes, though Raynaud's phenomenon is reversible on rewarming, but in severe disease, prolonged vasospasm can result in loss of digital pulp, stellate digital ulcer and eventually gangrene.

Q. What is the pathogenesis of tricolor response?

Ans: Read Table 196.1

Table 196.1: Tricolor response in Raynaud's phenomenon

Color	Mechanism
Pallor or whiteness	Digital ischemia due to vaso-constriction
Bluishness (cyanosis)	Local capillaries and venules dilate and cyanosis results from deoxygenated blood present in these vessels
Redness (Rubor)	Resolution of vasospasm and reactive hyperemia due to vaso-dilatation and return of blood flow imparts a bright red color to the digits

Note: Although tricolor response is a characteristic of Raynaud's phenomenon, but some patients may experience only pallor and cyanosis or only cyanosis.

Q. What is Raynaud's disease?

Ans: It is primary idiopathic Raynaud's phenomenon hence, it is diagnosed by exclusion.

It affects young females (20–40 years) and is confined to fingers more frequently than toes. Peripheral (radial, ulnar and pedal) pulses are normal.

The patients tend to have attacks of pain and paraesthesia with tricolor response which resolves completely in most of the cases or may improve spontaneously in about 15 percent cases, while in 30 percent cases it may progress.

Q. What are the common causes of Raynaud's phenomenon?

Ans:
1. Raynaud's disease (idiopathic)
2. Collagen vascular disease, e.g. SLE, scleroderma
3. Primary pulmonary hypertension
4. Cold injury or mechanical injury
5. Myeloproliferative disorders, e.g. leukemias, lymphomas
6. Thoracic outlet syndrome
7. Drugs, e.g. ergot alkaloids, beta blockers, methysergide, cisplastin

Q. What is the signification of occupational history in Raynaud's phenomenon?

Ans: Mechanical injury in certain occupation (i.e. polishing tools, vibrating tools, typing, drilling piano-playing) can lead to vasospastic (Raynaud's) phenomenon.

Q. Name some vasospastic conditions.
Ans:
- White finger syndrom • Chilblain
- Livedo reticularis • Erythromelalgia

Q. How would you investigate a case of Raynaud's phenomenon?

Ans:
- Complete hemogram, ESR
- Total immunoglobulin and immuno-globulin electrophoresis
- Urine exam
- Chest X-ray
- Renal and liver function test
- Test for antinuclear antibody
- Hand radiography
- Nail-fold capillaroscopy

Q. What is the treatment of Raynaud's phenomenon?

Ans: Most of the patients have mild attacks, do not need treatment except reassurance and protection of the body from exposure to cold by warm clothings, gloves and socks.
- *Drug treatment:* It is indicated in severe cases. The calcium channel blockers, e.g. nifedipine (10–30 mg tds) and diltiazem (30–90 mg tds) or nitrates decrease the frequency and severity of attacks. Postsynaptic alpha blockers, e.g. prazosin (1–5 mg tds), doxazosin and tetrazosin may be effective. Long-term use of reserpine (0.25–0.5 mg q.i.d.) therapy is not recommended due to adverse effects.

  Treatment with vasodilator prostaglandins 12 is under investigation.
- *Surgical sympathectomy* is helpful in those cases who are resistant to medical therapy and trophic changes interfere with work.

197

Scleroderma

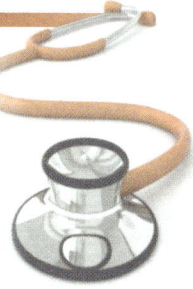

INSTRUCTION

- Perform general physical examination

SALIENT FEATURES

- Difficulty in opening the mouth

HISTORY

Ask for the following:

- History of tightness of fingers and face (present)
- History of Raynaud's phenomenon
- Puffy hands (fingers) and feet (toes)
- Fatigue, weakness
- History of dyspnea, dry cough (lung involvement)
- History of dysphagia (present), diarrhea, bloating and indigestion (GI involvement)
- Dryness of eyes
- History of joint pain/polyarthritis or muscular weakness (proximal myopathy)
- History of hypertension or renal failure or CHF

EXAMINATION

General Physical Examination (Fig. 197.1)

- Expressionless (mask-like) face (present)
- Absence of normal skin wrinkling (present)
- Pinched out nose or beaking of nose (present)
- Microstomia
- Telangiectasia of fingers (present), face, lips, tongue, etc.
- Inability to open the mouth (present)
- Skin is glossy and shiny (present)
- Pigmentation and depigmentation

Hands in scleroderma

- Sclerodactyly, e.g. skin is thick and tight bound on the fingers and cannot be lifted (Fig. 197.1B)
- Symmetrical puffy fingers
- Limitation of movements (extension and flexion of fingers) leading to contractures
- The fingertips may lose soft tissue (pulp atrophy present) due to sclerodactyly and develop digital ulcers (Fig. 197.1B) and scars

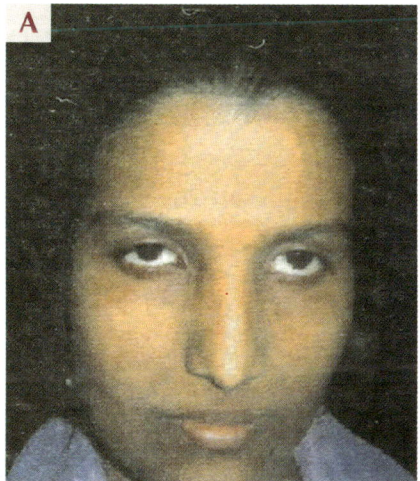

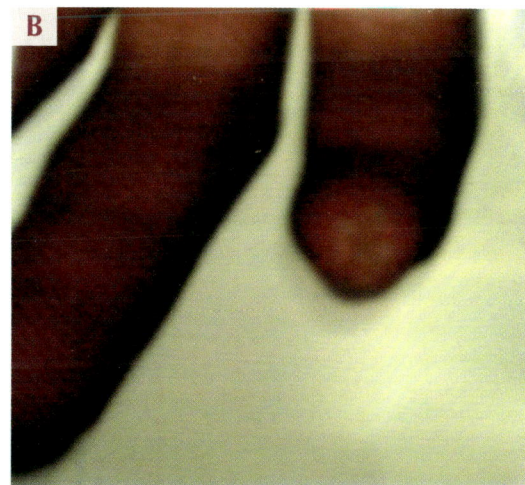

Fig. 197.1: Scleroderma. (A) Patient; (B) Sclerodactyly with sterillite fingertips

- Skin is dry, coarse but shiny with loss of hairs
- Nail fold changes include thrombi, blotchy telangiectasia (present)
- Digital infarcts and gangrene
- Pseudoclubbing (beaking of nails) may be present due to bone resorption of terminal phalanx

Relevant Other System Examination

N.B Tell the examiner that you would like to examine other systems which are likely to be involved in this condition.

- Examine the system likely to be involved, i.e.
  - CVS
  - Respiratory (bilateral basal crackles present)
  - Abdomen, e.g. liver for primary biliary cirrhosis

PROVISIONAL DIAGNOSIS

The patient has tightening of the skin over the fingers, sclerodactyly (finger pulp atrophy), beaking of nails, nail telangiectasia (lesion) caused by scleroderma (aetiology). He is finding difficulty in doing daily life activities and has dysphagia (functional status).

Q. What are the points in favor of your diagnosis?

Ans:
1. A young female with expressionless face and inability to open the mouth
2. Skin is thin, shiny, can not be lifted off the fingers
3. Sclerodactyly, digital ulcerations and infarct
4. Nails telangiectasia
5. Limitation of fingers movements
6. Dysphagia
7. Presence of bilateral basal crackles in the lungs

QUESTIONS AND ANSWERS

Q. What is scleroderma?

Ans: *Scleroderma* also called *systemic sclerosis* is a multisystem disorder of unknown etiology characterized by inflammatory, vascular and fibrotic changes in the skin, blood vessels and internal organs (chiefly GI tract, heart, lungs and kidneys). Immunological mechanism leading to vascular damage and stimulation of fibroblasts are considered responsible for it.

Q. What are the early and late skin changes in scleroderma?

Ans: I. *Early change*
- Pitting edema of hands, fingers, toes, feet, face and extremities
- Tightening of skin over the fingers and face, etc.

II. *Late change*
- Atrophy of pulps of fingers, hands, toes and feet leading to contractures/fibrosis
- Depigmentation

Q. What are the diagnostic criteria for scleroderma?

Ans: I. *Major criteria*
- Proximal scleroderma affecting metacarpophalangeal and metatarsophalangeal joints.

II. *Minor criteria*
- Sclerodactyly
- Digital tip pitting or loss of distal fingers pads
- Bilateral basal pulmonary fibrosis

Note: The major criteria plus two or more minor criteria clinch the diagnosis.

Q. What are the clinical manifestations of scleroderma?

Ans: The clinical manifestations are:

1. **Cutaneous**
   - Raynaud's phenomenon with puffy fingers (90% cases) is the presenting manifestation
   - Thickening of skin which is tightly bound to underlying subcutaneous tissues, e.g. extremities, face and trunk
   - Mat-like telangiectasia
   - Calcinosis cutis on pressure points

   Some of these features are included in CREST syndrome.

2. **Musculoskeletal**
   - Symmetrical polyarthritis
   - Carpal tunnel syndrome
   - Proximal muscle weakness or myopathy

3. **GI tract/Liver**
   - Esophageal hypomotility (e.g. heart burn, GERD, dysphagia)
   - Intestinal hypofunction, e.g. pseudo-obstruction, malabsorption, chronic constipation
   - Primary biliary cirrhosis

4. **Pulmonary**
   - Aspiration pneumonia/alveolitis
   - Fibrosis or interstitial lung disease
   - Restriction of chest movements (hidebound chest)

5. **Cardiac**
   - Pericarditis
   - Cardiomyopathy (restrictive)

- Conduction defects/arrhythmias
- Hypertension and left vetricular failure

6. Renal
- Hypertension, Renal failure

Q.   What are the types of scleroderma?

Ans: *Types/Subsets of Scleroderma:*

1. *Diffuse cutaneous scleroderma.* It involves skin of proximal and distal extremities, face and trunk. Visceral involvement occurs in early course of the disease.

2. *Limited cutaneous scleroderma or CREST syndrome.* It is characterized by *Calcinosis, Raynaud's phenomenon, Esophageal dysmotility, Sclerodactyly* and *Telangiectasia.* Skin involvement is limited to face and extremities distal to elbows. It has better prognosis.

3. *Systemic sclerosis* in which there is visceral involvement only without Raynaud's phenomenon or other skin manifestations is called *systemic sclerosis sine scleroderma, scleroderma sine scleroderma.*

Q.   Name the localized from of scleroderma.

Ans: Localized forms are:
- *CREST syndrome* (read as discussed above)
- *Morphea* (single or multiple plaques of skin induration)
- *En coup de-sabre* (e.g. linear scleroderma of one side of face. It may be associated with facial hemiatrophy)

Q.   What are the pulmonary manifestations of scleroderma?

Ans: Read clinical manifestations.

Q.   What are the cardiac manifestations of scleroderma?

Ans: Read clinical manifestations.

Q.   Name the drugs that produce scleroderma like illness.

Ans: Drugs are Bleomycin, Vinyl chloride, Pentazocine

Q.   What is mixed connective tissue disease (MCTD)?

Ans: It is an *overlap syndrome* comprising of features of SLE, scleroderma, polymyositis and rheumatoid arthritis. It is accompanied by high titres of circulating antibodies to nuclear ribonucleoprotein (NRNP) antigen.

Q.   What are the causes of anemia in scleroderma?

Ans:
- Iron deficiency combined with folate and vit. B_{12} deficiency due to GI tract involvement
- Anemia due to chronic disease
- Microangiopathic hemolytic anemia

Q.   What is the treatment of systemic sclerosis (scleroderma)?

Ans: The treatment is as follows:

1. Regular exercises to maintain flexibility of the limbs

2. *Drug treatment*
   - D-penicillamine (diminishes cross-linkage collagen)
   - Colchicine (inhibits procollagen conversion to collagen)
   - PABA
   - Vitamin E
   - Dimethyl sulphoxide

3. *Symptomatic treatment*
   - For reflux esophagitis (use mosapride or itopride)
   - For myositis — use steroids
   - For articular symptoms—use NSAIDs
   - Antibiotics for infection
   - ACE inhibitors for hypertension

4. *Treatment of Raynaud's phenomenon–* already described.

Q.   What are the uses of colchicine?

Ans: Uses are:
- Acute gout
- Familial Mediterranean fever
- Scleroderma
- Chromosomal study

Q.   What are the causes of death in scleroderma?

Ans: The fatal events in scleroderma are:

1. Cardiac failure
2. Renal failure
3. Respiratory failure

198

Subcutaneous Nodules/Swellings

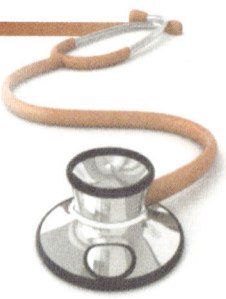

INSTRUCTION

- Perform general physical examination

SALIENT FEATURES

- Multiple swellings over the body

HISTORY

Ask for the following:

- History of rheumatic fever (fever with migratory polyarthritis) for rheumatic nodules
- History of deforming arthritis (RA) or gouty arthritis
- History of bacterial endocarditis
- History of skin eruptions following fever/drugs (erythema nodosum)
- Site of swellings for xanthomas
- Dietary history (vegetarian/non-vegetarian for cysticercosis)
- Family history of neurofibromatosis (present in this case)

EXAMINATION

General Physical Examination

- There are small, superficial palpable swellings, darker in color, non-tender, distributed all over the body (Fig. 198.1). They are soft in consistency and can be moved from side to side.
- There is no freckling of axillary and inguinal region
- 3–5 café au lait spots present over the trunk (in this case)
- Slit-lamp examination—normal
- No bony deformity (kyphoscoliosis)
- Check, pulse and BP for pheochromocytomas

Nervous System Examination

N.B Tell the examiner that you would like to examine nervous the system

- IInd and VIIIth cranial nerve normal. Fundus normal
- No evidence of paraplegia or any other neurological deficit.

PROVISIONAL DIAGNOSIS

The patient has multiple subcutaneous palpable swellings with café au lait spots (lesion) caused by neurofibromatosis called von Recklinghausen's disease (etiology). Patient is upset with the presence of disease in the family (functional status)

QUESTIONS AND ANSWERS

Q. **What von Recklinghausen's disease?**

Ans: von Recklinghausen's disease (type I neurofibromatosis) is characterised by multiple hypopigmented macules and neurofibromas resulting from mutations in NF1 gene on chromosome 17.

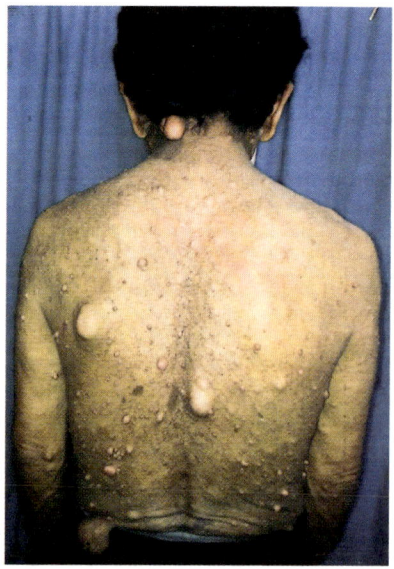

Fig. 198.1: Neurofibromatosis. Note the multiple subcutaneous swellings. Family history was positive in this case. He brought his child suffering from the disease with him

Q. What are the causes of subcutaneous swellings?

Ans: The causes are:

- Neurofibromatosis
- Rheumatoid nodules
- Rheumatic nodules
- Skin metastases from carcinomas
- Panniculitis (erythema nodosum)
- Xanthomas
- Leprosy
- Osler's nodes
- Cysticercosis
- Lipomas, fibromas
- Gouty tophi
- Calcinosis

Q. How would differentiate among common conditions producing subcutaneous nodules?

Ans: Read Table 198.1 for differential diagnosis of subcutaneous nodules.

Q. What do you understand by neurofibromas?

Ans: Neurofibromas are multiple benign tumors of the peripheral nerves, comprising of Schwann cells and fibroblasts. They are fixed to the nerves from which they arise, hence, can only be moved from side to side. They are soft, usually nontender (sometimes painful and tender) and exhibit the "*button-hole*" *sign, i.e.* they invaginate into the skin with pressure.

Q. What is neurofibromatosis? What are its types?

Ans: Neurofibromatosis is an inherited autosomal dominant condition characterized by neurofibromas and pigmented lesions of the skin, e.g. *café au lait spots* and phakomatosis (collection of neuroglial tissue) of retina.

Types:

1. *Neurofibromatosis type I (von Recklinghausen's disease)* is peripheral type of neurofibromatosis. Mutation of the neurofibromatosis gene I (NF1) causes it. The gene is situated on chromosome 17 that encodes a protein called *neurofibromin*. The features of the disease are:
   1. Multiple cutaneous or subcutaneous neurofibromas
   2. Compressive radioculopathy or neuropathy
   3. *Café au lait spots* (>6 in number and >1.5 cm in diameter)
   4. Hamartomas of iris (*Lisch nodules*)
   5. Axillary freckling
   6. Pseudoarthrosis of tibia
   7. Hydrocephalus, sclerosis, short stature, hypertension (pheochromocytomas), epilepsy and mental retardation may occur

2. *Neurofibromatosis type 2.* It is central type of neurofibromatosis. Mutation of gene NF2 causes it. The gene is situated over the chromosome 22 that encodes a protein called *neurofibromin 2, Schwannomin* or *merlin*. The features of this type of disease are:
   1. Bilateral acoustic Schwannomas
   2. Predisposition to development of meningiomas, gliomas and Schwannomas
   3. Cataract (juvenile posterior subcapsular lenticular opacity)
   4. Multiple café au lait spots
   5. Peripheral neurofibromas

Q. What is the diagnostic triad of neurofibromatosis?

Ans: The diagnostic triad of neurofibromatosis I include neurofibromas, cafe au-lait spots (Fig. 198.2) and Lisch nodules in iris.

Q. What are the diagnostic criteria for neurofibromatosis Type 2?

Ans:
- Bilateral 8th cranial nerve palsy confirmed by CT or MRI.
- A parent, sibling or child with neurofibromatosis type 2 and either unilateral 8th nerve mass of any two of the followings, i.e. neurofibroma, meningioma, schewannoma or juvenile posterior subscapular cataract.

Q. What are the common causes of café-aulait spots?

Ans:
- Neurofibromatosis
- Albright's disease (polyostotic fibrous dysplasia)
- Tuberous sclerosis
- Ataxia-telangiectasia
- Multiple endocrine adenomatosis type III
- Occasionally occur normally usually <3 in number
- *Watson's syndrome* (neurofibromatosis with pulmonary stenosis)

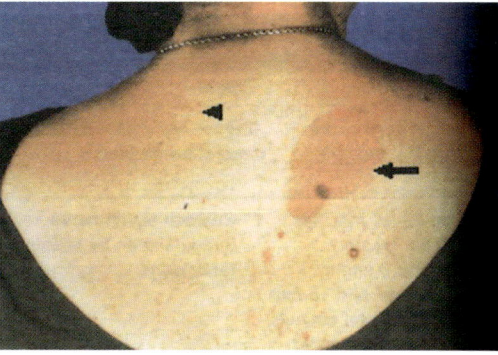

Fig. 198.2: Café au lait lesions neurofibromatosis

Cafe-au-lait spots are commonly seen on the trunk.

Q.   **What are the common sites of cutaneous neurofibromas? What is plexiform neurofibromatosis?**

Ans: Sites of cutaneous neurofibromatosis are:
- Sides of the neck
- Extremities

Plexiform neurofibromatosis refers to diffuse overgrowth of the skin and subcutaneous nerve trunks leading to a boggy swelling. The common sites are temple, upper eyelids and back of the neck. *Elephantiasis neurofibromatosa* is severe form of this variety involving the lower limbs.

Q.   **Is biopsy necessary to make diagnosis of neurofibroma?**

Ans: No. The diagnosis is made purely on clinical grounds.

Q.   **What is pachydermocele?**

Ans: It is a variety of neurofibromatosis on which coils of soft tissue hang around the neck.

Q.   **What are Lisch nodules? What is their significance?**

Ans: These are melanocytic hamartomas that appear as well defined dome-shaped swellings projecting from the iris and are clear or yellow, brown in color. They are seen on slit lamp examination. Their presence establishes the diagnosis of type I neurofibromatosis.

Q.   **What is phakomatoses? What are the conditions associated with it?**

Ans: Phakomatoses include a group of genetic disorders in which a variety of developmental abnormalities involve the skin, nervous system, retina and other organs. The causes are:
1. von Recklinghausen's disease
2. von Hippel-Lindau syndrome
3. Multiple endocrine neoplasia 1 (Werner's syndrome)
4. Retinoblastoma
5. Tuberous sclerosis
6. Sturge-Weber disease
7. Turcot's syndrome

These are also called *congenital or hereditary neurocutaneous syndromes.*

N.B Phakoma is seen as a grayish circular mass about the size of the half of the disk in the retina and is produced by collection of abnormal glial tissue.

Q.   **What is cutaneous cysticercosis?**

Ans: Read Table 198.1.

Table 198.1: Differential diagnosis of subcutaneous nodules

Type	Site	Characteristics	Associated features
Cutaneous neurofibromas (*molluscum fusrosum*)	• Side of neck • Extremities • Trunk	Small, superficial, soft palpable, skin colored or darker color dome-shaped nodules which can be pushed through a defect (*button-hole sign*) or diffuse plaques with knotty or wormy feel (plexiform neuro-fibromas)	• Café au lait macules (CALMS). These are light brown oral macules with defined margins. More than 6 (>1.5 cm in diameter) are diagnostic of neurofibromatosis • Freckling of axillary and inguinal regions • Lisch nodules on iris (slit lamp examination). Two or more are diagnostic • A parent, sibling or child with neurofibromatosis
Rheumatoid nodules	• Flexor and extensor tendons of hands, elbow, sacrum and Achilles tendon	These are periarticular, marble like nodules seen in seropositive patients of rhenumatoid arthritis	• Rheumatoid nodules may be seen in viscera, e.g. lungs, sclera and myocardium • Other skin lesion of rheumatoid arthritis, i.e. vasculitis, nail-fold infarct, palmar erythema may be present
Rheumatic nodules	Situated over the bony prominences or pressure points	They are small often tender nodules which are freely mobile	• Subcutaneous rheumatic nodule is a Jone's major criteria, is uncommonly seen • Other John's major criteria, e.g. carditis, e.g. carditis, polyarthritis, chorea, erythema marginatum may be present

Contd.

Table 198.1: Differential diagnosis of subcutaneous nodules

Type	Site	Characteristics	Associated features
Xanthomas	• Tendon xanthoms over extensor tendons • Eruptive xanthoma over the extensor surface, i.e. buttocks back, knee and elbows • Palmar xanthomas over the palmar and digital creases	They are yellowish orange, small or large (eruptive) subcutaneous swellings which may be itchy They are mobile	• They are present in children with familial hypertriglyceridemia/hypercholestrolemia • Xanthelasma over the eyelids may be present • Serum lipids are high • Family history is positive
Gouty tophi	• Around the joints of hands/feet, pressure points • Helix of car • Olecranon bursa • Achilles tendon • Forearm	They are yellow colored small, firm swellings which are tender and mobile	• Asymmetric polyarthritis involving small joints, i.e. feet (common) • Painful arthritis, worst at night, often occurs with redness (acute attack) • Systemic symptoms, e.g. fever • Serum uric acid high • Renal stones common
Cutaneous or Muscular Cysticercosis	• In muscle/skin any where in the body	Small firm nodules, nontender, mobile from side to side not above downward/muscular mobilities	• Patients are pork-eater • Other features of neurocysticercosis may be present (read case discussion of neurocysticercosis)
Skin metast-stases	• Any where	The are firm, skin coloured subcutaneous nodules, red to red-brown in color	• They occur due to hematogenous/lymphatic spread from internal malignancy, i.e. lung, colon, melanoma and oral cavity in men, breast, colon, lung in women
Panniculitis (erythema nodosum, erythema induration	• Shin is common site for erythema nodosum • Calf is common site for erythema induratum	Initially these nodules are red (erythematous) become blue as they resolve	• Patients have symptoms of systemic illness, i.e. fever, malaise, arthralgia or arthritis
Calcinosis	• Extremities and trunk	Wide spread cutaneous or subcutaneous nodules or plaque, firm, small	• Symptoms or signs of collagen vascular disease or CREST syndrome • Hypercalcemia/hyperphosphatemia

199

Tuberous Xanthomas

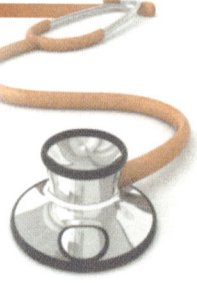

INSTRUCTION

- Perform general physical examination

SALIENT FEATURES

- Multiple swellings on the buttocks

HISTORY

Ask for the following:

- Family history of hyperlipidemia
- Premature coronary artery disease

EXAMINATION

General Physical Examination

- There are yellow colored tumor-like projections seen on the buttocks (Fig. 199.1)
- Look at the other tendons (patellar and Achilles) for xanthomas
- Look at the eyelids for xanthelasma. Look at cornea for arcus senalis
- Palpate all the vessels for atherosclerosis

Systemic Examination

Tell the examiner that you would like to auscultate the heart
- Auscultate the heart for aortic stenosis

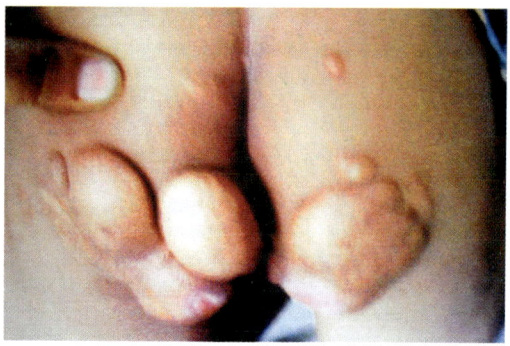

Fig. 199.1: Tuberous xanthomas around the buttocks

PROVISIONAL DIAGNOSIS

The patient has tuberous xanthomatosis (lesion) caused by hypercholesterolemia (aetiology).

QUESTIONS AND ANSWERS

Q. In which type of hypercholesterolemia they are seen?

Ans: They are seen in type III hypercholestero-lemia, rarely in type II and IV.

Q. At which age do these patients present?

Ans: Homozygous usually present at birth or during childhood. About 50% heterozygous present during childhood.

Q. What is Xanthomas? What are the types of xanthomatosis?

Ans: Xanthomas are yellow-colored cutaneous papules/nodules or plaques, commonly associated with hyperlipidemia (hyper-triglyceridemia), occur mainly on the extensor surfaces of the extremities and buttocks.

Five types of xanthomas are:
  i. *Eruptive xanthomas*
  ii. Xanthomas on the eyelids
  iii. Tendinous xanthomas seen on Achilles and extensor finger tendons
  iv. Palmar xanthomas seen on palmar creases, face, upper trunk and scars
  v. *Tuberous xanthomas:* They are seen over the large joints (elbow, wrist, knee, ankle) and buttocks. They are seen in patients with hypercholestrolemia due to prolonged cholestasis.

Q. What are the common causes of xanthomas?

Ans: *Common causes of xanthomas:*
  - Familial hyperlipidemia and hypercho-lesterolemia
  - Biliary cirrhosis or prolonged cholestasis
  - Uncontrolled diabetes mellitus

- Multiple myeloma or monoclonal gammopathy
- Hypothyroidism
- Nephrotic syndrome or chronic renal failure
- Obesity
- Drug induced hyperlipidemia

Q. **What is the basic defect in familial hypercholesterolemia?**

Ans: Autosomal dominant familial hypercholesterolemia is caused by mutation either in the gene encoding LPL receptor or in the gene encoding APO-B.

Recessive familial hypercholesterolemia results from mutations in the gene encoding an adapter protein involved in the internalization of the LPL receptor.

Q. **What do you understand by phytosterolemia?**

Ans: Phytosterolemia means accumulation of large amounts of plant sterols, is caused by increased absorption of dietary sterols and decreased biliary excretion. It is an inherited disorder (autosomal recessive) characterised by xanthomatas and premature cardiovascular events.

200

Eruptive Xanthomas

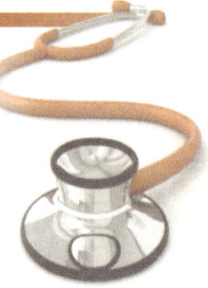

INSTRUCTION

- Take detailed history and perform general physical examination

SALIENT FEATURES

- A diabetic patient complains of multiple small swellings

HISTORY

Ask for the following:

- Duration and type of diabetes
- Status of lipids in blood or history of hyper-lipidemia
- *Eruptions:* Note the onset, duration, evolution, itching, etc.
- History of ischemic heart disease
- History of nephrotic syndrome, biliary cirrhosis, obesity, metabolic syndrome (secondary causes of hypertriglyceridemia)

EXAMINATION

General Physical Examination

- Multiple, yellow nodules seen over the extensor surfaces, i.e. buttocks (Fig. 200.1)

- Look for these nodules over back, knees and elbows

Systemic Examination

Tell the examiner that patient is diabetic, hence, you would like to examine other systems

- As patient is diabetic, look the complications, e.g. nephropathy, coronary artery disease, retino-pathy, vascular disease
- Examination of the fundus for lipaemia retinalis

PROVISIONAL DIAGNOSIS

The patient has eruptive xanthomas over the buttocks (lesion) caused by hypertriglyceridemia (aetiology). He is diabetic, hence, likely to have effects of hypertriglyceridemia, i.e. ischemic heart disease (functional status).

QUESTIONS AND ANSWERS

Q. **What are the causes of eruptive xanthomas?**
Ans:
- Type IV hyperlipidemia
- Familial hypertriglyceridemia
- Lipoprotein lipase deficiency
- Apolipoprotein CII deficiency

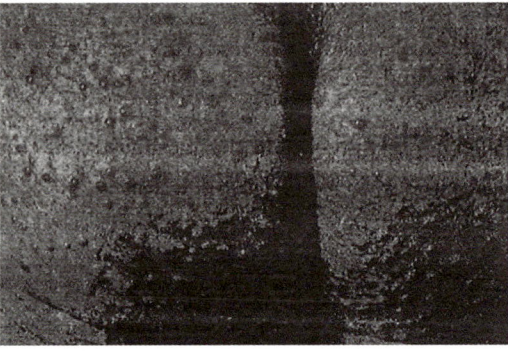

Fig. 200.1: Tuboeruptive xanthomas. Eruptive xanthoma on the buttocks of a patient with familial hypertriglyceridemia and hyperchylomicronemic syndrome

- Type I hyperlipidemia: Chylomicronemia
- Type V hyperlipidemia

Q.   How would you classify hypertriglyceridemia?

Ans: Read Table 200.1.

Q.   What is risk for patients with hypertriglyceridemia?

Ans: They are vulnerable to acute pancreatitis and hyperchylomicronemia.

Q.   How would you treat hypertriglyceridemia?

Ans: 1. Restriction of dietary fat, alcohol and simple sugars
2. Reduction of weight and exercise
3. Discontinue drugs (e.g. beta blockers)
4. Treat the secondary cause, if found
5. Niacin, fibrate, omega-3-fatty acids may be used

Table 200.1: Fredrickson classification of hyperlipoproteinemia

Type	Lipoprotein elevated	Triglyceride	Cholesterol	LDL Cholesterol	HDL Cholesterol	Xanthomas
I.	Chylomicrons	++++	+/++	↓	↓↓↓	Eruptive
IIa.	LDL	– –	+++	↑	↓	Tendinous or tuberous
IIb.	LDL and VLDL	++ to +++	++/+++	↑	↓	None
III.	Chylomicron and VLDL remnants	++ to +++	++/+++	↓	–	Palmar or tubero-eruptive
IV.	VLDL	– – to +	– –	↓	↓↓	None
V.	Chylomicrons and VLDL	++++	++/+++	↓	↓↓↓	Eruptive

201
Palmar (Planar) Xanthomas

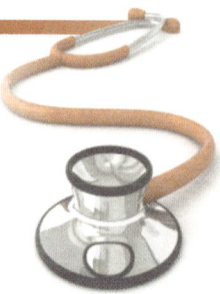

INSTRUCTION

- Perform the general physical examination

SALIENT FEATURES

- Multiple swellings over arms and trunk

HISTORY

Ask for the following:

- History of coronary artery disease
- Hyperlipidemia
- History of jaundice and pruritus

EXAMINATION

General Physical Examination

- There are small (tiny) yellow swellings over the palmar and digital creases which can easily be felt on rubbing the palms and cause difficulty during working.
- Look at other sites, i.e. arms (present; Fig. 201.1), trunk

Look for the following:

- Xanthelasma
- Tuberoeruptive xanthomas [elbow/knees (*see* Figs 199.1 and 200.1)]
- Signs of primary biliary cirrhosis (itching, jaundice)

PROVISIONAL DIAGNOSIS

The patient has planar xanthomas (lesion) caused by familial type III hyperlipidemia (aetiology).

QUESTIONS AND ANSWERS

Q. **Name common secondary causes of palmar (planar) xanthomas.**

Ans: 1. Primary biliary cirrohsis
2. Monoclonal gammopathy of myeloma or lymphoma

Q. **What is the histology of xanthomas?**

Ans: Xanthomas are collection of foamy histiocytes within the dermis. These cells have abundant and finely reticulated cytoplasm giving it a foamy appearance. Cholesterol, triglycerides and phospholipids are present within the cells. These foamy cells may often be surrounded by inflammatory cells and fibrosis.

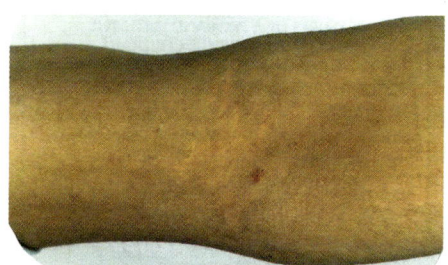

Fig. 201.1: Flat planar xanthomas are characteristic of patients with markedly reduced plasma high-density lipoprotein (HDL) cholesterol due to structural defects in the apolipoprotein (Apo) A-I gene. These xanthomas are usually present on the arms and trunk and have an orange hue

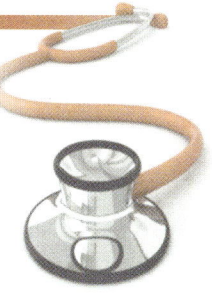

202

Xanthelasma

INSTRUCTION

- Perform general physical examination

SALIENT FEATURES

- Swellings over the upper eyelids

HISTORY

Xanthelasma commonly occurs in secondary hyperlipidemia, *hence ask for the following*:

- History of jaundice, pruritus, dark colored urine and pigmentation (primary biliary cirrhosis)
- History of diabetes, hypertension, obesity, metabolic syndrome
- Symptoms of myxedema
- Drug history (intake of oral contraceptive)

EXAMINATION

General Physical Examination

- There are yellow-colored nodules on the both upperlids particularly on inner canthus (Fig. 202.1)

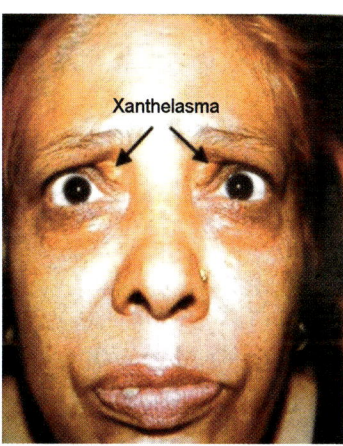

Fig. 202.1: Xanthelasma. Note the small round yellowish swellings over both upper lids (↓)

- Look for palmar and tendon xanthomas
- Look for corneal arcus
- Look for jaundice, pigmentation, scratch marks for primary biliary cirrhosis
- Look for symptoms and signs of complication of diabetes
- Check pulse and BP for hypertension, hypothyroidism
- Look for the signs of hypothyroidism (slow mentation, change in voice, facial swelling, non-pitting edema, slow pulse, constipation and delayed ankle jerks)

PROVISIONAL DIAGNOSIS

This patient has xanthelasma on the upper eyelids (lesion), the cause of which will be determined after lipid profile (aetiology).

QUESTIONS AND ANSWERS

Q. In which primary hyperlipidemia the xanthelasma are seen?

Ans:
- Type IIb (hyperlipidemia, increased cholesterol and triglyceride)
- Type IIa (hyperlipidemia with increased cholesterol only)
- Type III (hyperlipidemia with equal increase in cholestrol and triglyceride)

Q. Enumerate few common causes of secondary hyperlipidemia.

Ans: Diabetes mellitus, myxedema, nephrotic syndrome, cholestatic jaundice, alcoholism, oral contraceptive, etc.

Q. Name the classes of drugs used in treatment of hyperlipidemia.

Ans:
I. HMG–CoA reductase inhibitors, e.g. statins
II. Bile salt sequestrant resin, e.g. cholestyramine, colestipol, etc.
III. Cholesterol absorption inhibitor, e.g. ezetimibe

IV. Fibrates, e.g. gemfibrozil, bezafibrate, fenofibrate, etc.

V. Nicotinic acid derivatives, e.g. niacin, probucol

Q. **What would you advise to a patient with hyperlipidemia?**

Ans: 1. Life style modifications, e.g. exercise, weight reduction

2. Dietary modifications (low intake of fat in diet)

3. Avoidance of alcohol, smoking, estrogens and thiazides

4. Control of hypertension and diabetes

5. Lipid lowering agents

Q. **Are statins useful in patients with hypercholesterolemia and CAD?**

Ans: Yes, the statins in various trials have been shown to reduce significantly the need for coronary revascularisation and mortality in patients with coronary artery disease (CAD). The risk of stroke is also reduced.

Q. **What is the role of statins in patients with hypercholesterolemia and in coronary artery disease?**

Ans: A Scotland study had shown that treatment with pravastatin significantly reduced the incidence of MI and death from cardiovascular causes.

Q. **What is the role of statins in patients with CAD and average cholesterol levels?**

Ans: It has been shown by a major clinical study that pravastatin lowered rates of coronary events in majority of the patients with CAD who have average cholesterol levels.

Q. **What is the role of statins in hypertriglyceridemia?**

Ans: All statins (atorvastatin, simvastatin) reduce the triglyceride levels significantly

- Higher the triglyceride levels, greater is the effect

Q. **What are the side effects of statins?**

Ans: 1. Common side effects include GI upset, diarrhea, myalgia, hepatitis.

2. Rare side effects include myopathy, neuropathy, insomnia, bad dreams, difficulty in concentration.

Q. **What is the effect of food on statins? Why statins are given in the evening?**

Ans: • Lovastatin is best absorbed with food while provastatin is best absorbed with empty stomach.

- Statins are given at night because the endogenous synthesis of cholesterol is higher at night.

Q. **Which lipid lowering agent increases the HDL more?**

Ans: Nicotinic acid is usually added as a second drug to statin to lower the hypercholesterolemia and to increase HDL. It increases the HDL more (30%) than fibrates (10–15%) and resins (1–2%).

Q. **What is the role of statins in primary prevention of cardiac events?**

Ans: In the JUPITER trial (justification for the use of statins in primary prevention an Interventional Trial Evaluating Rosuvastatin), rosuvastatin significantly reduced the primary end points (nonfatal MI, nonfatal stroke, hospitalisation for unstable angina, arterial revascularisation and death from cardiovascular causes) in apparently healthy people with elevated LDL and high-sensitivity C-reactive protein.

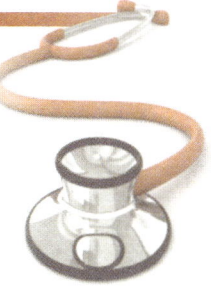

203

Lipoatrophy

INSTRUCTION

- Perform general physical examination

SALIENT FEATURES

- Visible pits over the abdomen and thighs

HISTORY

Ask for the following:

- History of intake of insulin (present)
- Past history of renal disease, i.e. edema and proteinuria (mesangiocapillary GN)
- History of HIV and treatment with antiretroviral drugs
- Family history

EXAMINATION

General Physical Examination

- There are small pits (depressed areas) located on the thighs (Fig. 203.1B) due to loss of subcutaneous fat
- Look at the abdomen and other sites for these pits. Pits are present over the abdomen (Fig. 203.1A)
- Look at the redistribution of fat (i.e. loss of fat in the limbs and from the face with accumulation of fat in the abdomen and back of neck (buffalo-hump appearance)
- History of erythema nodosum
- Manifestations of diabetes (present), renal disease, endocrinal disease, scleroderma

PROVISIONAL DIAGNOSIS

The patient has lipoatrophy (lesion) caused by subcutaneous insulin therapy (aetiology). Patient has disfiguring thighs (functional status).

QUESTIONS AND ANSWERS

Q. What are the conditions associated with lipoatrophy or lipodystrophy?

Ans: • Mesangiocapillary GN

- Scleroderma (localised)
- HIV (antiretroviral therapy)
- Morphea
- Relapsing panniculitis
- Familial
- Insulin therapy and insulin resistance syndromes

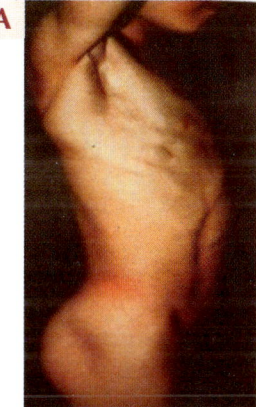

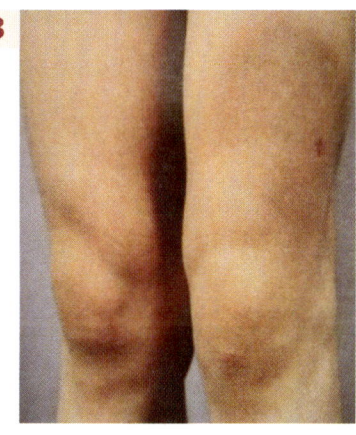

Fig. 203.1: Insulin induced lipoatrophy. Note the pits on; (A) Abdominal wall; (B) Thighs

Q. What is the mechanism of pathogenesis of this condition?

Ans: It occurs due to an immune reaction.

Q. How insulin can lead to lipoatrophy/lipo-hypertrophy at the sites of injection?

Ans: The precise pathogenesis is unknown, but repeated injection of insulin at one site can lead to it due to following plausible mechanisms.

- Immune reaction to insulin—a protein or excipients of the injection solution
- Injury from old insulin (unpurified)
- Local trauma due to repeated injection

Q. What advice do you give to this patient using insulin?

Ans: 1. The insulin should be changed to more pure (human) insulin.
2. The purified insulin should be injected directly into the atrophic area which often results in the restoration of the local contours.

Q. How insulin-induced lipoatrophy can be prevented?

Ans: Rotation/change of the injection site can prevent it.

Note: It can even occur with purified insulin.

Q. What is the relation of HIV with lipoatrophy/lipodystrophy/fat distribution?

Ans: The patient of HIV treated with antiretroviral therapy have been reported to have abnormal fat distribution, i.e. there is loss of fat or lipoatrophy of the extremities and face with adipose tissue accumulation in the central body parts, e.g. abdomen, back of neck (camel hump) and viscera. It is caused by HIV-I protease inhibitors, (previously thought) but now by nucleoside reverse transcriptase inhibitors via mitochondrial toxicity and lipid metabolism. Starvudine-based regimen have a higher prevalence than other regimens. In general, thymidine-based nucleoside analogues have been most associated with lipoatrophy while protease inhibitors are most associated with metabolic syndrome.

Q. Does lipodystrophy lead to insulin-resistance syndrome?

Ans: Leptin deficiency contributes to the insulin resistance and other metabolic abnormalities associated with severe lipodystrophy.

Leptin replacement therapy improve glycemic control and decrease triglycerides levels in patients with lipodystrophy and leptin deficiency.

Q. Name the familial lipoatrophy.

Ans: • Familial partial lipodystrophy
• Congenital generalised lipodystrophy, e.g. type 1 and type 2.

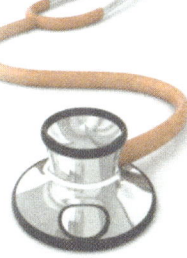

204 Necrobiosis Lipoidica Diabeticorum

INSTRUCTION

- Perform general physical examination

SALIENT FEATURES

- Skin lesion in a patient with diabetes

HISTORY

Ask for the following:

- This is a skin lesion seen uncommonly in patients with diabetes, therefore, ask about the history of diabetes
- History of hyperlipidemia, xanthomas
- Age and sex (common in females)

EXAMINATION

General Physical Examination

- Especially seen in females over the shin
- The lesions are sharply defined oval plaques seen on the front of leg (Fig. 204.1), arms and back
- The plaques are yellow in color, shiny, waxy with atrophic centres. The plaques have red margins with surrounding telangiectasia

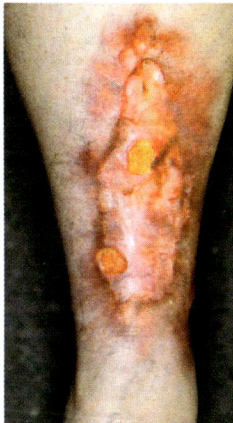

Fig. 204.1: Necrobiosis lipoidica diabeticorum

PROVISIONAL DIAGNOSIS

The patient has well defined yellowish waxy plaques with atrophic centres over the front of tibia (lesions) caused by diabetes mellitus (aetiology). The lesions are cosmetically disfiguring.

QUESTIONS AND ANSWERS

Q. What do you know about the term necrobiosis lipoidica diabeticorum?

Ans: It is a chronic granulomatous dermatitis of unknown aetiology seen in patients with diabetes mellitus.

Q. What is the histology of these lesions?

Ans: It is a disorder characterised by collagen degeneration followed by a granulomatous response (surrounded by epithelioid and giant cells), thickening of blood vessel walls and lipid deposition. The exact aetiology is unknown. In nut shell, necrobiosis lipoidica diabeticorum may be an antibody-mediated vasculitis with secondary collagen degeneration or microangiopathy of diabetes.

Q. Name the skin lesions seen on the shins.

Ans:
- Erythema nodosum
- Pre-tibial myxedema
- Diabetic dermopathy
- Erythema ab igne
- Livedo reticularis

Q. What are the dermatological manifestations of diabetes?

Ans:
1. Granuloma annulare
2. Pyogenic infections of skin (*carbuncles*)
3. Eruptive xanthomatas (read case discussion)
4. Xanthelasma (read it as case discussion)
5. Diabetic dermopathy
6. Lipodystrophy/lipoatrophy (read it as case discussion)

7. Leg ulcer, gangrene, diabetic foot
8. *Acanthosis* nigricans (read it as case discussion)
9. Anhydrosis/dry skin from autonomic neuropathy
10. Vulval candidiasis

Q.   What are the complications of this condition?

Ans: In necrobiosis lipoidica diabeticorum, the plaques (lesions) can become painful and ulcerate over the years. The squamous cell carcinoma can complicate it.

Q.   How would you confirm the diagnosis?

Ans: *By skin biopsy:* The biopsy specimen shows aggregates of lymphoid cells and palisading necrobiotic granuloma in the dermis.

Q.   How would you treat it?

Ans: Steps of treatment are:
 i. Good glycemic control
 ii. Whirlpool therapy, occlusive dressings, vasodilators (pentoxifylline)
 iii. Local steroid ointment
 iv. Excision and skin grafting
 v. Hyperbaric oxygen

Remember: Flare-ups are common. No treatment is effective.

205

Acanthosis Nigricans

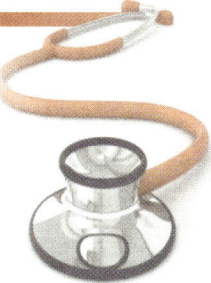

INSTRUCTION

- Perform general physical examination (GPE)

SALIENT FEATURES

- Skin outgrowths in axillae

HISTORY

Ask for the following:

- Age of the patient (> 40 years)
- Anemia, asthenia, anorexia, weight loss (malignancy stomach)
- Polyuria, polydipsia, polyphagia and weight loss (type I diabetes present)
- History or symptoms related to some endo crinal disease (Cushing's syndrome, polycystic ovaries, hyper or hypothyroidism)
- Patient is obese or non obese (BMI to be calculated, pigmented verrucous areas develop in the body folds of non obese persons indicate gastric cancer)

EXAMINATION

General Physical Examination

- *General appearance*; patient is cahexic, asthetic built, anemic or malnourished (this case)
- Black velvety outgrowths are seen in axillae (Fig. 205.1) neck, nipples, groin and face
- Presence of loose skin tags present at the site of skin lesions
- Rough palms and soles (*Tripe palms*)
- Filiform growth around the face, mouth and tongue suggest underlying neoplasm

PROVISIONAL DIAGNOSIS

The patient has typical velvety black pigmented outgrowths of skin in the axillae (lesion), could be due to diabetes (aetiology). Patient has uncontrolled status of diabetes (functional status)

QUESTIONS AND ANSWERS

Q. What is acathosis nigricans?
Ans: These are skin outgrowths due to hyperplasia, hyperkeratosis and slight pigmentation of the basal layer of epidermis (undulating epidermis with sharp peaks and valleys).

Q. What does acanthosis nigricans mean?
Ans: Acanthosis is hyperplasia of the stratum spinosum of the epidermis.

Q. What are its types?
Ans:
1. Benign
2. Malignant
3. Obesity-associated
4. Syndemic
5. Acral
6. Unilateral
7. Drug-induced
8. Mixed type

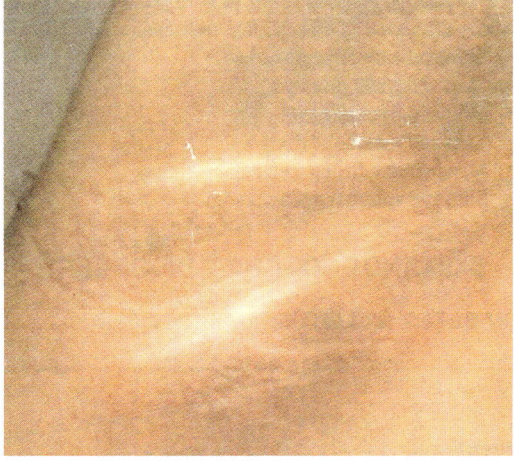

Fig. 205.1: Acanthosis nigricans in diabetes: Velvety, hypopigmented plaques in major flexures

Q. Name the various conditions associated with acanthosis nigricans.

Ans: Certain benign as well as malignant conditions are associated with it or can lead to it.

A. Benign conditions	B. Malignant conditions
• Diabetes mellitus	• Adenocarcinoma of
• Cushing's syndrome	stomach, GI tract,
• Acromegaly	genital tract (uterus,
• Obesity-associated	ovary), breast, lung and
	prostate
• Polycystic ovarian	• Rarely lymphoreticu-
disease	lar malignancies

Q. What is the relationship of acanthosis nigricans with malignancy?

Ans: Acanthosis nigricans may precede the neoplast by many years, may be associated with occult malignancy or manifest malignancy.

Q. What are the dermatological manifestations of internal malignancy?

Ans:
- Migratory thrombophlebitis
- Ichthyososis
- Dermatomyositis
- Tylosis or palmar hyperkeratosis
- Paget's disease of nipple
- Acanthosis nigricans

Q. What is the treatment of this condition?

Ans:
1. Medications, e.g. metformin, oral iso-tretinoin, topical retinoic acid, topical salicylic acid and oral fish oil (vit. A).
2. Laser therapy, e.g. Co laser and the long-pulsed Alexandrite laser.

206

Pityriasis Versicolor

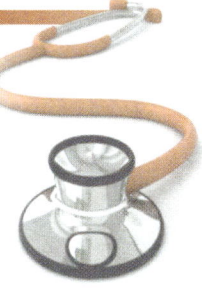

INSTRUCTION

- Examine the back of the patient

SALIENT FEATURES

- Hypopigmented macules with scales

HISTORY

Ask for the following:

- Profuse sweating
- Diabetes mellitus
- Pregnancy

EXAMINATION

- The skin lesions are well defined, hypopigmented macules with fine brawny scales of different shapes and sizes, present in front and back of the chest (Fig. 206.1), side of neck, face and upper arms
- There is no itching

Fig. 206.1: Pityriasis versicolor. Note the perifollicular hypopigmented macules with scales

PROVISIONAL DIAGNOSIS

The patient has hypopigmented maculas (lesion) caused by a parasite *M. furfur* — a sapropyhte yeast called pityrosporum orbiculare. It causes disfigurement (functional status).

QUESTIONS AND ANSWERS

Q. **What are the causes of hypopigmented macules?**

Ans: Following are the causes:

1. *Tuberculoid leprosy* (the hypopigmented macules are anesthetic)
2. *Vitiligo* (idiopathic or associated with other autoimmune disease)
3. *Pityriasis alba* and *pityriasia versicolor*
4. *Following burn* (History of burn)
5. *Tuberous sclerosis (Shagreen patch)*. There is history of epilepsy, low intelligence and sebaceous adenoma. It may be familial.
6. *Prolonged use of chloroquine* in rheumatoid arthritis and SLE
7. *Psoriasis*
8. *Albinism*

Q. **What are its precipitating factors?**

Ans: These are as follows:

- Profuse sweating
- Diabetes mellitus
- Pregnancy

Q. **How do you confirm the diagnosis?**

Ans: The diagnosis is confirmed by demonstration of fungal hyphe in the scraped scales treated with KOH (10% solution) taken on a slide and examined under the microscope.

Q. **What is ringworm? What are the characteristics of its lesions? How do you diagnose it? Describe the treatment.**

Ans: It is discussed separately, Case No. 223.

Q. Name the opportunistic fungal infections in HIV.

Ans: These are as follows:
- Cryptococcosis
- Mucormycosis
- Aspergillosis
- Candidiasis

Q. What is the treatment of P. versicolor?

Ans: The treatment includes:
- Maintain good personal hygiene.
- Topical sodium thiosulphate (25–40% solution) locally is inexpensive therapy used daily for 3 weeks.
- Selenium sulphate 2.5% locally at night and wash off in the following morning, 2–3 applications are adequate, weekly shampoo for 3–4 weeks should accompany.
- Topical antifungal solutions such as 1% clotrimazole, 2% miconazole, 1% tolnaftate and 2% ketoconazole are effective.
- For recurrence, weekly use of selenium sulphide or zinc pyrithionate shampoo are useful.

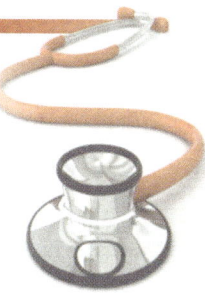

207

Lupus Pernio

INSTRUCTION

- Perform general physical and relevant systemic examination

SALIENT FEATURES

- Cough, dyspnea, chest pain

HISTORY

Ask for the following:

- Cough, dyspnea, chest pain or discomfort (present)
- Weight loss, fatigue, malaise, anorexia
- Fever, night sweats, arthralgias
- History of uveitis
- History of treatment with interferon-alpha (for hepatitis C infection)

EXAMINATION

General Physical Examination

- Indurated, blue-purple, swollen shiny plaques on the nose (present in this case), cheeks, lips, ears, fingers with telangiectasia around the plaques (Fig. 207.1) and knees
- Examine the neck, axillae, groins for lympha-denopathy
- Eye examination for uveitis, keratoconjunctivitis (ocular abnormalities)

Systemic Examination

Tell the examiner that you would like to examine respiratory system for sarcoidosis.

PROVISIONAL DIAGNOSIS

The patient has purple-blue plaques on the face (lesion) caused by sarcoidosis (aetiology) which is disfiguring to the patient (functional status).

QUESTIONS AND ANSWERS

Q. **What is differential diagnosis of lupus pernio?**
Ans: • Rhinophyma

- Lupus vulgaris
- Leprosy

Q. **What is sarcoidosis?**
Ans: It is multisystem disorder of unknown aetiology characterised by accumulation of T lymphocytes and mononuclear phagocytes, noncaseating epithelioid granulomas and derangement of normal tissue architect.

Q. **What are the skin manifestations of sarcoi-dosis?**
Ans: • Lupus pernio
- Erythema nodosum
- Maculopapular eruptions
- Sarcoid plaques over limbs, shoulder, buttocks and thighs

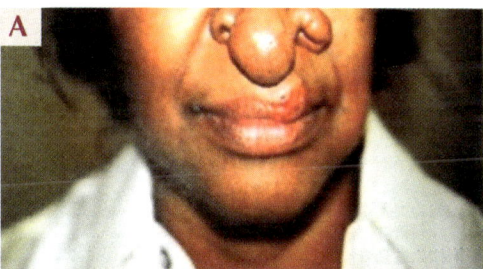

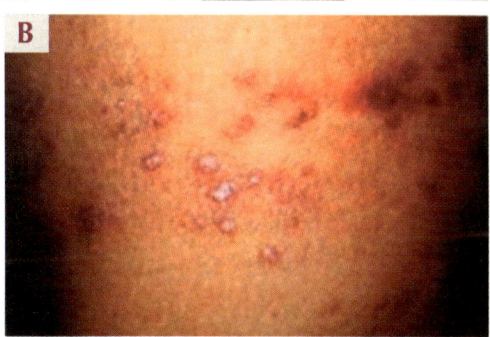

Fig. 207.1: (A) Lupus pernio plaque on the nose in a patient with sarcoidosis; (B) Telangiectasia over and plaques

- Subcutaneous nodules
- Old surgical scars infiltration

Q. What are the clinical presentations of sarcoidosis?

Ans: The presentations are:

1. *Asymptomatic disease* detected on routine examination

2. *Acute* or *subacute sarcoidosis* presents in young age (3rd decade) characterised by hilar lymphadenopathy, parotid enlargement, erythema nodosum and general constitutional symptoms. It includes two syndromes:
   - i. Lofgren's syndrome
   - ii. Heerfordt-Waldenstrom syndrome

3. *Chronic sarcoidosis* has late age of onset (5th decade), insidious in nature characterised by fatigue, dyspnea, polyarthritis and lupus pernio.

Q. What are the organs commonly involved in sarcoidosis?

Ans: The lungs, skin, eyes, lymph nodes, peripheral nerves. Heart, kidneys, nervous system, liver and other organs are uncommonly involved.

Q. What is the treatment of lupus pernio?

Ans: Monthly intralesional triamcinolone injection, topical and systemic steroids, hydroxychloroquine, allopurinol, thalidomide and tranilast.

Q. What are the ocular manifestations of sarcoidosis?

Ans:
1. Anterior uveitis
2. Retinal vasculitis
3. Keratoconjunctivitis sicca syndrome
4. Choroidal and optic nerve granulomata

Q. What is Lofgren syndrome?

Ans: It is seen in Scandinavian and Irish females, consists of erythema nodosum, bilateral hilar lymphadenopathy and polyarthritis.

Q. What is Heerfordt-Waldenstrom syndrome?

Ans: It is characterised by fever, parotid enlargement, anterior uveitis and facial nerve palsy.

Q. What is the source of raised ACE (angiotensin converting enzyme) in sarcoidosis?

Ans: Epithelioid cells of sarcoid granuloma.

Q. What is the pathogenesis of sarcoidosis?

Ans: The cardinal pathogenic feature is interaction between CD4 T cells with antigen-presenting cells to initiate the formation and maintenance of noncaseating granuloma.

Q. What are the manifestations of neuro sarcoidosis?

Ans:
1. Cranial nerve (7th) palsy
2. Optic nerve dysfunction, papilledema
3. Palatal dysfunction
4. Hearing abnormalities
5. Chronic meningitis

Q. What are the cardiac manifestations of sarcoidosis?

Ans:
1. Arrhythmias and conduction blocks
2. Cardiac dysfunction (left ventricular wall motion abnormalities)
3. Papillary muscle dysfunction
4. Pericarditis
5. Congestive heart failure
6. Cor pulmonale secondary to chronic pulmonary fibrosis

Q. How would you investigate this case?

Ans:
- *Full blood counts and ESR:* There can be leucopenia with eosinophilia
- *Chest X-rays* for hilar lymphadenopathy and lung parenchymal involvement
- *Slit-lamp examination* of eyes
- *Kveim's test* (with cultured antigens in the spleen). It is not recommended commonly due to risk of viral infection transmission
- *Serum Angiotensin Converting Enzymes (ACE) levels* are raised in 40% cases
- *Lung function tests* show restrictive lung defect
- *Bronchoalveolar lavage* for lymphocytes (high CD4 and CD8 ratio)
- *Serum calcium levels* are high
- *Gallium lung scan*
- *Lung biopsy* which confirm the diagnosis. Typical non-caseating granulomas with fibrosis (interstitial lung disease) is a characteristic histological feature

Q. How would you treat sarcoidosis?

Ans:
- Acute sarcoidosis regresses spontaneously and does not recur, hence, no treatment is required.
- Chronic sarcoidosis is treated with corticosteroids. Immunosuppressive drugs are used when the corticosteroid therapy is ineffective.

208

Venous Ulcer

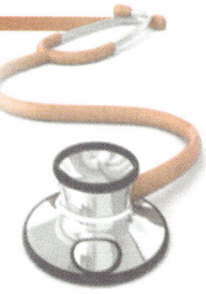

INSTRUCTION

- Perform general physical examination

SALIENT FEATURES

- An ulcer over the right leg

HISTORY

Ask about the following:

- History of prolonged standing
- History of varicosity of veins and duration
- Past history of DVT and venous thromboembolism
- Is this ulceration has occurred for the first time or recurrent?
- Is ulcer painful or painless (neuropathic cause)?
- History of rheumatoid arthritis

EXAMINATION

General Physical Examination

- A large ulcer is present on the medial aspect of right ankle joint extending on to the lower leg, irregular in shape, 10 × 7 cm in size. There is sprouting granulation tissue at the base of the ulcer.
- There is serosanguinous foul smelling discharge from the ulcer. The ulcer is secondarily infected (Fig. 208.1).
- The surrounding skin around the ulcer is pigmented (blackish discoloration) with varicosities of veins in the leg. There is white atrophy with scars in the overlying skin.
- On palpation, the ulcer was not painful. There is no evidence of chronic ischaemia (pulses were normal) gangrene or neuropathy (loss of sensation).
- Varicosities in the form of thread veins with perforator incompetence in the lower leg is noted on multiple tourniquet test. Perthes test was negative. Homan's sign was negative.
- There is no evidence of saphenofemoral or saphenopopliteal junction incompetence.

- Test the range of movements of right knee and ankle (normal in this case).
- Test the sensations to exclude peripheral neuropathy (normal in this case).

PROVISIONAL DIAGNOSIS

The patient has a large venous ulcer right leg (lesion) caused by varicosities of veins (aetiology). There is pigmentation and stereotactic dermatitis (functional status).

QUESTIONS AND ANSWERS

Q. **What are the common causes of ulcers on the lower extremity?**

Ans:
- Diabetic neuropathy/diabetic foot
- Arterial insufficiency
- Cardiovascular disease with embolism
- Sickle cell crisis/sickle cell anemia
- Vasculitis
- Traumatic ulcer

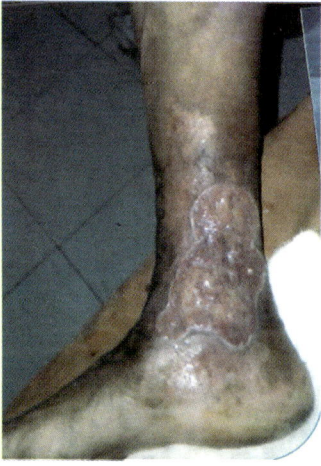

Fig. 208.1: Varicosities and venous ulcer

- Pyoderma gangrenosa
- Skin malignancy
- Autoimmune disease, e.g. Felty syndrome

Q. **What is the cause of white atrophy of the skin?**

Ans: This is due to hyalinization of the skin vessels leading to scarring in the overlying skin.

Q. **What is the pathogenesis of venous ulcer?**

Ans: This is due to chronic varicosity of veins with disturbed venous flow pattern combined with stasis of blood leading to rise in venous pressure, atrophy of skin and inflammation resulting in ulceration.

Q. **What is the cause of pigmentation around the ulcer?**

Ans: It is due to deposition of hemosiderin and extravasation of blood from the dilated varicose veins.

Q. **Does skin changes in presence of varicose vein indicate chronic venous insufficiency?**

Ans: Yes. Chronic venous insufficiency with disturbed venous flow pattern are responsible for skin changes.

Q. **What are the factors which produce chronic venous insufficiency and varicosity of veins?**

Ans: Two factors, e.g. *hydrostatic pressure* in the veins and *hydrodynamic pressure* generated by the contractions of skeletal muscles try to generate high pressure during standing and muscular activity which is released by the third factor called *venous valve competence.* If venous valves are competent, then venous blood flows towards the heart, thus, emptying the deep and superficial venous systems. If the valves in the perforator veins (connecting the two venous systems) are incompetent, then higher pressure generated in the deep venous system during muscular contractions is transmitted to the superficial venous system making them prominent, dilated and tortuous.

Q. **What is gravitational (static) eczema?**

Ans: Gravitational eczema occurs in middle or old aged persons with venous insufficiency or as a result of venous hypertension. History of deep vein thrombosis or presence of superficial varicose veins are usual features. This occurs around the ankle (Fig. 208.2). The signs of venous insufficiency (red or bluish discolouration, loss of hair, induration, pigmentation due to hemosiderin deposition and ulceration) are associated with eczema (itching, oozing and atrophy).

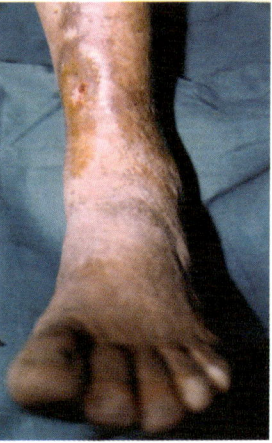

Fig. 208.2: Gravitational eczema due to chronic venous stasis

209

Arterial Leg Ulcer

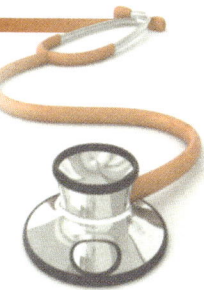

INSTRUCTION

- Perform general physical and relevant systemic examination

SALIENT FEATURES

- An ulcer over the big toe and toes

HISTORY

Ask for the following:

- History of intermittent claudication
- History of underlying cardiovascular and cerebrovascular disease
- History rest pain
- History impotence
- History of trauma or presence of deformity
- History of diabetes and chronic renal failure (CRF)

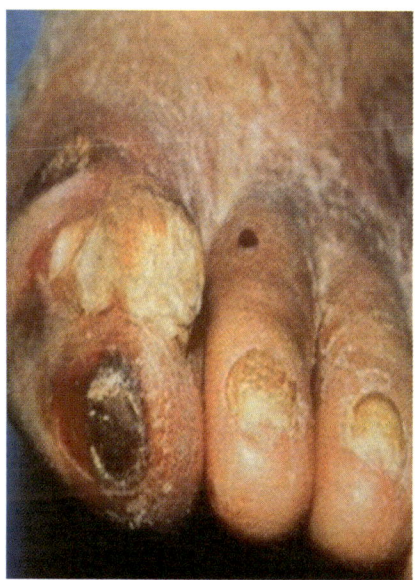

Fig. 209.1: Necrotic arterial foot ulcers

EXAMINATION

General Physical Examination

- A well circumscribed, tender, punched out ulcer over the plantar surface of first (big toe) and other toes metatarsal (these are the areas where pressure is sustained and perfusion is poor)
- The skin is cold and atrophic. There is no callus, pigmentation may be present
- Loss of hair. Nails are thickened
- Peripheral pulses are not palpable (tibialis anterior in this case) or diminished (diabetes, atherosclerosis, CRF)
- There is pallor of the foot on elevation and dusky rubor on dependency (absent in this case)
- Sluggish filling of the capillaries

Systemic Examination

- Tell the examiner that you would like to examine CVS, cerebrovascular and renal system.

PROVISIONAL DIAGNOSIS

The patient has arterial ulcers (lesion) caused by vascular insufficiency (aetiology).

QUESTIONS AND ANSWERS

Q. **Enumerate some common causes of leg ulcers.**

Ans:
- Venous ulcer
- Arterial ulcer (Buerger's disease, atherosclerosis)
- Neuropathic ulcer (diabetes, leprosy)
- Vasculitic ulcers (RA, SLE, pyoderma gangrenosa)
- Sickle cell anemia, spherocytosis
- Malignant ulcer (skin cancer)
- Traumatic

Q. **What is differential diagnosis of arterial ulcer?**

Ans: Two common ulcers, e.g. venous and neuropathic are to be differentiated (Table 209.1).

Table 209.1: Differentiation between various trophic ulcers

Feature	Arterial ulcer	Venous ulcer	Neuropathic ulcer
• Site	Toes, feet in areas of trauma	Around the ankle	Pressure points with diminished sensations as in diabetes
• Skin around the ulcer	Cold, atrophic, No callus, pigmented	Pigmented	Calloused
• Pain	Severe	Not severe	Absent
• Associated gangrene	May be present	Absent	Absent
• Peripheral pulses	Diminished, pallor of foot on elevation, dusky rubor on dependency	Peripheral pulses present Edema is also present pitting	Pulses are present
• Sensations	Normal	Normal may be present.	Diminished/absent, Burn marks
• Jerks	Normal	Normal	Ankle jerk absent

Q. How would you investigate this case?

Ans: 1. *Plain X-ray* of the area for calcification of artery

2. *Doppler ultrasonography* to define arterial involvement and its severity

3. *Measurement of segmental limb pressure.* An ankle-brachial pressure index <0.6 indicate arterial compromise

4. *Magnetic resonance angiography* for narrowing and stenosis of the leg arteries

Q. How would you treat arterial ulcers?

Ans: • Avoidance of precipitating factors, e.g. smoking, obesity

• Control of diabetes and HT (hypertension)

• Keep the limb warm

• Feet—chiropodist and foot care. Use of appropriate foot-wear

• *Regular exercise* to promote collaterals

• Low dose aspirin

• Surgery—balloon dilatation of limb vessel in occlusive arterial disease

• Bypassed prosthetic vascular grafts or autologous vein grafts in non-healing ulcers

Q. What is Buerger's disease?

Ans: Read it as a separate case report in cardiovascular system.

210

Psoriasis

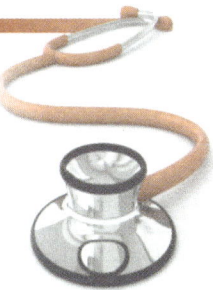

INSTRUCTION

- Perform general physical examination

SALIENT FEATURES

- Itchy skin lesions

HISTORY

Ask about the following:

- History of itching, pain, bleeding, flexural intertrigo
- Nail changes (onycholysis, pitting and thickening of nail plate)
- Ask about precipitating factors, e.g. skin trauma, winter season, emotional stress, infection, pregnancy, URC, etc.
- Drug history, e.g. betablockers, lithium, carbazepine, calcium channel blockers, penicillin
- History of joint pains (*psoriatic arthropathy*)
- Family history

EXAMINATION

General Physical Examination

- The patient has well-demarcated salmon pink plaques with silvery white scales over extensor surfaces, scalp, navel and natal cleft. The skin lesions are itchy (Fig. 210.1)
- There is moist red surface on removal of scales (*bulkeley's membrane*)
- *Auspitz's sign* is positive (in this case), i.e. there is bleeding on removal of silvery scales from the plaques
- New skin lesion present at the site of trauma (*Koebner's phenomenon*)
- *Nails.* Look at the nails for pitting and onycholysis (separation of nail plate from the bed)
- *Joints* (small joints of hands/feet) for psoriatic arthropathy

PROVISIONAL DIAGNOSIS

The patient has silvery white scaly lesions of skin with nail pitting (lesion) caused by psoriasis (aetiology). There is considerable itching (functional status).

Q. **What are the points in favor of your diagnosis?**
Ans:
- Typical silvery white scaly lesions
- The lesions are pruritic
- There is moist red surface on removal of scales
- Auspitz sign is positive
- Presence of nail changes, i.e. oncholysis, pitting of nail plates, subungual hyper-keratosis with discoloration

QUESTIONS AND ANSWERS

Q. **What is its incidence?**
Ans: It affects 1–2% of the population.

Q. **What is differential diagnosis?**
Ans: Psoriasis has to be differentiated from mycosis fungoides (read it as separate case).

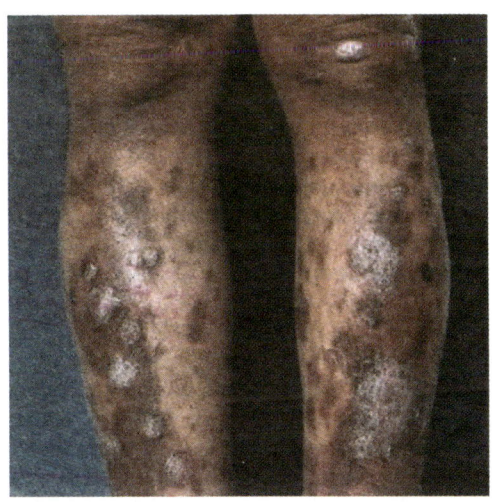

Fig. 210.1: Chronic plaque psoriasis. Note the plaques with silvery-white scales on extensor surfaces of legs

Q. Name the common scaly lesions of the skin.

Ans: Common scaly lesions are:
- Psoriasis
- Seborrheic dermatitis
- Eczema
- Ringworm
- Pityriasis (all the varieties)
- Lichen planus
- Exfoliative dermatitis

Q. What do you understand by psoriasis?

Ans: It is a common chronic inflammatory skin disorder clinically characterised by red erythematous plaques covered with silvery white scales.

Q. What are the various clinical types of psoriasis?

Ans: 1. Numular/chronic plaque psoriasis
2. Guttate psoriasis
3. Exfoliative/erythrodermic psoriasis
4. Pustular type (palmoplantar psoriasis)
5. Generalised pustular
6. Genital type
7. Flexural type
8. Scalp psoriasis
9. Psoriasis unguis (nail psoriasis)

Q. What are the characteristics of psoriatic lesion?

Ans: The characteristics of psoriatic lesions are:
1. Classic lesion is a well defined erythematous plaque covered with silvery-white adherent scales.
2. The lesions are distributed over the extensor surfaces (e.g. knees, elbows, buttocks), may also involve scalp, hands, palms and soles.
3. The skin lesions are pruritic.
4. Traumatized areas often develop lesions of psoriasis by local spread (*Koebner's phenomenon*).
5. On grattage, characteristic coherence of scales can be seen as if one scratches a wax candle (*signe de la tache de bougie*).
6. Scrapping or removal of scales leaving behind punctate bleeding spots (*Auspitz's sign*) is diagnostic.
7. Associated findings include psoriatic arthritis and nail changes (onycholysis, pitting or thickenings of nail plate with accumulation of subungal debris).

Q. What is its etiology?

Ans: Following are causes:
1. *Genetic basis:* Psoriasis occurs in families (50% patients with psoriasis have positive family history). HLA studies have shown increased frequency of HLA-B12, HLA-B17 and HLA-BW16 in the affected patients. Twin studies report 70% concordance rate among monozygotic twins.
2. *Immunological basis:* Evidence has accumulated indicating a role of T cells in pathophysiology of psoriasis. There is persistent activation of T cells by the antigen as a result of auto-reactivity or by the cytokines such as interleukin 2 released from keratinocytes during chemical/physical or UV injury.
3. *Precipitating factors:* Skin trauma, winter season, emotional stress, depression, infection (streptococcal/HIV), pregnancy and upper respiratory infection precipitate it.
4. *Drugs:* Beta blockers, NSAIDs, lithium, calcium channel blockers, chloroquine, valproate, carbamazepine, clonidine, penicillin, tetracyclines, glibenclamide and topical coal tar precipitate psoriasis.

Q. What is psoriatic arthropathy (PA)?

Ans: It is an inflammatory arthritis that occurs in 5 to 10 percent of patients with psoriasis with negative rheumatoid factor (seronegative arthritis). It is commonly associated with HLA-B27. Five distinct types recognized are:
1. *Oligoarticular PA* (asymmetrical involvement of joints of fingers). This is commonest type (38%)
2. *Rheumatoid type* (Fig. 210.2)
3. *Classical psoriatic arthropathy* this is arthritis involving the distal interphalangeal joints (16%)
4. *Psoriatic spondylitis* (*sacroilitis* and/or *spondylitis*)
5. *Arthritis mutilans* (severe destructive arthritis 5%)

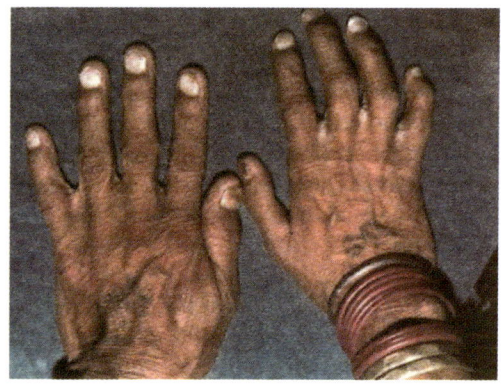

Fig. 210.2: Psoriatic arthropathy. Note the involvement of small joints of the hands with nail changes in a patient with psoriasis

Q.   What are the dermatological causes of pitting nails?

Ans: • Psoriasis unguis   • Alopecia areata
        • Eczema

Q.   Name the skin diseases precipated by trauma (positive Koebner's phenomenon).

Ans: • Psoriasis   • Viral warts
        • Lichen planus

Q.   What are the histological changes in psoriasis?

Ans: Following are the changes:
- Hyperkeratosis and parakeratosis
- Absence of granular layer
- Hyperplasia of stratum malpighii
- Dilated and tortuous blood vessels in dermal papillae
- Microabscesses of *Munro* in the horny layer

Q.   How will you investigate a case with psoriasis?

Ans: Following are the investigations:
- *TLC, DLC* for an evidence of infection
- *Rheumatoid* factor
- *Skin scrappings* and *nail clippings* may be examined for tinea (fungal infection has to be differentiated from psoriasis)
- *Skin biopsy*. It is rarely required
- *X-rays of hands* and feet may show fish tail or "pencil-in-cup" deformity if joints are involved. Subarticular erosions and later cystic destruction of bones may occur. Sacroilitis may occur

Q.   How will you treat such a case?

Ans: • Triggering factors should be found out and eliminated
        • Good diet with supplementation of iron and folate
        • Any focus of infection may be treated with antibodies
        A. *Topical treatment:* It consists of:
           1. *Dithranol (anthralin).* Ingram regimen consists of coal tar bath, exposure to UV rays and application of anthralin (0.1 to 0.8%) in Lassar's paste to psoriatic plaques
           2. Crude coal tar preparation with keratolytic salicylic acid is used as an ointment. It may be combined with UV light or anthralin as described above
           3. *Local steroid ointments*
           4. *Vitamin D analogue (calcipotriol)* is used locally
           5. *Topical preparation* of retinoid acid derivatives (0.1%)
           6. Systemic therapy plus/*Tazarotene-a retinoid* is used as 0.1% gel

B. *Systemic therapy*

   Indications for systemic therapy
   - Failure of tropical therapy
   - Extensive plaque psoriasis in the elderly
   - Generalized pustular or erythrodermic psoriasis
   - Severe psoriatic arthropathy

PUVA therapy: Administration of psoralens (p stands for Psoralens) and subsequent long wave UVA radiation is called PUVA therapy. Oral psoralens (8-methoxy psolarens) is followed 2 hours later by UVA therapy. Two to four sittings per week are necessary (total 10–20 sittings). UVB is useful in winter season.

Other drugs used are:
1. Methotrexate and cyclosporin
2. Mycophenolate Mofetil
3. Oral retinoids (etretinate, treatinoin)
4. Oral corticosteroids may be used judiciously in refractory psoriasis, psoriatic arthropathy and in erythrodermic form of psoriasis.
5. NSAIDs are used for arthropathy.

   Novel approach: Anti-CD4 monoclonal antibody. It is a novel approach.

211

Scabies

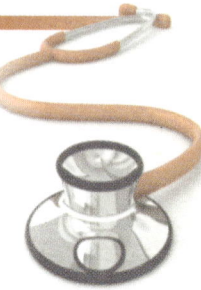

INSTRUCTION

• Examine the patient's hands

SALIENT FEATURES

• Severe itching

HISTORY

Ask for the following:

• History of itching (pruritus) over wrists, forearms and arms, axillae and in-between fingers (present)
• Is itching more at night or hot bath?
• History of involvement of many members of the family due to sharing of bedding, towels (present in this case)

EXAMINATION

Examination of the Hands

• Papulovesicular lesions are seen between fingers (Fig. 211.1) and axillae. These lesions are itchy. Burrows/tunnels are also seen between the fingers which indicate the entry point of the parasite (Fig. 211.2)

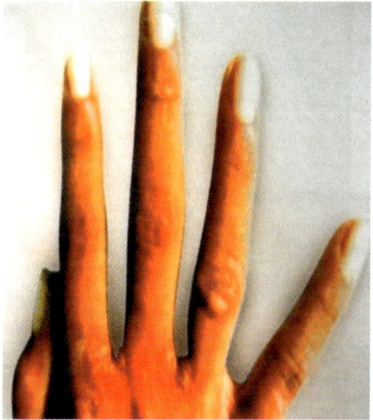

Fig. 211.1: Infected scabies

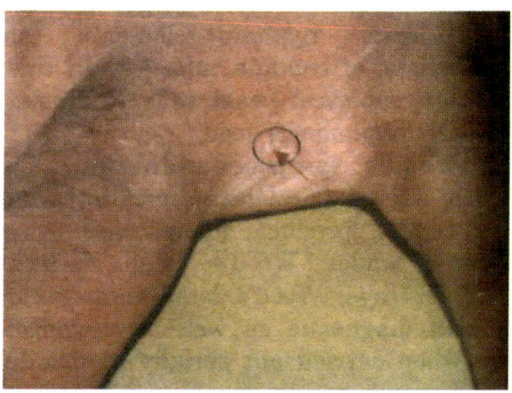

Fig. 211.2: A burrow at the site of entry of mite

PROVISIONAL DIAGNOSIS

The patient has papulovesicular, itchy lesions between the fingers, axillae and forearm (lesion) caused by scabies (aetiology), a contagious disease. This has spread to involve other family members (functional status).

QUESTIONS AND ANSWERS

Q. **What are the points in favor of your diagnosis?**

Ans: The points are:
  • Pruritus and polymorphic skin lesions at characteristic locations
  • Burrows or comedones
  • Itching is nocturnal, also occurs after a hot bath
  • History of involvement of several members of the family due to household contact

Q. **How would you confirm your diagnosis?**

Ans: • Biopsy or scrappings of papulovesicular lesions for mite, its eggs or fecal matter will confirm the diagnosis

- Burrows unroofed with a sterile needle or scalpel blade and scrapings taken and transferred to a glass slide on which 10% potassium hydroxide is kept. The slide is then examined under microscope for mite, its eggs or its fecal pellets which will confirm the diagnosis.

Q. How is scabies caused? How does it get transmitted?

Ans: The scabies is caused by infestation by an ectoparasite—*Sarcoptes scabiei*, a human itch mite. Gravid female mites burrow beneath the skin (stratum corneum) for a month, depositing the eggs. Nymphs hatch out from these eggs and mature into adults on the surface of the skin, where they mate and subsequently reinvade the skin of the same or another person.

Transfer of newly fertilized female mites from person to person by intimate personal contact is the mode of transmission of scabies. Medical practitioners are, therefore, at particular risk of infestation.

The crowding, uncleanliness, promiscuity are the precipitating factors. Transmission via sharing of the contaminated bedding, clothing, towel is infrequent because these mites cannot survive more than a day without host contact.

Outbreaks occur in nursing homes, mental institutions and hospitals.

Q. What is pathognomonic lesion of scabies? What is its characteristic distribution? Which areas are spared?

Ans: *Burrow or tunnel* is the pathognomonic lesion. Burrows (Fig. 211.2) appear as dark wavy lines in the epidermis caused by tunnelling of the mite in the skin and end in a small pearly bleb that contains the female mite.

The Characteristic Distribution of Burrows:

The areas involved are:
- Webs of the fingers, volar aspect of wrist, ulnar border of forearm and arms, anterior axillary folds
- Scrotum, penis, vulva, groin and medial aspects of thigh and webs of toes

Areas spared are:

Face, scalp, neck, palms and soles.

Q. Name the various lesions in scabies.

Ans: Various lesions are:
- Typically burrows seen as wavy lines
- Small papules and pustules often accompanied by eczematous plaques
- Pustules or nodules

- Crusted scabies and prominent fissuring can occur due to bacteremia in AIDS patients

Q. What is non-itchy (Norwegian) scabies?

Ans: Features of non-itchy scabies are:
- *Crusted (or Norwegian) scabies* (Fig. 211.3) is a non-itchy scabies. It results from hyperinfestation with thousands or millions of mites, the predisposing conditions being steroids use, immunocompromised state and neurological or psychiatric illness (mentally retarded patients).

Q. Why is the itch nocturnal in scabies?

Ans: The mites need a warm environment to move, hence, when patient retires in a warm bed at night, the mites start moving within the burrows and cause itch.

Q. Which skin conditions lead to itching?

Ans: The conditions are:
- Scabies
- Psoriasis
- Insect bite
- Ringworm
- Pediculosis
- Lichen planus
- Eczematous dermatitis
- Urticaris
- Dermatitis herpetiformis

Q. What are the medical causes of generalized pruritus?

Ans: Medical causes are:
- Cholestasis (obstructive jaundice)
- Chronic renal failure (CRF)
- Polycythemia rubra vera
- Systemic anaphylaxis
- Carcinoid syndrome
- Systemic mastocytosis

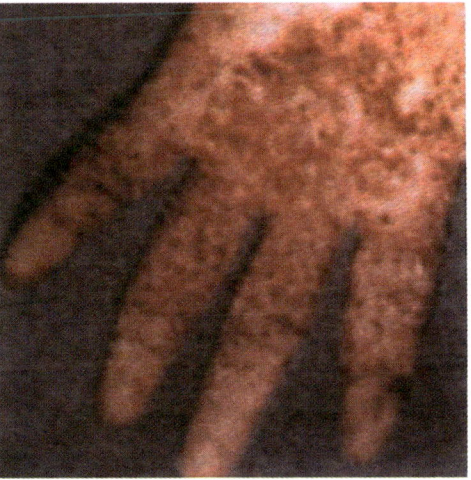

Fig. 211.3: Crusted scabies (Norwegian scabies)

- Thyrotoxicosis
- Diabetes mellitus
- Drug-induced
- Psychogenic
- Pregnancy

Q. What are the complications of scabies?

Ans: Common complications of scabies are:

- *Superinfection,* e.g. pyoderma
- *Acute glomerulonephritis* due to sensitization to nephrogenic strains of streptococci (superinfection)
- *Eczematous dermatitis* due to prolonged itching or sensitization from parasite
- *Complications due to treatment,* e.g. *sulphur dermatitis*

Q. How do you treat scabies?

Ans:
- Family contacts to be screened and treated simultaneously
- Secondary infection is treated by antibiotics
- Medicine used and instructions given to the patient are:

Medicines used:

1. Twenty-five percent benzylbenzoate
2. Unguentum sulphur
3. Gamma benzene hexachloride (1%)—not to be used in pregnant women and infants
4. Monosulfiram used as soap
5. Topical thiabendazole
6. Permethrin (5% cream)
7. Malathione (0.5%)
8. Ivermectin (200 mg/kg/orally as a single dose). Patients with crusted scabies (Norwegian variety) require two or more doses of ivermectin.

Methods used:

Patient is advised to take bath with soap and H_2O. During bath, patient must scrub his body to open the burrows and then allow the skin to dry. Now apply the specific medicine from the neck to foot for 3 consecutive days. Patient should take bath daily and wear fresh garments. Clean or autoclave the bed sheets and used garments.

- Antihistamines and calamine lotion may be used to relieve itching.
- Patient's nail should be cut properly. His daily used articles (towel, pillow, bed sheet) to be kept separately.

212

Hairy Leukoplakia

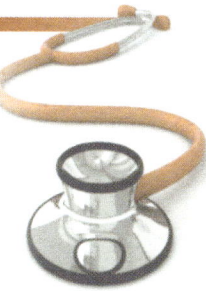

INSTRUCTION

- Perform general physical examination

SALIENT FEATURES

- Pain during deglutition

HISTORY

Ask for the following:

- History of sore tongue, pain during deglutition (present)
- History of change in voice
- History of cracking of lips or fissuring of tongue
- History of HIV and treatment, if being received
- History of drugs, e.g. steroids, immunosuppressive

EXAMINATION

General Physical Examination

- Hairy white lesions on the lateral margins of the tongue (Fig. 212.1). The lesions are corrugated and has vertical lines with fine thick hairy projections
- Gums are normal
- Mucous membrane of oral cavity is normal
- No angular stomatitis, no cheilosis
- No evidence of oral candidiasis

PROVISIONAL DIAGNOSIS

The patient has typical hairy white lesions on lateral aspect of the tongue (lesion) due to oral hairy leukoplakia caused by Epstein-Barr virus (aetiology). It is precancerous condition (functional status).

QUESTIONS AND ANSWERS

Q. **What is the cause of lesion?**
Ans: It is caused by Epstein-Barr virus.

Q. **What is its significance?**
Ans: *First:* These lesions are highly suggestive of

HIV infection in patients who have no other obvious cause of immunodeficiency.
Second: This has higher rates of progression to AIDS.

Q. **What are the common oral manifestations of AIDS?**
Ans: 1. Oral candidiasis
2. Hairy leukoplakia
3. Acute necrotising ulcerative gingivitis
4. Necrotising ulcerative periodontitis
5. Necrotising stomatitis
6. Aphthous ulceration
7. Warts
8. Kaposi's sarcoma on hard palate

Q. **What is histopathology of oral leukoplakia?**
Ans: The histopathological changes include:
- Hyperplasia and ballooning of prickle cells (acanthosis)
- Hyperkeratosis
- Depletion of Langerhans cells

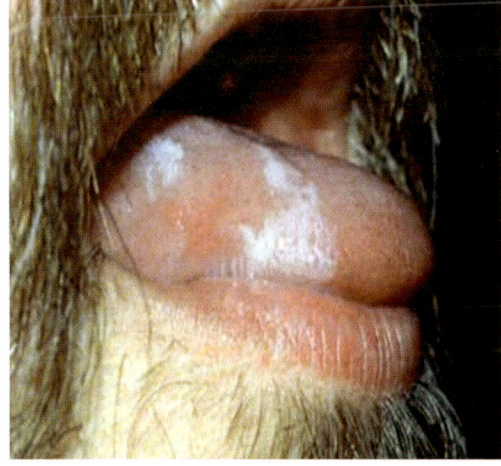

Fig. 212.1: Hairy leukoplakia of the tongue in a patient with AIDS

Q. **What is the cause of dark colored tongue in this condition?**

Ans: Dark-colored tongue is due to deposition of porphyrin pigment by the bacterial metabolism.

Q. **How would you confirm the diagnosis?**

Ans: By biopsy.

Q. **How would you treat it?**

Ans: The lesions may sometimes resolve spontaneously, hence, treatment is seldom indicated.

Anti-viral drugs, e.g. ganciclovir or acyclovir may be helpful to relieve discomfort. Podophyllin and retinoin have been used.

213

Kaposi's Sarcoma

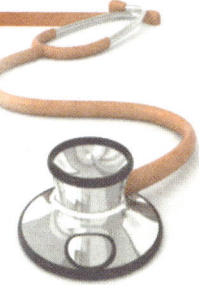

INSTRUCTION

- Perform general physical examination

SALIENT FEATURES

- Patient is a case of HIV on treatment

HISTORY

Ask for the following:

- Ask about the history of HIV
- Drug history, e.g. steroids, immunosuppressive
- History of dysphagia, mouth pain, change in voice
- History of oral lesions, e.g. angular chlorosis, raw tongue, aphthous ulcers, oral candidiasis, gingivitis, etc.

EXAMINATION

General Physical Examination

- Purplish non-blanching papular or nodular lesions either solitary or in crops present on the limbs (Fig. 213.1B), mouth, pinnae, nose, palate (Fig. 213.1A) and eyelids

PROVISIONAL DIAGNOSIS

The patient has lesions suggestive of Kaposi's sarcoma (lesion) caused by human herpes virus 8 (aetiology) in patients with AIDS.

QUESTIONS AND ANSWERS

Q. **What are the clinical types of Kaposi's sarcoma?**

Ans: I. *Classical KS or Epidemic type:* It is found in Jews, indolent in nature, found on the legs of old men, not fatal.

II. *Endemic type (African variety):* This is an aggressive invasive tumor, occurs in children and young men. It can be fatal.

III. *AIDS Associated KS:* It is found in patients with AIDS and more common

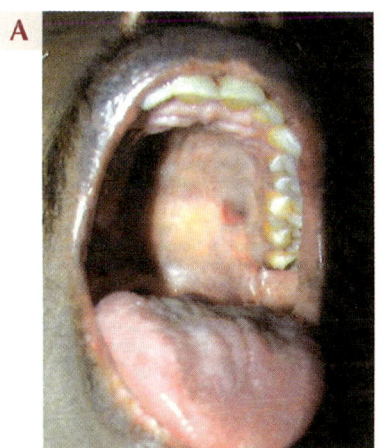
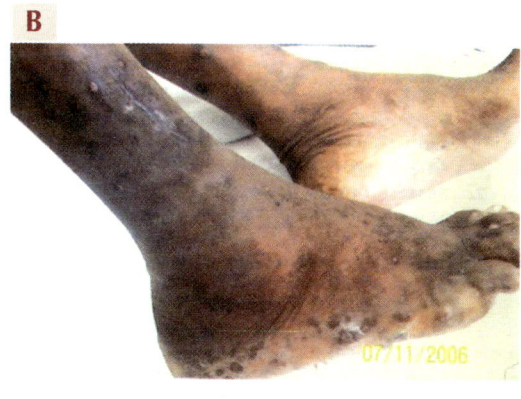

Fig. 213.1: Kaposi's sarcoma (KS) in HIV-positive immunocompromised patient. (A) Kaposi's sarcoma on the left side of the hard palate; (B) Kaposi's sarcoma of leg with brawny edema and hyperpigmentation of the skin

in homosexuals. The cutaneous lesions respond to interferon-alfa and cytotoxic chemotherapy. Some patients may develop second malignancy such as lymphoma.

IV. *Transplantation Associated KS:* It occurs in patients receiving high-dose immuno-suppressive therapy. These usually regress when therapy is stopped. Transmission of human herpes virus 8 infection occurs from renal transplant donor to recipient and is a risk factor.

Q. **What is the aetiology of KS?**

Ans: Human herpes virus 8 infection is implicated in its aetiopathogenesis because 70 to 100% of patients with KS have antibodies to this virus (1–3% persons in general population may have these antibodies).

Q. **What is the histopathology of Kaposi's sarcoma?**

Ans: The characteristic features of KS comprise spindle-shaped stroma cells with irregular slit like space filled with RBCs and lined by endothelium interwined with normal vascular channels.

Q. **How would you treat KS in patients with HIV infection?**

Ans: 1. Antiretroviral therapy especially regimen of zidovudine. Retinoic acid is a promising alternative.
2. Localised lesions respond to radio-therapy, cryotherapy, surgical excision, intralesional vinblastine, bleomycin or interferon-alfa.
3. Systemic treatment with interferon-alfa.
4. Radiation therapy.
5. Marrow sparing chemotherapy (e.g. bleomycin, vincristine or low-dose dox-orubicin) is used when other treatment fails in aggressive KS.

Q. **What are the differences between classical KS and KS in immunocompromised persons?**

Ans: Read Table 213.1.

Table 213.1: Clinical features of Kaposi's sarcoma

	Classical KS	KS in Immunocompromised
Epidemiology	• Elderly jews (classical KS) • Africans (endemic KS)	Common in HIV-positive homosexuals (epidemic KS)
Site	Cold parts (feet, ankles, hands, ear, nose)	Anywhere, frequent on upper trunk, head and neck. Oral mucosal lesions frequent (Fig. 213.1A)
Morphology	Dark blue to purple macules, tumors ulcerate and fungate	Bruise-like macules, nodules and plaques
Prognosis	Not so bad	Poor

214

Mycosis Fungoides

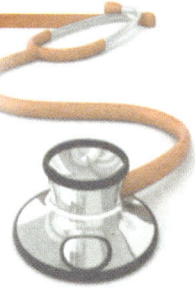

INSTRUCTION

- Perform general physical examination

SALIENT FEATURES

- Skin lesions around buttocks and pruritus

HISTORY

Ask about the following:

- Age of the patient (middle to old age)
- Itching
- Neck/inguinal swellings
- Multiple skin nodules

EXAMINATION

General Physical Examination

- There are brownish red, pruritic plaques present on the back and buttocks of this patient (Fig. 214.1)
- There is neck or inguinal lymphadenopathy (present)

PROVISIONAL DIAGNOSIS

The patient has brownish pruritic plaques with lymphadenopathy (lesions) suggestive of mycosis

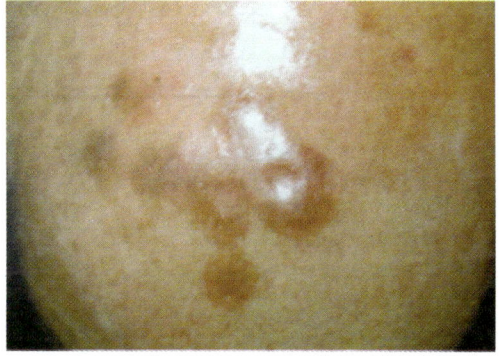

Fig. 214.1: Mycosis fungoides. Note the erythematous ulcerated nodule

fungoides (aetiology). The patient is disturbed by pruritus.

QUESTIONS AND ANSWERS

Q. What is differential diagnosis?
Ans: Psoriasis is the other condition which produces silvery white scaly pruritic plaques with red margins.

Q. What is mycosis fungoides?
Ans: The name implies mushroom-like growths on the skin, but these are rare. It is defined as lymphomatous invasion of the skin by T lymphocytes (CD4+), hence, it is a variant of cutaneous T cell lymphoma.

Q. What are the stages of cutaneous T cell lymphoma?
Ans: Stage I: Eczematoid or psoriasiform erythematous lesions
Stage II: Plaques lesion (infiltrative lesions)
Stage III: Nodules, ulcers (Fig. 214.1) and tumors formation
Stage IV: Lymphadenopathy with or without systemic involvement

Q. What is sezary syndrome?
Ans: It is an erytherodermic variant of cutaneous T cell lymphoma, where the area of skin infiltration is more and 10% or more large mononuclear cells appear in the blood accompanied by lymphadenopathy. It is resistant to treatment. Extracorporeal photopheresis (it consists of oral administration of psolarens with exposure of a lymphocyte enriched blood fraction to ultraviolet A light and reinfusion of these cells into the patient) has shown promising results.

Q. How would you confirm the diagnosis of mycosis fungoides?
Ans: Skin biopsy.

Q. Where does mycosis fungoides disseminate?
Ans: It disseminates to lymph nodes, liver, spleen, lungs, bones and kidneys.

Q. How would you treat this condition?

Ans: Topical steroids, chemotherapeutic agents, PUVA therapy and electron-beam radiotherapy have been used since long.

Now other approaches to treat it include acyclovir, interferons, pentostatin, monoclonal antibodies against T cell antigen and extracorporeal photopheresis.

215

Systemic Mastocytosis

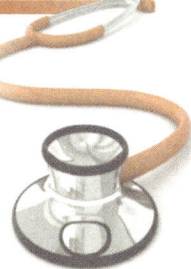

INSTRUCTION

- Perform general physical examination

SALIENT FEATURES

- Recurrent flushing and episodes of diarrhea

HISTORY

Ask for the following:

- Recurrent flushing, sweating, diarrhea, headache
- Pruritus, palpitations, vascular collapse
- Urticaria with pruritus on trauma, rubbing or exposure to heat [urticaria pigmentosa (Fig. 215.1)]
- Retrosternal burning or pain, vomiting (histamine induced gastric secretion)
- Recurrent abdominal pain (gastric erosions, peptic ulcerations)
- Bleeding, anemia
- History of repeated cough and wheezing

EXAMINATION

General Physical Examination

- There is flushing of face (present)

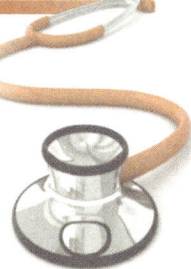

Fig. 215.1: Urticaria pigmentosa due to systemic mastocytosis

- There is reddish-brown macular lesions with telangiectasia (urticaria pigmentosa) which become pruritic on trauma, rubbing or exposure to heat (*Darier's sign*)
- BP shows wide pulse pressure or low BP
- No hepatosplenomegaly (to rule out leukemia)
- Chest shows wheezing (present)

PROVISIONAL DIAGNOSIS

The patient has urticaria pigmentosa, flushing of face, wheezes in the chest (lesion) caused by systemic mastocytosis (aetiology). Patient is disturbed by pruritus (functional status).

Q. **What are the points in favor of your diagnosis?**

Ans: 1. Recurrent flushing of face on exposure to heat. Recurrent abdominal pain
2. Urticaria with pruritus
3. Reddish-brown macular lesions with telangiectasia (urticaria pigmentosa)
4. Wide pulse pressure
5. Wheezing in the chest

QUESTIONS AND ANSWERS

Q. **What is urticaria pigmentosa?**

Ans: It is a cutaneous manifestation of systemic mastocytosis characterised by reddish brown macules with telangiectasia which is pruritic on rubbing or exposure to heat.

Q. **What do you know about systemic masto-cytosis?**

Ans: It is defined as mast cell hyperplasia in bone marrow, skin, GI tract, liver and spleen. It occurs in younger age and common in males.

Q. **What are the causes of flushing of face?**

Ans: • Systemic mastocytosis
- Carcinoid syndrome
- Drug induced

- Carbon monoxide poisoning
- Cushing's syndrome

Q. How would you classify systemic masto-cytosis?

Ans: I. Cutaneous mastocytosis (urticaria pigmentosa or variants)

II. Indolent systemic mastocytosis

III. Systemic mastocytosis with an associated clonal non-mast cell lineage disease

IV. Aggressive systemic mastocytosis

V. Mast cell leukemia

VI. Mast cell sarcoma

Q. What are the chemical mediators released by mast cells?

Ans: Histamine, prostaglandin-D, leukotrienes, heparin, etc.

Q. What investigations would you advise?

Ans: 1. Urinary histamine (increased)

2. Serum tryptase levels (elevated)

3. Coagulation profile. It is disturbed due to release of heparin by the mast cells

4. Bone marrow biopsy for confirmation (there is mast cell infiltration of the bone marrow)

5. Immunohistochemical analysis with monoclonal antibodies against mast cell markers tryptase and CD117.

Q. How would you treat it?

Ans: Treatment is symptomatic.

i. Antihistamines are used for pruritus and flushing

ii. H_2 blocker or proton pump inhibitors for gastric hypersecretion

iii. Oral cromolyn sodium for diarrhea, abdominal pain

iv. NSAIDs are used for headache, flushing not responsive to antihistamines

v. Interferon-alfa has been used for patients with aggressive disease

vi. Imitinib has shown promising results

vii. Hydroxyurea to reduce mast cell lineage progenitors

216

Urticaria

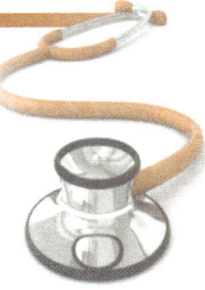

INSTRUCTION

- Perform general physical examination

SALIENT FEATURES

- Complains of pruritus following insect bite

HISTORY

Ask about the following:

- Ask about the physical agents that can precipitate it, i.e. cold, sunlight (solar rays), exercise, hot shower, pressure
- Drug precipitants, e.g. salicylates, NSAIDs, morphine, codeine, penicillin, sulphonamides
- Food allergens, e.g. strawberries, seafood, nuts, chocolate
- Blood products
- Bee and wasp stings (insects bite)
- Helminth infestations (history of expulsion of round worm)
- Viral infections and fibrile illnesses
- History of recurrent angioedema
- Obtain a history of atopy
- Inhalation of pollens, moulds, fungi or animal danders
- History of connective tissue disorder (SLE, SJögren's syndrome)

EXAMINATION

General Physical Examination

- There are typical wheal and flare lesions which are pink, smooth, edematous and ring shape with central clearing distributed over trunk, (Fig. 216.1) extremities and genitalia
- These lesions are itchy, hence, scratch marks are present (in this case)
- There is no associated respiratory difficulty or wheezing or respiratory obstruction
- The lesions are in crops (present in different stages of evolution, i.e. some are old, fading while others are fresh and red)

PROVISIONAL DIAGNOSIS

The patient has typical wheal and flare eruptions (lesion) caused by chronic urticaria and dermatographism (aetiology). There is severe itching (functional status).

QUESTIONS AND ANSWERS

Q. **What is chronic urticaria?**
Ans: It is defined as occurrence of daily or almost daily widespread pruritic wheals for at least 6 weeks duration. The causes include urticarial vasculitis due to collagen vascular disease and physical urticaria.

Q. **What is dermatographism?**
Ans: It is the presence of linear, itchy wheals, surrounded by bright red flare at the site of scratching called "wheal and flare lesions".

Q. **What are the causes of urticaria.**
Ans: Causes of urticaria are:
   I. *Primary cutaneous disorders*
      A. Acute and chronic urticaria (inhaled/ ingested allergens)

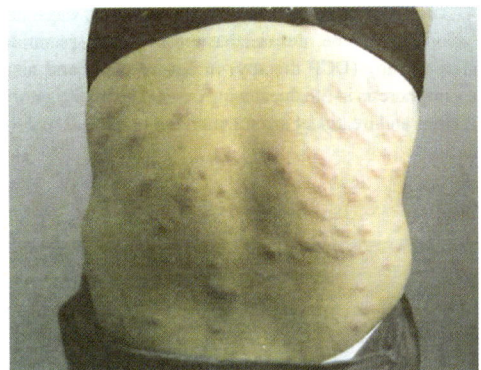

Fig. 216.1: Chronic urticaria. Note the pale pink edematous wheals with surrounding flare (wheal and flare lesions)

B. Physical urticaria
  - Dermatographism
  - Solar urticaria
  - Cholinergic urticaria
C. Angioedema (hereditary or acquired)

II. *Systemic Diseases*
  - Urticarial vasculitis
  - Hepatitis B and C infection
  - Serum sickness
  - Angioedema (hereditary or acquired)

Q.   What is angioedema?

Ans: Angioedema like urticaria is also a type I hypersensitivity reaction characterised by localised nonpitting edema involving the deeper layers of skin and subcutaneous tissue.

Q.   What are the complications of acute urticaria?

Ans: Anaphylactic shock, bronchospasm and angioedema are immediate complications.

Q.   Name the systemic disorders associated with chronic urticaria.

Ans: Hashimoto's thyroiditis and Graves' disease.

Q.   How would you investigate such a case?

Ans:
1. Blood counts for eosinophilia
2. Stool for parasite (ova)
3. Challenging test with the suspected allergen in physical urticaria
4. Serum complement C_4 levels
5. Thyroid function tests for antibodies

Q.   How would you treat chronic urticaria?

Ans:
  - Identify the trigger and try to remove it or treat it
  - Antihistamines for pruritus
  - H_2 and H_1 receptors antagonists
  - Leukotriene antagonists (montelukast and zafirlukast)
  - Corticosteroids where antihistamines show poor response
  - Cyclosporin as an immunosuppressive therapy for immunological chronic urticaria
  - Avoid the drugs, e.g. aspirin, NSAIDs, ACE inhibitors, macrolide antibiotics and antifungal (imidazole group)

217

Tuberous Sclerosis

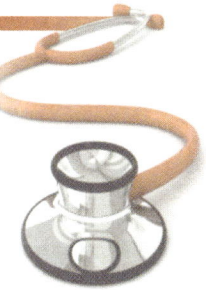

INSTRUCTION

- Perform general physical examination
- Examine relevant system

SALIENT FEATURES

- Skin lesions with seizures

HISTORY

Ask for the following:

- Family history (autosomal dominant disease)
- Seizures (recurrent)
- Mental retardation since childhood
- Skin lesions since childhood

EXAMINATION

General Physical Examination

- There are angiofibromas (ash-leaf macules/papules/nodules) distributed over the face in a butterfly distribution (Fig. 217.1A). These tumors are vascular and fibrous in origin
- There are also flesh colored patches (leathery thickenings) that are firm and plaque like present on the back [shagreen patches (Fig. 217.1B)] in lumbosacral region

- The macular hypopigmented leaf-like lesion (ash-leaf) seen on the trunk that are easily detected by wood's light
- Subungal fibromas absent
- Examine the fundus (retinal glial hamartomas)

PROVISIONAL DIAGNOSIS

The patient has adenoma sebaceum (lesion) caused by tuberous sclerosis (etiology). The patient has mental retardation (low IQ) and seizures (functional status).

QUESTIONS AND ANSWERS

Q. **What is the genetic defect in tuberous sclerosis?**

Ans: Tuberous sclerosis is an autosomal dominant disorder characterised by gene mutations of gene TSC1 and TSC2 located on chromosome 9.

Q. **What are the various lesions in tuberous sclerosis?**

Ans: 1. CNS hamartomas
2. Retinal angiolipomas

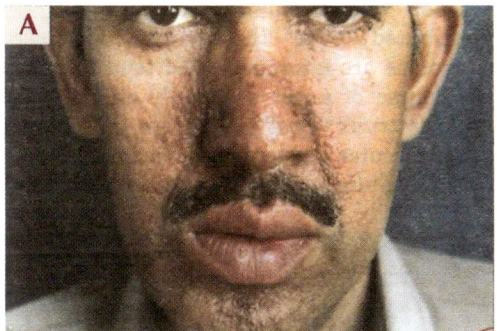
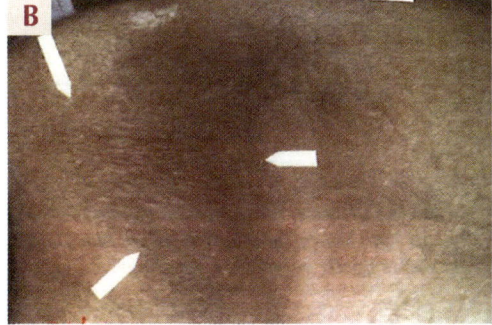

Fig. 217.1: Tuberous sclerosis. (A) Adenoma sebaceum over the side of the mouth and nose; (B) Shagreen patch—a flesh-colored tumor over the back

3. Cardiac rhabdomyomas and pulmonary myomas
4. Cysts in liver and kidneys

Q. **What is prevalence of this disease?**

Ans: Population based studies estimate a frequency of I in 12,000 to I in 14,000 children below the age of 10 years.

Q. **What is the sequence of appearance of clinical manifestations of tuberous sclerosis?**

Ans: 1. Hypopigmented macules (ash-leaf spots, cortical tubers and cardiac rhabomyomas and renal cysts are present since infancy or early childhood).
2. Shagreen patch is identified only in early childhood.

3. Adenoma sebaceum, CNS gliomas and angiomyolipomas are seen in childhood and adolescence.
4. Ungual fibromas appear after puberty.

Q. **What could be the cardiac manifestation of tuberous sclerosis?**

Ans: Due to cardiac rhabdomyomas, there can be outflow tract obstruction, murmurs and arrhythmias

Q. **What is the cause of seizures in tuberous sclerosis?**

Ans: CNS hamartomas, CNS gliomas and cortical tubers are the causes of neurological manifestations including epilepsy.

218

Malignant Melanoma

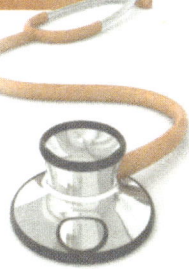

INSTRUCTION

- Look at the skin lesion and perform general physical examination

SALIENT FEATURES

- Recent change in the size of mole

HISTORY

Ask for the following:

- Family history
- Make the following enquiries about the mole:
  - i. Is there any change in color?
  - ii. Does the mole itch?
  - iii. Is there any change in size, shape or morphology of mole?
  - iv. Does your skin has freckles or tendency to freckling?

EXAMINATION

General Physical Examination

- There is asymmetrical, hyperpigmented mole with irregular spreading borders as if pigment is leaking into the surrounding skin (Fig. 218.1)
- This mole is raised from the surface as compared to other moles
- It shows color variegation
- There is no bleeding or ulceration
- There is no regional lymphadenopathy or hepatomegaly

PROVISIONAL DIAGNOSIS

The patient has a large pigmented mole suggestive of malignant melanoma (lesion) which is a malignant tumor arising from the melanocytes (etiology). It is spreading and increasing in size (functional status).

QUESTIONS AND ANSWERS

Q. **Why do you call it malignant?**
Ans: • The lesion (mole) has been persisting for sometimes.

- There is recent change in size, color and has adopted infiltrating nature.
- It is itchy now.
- It fullfils the ABCDE mnemonic about malignant melanoma (read it as a question).

Q. **What are the different types of malignant melanoma?**

Ans: a. **Superficial spreading melanoma:** It is commonly seen on the trunk as an elevated hyperkeratotic pigmented lesion existing for sometimes, it displays inflammation at the periphery. Elevated nodules and serosanguinous oozing arouse the suspicion.

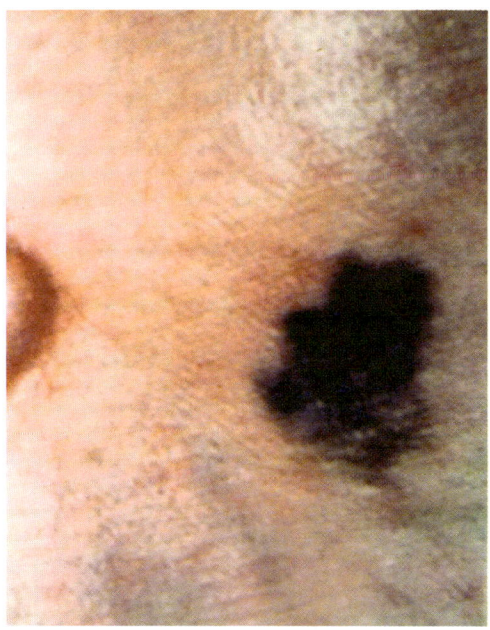

Fig. 218.1: Malignant melanoma. Note the irregular hyperpigmented mole which has variegation of color

b. **Nodular melanoma:** It is more common in males, develops as a pigmented nodule with no preceding *in situ* phase. It is usually seen on the head, neck and trunk. The prognosis is poor.

c. **Acral lentiginous melanoma** occurs on the palms and soles and is the most common type in the Chinese and Japanese.

d. **Lentigo maligina** (*in situ changes of malignancy only*) and **lentigo maligna melanoma** occurs most often on the exposed skin in elderly. A speckled macular lentigo maligina may have been present for many years before a nodule of invasive melanoma appears within it.

Q. **What is ABCDE mnemonic about malignant melanoma?**

Ans: All changing pigmented lesions deserve careful examination for malignant melanomas remembering its 'ABCDE' characteristics (*see* the box).

ABCDE Characteristics of Malignant Melanoma

A — Asymmetric

B — Border irregular and infiltrating

C — Color irregularity

D — Diameter > 0.6 cm

E — Elevation irregular

Q. **What are predisposing factors?**

Ans: 1. Presence of pre-existing nevus for long duration (dysplastic nevus), freckles and melanocytic nevi
2. Sunlight
3. Positive family history

Q. **What is the role of genetics in malignant melanoma?**

Ans: There is mutation or deletion of tumor suppressor gene p16 in this condition. Other genes associated with this condition are CMMI on chromosome Ip36 and CDK4 on chromosome 12q14.

Q. **What are the patterns of growth of malignant melanoma? What is their significance?**

Ans: Read Table 218.1

Table 218.1: Pattern of growth and significance

Pattern	Significance
1. Radial or horizontal growth within epidermis and dermis	The tumour does not have the capacity to metastasize
2. Vertical growth downwards deep into the dermis as an expansile mass lacking cellular growth	There is emergence of clones of cells with metastatic potential, hence, can spread to other tissues (lymph node and liver)

Q. **What are the prognostic indicators in malignant melanoma?**

Ans: 1. Tumour thickness. Deeper the tumor, the more likely is metastasising
2. Level of invasion (superficial or deep)
3. Sex of the patient (male sex)
4. Anatomical location (melanomas in thorax, upper arms, neck and scalp show a higher risk)

Q. **How would you treat such lesions?**

Ans: Surgical excision is the treatment of choice.
- Excision biopsy with a 2 mm margin is recommended for suspected lesions
- In biopsy proven cases, a wider excision is recommended depending on the thickness of tumor
- Elective lymph node dissection is controversial. In general, it is indicated in melanomas of intermediate thickness with enlargement of regional lymph nodes (stage II melanoma)
- Intralesional avirulent HSV, interferon alpha and vaccine are being tried with promising results to reduce recurrences
- For disseminated disease, chemotherapy is used. Radiotherapy is only palliative therapy for recurrences

Q. **How do you stage malignant melanoma?**

Ans: The clinical stages are:

Stage I: Primary skin lesion only

Stage II: Regional lymph nodes involved

Stage III: Distant metastasis (nodal or visceral)

The stage I has the best prognosis (5 yrs survival in 75% patients)

219

Atopic Dermatitis

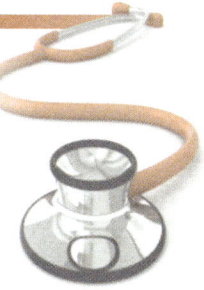

INSTRUCTION

- Perform general physical examination

SALIENT FEATURES

- Itchy and discharging skin lesions

HISTORY

Ask for the following:

- Personal or family history of atopy (asthma, hay fever, atropic dermatitis, gastrointestinal or food allergy)
- History of itching (present)
- History of discharge from the lesions (weeping eczema) is also present

EXAMINATION

General Physical Examination

- Scratch marks or excoriation of skin (present)
- Hyperpigmented or hypopigmented lichenified lesions in flexures (face, neck, trunk, feet (Fig. 219.1), wrist, popliteal folds)

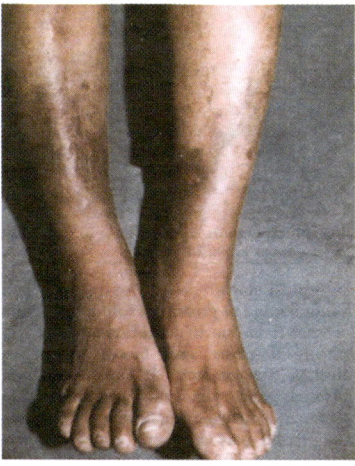

Fig. 219.1: Chronic eczematous dermatitis

PROVISIONAL DIAGNOSIS

The patient has itchy, discharging skin lesions called chronic dermatitis (lesion) caused by atopy (there is family history of asthma and rhinitis). The patient has severe pruritus (functional status).

QUESTIONS AND ANSWERS

Q. What is atopic eczema/dermatitis?

Ans: Atopic dermatitis is chronic pruritic skin disorder of unknown aetiology associated with personal or family history of atopy and a typical distribution and morphology. Itching is severe, distressing and there is tendency for lichenification and frequently raised levels of IgE.

Q. What is its prevalence?

Ans: It is estimated that about 3% infants and about 10% of school-going children suffer from atopic dermatitis.

Q. What are the common causes of pruritus?

Ans: *Skin conditions:*

- Scabies
- Urticaria
- Insect bite (e.g. flee, bed-bug)
- Atopic eczema
- Allergic reactions

Systemic disorders:

- *Metabolic disorders*, e.g. hyperthyroidism
- *Malignant disease*, e.g. chronic lymphatic leukemia, lymphoma, some carcinomas
- *Hematological disease*, e.g. polycythemia, vera
- *Renal disease*, e.g. chronic renal failure
- *Liver disease*, e.g. cholestasis, particularly primary biliary cirrhosis
- *Miscellaneous*, e.g. senile pruritus, drug (opiates)

Q. What are the stages of atopic dermatitis?

Ans: There are three age-related stages as follows:
Infantile stage (Infant <1 yr): The eczema is

acute with pruritic papular vesicular oozing lesions distributed over the face and trunk. The napkin area is mostly spared.

Childhood stage (2–12 yrs): The rash becomes settled on the back of the knees, front of elbows, wrists and ankles. There is intense itching.

Adults (puberty onwards): The face and trunk are common sites of involvement. Lichenification is common. Discoid pattern of eczema may be seen on hands and feet.

Q.   **What are the diagnostic criteria for atopic eczema?**

Ans: Read Table 219.1

Q.   **What is the immunological basis of atopic dermatitis?**

Ans: **Immunological abnormalities:** Raised IgE levels occur in 80% individuals. There is defect in cell-mediated immunity in some patients. Infections are common due to defects in neutrophils and monocytes chemotaxis.

Q.   **What is the genetic basis of this disorder?**

Ans: Two major genetic defects are:
  i. Genes encoding epidermal and other epithelial structural proteins
  ii. Genes encoding major elements of immune system

Q.   **Name the exacerbating factors.**

Ans: **Exacerbating factors:** Non-specific, e.g. heat, humidity, dryness of skin and contact with woolen clothes may causes flare-up of the disease, hence, are to be avoided. Irritation may occur following contact with food or animal saliva in a sensitised individual.

Table 219.1: Hanifin and Rajka's diagnostic criteria for atopic dermatitis

A. Major criteria (*must have 3 or more*)

- Pruritus
- Typical morphology and distribution, i.e.
    - Facial and extensor involvement in infants and children
    - Flexural lichenification in adults
- Dermatitis, e.g. chronic or relapsing
- Positive family history of atopy (e.g. hay fever, asthma, rhinitis, atopic dermatitis)

B. Minor criteria (*must have 3 or more*)

• Cataract	• Infections
• Cheilitis	• Itching when sweating
• Conjunctivitis, recurrent	• Keratoconus
• Facial pallor/erythema	• Keratosis pilaris
• Food intolerance	• Nipple dermatitis
• Hand dermatitis	• Orbital darkening
• Ichthyosis	• Palmar hyperlinearity
• High IgE level	• Pityriasis alba
• Positive type I hypersensitivity on testing	• White dermographism
• Xerosis	• Wool intolerance

220

Herpes Labialis

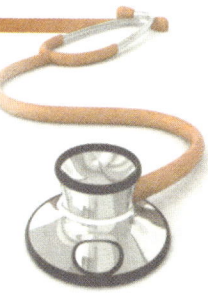

INSTRUCTION

- Perform general physical examination

SALIENT FEATURES

- Ulcerations of the lips and mouth with difficulty in swallowing

HISTORY

Ask for the following:

- Pain, itching, burning around or inside the mouth
- Vesiculations of the lesion (present)
- Sore mouth with odynophagia (present)
- Fever, myalgia
- Swelling and pain in the gums
- Ulceration of the mouth present and gums
- Pain in fingertips (whitlow)
- History of flu-like symptoms, fever, confusion and speech and behaviours disturbance (encephalitis or meningitis)
- History of genital infection (vulvovaginitis, cervicitis)

EXAMINATION

General Physical Examination

- The patient has multiple vesicles with a erythematous base on the lips and around the mouth (Fig. 220.1). Mouth ulceration present.

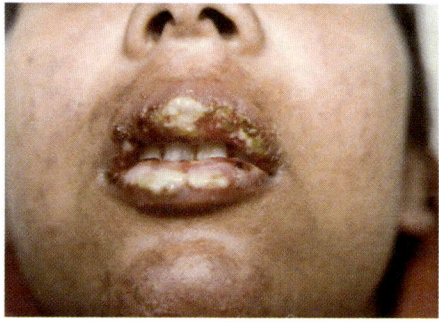

Fig. 220.1: Herpes labialis

- There are no vesicles over the tongue, palate (soft and hard), gums and pharynx
- No neck lymphadenopathy
- No genital involvement

Systemic Examination

- Tell the examiner that you would like to examine CNS
- CNS is normal

PROVISIONAL DIAGNOSIS

The patient has small vesicles around the mouth (lesion) caused by herpes simplex (labialis) virus I (aetiology) which is causing severe itching and bleeding (functional status).

QUESTIONS AND ANSWERS

Q. What are the clinical manifestations of Herpes Simplex Virus I (HSV1) infection?

Ans: 1. Herpes labialis (cold sore)
2. Keratoconjunctivitis
3. Gingivostomatitis, mouth ulcers
4. Encephalitis
5. Finger infection (whitlows)

Q. What are the clinical manifestations of HSV2 infection?

Ans: HSV2 causes genital infection (vulvovaginitis, cervicitis), neonatal infection (congenital malformations).

Q. What are the complications of herpes infections?

Ans: 1. Erythema multiforme and Stevens-Johnson syndrome (rare)
2. Dissemination of infection in immunocompromised persons
3. Esophagitis and proctitis, hepatitis, pneumonia in those with AIDS or immunosuppression
4. Keratitis, scarring and impaired visual acquity

5. Herpes simplex encephalitis (temporal lobe encephalitis)
6. Herpes gladiatorum in wrestlers (infection of skin)
7. Neonatal CNS infection
8. CNS complications include aseptic meningitis, radiculomyelopathy, benign lymphocytic meningitis (Mollaret's meningitis)
9. Bell's palsy. An association between HSV1 and Bell's palsy is established
10. Febrile neutropenia, chronic urticaria, perinephric abscess

Q.   What is the pathogenesis of herpes simplex infection?

Ans: The portal of entry of HSV1 is through breaks in the mucosa or skin. It then attaches and enters the epithelial cells to replicate. From here, it is taken up by free sensory nerve endings at the dermis and transported to sensory ganglion. The primary lesion goes undetected. After recovery from the primary (initial) lesion, the virus remains dormant in the sensory ganglion for rest of the life of the person. Periodically it gets reactivated by stress, trauma, radiation and travels down the sensory nerves to the skin or mucosa to produce the lesion.

Viral shedding from the lesions occurs for weeks and months which is the cause of transmission to other contacts (sexual partners). HSV1 can also be transmitted from mother to infant at the time of delivery.

Q.   What are the risk factors for HSV transmission?

Ans: 1. Female gender
2. Sexually transmitted infections
3. An increased number of sex partners
4. Contact with commercial sex workers
5. Lower socioeconomic status
6. Young age at first sexual activity

Q.   How would you confirm your diagnosis?

Ans: 1. *Scrappings from the lesions* stained with Wright, Giemsa (Tzanck preparation) or Papanicolaou's stain will demonstrate the giant cells or intranuclear inclusions of herpes infection
2. *Tissue cultures* for isolation of virus
3. Detection of HSV1 antigen from the scrappings
4. Herpe select HSV1 and HSV2 by *Enzyme-linked immunosorbent assay* and HSV1 and HSV2 *immunoblot test*

Q.   How would you treat HSV1 infection?

Ans: 1. Acyclovir, valaciclovir, foscarnet for muco-cutaneous infection
2. I.V. acyclovir for HSV encephalitis
3. Idoxuridine, topical vidarabine for eye infections
4. High dose vidarabine and acyclovir for neonatal infection

Q.   How will you treat herpes labialis?

Ans: Acyclovir cream locally is quite effective.

Q.   How would you confirm HSV encephalitis?

Ans: By PCR of CSF to detect HSV DNA.

221

Herpes Zoster

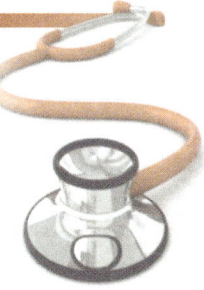

INSTRUCTION

- Perform general physical examination

SALIENT FEATURES

- Unilateral peripheral chest pain and skin lesion

HISTORY

Ask for the following:

- Pain and irritation around the lesions, i.e. around the nose and eyes (herpes zoster ophthalmicus) and in the lower thoracic (present in this case) and abdominal dermatomes (postherpetic neuralgia)
- Age of the patient
- Facial palsy, lesions around the external ear, vertigo, tinnitus, deafness, etc. (Ramsay Hunt syndrome)
- Presence of an underlying immunocompromised state (zoster infection is seven times more common in homosexual men with HIV than in HIV negative persons)
- History of SLE on steroids and immunomodulators (they are more prone to zoster infection)
- Patients of multiple myeloma receiving bortezomib therapy

EXAMINATION

General Physical Examination

- There is a group of vesicular eruptions in the thoracic dermatomes (Fig. 221.1). There is excoriation and itching
- There is no enlargement of regional lymph nodes (axillary or inguinal)
- No lesion around the eye, nose or ear

PROVISIONAL DIAGNOSIS

The patient has groups of vesicular eruptions along 9th to 11th thoracic dermatomes (lesion) caused by herpes zoster (etiology). Patient has severe local pain (functional status).

QUESTIONS AND ANSWERS

Q. Where are the vesicles formed in herpes zoster infection?

Ans: Prickle cell layer of the epidermis as a result of balloon degeneration of cells and serous exudation.

Q. What are the clinical hallmarks of herpes zoster infection?

Ans: 1. It starts as macules, then forms vesicles and then pustules
2. The lesions have dermatological distribution
3. Severe pain associated with fever and malaise followed by a rash a few days later

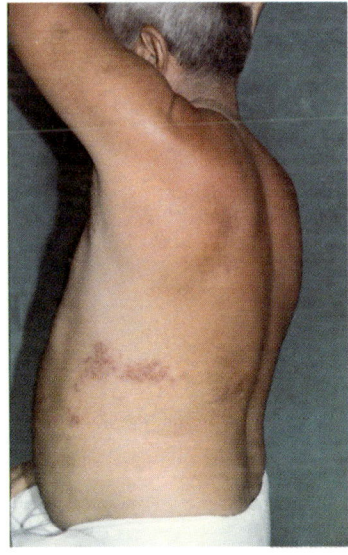

Fig. 221.1: Herpes zoster. Note the vesicular eruptions along the thoracic dermatomes which were the cause of his chest pain

Q. Which nerve is affected when the lesions are present around the nose?

Ans: The ophthalmic (Ist) division of the 5th (trigeminal) cranial nerve.

Q. What is Ramsay Hunt syndrome?

Ans: Facial palsy, lesions of the external ear with or without tympanic membrane involvement, vertigo and tinnitus or deafness signify geniculate ganglion involvement called Ramsay Hunt syndrome.

Q. What are the complications of herpes zoster?

Ans: 1. Postherpetic neuralgia (Fig. 221.2)
2. Herpes zoster ophthalmicus
3. Aseptic meningitis
4. Peripheral motor neuropathy, phrenic nerve palsy
5. Myelitis, encephalitis, cerebellitis (rare)
6. Stroke
7. Bacterial skin superinfections
8. Ramsay Hunt syndrome
9. Bell's palsy
10. Acute retinal necrosis

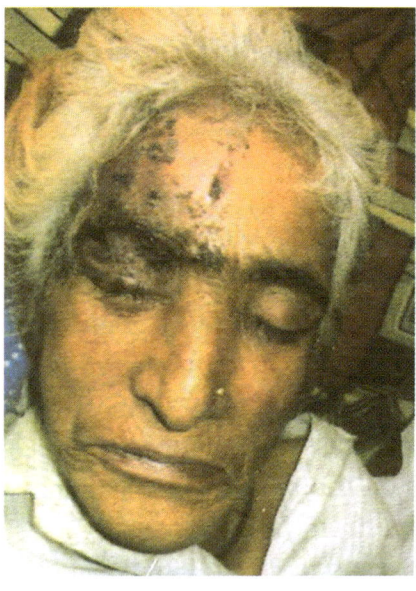

Figs. 221.2: Postherpetic neuralgia. Note the typical vesiculopapular lesion (healing) that was associated with severe pain over the right forehead

Q. What are the features of herpes zoster in patients with HIV infection?

Ans: It is usually unidermatomal and uneventful, but may be multi-dermatomal, disseminated, recurrent or persistent infection in the form of hyperkeratotic nodular lesions.

Q. How would you confirm your diagnosis?

Ans: The diagnosis is confirmed by rising viral titres and isolation of the virus from the blister (The Tzanck smear demonstrates giant cells and viral inclusions when material scrapped from the vesicle is stained with Wright's stain).

Diagnosis of neurological complications require detection of VZV DNA or anti-VZV IgG in CSF or VZV DNA in tissue.

Q. How would you manage this case?

Ans: 1. *Local soothing agent*, e.g. calamine lotion locally
2. *Pain* will be relieved either by topical capsaicin, lignocaine patch or by oral gabapentin, pregablin and amitriptyline
3. *Antiseptic powder* to be sprinkled to prevent secondary infection
4. *Antiviral therapy* (aciclovir, famciclovir, famiclovir) for faster healing and to reduce incidence and intensity of post-herpetic neuralgia
5. *Interferon* is found to be effective in limiting zoster infection in cancer patients

Q. What is the role of vaccination?

Ans: Vaccination in older persons > 60 yrs has been useful to reduce incidence of herpes zoster infection, its severity and chances of complications.

Q. How would you prevent this condition?

Ans: Immunoglobulin is indicated for protection in immunocompromised patients after zoster infection and for women in pregnancy exposed to zoster infection.

Q. What are the CNS complications of herpes zoster in patients with AIDS?

Ans: 1. Multifocal encephalitis, ventriculitis
2. Vasculopathy (vasculitis of meningeal vessels)
3. Focal necrotizing myelitis
4. Acute severe cerebellitis
5. Acute hemorrhagic meningomyeloradiculopathy

222

Seborrheic Dermatitis

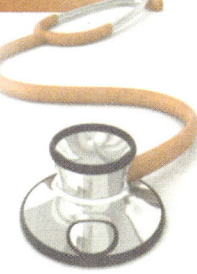

INSTRUCTION

- Perform general physical examination

SALIENT FEATURES

- Itching over the scalp and back

HISTORY

Ask for the following:

- History of scalp dandruff (present)
- History of itching (present)
- History of underlying parkinsonism, stroke and HIV (it is common in these conditions)

EXAMINATION

- Greasy scales overlying the erythematous plaques in the interscapula region (Fig. 222.1A)
- There were also patches of greasy scaly lesions over the face (eyebrows, eyelids, nasolabial folds) and ear
- There is no involvement of submammary folds and gluteal crafts
- There can be dandruff over the scalp (white scales are shown in a child with seborrheic dermatitis (Fig. 222.1B)
- The patient has features of parkinsonism

PROVISIONAL DIAGNOSIS

There is seborrheic dermatitis (lesion) in a patient with parkinsonism. The condition is cosmetically unacceptable to the patient (functional status).

QUESTIONS AND ANSWERS

Q. What is the etiology of this condition?

Ans: This is a genetically predisposed condition mediated by several factors including poor nutritional status, infection (*Malassezia furfur*) and hormones (androgens).

Q. Name adult clinical variants of this condition.

Ans: Adult variants are:

1. Pityriasis capitis (dandruff)
2. Blepharitis
3. Pityriasiform seborrheic dermatitis involving trunk and limbs (rare)
4. Flexural seborrheic dermatitis involving body folds (breast folds, thighs axillary folds, groins, genitalia and intertriginous area)
5. Pitirosporum (malassezia) folliculitis in immunocompromised hosts

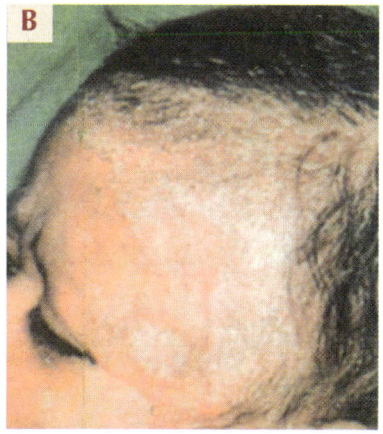

Fig. 222.1: (A) Seborrheic dermatitis. Note the erythematous plaques with greasy scales in the interscapular region in a patient with parkinsonism; (B) Seborrheic dermatitis over the head in a child

6. Erythroderma (exfoliative dermatitis)—a generalised variety with systemic manifestations

Q. Name the infantile variant.

Ans:
1. Scalp seborrheic dermatitis (cradle cap) on the scalps of infants
2. Leiner's disease (a poorly defined entity)
3. Pityriasis amiantacea (asbestos like scales adhering to the scalp hairs). It is associated with psoriasis, atopic dermatitis or tinea capitis

Q. What is HIV-related seborrheic dermatitis?

Ans: It is severe, diffuse and inflammatory seborrheic dermatitis that occurs in patients with HIV when CD4 count is $< 400 \times 10^6$ cells/l.

Q. How would you treat it?

Ans: The skin lesions are treated by:
1. Topical antifungal shampoos, creams, gels and ointment containing ketoconazole, bifonazole
2. Topical glucocorticoids
3. Shampoos containing coal tar and salicylic acid
4. Selenium sulphide shampoo for scalp lesion
5. Eyelids margin respond to cleaning of lid margins with undiluted Johnson and Johnson baby sampoo using a cotton swab
6. Topical tacrolimus ointment
7. Topical lithium (succinate and gluconate) is also effective as an alternative therapy

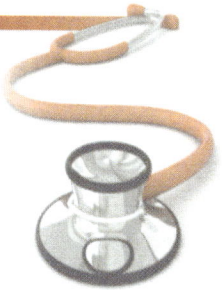

223

Dermatophytosis (Ringworm)

INSTRUCTION

• Examine the skin of the patient

SALIENT FEATURES

• Scaly skin lesion over the head

HISTORY

Ask for the following:

• Hypo or hyerpigmented macules with scaling over trunk, face and extremities
• History of seborrheic dermatitis (it predisposes to fungal infections)
• History of itching (present over scalp and body)
• History of involvement of many family members (it is contagious)
• Moist skin (bathing and perspiration perpetuate it)

EXAMINATION

• Velvet pink macules with fine scales over the scalp (Fig. 223.1)
• Large confluent areas are also seen

PROVISIONAL DIAGNOSIS

The patient has Tinea capitis (lesion) caused by mild superficial fungal infection of the skin (aetiology). There is itching (functional status).

QUESTIONS AND ANSWERS

Q. **What do you understand about Tinea capitis?**
Ans: Tinea capitis refers to fungal involvement (ring worm) of scalp and hair (Fig. 223.1). The organism most commonly is *Microsporum canis*, which is transmitted from the coats of dogs and cats. It occurs commonly in children as adults are protected due to fungistatic properties of sebum.

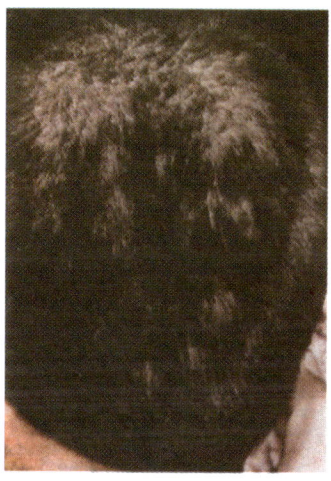

Fig. 223.1: Tinea capitis

There are 4 different types of T. capitis:
i. *Non-inflammatory:* Circular patches
ii. *Inflammatory:* Boggy soft mass
iii. *Black dot variety (Trichophyton species infection):* There is invasion of hair shaft
iv. *Favus (Trichophyton sp. infection):* This is more widespread and severe infection

Q. **Name the conditions with superficial and subcutaneous fungal infection of the skin?**
Ans: Read Box 1.

Box 1: Fungal infection of the skin	
Clinical condition	**Causative organism**
A. Superficial and subcutaneous infection	
• Pityriasis	*Pityrosporon* versicolor *orbiculare*
• Dermatophytosis	*Dermatophytes*
• Candidiasis	*Candida albicans*
• Mycotic mycetoma	*Madurella mycetomii*
• Rhinosporidiosis	*Rhinosporidium seeberi*
• Sporotrichosis	*Sporothrix schenckii*

Q. **What is Tinea barbae?**

Ans: **Tinea barbae** (dermatophytosis of beard and moustache) presents with perifollicular pustules, papules, erythema, crusting, seropurulent discharge and easy pluckability of hairs of the beard and moustache. There is alopecia on healing.

Q. **What is *Tinea corporis* and *Tinea cruris*?**

Ans: *Tinea corporis* is fungal infection on glabrous skin with exclusion of palms, soles and groin and *Tinea cruris* is fungal infection of groins (Fig. 223.2). Both present as annular lesions with erythematous and vesicular or scaly borders with central clearing on the trunk and limbs. The waist is common site for chronic and indolent lesions especially in obese women and the causative fungus is *Tinea rubrum*. *Tinea cruris* (causative organism— *T. cruris*) involving the groin is frequently seen in males with chronic infection. Secondary bacterial infection with maceration may supervene.

Q. **What is Tinea pedis? and Tinea manum?**

Ans: **Tinea pedis** is fungal infection of the soles and **Tinea manum** is fungal infection of palms. Both present with fissuring, scaling or maceration in the interdigital areas over the soles (pedis) and palms (manum). The inflammatory type manifests as clear vesicles which later become seropurulent. When there is involvement of web spaces alone, it is called *intertriginous variety*.

Tinea unguium (involvement of nails) (Fig. 223.3): Asymmetrical nail involvement is seen in the form of discoloration, chalky deposits, subungual hyperkeratosis and fragmentation or partial separation of nail plates. Great toe nails are commonly involved than finger nails. Untreated Tinea unguium is the most common cause of failure and relapses of tinea on other parts of the body.

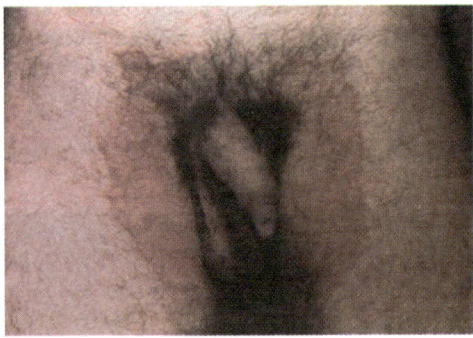

Fig. 223.2: Tinea cruris—fungal infection of groin

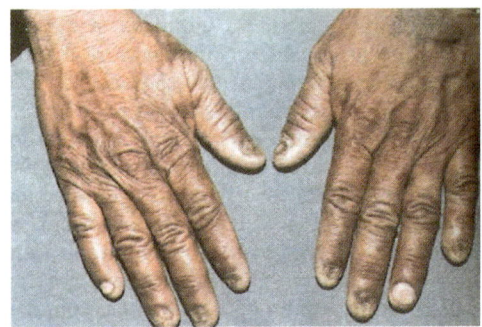

Fig. 223.3: Tinea unguium. Note the thickening and discolouration of nail plates oncholysis is frequent

Q. **How would you investigate a patient with tinea (fungus) infection?**

Ans: 1. *Potassium hydroxide mount 10%:* The fungi will be seen as long refractile, branched and separate hyphae

2. *Wood's lamp examination:* The lesions of tinea produce fluorescence when examined under Wood's lamp. This examination has diagnostic as well as prognostic value

3. Slide agglutination test

4. Culture on Sabourand's medium

Q. **How would you treat tinea infection?**

Ans: 1. **Topical antifungal agents:** They are used for local application and are time-tested and effective. They are:

- Benzoic acid (whitefield ointment) compound

- *Imidazoles*
  - Clotrimazole (1% cream, solution, powder and 100 mg, 200 mg, 500 mg vaginal pessary)
  - Miconazole (2% cream, solution, powder, vaginal pessary)
  - Econazole (1% cream)
  - Ketoconazole (2% cream and shampoo)

- *Allylamines*
  - Gention violet
  - Povidone iodine

- *Miscellaneous*
  - Olamine, nystatin, halopeogin, gention violet, selenium sulphide shampoo, sodium thiosulphate solution, etc.7

Sodium thiosulphate, zinc pyrithione and selenium sulphite shampoo (half diluted) are exclusively used for treatment of tinea versicolor. All these medications are applied locally thrice weekly 10–30 minutes before bath for about 15 applications.

2. **Systemic antifungal agents:** The classification of antifungal agents is given in Box 2.

3. **General measures**
   - Correction of contributory factory, e.g. diabetes, HIV, hot humid environment, occlusive clothing and foot ware.

Box 2: Classification of systemic antifungal agents

1. *Antibiotics*
   - Polyenes — Amphotericin B, nystatin, natamycin
   - Benzofuran — Griseofulvin
2. *Antimetabolites*, *e.g.* Flucytosine
3. *Azoles*
   - Imidazole — Ketoconazole
   - Triazoles — Fluconazole, traconazole
4. *Allylamines* — Terbinafine

Molluscum Contagiosum

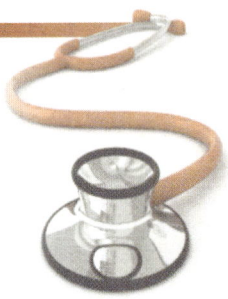

INSTRUCTION

- Examine the skin lesions

SALIENT FEATURES

- Skin lesions around the genitalia

HISTORY

Ask for the following:

- Ask the patient whether such lesions are present elsewhere
- History of sexual contact
- History of HIV

EXAMINATION

Examination of Skin and Genitalia

- Multiple rounded umbilicated pearly white plaques about 2–5 mm in diameter are present (Fig. 224.1) on the flexural surface of the skin

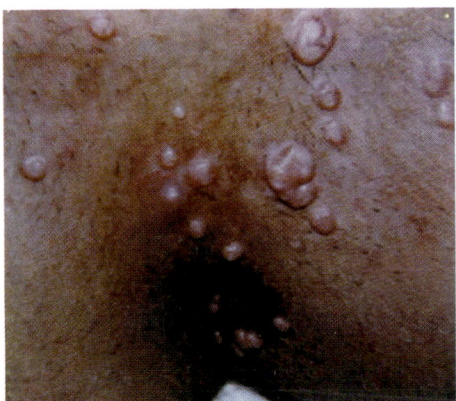

Fig. 224.1: Molluscum contagiosum in an adult. Note the umbilicated pearly white plaques. It is a sexually transmitted variety caused by pox virus

- Examine such lesions on face, trunk, hands and genitals

PROVISIONAL DIAGNOSIS

The patient has molluscum contagiosum (lesion) which is caused by pox virus (aetiology).

QUESTIONS AND ANSWERS

Q. How do these lesions spread from one part to another?

Ans: By autoinfection. Irritation over the surrounding skin induces scratching and further spread of infection.

Q. How does the infection spread from one patient to another?

Ans: By direct contact but in adults it is commonly transmitted by sexual contact.

Q. What is the histopathology of these lesions?

Ans: Cellular proliferation of the lower parts of stratum malpighii produces multiple pear-shaped lobules which compress the papillae which appear as septae between lobules. Many cells of the stratum corneum and granulosum contain large inclusion bodies called *"molluscum bodies"*. Numerous virions are present within the molluscum bodies.

Q. How would you treat these lesions?

Ans: Patient should be investigated for HIV status before treatment. The treatment includes:

1. Physical expression by squeezing
2. Curettage or cryotherapy
3. Cauterisation using trichloroacetic acid, podophyllin or phenol or silver nitrate
4. Topical cidofovir may be used in severe molluscum contagiosum in immuno-deficient individuals.

Acne Vulgaris

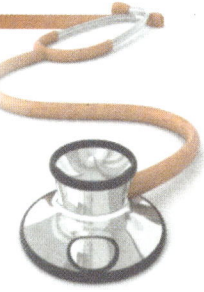

INSTRUCTION

- Examine the face of this patient

SALIENT FEATURES

- Disfigurement of face

HISTORY

Ask for the following:

- Use of steroids, androgenic steroids, INH
- Use of excess hair oil (greasy skin)
- History of local trauma, premenstrual tension (exacerbate the disease)
- Occupational exposure to oil, waxes
- Ask profession of the patient (common in professional violin player)

EXAMINATION

- Comedones or black heads caused by keratotic plugging of hair follicles, i.e. the hallmark of acne are present on the cheeks (Fig. 225.1)
- Look for these lesions at other sites, i.e. neck, trunk, chest, upper back and upper arms. (These are the areas where sebaceous glands are abundant.)

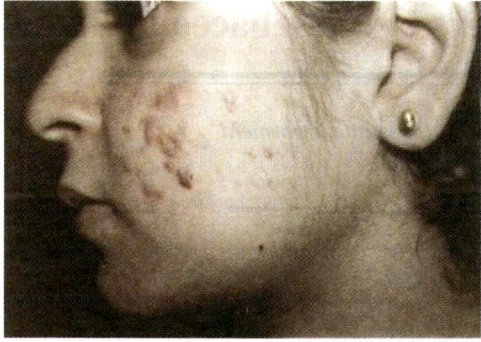

Fig. 225.1: Acne vulgaris

- Look for closed comedones (white heads), cysts (large deeper masses of retained sebum)
- There is associated scarring (ice pick scars)
- Skin over the face is greasy

PROVISIONAL DIAGNOSIS

The young girl has black heads on the face with greasy skin (lesion) called acne vulgaris (etiology). It is cosmetically unacceptable to the patient (functional status).

QUESTIONS AND ANSWERS

Q. **What is the causative organism in acne?**
Ans: An anaerobic diphtheroids called *Propionibacterium acne (P. acne)*

Q. **What do you know about the pathogenesis of acne?**
Ans: Hypercornification of pilosebaceous duct and subsequent blockage, excessive sebum production and colonisation of *P. acne* play role in the development of these lesions.

Table 225.1: Sequence of events in acne vulgaris

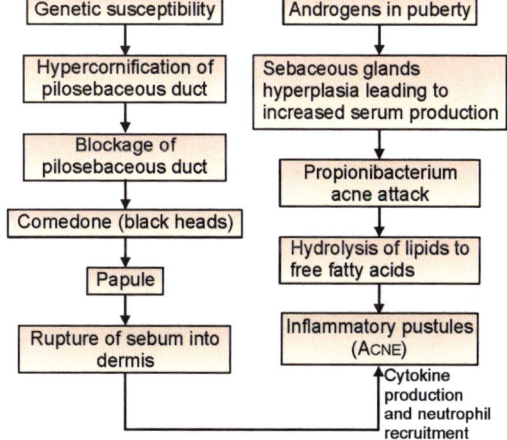

Q. How would you grade acne?
Ans: • Lesions (inflammatory or non inflammatory) are graded into severity
- **Mild disease (Grade I):** Comedones and few papules
- **Moderate disease (Grade II):** Comedones, papules and few pustules
- **Severe disease (Grade III):** Mainly pustules, abscesses and nodules
- **Cystic disease (Grade IV):** Cysts, nodules and widespread scarring

Q. What are the exacerbating factors?
Ans: 1. Oils, waxes, cosmetics
2. Sports helmet, bra strap, turtle necks head gear, strapping across shoulders or trunk
3. Professional violin players
4. Premenstrual tension
5. Excessive sweating (perspiration)

Q. What are the variants of acne?
Ans: 1. **Infantile acne or acne neonatorum.** It occurs in newborns, mostly males, around 3 months of age due to either maternal androgens or transplacental stimulation of the infant's adrenals. It may last upto 3 yrs and may be forerunner of severe acne in adolescents. The lesions are often seen on the nose and cheeks.
2. **Acne conglobate** (Fig. 225.2). It is common in men during late puberty and continues into later life. It is severe form of the disease characterised by comedones, papules, pustules, nodules and cysts with many abscesses and sinuses. This is disfiguring acne due to scarring (Fig. 225.2).
3. **Acne fulminans.** It is a type of conglobate acne accompanied by fever, tachycardia, joint pains and raised ESR.

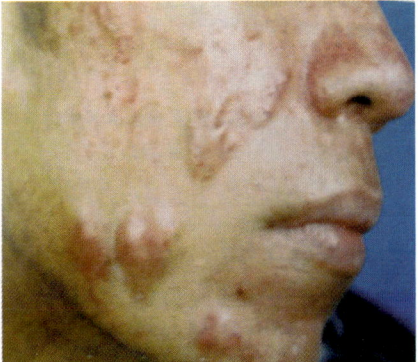
Fig. 225.2: Acne conglobate

4. **Acne excorice.** It manifests as denuded areas caused by picking and is seen most often in young females (teenage girls). The excoriation have an emotional basis. The lesions usually leave behind scarring.
5. **Exogenous acne (occupational acne).** Many oils and tars produce acneiform eruptions at the site of contact with the skin, therefore, this type of acne occurs at unusual sites. It is seen in industrial workers exposed to oils, waxes and chlorinated hydrocarbons.
6. **Drug-induced acne.** It results from treatment with corticosteroids, androgenic steroids, lithium, oral contraceptives, antiepileptics (phenytoin) and isoniazid.
7. **Acne associated with virilisation or adrenal hyperplasia.** Acne may be associated with secreting tumor of the adrenals, ovaries or testes. It is nonclassic cystic acne refractory to treatment seen in patients with congenital adrenal hyperplasia.

Q. How would you investigate?
Ans: 1. Bacterial swab for culture to exclude pyogenic infection (anaerobic infection or gram-negative folliculitis).
2. Endocrinal assessment is needed to exclude endocrinal cause of acne.

Q. How would you treat it?
Ans: *Local measures:*
- Regular washing with acne soap to remove grease
- Topical applications with antibacterial agent (tetracycline or clindamycin) benzoyl peroxide and common drug—tretinoin retinoic acid (Vit. A derivative) are cornerstone of local treatment. They are irritating drying preparations, hence to be used at night
- Avoid steaming and sauna baths

Systemic measures:
- **Oral low dose antibiotics.** The broad spectrum antibiotics are currently used widely in the treatment of acne. Tetracyclines (250 mg 6 hourly), doxycycline, minocycline are given for a longer period of 6 months
- To reduce sebum overproduction, systemic oestrogen and androgens, isotretinoin and spironolactone are given
- *Isotretinoin* and corticosteroids may be used to reduce inflammation
- Physical or surgical methods, i.e. comedones extraction, dermabrasion, chemical peeling, laser resurfacing, pulsed-dye laser treatment and punch grafts.

226

Rosacea

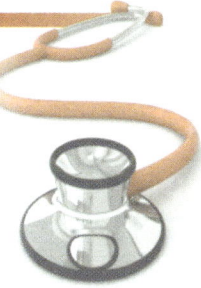

INSTRUCTION

- General physical examination

SALIENT FEATURES

- Facial flushing

HISTORY

Ask about the following:

- Age of onset
- Intermittent facial flushing/erythema
- Exacerbation of flushing/blushing by alcohol, coffee and spicy foods, hot drinks, etc.
- History of throbbing headache (unilateral, vasodilatation)

EXAMINATION

General Physical Examination

- There are dome-shaped papules and pustules, but no comedones over the blush area of face,

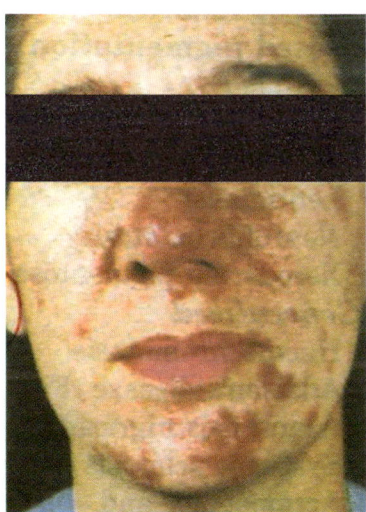

Fig. 226.1: Rosacea

i.e. lower half of face, cheeks, nose and chin (Fig. 226.1)
- No blepharitis, conjunctivitis, iritis, episcleritis and keratitis
- There is no rhinophyma or whiskey nose or run blossom (irregular thickening of the skin of the nose with enlarged follicular orifices caused by hyperplasia of sebaceous glands and hyperplasia of connective tissue)

PROVISIONAL DIAGNOSIS

The patient has a red patch (flushed area) over the face with papules and pustules (lesion) caused by rosacea (etiology) which is cosmetically not acceptable (functional status).

QUESTIONS AND ANSWERS

Q. How would you differentiate rosacea patch from SLE patch?

Ans: Both rosacea and SLE produce red erythematous patch over the face, but rosacea patch is associated with papules and pustules not the SLE patch.

Q. What are the precipitants for rosacea?

Ans: Warm atmosphere, hot drinks, spicy food, emotional upset and alcohol are known precipitants.

Q. What are the various types of rosacea?

Ans: Four subtypes of rosacea are described:
1. Erythema telangiectatic
2. Papulopustular
3. Rhinophymatous
4. Ocular

Q. How would you distinguish rosacea from acne?

Ans: Read Table 226.1.

Table 226.1: Distinguishing features between rosacea and acne

Feature	Rosacea	Acne
Age	Middle and older age	Younger age
Lesion	The lesion has vascular hue, i.e. red, erythematous with telangiectasia	These are papules and pustules
Comedones	Absent	Present

Q.   **What are the causes of red face in an adult?**

Ans: This question has been answered already under mastocytosis

- SLE producing malar rash
- Dermatomyositis
- Seborrheic dermatitis
- Perioral dermatitis
- Carcinoid syndrome
- Drug-induced (hydralazine)
- Mastocytosis

Q.   **How would you treat such a patient?**

Ans:
- Avoid precipitants as discussed
- Use sunscreen to avoid photo damage
- For mild cases, topical metronidazole gel is effective
- For moderate to severe cases, oral tetracycline or erythromycin in anti-acne doses are given and repeat courses are often necessary
- Isotretinoid for resistant cases
- Electrolysis or pulse-dye laser therapy for telangiectasia
- Surgical removal of rhinophyma

227

Dermatitis Herpetiformis

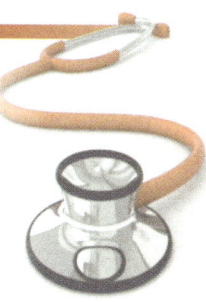

INSTRUCTION

- Examine the abdomen

SALIENT FEATURES

- Diarrhea with skin lesions

HISTORY

Ask about the following:

- History of chronic diarrhea (present)
- Remissions and exacerbations of symptoms
- History of hypersensitivity to rye, oat and barley and wheat (present)
- Time of appearance of rash after diarrhea episode
- Whether the rash itches?
- History of hypothyroidism (look for signs of hypothyroidism)

EXAMINATION

General Physical Examination

- Erythematous, dry itchy urticarial plaques, vesicles and crusts on the extensor surfaces of elbows, knees, shoulders and buttocks and back

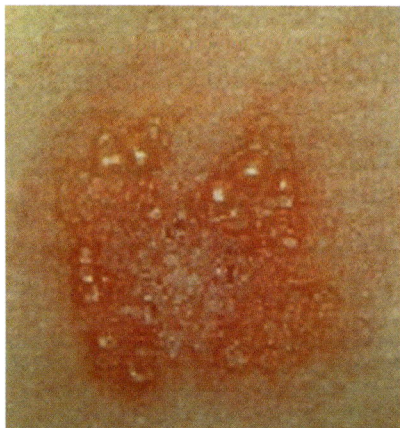

Fig. 227.1: Dermatitis herpetiformis

- The rash is bilaterally symmetrical
- Look for the similar region on other sides, i.e. face, scalp, neck, legs, etc.
- Look for the deficiency signs of vitamins and minerals

Abdominal Examination

- No organomegaly/ascites

PROVISIONAL DIAGNOSIS

The patient developed itchy vesicles on elbows following episodes of diarrhea (lesion) caused by dermatitis herpetiformis (etiology). The lesions are itchy (functional status).

QUESTIONS AND ANSWERS

Q. What is differential diagnosis?
Ans: Scabies is an another condition which produces such type of lesions, but the burrows are its characteristic features.

Q. What is the cause of diarrhea in your case?
Ans: Coeliac disease may be the cause since it is the common association with dermatitis herpetiformis.

Q. Name the gluten-containing foods.
Ans: Wheat, barely, oat and rye.

Q. Which food is permitted to gluten-sensitive patients?
Ans: Rice and maize.

Q. What are the extracutaneous manifestations of dermatitis herpetiformis?
Ans: Coeliac disease, lymphoma and hypothyroidism can be associated.

Q. What is the relation of dermatitis herpetiformis to coeliac disease?
Ans: It is a cutaneous variant of coeliac disease, occurs in <10% patients. On the other hand,

all patients with dermatitis herpetiformis have evidence of coeliac disease on intestinal biopsy, though it may not be clinical evident.

Q. **How would you investigate?**

Ans: 1. *Skin biopsy:* Fibrin and neutrophils accumulate at the dermal papillae leading to microabscesses. There is leucocytic infiltration of subepidermal vesicles. Immuno fluorescence demonstrate immunoglobulin A deposition in dermal papillae

2. *Anti-endomysium antibodies* in the blood is present in all cases

3. *Jejunal biopsy* may show subvillus atrophy with lymphocytic infiltration in the epithelium

4. *Therapeutic test*. Dapsone dramatically reduces itching in 72 hours providing confirmation before biopsy report

5. $HLA - B_8$ and $HLA - DRW_3$ are positive in 80%

Q. **How would you treat it?**

Ans: • Gluten restricted or gluten free diet
• Dapsone and sulfapyridine are effective. Neither of them is indicated in presence of G6PD deficiency. Treatment is lifelong

Q. **Is it advisable to add oat to the diet for dermatitis herpetiformis?**

Ans: Yes, moderate amount of oats can be ingested as they do not contain gliadin, but do have avenin. Avenin constitute 5–15% of protein and is as toxic as gliadin, but a good amount of oats would need to be ingested to bring about an equivalent effect.

Q. **What is gluten?**

Ans: Gluten is a protein component that persists following the removal of water and starch from defatted flour. Gliadin is an active ingradient of gluten flour. There are 4 gliadin fractions (α, β, γ and ω) out of which α-gliadin is injurious to intestine.

In dermatitis herpetiformis, IgA and IgG anti-gliadin antibodies are found in the dermal papillae on immunofluorescene.

Q. **What is the role of gluten free diet in dermatitis herpetiformis?**

Ans: Skin lesions as well as subclinical malabsorptive enteropathy improve slowly on withdrawal of gluten from the diet (gluten-free diet) and there are reduced chances of development of intestinal lymphoma. There may be even complete resolution of lesions (skin and intestinal lesions).

228

Pyoderma Gangrenosa

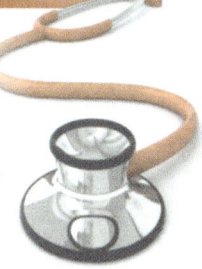

INSTRUCTION

- Look at the patient skin lesions
- Perform relevant systemic examination

SALIENT FEATURES

- Skin lesions in a patient with loose motions with blood and mucus

HISTORY

Ask about the following:

- History of diarrhea, tenesmus, pain in abdomen (inflammatory bowel disease)
- History of polyarthritis (rheumatoid arthritis present)
- History of leukemia and multiple myeloma

EXAMINATION

- Necrotic ulcer with overhanging purplish edges usually seen over the lower limbs (Fig. 228.1) or trunk
- Look at the mouth for mouth ulcers
- Anal examination for fissures, fistula, anorectal abscess. Skin tag (hemorrhoids)
- Extraintestinal manifestation of inflammatory bowel disease, i.e. iritis, scleritis, polyarthritis, aortic or mitral regurgitation, sclerosing cholangitis, peri hepatitis, etc.
- Deformities due to rheumatoid arthritis (present, Fig. 228.1)

PROVISIONAL DIAGNOSIS

There are necrotic skin ulcers over the limbs (lesion) probably due to rheumatoid arthritis (etiology).

QUESTIONS AND ANSWERS

Q. **What are the causes of necrotic ulcers simulating pyoderma gangrenosa?**
Ans: 1. Vascular occlusive or venous ulcers
2. Vasculitis

3. Infection with ulceration
4. Malignant ulcers
5. Exogenous tissue injury
6. Inflammatory skin disorders

Q. **What are the causes of pyoderma gangrenosum?**
Ans: • Ulcerative colitis
- Crohn's colitis
- Chronic active
- Hepatitis
- Multiple myeloma
- Rheumatoid arthritis (in this case)
- Leukemia (acute and chronic myeloid)
- Polycythemia vera
- Gammopathy

Q. **How would you investigate this case?**
Ans: 1. *Skin biopsy* for histopathology and culture (for bacteria, virus and fungus).

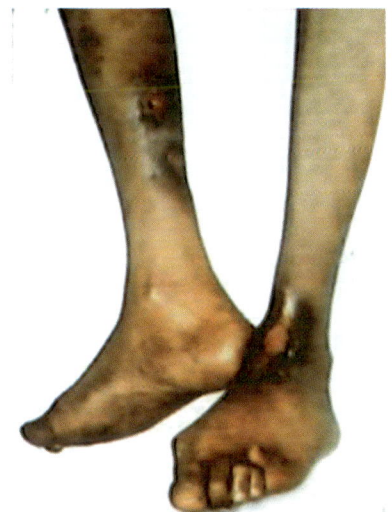

Fig. 228.1: Pyoderma gangrenosa in a patient with rheumatoid arthritis. Note the deformities of the toes due to RA

The skin biopsy shows necrosis of epithelium with neutrophilic infiltration

2. *GI tract studies*, e.g. sigmoidoscopy/ colonoscopy or radiology
3. *Serum protein electrophoresis*
4. *Antinuclear antibodies* (ANA), anti-neutrophil cytoplasmic antibodies (ANCA), rheumatoid factor (RF) and antiphospholipid antibodies

5. Complete blood count and bone marrow examination
6. X-rays joint for rheumatoid arthritis

Q. How would you treat these lesions?

Ans: 1. Intralesional steroids
2. High-dose steroids
3. Treatment of the underlying cause
4. Dapsone therapy is quite helpful
5. Topical ointments and dressings

229

Sturge-Weber Syndrome

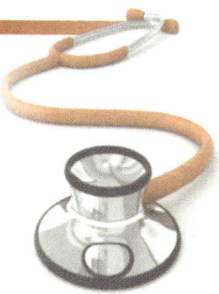

INSTRUCTION

- Look at the skin of face
- Perform relevant systemic examination

SALIENT FEATURES

- Skin lesions with epilepsy

HISTORY

Ask about the following:

- History of seizures (focal or generalised)
- History of hemiparesis/Hemianesthesia/ Hemianopia
- Glaucoma (ipsilateral)
- Mental insufficiency (Low IQ)

EXAMINATION

- There is port-wine stain over the left side of the face in the distribution of 1st and 2nd division of 5th cranial nerve (Fig. 229.1A)
- Hypertrophy of the involved area of the face and upper lip
- Look for hemangiomas of episclera and iris
- Fundus examination for choroidal hemangiomas
- BP (for pheochromocytoma)

PROVISIONAL DIAGNOSIS

The female patient has port-wine stain on the whole left side of the face and convulsions (lesion) probably caused by Sturge-Weber syndrome (etiology) which is unacceptable to this patient (functional status).

QUESTIONS AND ANSWERS

Q. Does inheritance play any role in this syndrome?
Ans: No. It occurs sporadically in both sexes.

Q. What are the neurological manifestations of this syndrome?
Ans: 1. Jacksonian (focal) epilepsy
2. Contralateral hemiparesis, hemianopia, hemianesthesia
3. Mental retardation (low IQ)

Q. What are the ocular manifestations of this syndrome?
Ans: This is a syndrome of phacomatosis with choroid angiomas, glaucoma, buphthalmos, optic atrophy.

Q. What is the histology of skin lesion?
Ans: This is a tumor consisting of dilated capillary vessels (capillary hemangioma) in the outer dermis.

Q. Does port-wine stain over the face carry any significance?
Ans: Yes. Patients who have port-wine stain in the distribution of 1st and 2nd division of trigeminal nerve are likely to have neuro-ophthalmological manifestations.

Q. What would you find on CT scan in a patient of Sturge-Weber syndrome with epilepsy?
Ans: Gyral calcification with underlying atrophy of cerebral hemisphere is a characteristic finding (Fig. 229.1B).

Q. How would you manage the skin lesion?
Ans: Photothermolysis and pulsed-dye laser therapy are treatment of choice for most port-wine stains.

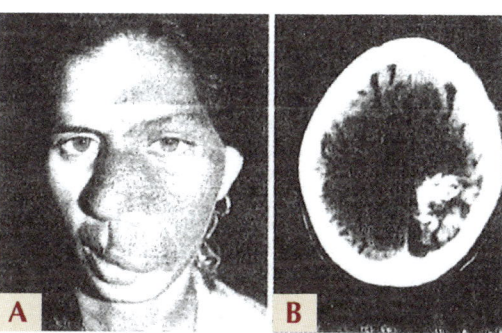

Fig. 229.1: Sturge-Weber syndrome. (A) Port-wine stain (capillary hemangioma) of left side of face; (B) CT scan of the patient shows gyral calcification in the same patient. Patient had epilepsy for more than 10 years

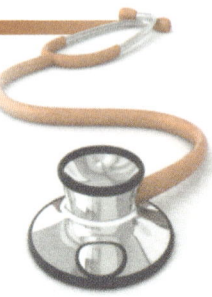

230

Thrombophlebitis Migrans

INSTRUCTION

- Look at the patient's arms and legs
- Perform relevant systemic examination

SALIENT FEATURES

- Pain and tenderness over a limb with visible veins

HISTORY

Ask about the following:

- Time of onset, course of the lesions
- Pain and tenderness of skin lesions
- Are the lesions stationary or migratory?
- History of I.V. infusions at different sites including legs
- Use of oral contraceptive
- Decrease appetite, weight, weakness, cachexia of malignancy (gastric or pancreatic)

EXAMINATION

Examination of arms and legs

- There is painful superficial thrombophlebitis of upper limb (Fig. 230.1)
- The veins are tenderness on palpation

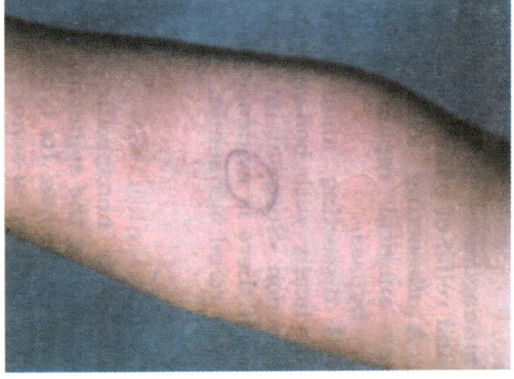

Fig. 230.1: Thrombophlebitis migrans

Systemic Examination

- Respiratory system is normal
- *Gastrointestinal system.* There is no organomegaly

PROVISIONAL DIAGNOSIS

The patient has migratory superficial thrombophlebitis (lesion) caused by some internal malignancy (aetiology) which is to be investigated.

QUESTIONS AND ANSWERS

Q. Name the disease where thrombophlebitis is a prominent sign.

Ans: Thromboangitis obliterans (Buerger's disease).

Q. Is superficial thrombophlebitis associated with DVT?

Ans: It can be associated with DVT in some cases, but pulmonary embolism is rare as the thrombus is adherent and nondetachable.

Q. How do I.V. catheter/needles cause thrombophlebitis?

Ans: Repeated needling of veins or prolonged duration of I.V. catheter can lead to thrombophlebitis.

Q. What are the dermatological manifestations of pancreatic disease?

Ans: 1. Panniculitis
2. Bronze pigmentation due to hemochromatosis
3. Cutaneous hemorrhage (Grey Turner's signs and Cullen's signs) of acute hemorrhagic pancreatitis
4. Necrolytic migratory erythema of glucagon secreting tumor

Q. What is the relationship between cancer and venous thromboembolism?

Ans: Cancer risk is 3–4 times increased in patients with venous thromboembolism. This risk becomes lower if patient has been treated with anticoagulants especially for 6 months. Patient with cancer are predisposed to thromboembolism because they are often at bedrest or immobilised, and tumor may obstruct or slow the blood flow. In addition, clotting may be promoted by release of procoagulants and cytokines from tumor cells or associated inflammatory cells or by platelet adhesion or aggregation.

Q. **Which malignancies are associated with migratory thrombophlebitis?**

Ans: The most common cancers with thrombophlebitis include that of lung, pancreas gastrointestinal breast varies, lymph nodes brain and genitourinary tract.

Q. **How would you treat superficial phlebitis?**

Ans:
- To relieve pain and swelling, local heat, NSAIDs and elevation of leg is sufficient
- Find out the underlying cause (e.g internal malignancy) and treat it accordingly.
- Antibiotic for septic thrombophlebitis. Excision of the involved vein up to uninvolved vein may be attempted in severe septic thrombophlebitis
- When there is risk of pulmonary embolism, division and ligation of the vein may be attempted

231

Lichen Planus

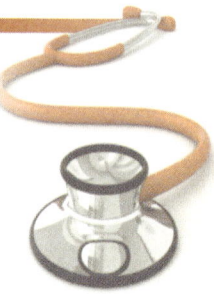

INSTRUCTION

- Look at the patients's skin
- Perform relevant system examination

SALIENT FEATURES

- Papular lesions over the trunk with severe itching

HISTORY

Ask about the following:

- Full drug history (a large number of drugs, e.g. diuretics, heavy metals, antimalarials anti-hypertensive, antidiabetics and proton pump inhibitors)
- Occupation of the patient (common in persons having contact with color film developer)
- Hepatitis C (jaundice or raised enzyme)

EXAMINATION

Skin Examination

- Pruritic, violaceous, flat-topped papules with fine white streaks and symmetric distribution are seen on the wrists, feet and trunk (Fig. 231.1)

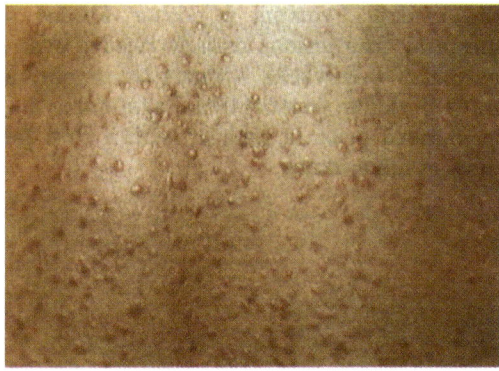

Fig. 231.1: Lichen planus (perifollicular violaceous papules over the trunk)

- Look into the mouth (buccal mucosa, tongue, gums or lips) for a lace-like pattern of white lines and papules. They are not present in this case
- Examine the scalp for scarring alopecia
- Examine the nails for longitudinal ridging, pterygium formation, nail dystrophy, nail loss
- Look for eruptions on genitalia also (penis)
- Look for eruptions that appear along the linear scratch marks (Koebner's phenomenon). Scratch marks are present in this case

PROVISIONAL DIAGNOSIS

The patient has purplish flat-topped papular eruptions (lesion) caused by Lichen planus (etiology) with several scratch marks indicating severe pruritus (functional status).

QUESTIONS AND ANSWERS

Q. What are the points in favor of lichen planus?

Ans: 1. Typical skin lesions (purplish flat-topped papules)
2. Symmetric distribution of skin lesions over the trunk
3. Scratch marks are present
4. Mucosal lesions

Q. What are the causes of white lesions in the mouth?

Ans: • Leukoplakia
• Aphthous stomatitis
• Secondary syphilis (mucous patches)
• Candidiasis (oral thrush)
• Squamous cell papilloma

Q. What are the causes of ulceration in the mouth?

Ans: 1. Aphthous ulceration
2. Behçet's syndrome
3. Erosive lichen planus

4. Stevens-Johnson syndrome

5. Recurrent herpes simplex (HSV1)

6. Pemphigus vulgaris

Q. Name the drugs which can cause lichen planus.

Ans: Sulphonamides, diuretics (thiazides), beta-blockers, ACE inhibitors, quinine NSAIDs methyldopa, chlorpropamide and proton pump inhibitor.

Q. What is the incidence of squamous cell carcinoma in erosive oral lichen planus?

Ans: About 5%.

Q. How would you confirm the diagnosis?

Ans: Biopsy of the skin of oral lesion is subjected to histopathology and immunofluorescence study.

Q. How would you treat these lesions?

Ans: 1. Topical corticosteroids or tacrolimus crew or intralesional steroids

2. General measures include psoralen plus PUVA, isotretinoin dapsone

3. Ultraviolet light for pruritus

4. For mucous lesion steroids or cyclosporine "Swish and Spit"

232 Lichen Simplex Chronicus (Neurodermatitis)

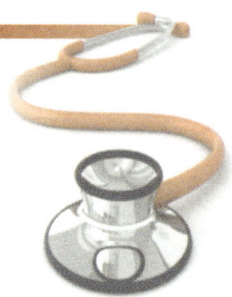

INSTRUCTION

- Look at the patient's skin

SALIENT FEATURES

- Pruritus over the legs

HISTORY

Ask about the following:

- Pruritus and eczema

EXAMINATION

Examination of Skin

- Well-circumscribed plaques which are lichenified with dry thickened skin on foot and ankles (Fig. 232.1)
- Several scratch marks are present (scratching perpetuate the cycle)
- Look for these lesions at other sites, i.e. wrists, nape of neck, perineum, etc.

PROVISIONAL DIAGNOSIS

The patient has lichen simplex chronicus (lesion) which is caused by chronic itching, scratching or rubbing (etiology). It is disturbing to the patient (functional status).

QUESTIONS AND ANSWERS

Q. What is pruritus?
Ans: It is an unpleasant sensation that provokes a desire to scratch.

Q. What is the pathway of pruritus/itch?
Ans: Itch has central as well as peripheral pathway similar to pain. It may originate centrally (cholestasis induced) or peripherally due to irritation of afferent pathway in the skin. It travels to higher centres through the spinothalamic tract to thalamus similar to pain.

Q. How would you classify itch?
Ans: Itch is classified depending on its central or peripheral origin.

I. *Proprioceptive itch.* It originates from the dryness or inflammation of the skin, is transmitted via C nerve fibres. The itch caused by insect bites, scabies, etc. are its examples.

II. *Neuropathic itch.* The cause of itch lies near to the afferent pathway (afferent neurons) of itch for example, post herpetic neuralgic, itch of multiple sclerosis and brain tumor.

III. *Neurogenic (central) itch.* It originates centrally without any evidence of central pathology, for example itch caused by obstructive jaundice through opioid "μ" receptors.

IV. *Psychogenic itch* as in delusional state.

Q. How would you treat this condition?
Ans: 1. As scratching perpetuates the cycle, hence, break the *scratch-itch-scratch cycle* by antihistamines or antipruritic agents
2. High-potency steroids
3. Protection of the area from irritation. Apply some antipruritic cream
4. Antidepressants at night

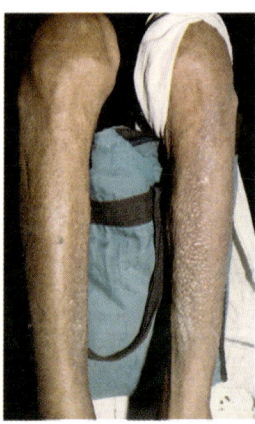

Fig. 232.1: Lichen simplex chronicus

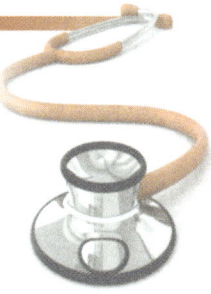

233

Pemphigus

INSTRUCTION

- Examine the patient is skin
- Perform relevant systemic examination

SALIENT FEATURES

- Denuded skin with exudation

HISTORY

Ask about the following:
- Onset of bullous eruptions
- History of mouth ulceration (mucosal involvement)
- Drug history, e.g. penicillins ACE inhibitors, NSAIDs, rifampicin, levodopa, propranolol, etc.
- History of fever, malaise
- History of dehydration (dry tongue)

EXAMINATION

Examination of Skin
- Bullous eruptions (Fig. 233.1) are present

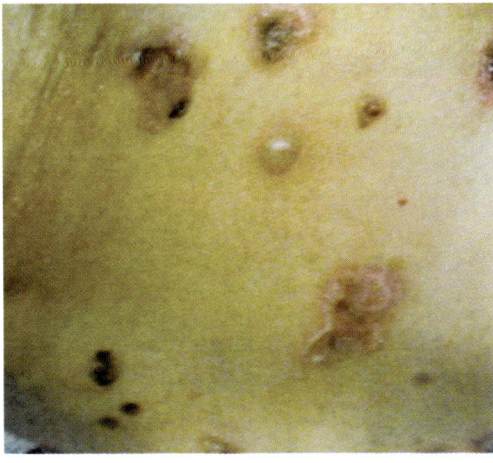

Fig. 233.1: Pemphigus vulgaris

- Flaccid blisters, moist eroded lesions appear after rupture of blisters (present)
- *Nikolsky's sign* is positive (Lateral pressure on normal skin near the active lesion results in new bulla formation)
- *Bulla spread sign* may or may not be present (i.e pressure applied over pre-existing bulla results in further spread)
- Look for signs of dehydration if larger areas of the skin involved (dehydration is present)

PROVISIONAL DIAGNOSIS

The patient has bullous eruptions (lesion) caused by pemphigus vulgari—an autoimmune blistering disease (etiology). There is wide spread denuded skin with exudation resulting in mild dehydration (functional status).

QUESTIONS AND ANSWERS

Q.   **What is a bulla? What is a vesicle?**
Ans: A circumscribed vesicle larger than 0.5 cm in diameter, containing fluid is called a *bulla*. Cutaneous blister less than 0.5 cm in diameter is called a vesicle

Q.   **What is pemphigus?**
Ans: Pemphigus refers to a group of autoimmune bullous disorders of skin and mucous membranes characterised by intradermal blisters formation.

Q.   **What are the various types of pemphigus?**
Ans: Pemphigus may be divided into two types, i.e.
   I. *Pemphigus vulgaris.* Blisters occur in the deeper epidermis
   II. *Pemphigus foliaceous.* This is superficial form of pemphigus where the blisters occur in superficial layer of epidermis (Fig. 233.2)
   III. Pemphigus erythematosus
   IV. Paraneoplastic pemphigus

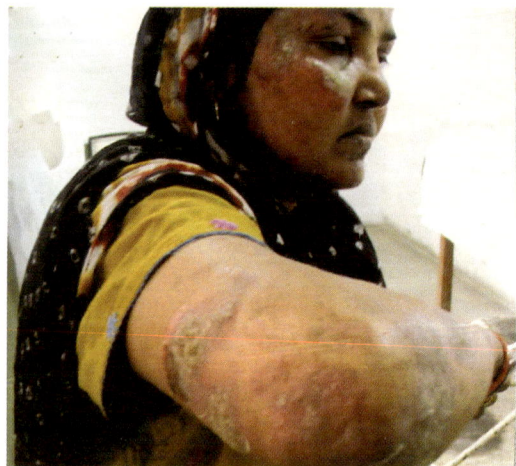

Fig. 233.2: Pemphigus foliaceous. There is extensive scaling and crusting over the face and arm with no blister

Q.   What is immunology of pemphigus?

Ans: The hallmark of pemphigus is formation of IgG anibodies against the keratinocyte cell membrane as demonstrated by direct immunofluorescence on skin biopsy. There is direct correlation between circulating antibodies and the disease activity. Patients with mild localised disease or disease in remission mostly have negative immuno-flourescence.

Q.   Name a few blistering conditions.
Ans:

Common	Uncommon
• Insect bites, drugs, burns, impetigo, contact dermatitis	• Pemphigus
	• Dermatitis herpeti-formis
• Staphylococcal scalded skin syndrome	• Immunoglobulin A mediated diseases
	• Bullous erythema multiforme
	• Epidermolysis bullosa
	• Porphyria cutanea tarda
	• Paraneoplastic pemphigus

Q.   What are metabolic causes of bullous erup-tions?

Ans: 1. Diabetic bullae, Tense bullae with clear fluid arise on normal skin on distal extre-mities

2. Porphyria cutanea tarda
3. Porphyria variegata
4. Pseudoporphyria (drug induced bullous photosensitivity)
5. Bullous dermatosis of hemodialysis

Q.   What are the characteristics of pemphigus vulgaris?

Ans: 1. It is an autoimmune blistering disorder

2. Pemphigus vulgaris is characterised by bulla formation in mucous membrane and deeper layer of epidermis
3. Nikolysky's sign is positive
4. Immunofluorescence shows intercellular deposition of IgG in the epidermis
5. Biopsy shows disruption of epidermal intercellular connection (acanthocytosis)

Q.   What are the characteristics of bullous pemphigoid?

Ans: 1. It is subepidermal blistering disease of old persons. Mucous membrane is not involved. It is relatively a benign con-dition

2. Tense bulla usually appear on flexural areas and trunk which usually do not rupture easily
3. Immunoelectron microscopy shows de-posits of IgG and C_3 in the basement membrane
4. Clinical course comprises of exacerbations and remissions
5. Immunosuppressive therapy, (steroids, immunosuppressive drugs) mycopheno-late mofetil, rituximab and I.V. immuno-globulins induce remission

Q.   What do understand by epidermolysis bullosa?

Ans: It comprises a group of genetically deter-mined disorder characterised by blistering of the skin after minimal trauma which lead to skin fragility.

234

Maculopapular Eruption/Rash

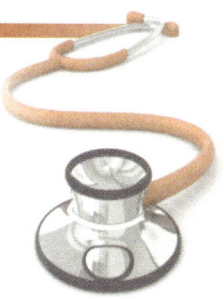

INSTRUCTION

- Perform general physical examination after taking detailed history

SALIENT FEATURES

- A widespread rash over the whole body following fever

HISTORY

Ask about the following:
- Presence of itching
- Onset and progression of rash. How did it evolve?
- History of taking drugs (take full history of drugs being taken or taken in the past)
- History of fever (viral exanthem)
- History of pain in the mouth or mouth ulcerations (mucous membrane involvement)

EXAMINATION

General Physical Examination
- There is reddish brown maculopapular eruption or rash spread over the trunk [front, back, chest and limbs (Fig. 234.1)]
- Check the mucous membrane for rash
- Examine the lymph nodes for enlargement (glandular fever)
- Examine the hemorrhage (hemorrhagic rash appear in dengue fever)
- Check the BP (hemorrhagic shock syndrome)

PROVISIONAL DIAGNOSIS

The patient has maculopapular rash (lesion) caused by dengue fever (aetiology) which resolves on recovery (functional status).

QUESTIONS AND ANSWERS

Q. What is your differential diagnosis?
Ans: Most of the conditions associated with fever and rash come into its differential diagnosis.

1. Drug induced fever and rash
2. Glandular fever, dengue fever
3. Viral exanthems (measles and rubella)
4. Pustular psoriasis
5. Erythroderma
6. Lyme disease
7. Secondary syphilis
8. Sweet's syndrome

Q. List the causes of rash with lymphadenopathy.
Ans: 1. Glandular fever
2. Hodgkin's lymphoma
3. HIV infection

Q. What are the clinical characteristics of drug induced rash?
Ans: The diagnostic clues to drug induced rash are:
1. Rash is atypical of known skin disease
2. History of hypersensitivity to drug
3. Past history of drug eruption to suspected drug
4. History of drug known to produce rash

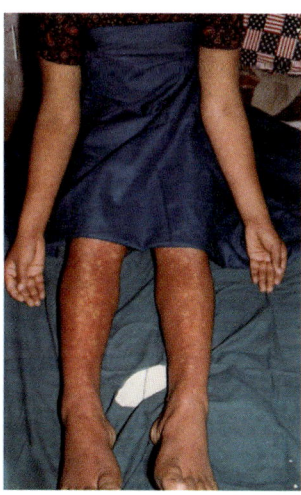

Fig. 234.1: Maculopapular rash in dengue fever

5. Asymmetric eruption which corroborates with the fixed recognised pattern caused by one of the prescribed drugs

Q. **What do you mean by fixed drug eruptions (Fig. 234.2)?**

Ans: Bright red annular lesions or even blisteral plaques appear on the body (face, hands, trunk and genitalia) following drug administration. The lesions may be itchy or produce burning discomfort. The lesions are fixed in site and appear within hours of offending drug. They will appear at exactly the same sites if drug is given again at another time. Post inflammation is a characteristic feature.

Phenolphthalein, tetracyclines, phenacetin, sulphonamides, salicylates and oral contraceptives are known to cause them.

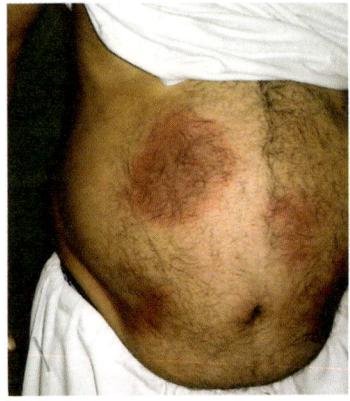

Fig. 234.2: Fixed drug eruptions over the abdomen due to sulphonamide (cotrimoxazole)

235

Vitiligo

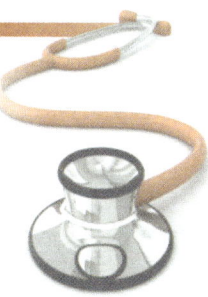

INSTRUCTION

- Perform general physical examination

SALIENT FEATURES

- White patches all over the body

HISTORY

Ask about the following:

- Age of onset
- Family history
- History of autoimmune conditions, e.g. thyroid disorders (hypo or hyperthyroidism, Hashimoto's thyroiditis), Addison's disease, diabetes mellitus type I, pernicious anemia

EXAMINATION

General Physical Examination

- Hypopigmented patches (Fig. 235.1) are symmetrically distributed over face, chest and wrists (in this case)

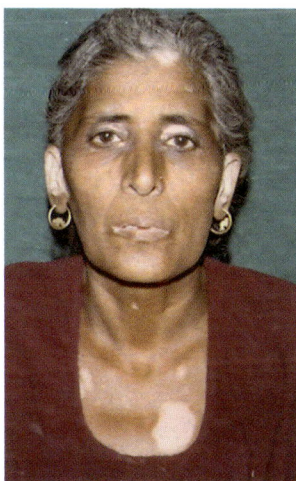

Fig. 235.1: Vitiligo

- White hairs in vitiliginous area (present)
- Some spontaneous repigmentation in the sun-exposed regions
- Look at the scalp for alopecia and white hair (present)
- Look for scratch marks (*Koebner's phenomenon*)

PROVISIONAL DIAGNOSIS

The patient has vitiligo (lesion), which is an auto-immune skin disorder (etiology) and can be disfiguring cosmetically (functional status).

QUESTIONS AND ANSWERS

Q. **Name some autoimmune diseases associated with vitiligo.**
Ans: They are classified as:
   I. *Primary hyperpigmentary disorders*, e.g. vitiligo, albinism and piebaldism. In these disorders pigment cells (melanocytes) are destroyed.
   II. *Secondary hypopigmentary disorders* called leukoderma which may complicate many skin conditions such as atopic dermatitis, lichen planus, psoriasis, DLE and lichen simplex chronicus.

Q. **What are the various types of vitiligo?**
Ans: I. *Segmental vitiligo.* Most of the patients have one patch or a unilateral distribution that match a dermatome.
   II. *Nonsegmental vitiligo. These are* white patches which are symmetric and increase over time with precipitating factors such as stress or a sympathetic neurogenic disturbance.

Q. **What is piebaldism?**
Ans: It is a congenital (autosomal dominant) hypomelanosis disorder in which areas of hypomelanosis contain normally pigmented and hyperpigmented macules of various sizes. The hypopigmented areas are symmetrically distributed over the forehead

trunk and extremities. The lesions enhance under wood's lamp. There is defect in migration of melanoblasts from neural crest to ventral skin or mutation within proto-oncogene encoding tyrosine kinase.

Q. How would you confirm the diagnosis?

Ans: *Wood's accentuates.* Wood's light accentuates epidermal pigmentation and highlights hypopigmentation. Hypopigmentation as seen in vitiligo enhances with Wood's lamp examination whereas post inflammatory hypopigmentation does not.

Q. What is the histopathology of vitiligo?

Ans: In vitiligo, there is partial or complete loss of melanocytes in the epidermis.

In contrast, some forms of albinism have melanocytes which lack melanin pigment because of genetic defect in tyrosinase enzyme.

Q. What is the aetiology of vitiligo?

Ans: The various theories of aetiopathogenesis are:

1. *Autoimmune theory.* There is auto immune destruction of melanocytes by cell mediated immunity (antibodies directed against melanocytes)
2. Self-perpetuating destruction by inter-mediates of melanin
3. Neurohumoral mechanism of destruction of melanocytes

Q. Name few common clinical conditions associated with hypopigmentation of skin.

Ans: 1. Hypopituitarism
2. Phenylketonuria, homocystinuria
3. Leprosy
4. Post-burns, post-inflammatory, etc.
5. Radiodermatitis
6. Tuberous sclerosis (Ash-leaf spots)
7. Leucoderma following lichen planus, lichen simplex chronicus, discoid lupus
8. Chemical leukoderma

Q. What is chemical leucoderma?

Ans: It is a hypopigmentary condition in which white patches appear on hands due to exposure to chemicals that selectively destroy melanocytes particularly phenols and cate-chols. Satellite lesions may also appear in areas not exposed to chemicals. These lesions appear more chalky white under wood's lamp.

Q. What are the complications of vitiligo?

Ans: 1. Actinic keratosis
2. Skin cancer

Q. How would you manage such patients?

Ans: 1. In secondary hypopigmentation, repig-mentation may occur spontaneously. Cosmetics such as Covermark and Dermablend are highly effective for concealing the disfiguring lesions.
2. If < 20% of the skin is involved, topical tacrolimus 0.1% twice daily is the first line therapy. A superpotent steroid may also be used.
3. With 20–25% involvement, narrowband UVB or oral PUVA is best.
4. Newer techniques such as epidermal autografts and cultural epidermis com-bined with PUVA therapy give hope for surgical correction of vitiligo.

236

Lupus Vulgaris

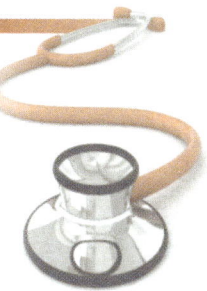

INSTRUCTION

- General physical examination
- Perform the relevant system

SALIENT FEATURES

- Skin lesion over the face

HISTORY

Ask about the following:

- History of prolonged, fever, night sweats, malaise, decreased appetite
- History of BCG vaccination
- Onset and progression of the lesion
- Site of the lesion (e.g. face is commonly involved, but in India, buttocks, thighs, legs and upper extremities are commonly affected)
- History of lymph nodes enlargement
- History of cough, hemoptysis, dyspnea and chest discomfort

EXAMINATION

General Physical Examination

- Red-brown nodules which look like apple-jelly when pressed with slide are present on cheeks (in this case)
- Erythema, scaling and scarring plaques are seen (Fig. 236.1)
- In severe cases, cutaneous tissue appears *gnawed* hence, the term lupus (meaning '*wolf*')
- No lymphadenopathy

Systemic Examination

- *Respiratory system:* No lung lesion or pleural effusion

PROVISIONAL DIAGNOSIS

The patient has lupus vulgaris over the face (lesion) caused by tuberculosis (etiology) which is disfiguring (functional status).

QUESTIONS AND ANSWERS

Q. **What are the causes of red-brown granulomatous lesion over the face?**

Ans: 1. Sarcoidosis (lupus pernio)
2. Foreign body granulomas
3. Late secondary syphilis
4. Lupus vulgaris

Q. **What is lupus vulgaris?**

Ans: Lupus vulgaris is a form of skin tuberculosis that is seen in previously infected and sensitized persons. There is often an active tuberculosis elsewhere either in lungs or lymph nodes.

Q. **How would you classify tuberculosis of the skin?**

Ans: It is classified as follows:
  I. *Primary tuberculosis*
  - Tuberous chancre
  - Miliary tuberculosis of skin

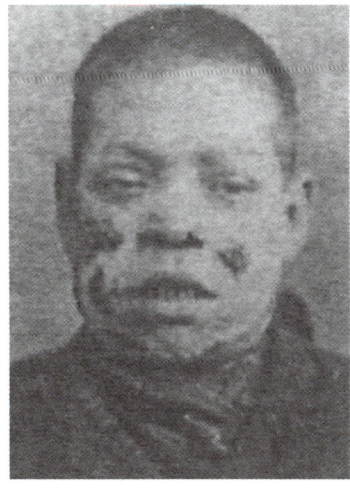

Fig. 236.1: Lupus vulgaris. Note the scaling and scarring plaques

II. *Reactivation tuberculosis*
- Lupus vulgaris
- Tuberculosis verrucosa cutis

III. *Tuberculides*
- Papulonecrotic
- Lichen scrofulosorum

Q. What are the skin lesions in reactivation tuberculosis?

Ans: Skin lesions in reactivation tuberculosis depends on the level of immunity, i.e.
1. Mild lesion *(lupus vulgaris)*
2. Moderate lesion *(tuberculosis verrucosa cutis)*
3. Extensive lesion *(scrofuloderma)*
4. Widespread and extensive lesion *(tuberculosis orofacial)*

Q. What is tuberculosis verrucosa cutis?

Ans: It is an occupational hazard in persons handling tubercular tissue, e.g. veterinary surgeons, morgue attendants, pathologists, butchers and anatomists. It appears as dull red deep seated papules or nodules that enlarge gradually and become warty and verrucous. Pus may be discharged and crusts may form.

Q. What is Scrofuloderma?

Ans: This type of tuberculosis occurs due to an extension of the infection into the skin from an underlying focus usually the lymph nodes and occasionally from the underlying tuberculosis of the bone or joint. It commonly follows cervical or axillary lymphadenopathy where the underlying lymph nodes enlarge and overlying skin gets infected, breaks down to form discharging sinuses. The ulcers are soft with undermined edges and heal by linear cord-like scars.

Q. What is tuberculides?

Ans: These are skin eruptions which are symmetrically distributed, represent a hypersensitivity reaction in the skin to hematogenous spread of miliary tuberculosis from an infected internal focus into the skin of a person who has high degree of immunity. The lesions are:
1. Papulonecrotic tuberculides
2. Lichen scrofulosorum
3. Erythema induratum or Brazin's disease

Q. What is swimming pool granuloma?

Ans: It is mycobacterial (*M. marinum*) infection of the skin, involves a digit, hand or forearm which gets traumatized against the side of aquarium during swimming or cleaning. The patient presents with chronic papular lesion (granuloma) on the abraded skin with scaling.

237

Onycholysis

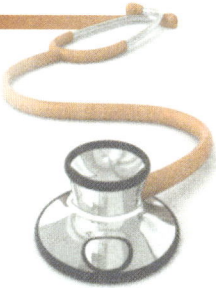

INSTRUCTION

- Examine the patient's hands

SALIENT FEATURES

- Nails changes

HISTORY

Ask about the following:

- Exposure to detergents, alkalis and keratolytic agents and demeclocycline (they induce photolysis)
- History of psoriasis
- History of hyperthyroidism or diabetes
- History of fungal nail disease (nail gets snagged in the clothing or discolored nails)

EXAMINATION

Examination of Hands

- There is distal separation of nail plates from the nail beds (Fig. 237.1)

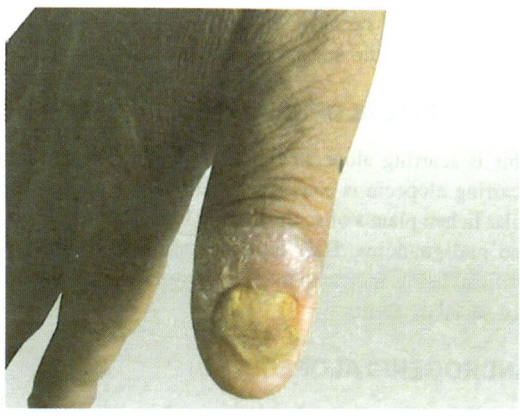

Fig. 237.1: Nails show onychodystrophy, onycholysis and subungual hyperkeratosis with psoriasis of the adjacent skin

- Look at the finger nails (nails are thickened, white nails with scaling under the free edge of nail in fungal disease). Nails are white, green or black, e.g. discoloring of nails occurs in fungal infection
- Check the nails for pitting and silvery white plaques (psoriasis present)
- Look at the immunodeficiency state, e.g. HIV disease, diabetes, etc.
- Check the neck for goitre (Graves' disease, hypothyroidism)

PROVISIONAL DIAGNOSIS

This patients has onycholysis without fungal nail disease (lesion) caused by psoriasis (aetiology).

QUESTIONS AND ANSWERS

Q. What are plummer nails?

Ans: This refers to onycholysis that occurs in thyrotoxicosis and involves the fourth finger.

Q. What are the nail changes in psoriasis?

Ans: Involvement of nails in psoriasis produce friable 'thimble pitting', onycholysis and subungual hyperkeratosis. All the changes are present in this case.

Q. What do you understand by the term onychomycosis?

Ans: It means fungal infection of nails (Fig. 237.2). It is characterised by discoloration of nails (white/yellow/brown patches or streaks), onycholysis, subungual hyperkeratosis and nail plate thickening.

Q. What are the causative organisms for onychomycosis?

Ans: 1. Dermatophytes (ringworm, Tinea unguium), e.g. Trichophyton rubra, T. interdigitale
2. Yeasts (Candida albicans)
3. Nondermatophytes (moulds), e.g. Fusarium

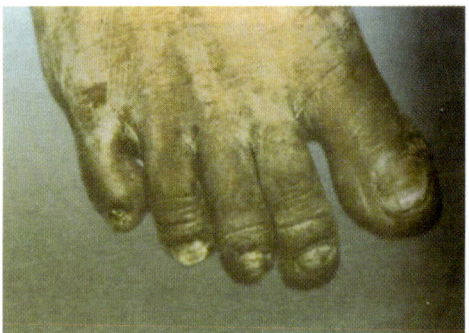

Fig. 237.2: Onychomycosis

Q. What are the causative organism for bacterial nail infection?

Ans: *Pseudomonas aeruginosa* and *Staph. aureus* (paronychia or whitlow).

Q. What are the patterns of fungal nail involvement?

Ans: 1. Distal lateral subungual onychomycosis
2. Superficial white onychomycosis
3. Total dystrophic onychomycosis

Q. How would you confirm the diagnosis of fungal nail infection?

Ans: Confirmation is done by microscopic examination of nail scrapings taken with a blunt scalpel as proximally as possible.

Q. How would you manage onycholysis?

Ans: • Manicure and debridement
• Avoidance of exposure to detergents bleaches and alkalis
• Intradermal steroids near the nail matrix
• Non-surgical removal of dystrophic nails
• Treat the underlying cause

238

Nail Changes

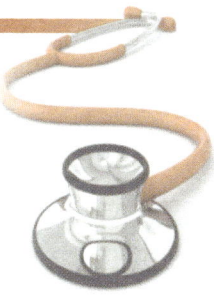

INSTRUCTION

- Examine the nails of the patient
- Perform relevant systemic examination

SALIENT FEATURES

- Patient has habit of nail biting

HISTORY

Ask for the following:

- Age of the patient. Terry's nails can occur in elderly
- Nutrition of the patient, e.g. poor nutrition due to less intake, malabsorption or systemic disease. Pale transverse band across the nail indicate edema of nail bed, seen in malnutrition
- History of cirrhosis of the liver, Wilson's disease
- CHF (congestive heart failure)
- Chronic renal failure
- Fungal nail infection
- Poisoning, e.g. arsenic
- Vasculitis
- Personality disorder (nail biting)

EXAMINATION

Examination of Nails

I. *Look for following abnormalities of nails*

- *Thimbling of nails* in nail biters (Fig. 238.1)
- *Splinter hemorrhage* seen following minor trauma, vasculitis, and SABE
- *Nail-pitting* occurs in psoriasis and eczema
- Koilonychia is seen in iron deficiency anemia
- Platonychia occurs either as congenital abnormality or seen in iron deficiency
- Onycholysis is seen following trauma, also occurs in psoriasis, lichen planus and ringworm infection, fungal nail diseases and thyrotoxicosis
- Transverse ridging occurs in acute illness and zinc deficiency
- White lines (transverse lines across the nails) called *Mee's lines* (Fig. 238.2), are seen in arsenic poisoning and vasculitis

- Absent nails occur in nail patella syndrome
- Fungal infection produces discoloration of nails (white, yellow, brown, black, etc.) with onycholysis
- Red-half moon (red lunula) shape nails are seen in CHF
- Blue half moon (blue lunula) nails are seen in copper sulphate poisoning and Wilson's disease
- Half and half nails are seen in chronic renal failure

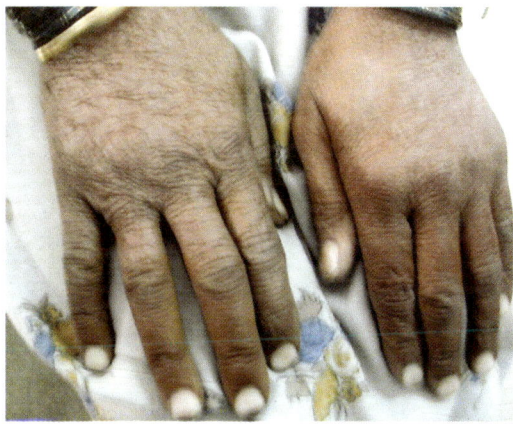

Fig. 238.1: Nail changes. Thimbling of nails in nail biters

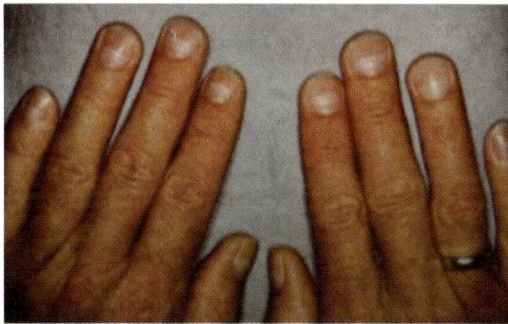

Fig. 238.2: Mee's lines in arsening of poisoning

- Beau's lines are transverse depression occuring in severe systemic illness and malnutrition (Fig. 238.3)
- Leukonychia [white nails (Fig. 238.4)] are seen in cirrhosis of the liver
- Clubbing of the fingers occurs in a variety of respiratory, cardiac and GI tract diseases (discussed as a separate case)

II. Look for disorders of nail fold

- Nail fold telangiectasis occurs in collagen vascular diseases
- Paronychia occurs in bacterial infection. It causes swelling and inflammation of lateral nail folds

III. Disorders of hyponychium (distal region of nail bed)

- Subungal angiofibromas are seen in tuberous sclerosis
- Warts

Systemic Examination

- Examine abdomen for liver and kidney disease
- Cardiovascular system for CHF

PROVISIONAL DIAGNOSIS

The patient is a habitual nail biters has developed thimbled nails (lesion) due to a personality disorder (aetiology). Patient is psychologically disturbed (functional status).

QUESTIONS AND ANSWERS

Note: They are covered in the examination

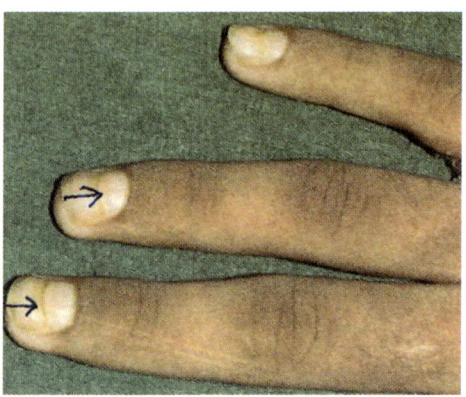

Fig. 238.3: Beau's lines: Transverse groove present in nails

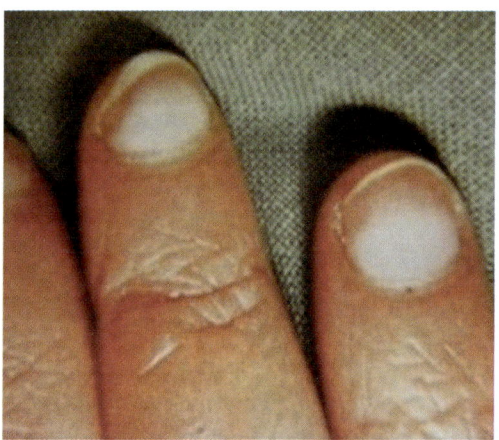

Fig. 238.4: Leukonychia in a patient with cirrhosis of liver

239

Diabetic Retinopathy

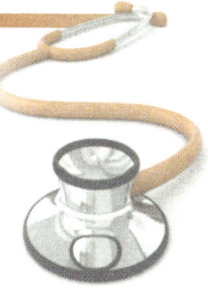

INSTRUCTION

• Examine the fundus of this patient who is diabetic

SALIENT FEATURES

• Patient is hypertensive and complains of diminished vision

HISTORY

Ask about the following:

• Age of onset, duration and course of diabetes
• Gradual or sudden loss of vision
• History of floaters
• Associated complications, e.g. neuropathy, nephropathy, hypertension (present)

EXAMINATION

Fundus (Fig. 239.1) shows:
• Dot and blot hemorrhages
• Microaneurysms
• Hard exudates
• Cotton wool spots

PROVISIONAL DIAGNOSIS

The patient has dot and blot hemorrhages, microaneurysms and hard exudates (lesion) caused by background diabetic retinopathy (aetiology) without any effect on visual acuity (functional status).

QUESTIONS AND ANSWERS

Q. **What is background diabetic retinopathy?**

Ans: It is nonproliferative retinopathy in diabetes, represents the earlier stage of retinal involvement. It is characterised by following changes:

    1. Microaneurysms, blot hemorrhages (dot and blot appearance)
    2. Hard exudates

    3. Retinal edema including macular edema due to leakage of proteins, lipids or red cells into the retina

Q. **What are the symptoms and signs of background retinopathy?**

Ans: It is mostly asymptomatic but when macular edema (maculopathy) occurs, visual acuity gets affected.

Q. **What is the earliest change in diabetic retinopathy?**

Ans: An increased capillary permeability is the earliest change. This is demonstrated by leakage of fluorescent dye into the vitreous or fluorescene-angiography.

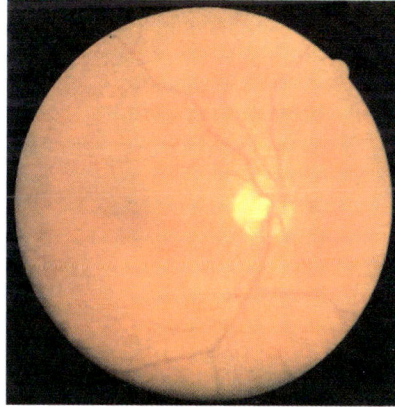

Fig. 239.1: Diabetic retinopathy: Background changes and cotton-wool spots. In addition to scattered microaneurysms and hemorrhages, there are several cotton-wool spots. Two of these lesions can clearly be seen in the upper pole of the eye, with a third less distinct cotton wool spot close to a hemorrhage near the upper margin of the film. A fourth cotton wool spot is present at the lower left margin of the photograph. The veins are neither unduly dilated nor variable in calibre. There is no arterial narrowing hence, this appearance falls short of being labelled 'preproliferative'. These cotton-wool spots had resolved when the eye was examined 6 months later

Q. **What are the symptoms and signs of diabetic maculopathy?**

Ans: When macula gets involved, the central vision suffers and patient finds difficulty in reading small print (newspaper) or seeing road signs.

Q. **What do you understand by the term pre-proliferative diabetic retinopathy?**

Ans: Before proliferative retinopathy (proliferation of new capillaries), a preproliferative phase often occurs in which arterial ischemia is characterised by:
- Cotton-wool spots (small infarcted areas of retina)
- Venous dilatation
- Arteriolar narrowing
- Hemorrhage, large dark blots

Q. **What is the cause of preproliferative retinopathy? How does it manifest?**

Ans:
- It is caused by retinal hypoxia
- It is asymptomatic unless macula is involved (central vision lost)

Q. **What do you understand by the term proliferative diabetic retinopathy?**

Ans: The appearance of neovascularisation is the hallmark of proliferative diabetic retinopathy. These new vessels appear near the optic disc and/or macula and rupture easily leading to vitreous hemorrhage, fibrosis and finally retinal detachment.

Q. **What is the prevalence of retinopathy in diabetes?**

Ans: The overall prevalence is about 25%. It is more prevalent in type 1 diabetics (40%) than type 2 diabetics (20%).

Q. **What is the relationship of duration of diabetes and retinopathy?**

Ans: After 10–15 yrs, 25–50% of patients with type 1 diabetes have signs of retinopathy. After 15 yrs, this prevalence increases to 75–90% and after 30 yrs, all the type 1 diabetics (100%) have retinopathy.

In type 2 DM, the nonproliferative retinopathy is 60% after 16 yrs.

Q. **What are the bad prognostic factors for diabetic retinopathy?**

Ans: 1. Hypertension   2. Chronic renal failure
3. Anemia   4. Pregnancy
5. Uncontrolled
   state

Q. **What is the effect of pregnancy on diabetic retinopathy?**

Ans: Retinopathy can progress rapidly in pregnant diabetic patients, hence, meticulous control of diabetes in indicated.

Q. **What is the pathogenesis of neovascularisation (neoangiogenesis) of retina?**

Ans: Production of certain angiogenic factors by ischemic and hypoxic retina and recently vascular endotherial growth sectors (VEGF) have been implicated in neovascularisation, that is why inhibitors of VEGF such as revacizumab, ranibizum, VEGF Trape-Eye have found place in the treatment of proliferative retinopathy.

Q. **What is the role of ACE inhibitors or ARBs in diabetic retinopathy?**

Ans: Blockage of renin-angiotensin system by either ACE inhibitors or ARBs slows the progression and advancement of diabetic retinopathy independent of nephropathy.

Q. **How would you treat background retinopathy?**

Ans: It is treated by argon laser photocoagulation applied directly to the leaking microaneurysms as well as grid photocoagulation applied to the diffused areas of leakage and thickening.

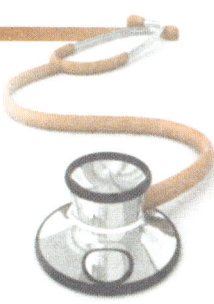

240

Hypertensive Retinopathy

INSTRUCTION

- Examine the fundus of a patient who is hypertensive

SALIENT FEATURES

- History of hypertension
- No ocular symptoms

HISTORY

Ask about the following:

- Age of onset and duration of symptoms
- History of dyspnea, palpitation, edema feet
- History of associated complications of hypertension
- History of diabetes, metabolic syndrome

EXAMINATION

- BP is high 170/110 mmHg

Fundus Examination (Fig. 240.1)

- It shows, AV nipping, arteriolar narrowing, flame shaped and blot hemorrhages
- Macular star (Fig 240.1)

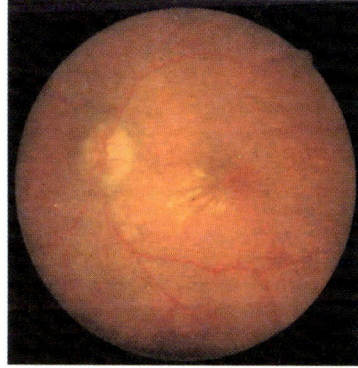

Fig. 240.1: Hypertensive retinopathy. There is narrowing of retinal arterioles which vary in calibre. Arteriovenous nipping is present below the disc. Flame shaped hemorrhages are seen. Macular star is prominently seen

- Cotton-wool exudate not seen
- Papilledema is not present

Systemic Examination

- Tell the examiner that you would like to examine CVS as patient's BP is high
- Cardiovascular examination for cardiomegaly and CHF
- Respiratory system for basal crackles

PROVISIONAL DIAGNOSIS

The patient has flame-shaped hemorrhage with macular star (lesion) caused by hypertensive retinopathy (etiology).

QUESTIONS AND ANSWERS

Q. How would you classify hypertensive retinopathy?

Ans: *Keith-Wagener* based on clinical findings of hypertension and atherosclerosis, classified fundus changes into 4 grades:

Grade I: Arteriolar narrowing

Grade II: Irregular calibre of arterioles, arteriolar-venous nipping

Grade III: Cotton-wool exudate and flame shaped hemorrhages and retinal edema

Grade IV: Papilledema

Q. What are the common causes of cotton-wool exudate?

Ans: • HIV infection per se
- Anemias
- Leukemias
- Infective endocarditis
- Diabetic retinopathy

Q. Name few common causes of hypertension.

Ans: 1. *Renal diseases,* e.g. glomerulonephritis, chronic pyelonephritis, polycystic kidneys and renal artery stenosis

2. *Endocrinal diseases,* e.g. Cushing's syndrome, Conn's syndrome, *pheochromocy-*

toma, acromegaly, myxedema, congenital adrenal hyperplasia

3. *Drug-induced,* e.g. oral contraceptives, NSAIDs

4. *Collagen vascular diseases,* e.g. PAN, SLE

5. *Toxemia of pregnancy* or pregnancy induced hypertension

6. *Coarctation of aorta*

Q. What do you mean by hypertensive urgency and hypertensive emergency?

Ans: *Hypertensive urgency.* It is a state of elevated BP (>200/120 mm Hg) which is not associated with severe symptoms or end-organ involvement. BP in these patients can be reduced by oral anti hypertensive on outpatient basis.

Hypertensive emergency. It is a state of severely elevated BP (>220/130 mm Hg) with symptoms and signs of end-organ damage (e.g. stroke, stage III and IV hypertensive retinopathy, MI, renal failure). These patients require hospitalisation for control of BP with parenteral antihypertensive.

Q. What is the relationship between hypertensive retinopathy and morbidity?

Ans: I. *Neurological morbility.* A population-based cohort study of atherosclerosis risk, incident stroke events were more common (2–4 times) in participants with retinopathy than in participants without hypertensive retinopathy. These were independent of other risk factors, i.e. diabetes, lipid abnormalities and other risks.

Hypertensive retinopathy is also associated with decline in cognitive function and lacunar infarcts (infarct-related dementia), cerebral atrophy and stroke mortality.

II. *Cardiovascular morbidity.* Hypertensive retinopathy is linked with coronary artery stenosis and with incident heart disease events such as MI and heart failure.

III. *Other morbidities.* Retinopathy itself is associated with morbidities due to other end organ damage, e.g. renal failure, left ventricular hypertrophy and micro-albuminuria.

241

Papilledema

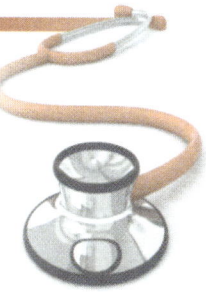

INSTRUCTION

- Examine the fundus of this patient

SALIENT FEATURES

- Patient is hypertensive, complains of narrow field of vision

HISTORY

Ask about the following:

- Headache, vomiting, blurring of vision
- Transient visual disturbances
- Barrel-shaped (tunnel-shape) vision
- Diplopia
- History of ingestion of drugs known to produce papilledema, i.e. steroids, hypervitaminosis A
- History of hypoparathyroidism
- History of brain tumor, trauma to head (subdural hematoma)
- History of delivery, post puerperal period, oral contraceptives (dural sinus thrombosis)
- Hypertensive hemorrhage, subarachnoid hemorrhage
- COPD (CO_2 narcosis)
- Anemia, leukemia
- Multiple sclerosis
- Orbital infection

EXAMINATION

Fundus Examination (Fig. 241.1)

It shows swelling of optic discs on both sides. There are soft exudates and hemorrhages.

Systemic Examination

- Tell the examiner that you would like to examine CNS.

PROVISIONAL DIAGNOSIS

The patient has bilateral papilledema (lesion) probably due to benign intracranial hypertension (etiology).

QUESTIONS AND ANSWERS

Q. What do you understand by the term papilledema?

Ans: Papilledema means swelling of the optic disc/head as seen on ophthalmoscopy. The swollen disc is pink and hyperemic. Disc vessels are clearly visible, more numerous, curve over the borders of the disc. The physiological disc cup is full and margins of the disc are blurred.

Q. What is the earliest sign of papilledema on fundus examination?

Ans: The earliest sign seen on ophthalmoscopic examination is venous dilatation, engorgement and loss of venous pulsations.

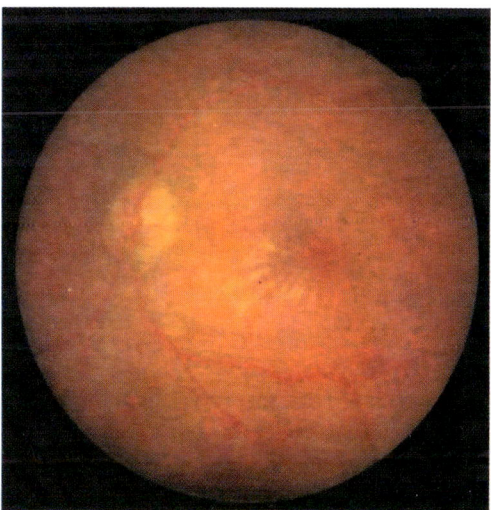

Fig. 241.1: Hypertensive retinopathy and papilledema. The optic disc is pink with the optic cup obliterated. The appearance of papilledema is confirmed by the dilatation of the veins, loss of venous pulsations and obliteration of arterioles. There are hemorrhages around the disc

Q.   List few common causes of papilledema.
Ans: Read Box 1.

Box 1: Causes of papilledema

I. *Raised intracranial tension*
- Brain tumor or abscess
- Meningitis, obstructive hydrocephalus
- Subdural hematoma, subarachnoid hemorrhage
- Dural sinus thrombosis

II. Cerebral edema
III. Malignant hypertension (hypertensive crisis)
IV. Blood disorders, e.g. anemia, leukemia, polycythemia
V. Respiratory diseases, e.g. COPD (CO_2 narcosis)
VI. Hypervitaminosis A
VII. Superior vena cava obstruction
VIII. Hypoparathyroidism

Q.   What do you understand by the term papillitis (optic neuritis)?
Ans: Optic neuritis/papillitis results from inflammatory, demyelinating or vascular disease leading to marked loss of vision.

Q.   What are the differences between papillitis and papilledema?
Ans: Read Table 241.1

Table 241.1: Papillitis vs papilledema

Papillitis	Papilledema
• Eye movements are painful	They are painless
• Usually unilateral	Usually bilateral
• Ocular tenderness on compression present	No tenderness
• Visual acuity is considerably reduced irrespective to degree of swelling of the disc	Visual acuity is slightly reduced
• Visual field defect is usually central particularly for red and green	Peripheral constriction or enlargement of blind spot
• Marcus Gunn pupil may be present	Marcus Gunn pupil is absent

---

Q.   What are the causes of papillitis?
Ans: 1. Papillitis/optic neuritis due to multiple sclerosis
2. Inflammation of disc
3. Degeneration (Leber's optic atrophy)
4. Vascular disorders of nerve head
5. Malignant infiltration

Q.   What are the causes of swelling of the disc?
Ans: • Papilledema
- Papillitis

• Drusen
• Malignant infiltration of nerve head

Q.   What is pseudopapilledema?
Ans: Pseudopapilledema means congenitally elevated disc secondary to hyaloid tissue (drusen) or hyperopia.

Q.   What is Marcus Gunn pupil?
Ans: It is pupil that shows better constriction to an indirect stimulus than to direct light, indicating a relative afferent pupillary defect.

Q.   What are the clinical characteristics of benign intracranial hypertension?
Ans: 1. Patient is alert but has all features of raised intracranial pressure, i.e. headache, vomiting, visual disturbance and papilledema
2. No localising signs except 6th nerve palsy (false localising sign)
3. CSF pressure is raised
4. Normal ventricles and normal CT/MRI study

Q.   What is Foster-Kennedy syndrome?
Ans: It is unilateral papilledema with or without secondary optic atrophy on the other side. It indicates a tumor on the side of optic atrophy arising either from olfactory lobe, frontal lobe or the pituitary grand.

Q.   What are the stages of papilledema?
Ans: **Stage I:** Venous dilatation and tortuosity
Stage II: Optic cup becomes pinker and less distinct vessels seem to disappear quickly on the surface of the disc
Stage III: Blurring of the disc on nasal side
Stage IV: The whole disc becomes suffused and elevated. The margins get blurred and vessels appear to emerge from the swollen disc. The optic cup is full and there are hemorrhages around the disc.

Q.   What is the type of field defect in papilledema?
Ans: There is enlargement of blind spot with peripheral constriction of the visual field (barrel-shape vision) with gradual loss of visual acuity.

Q.   What is the treatment of benign raised intracranial pressure (pseudotumor cerebedi)?
Ans: • Discontinue steroids if being used
- Diuretics, carbonic anhydrase inhibitor
- Weight reduction
- CSF drainage by serial lumber punctures, lumboperitoneal shunt
- Optic nerve fenestration, subtemporal decompression

242

Optic Atrophy

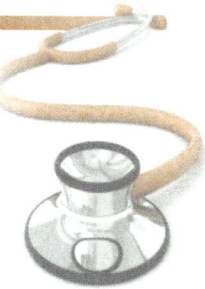

INSTRUCTION

- Examine the eyes of this patient
- Perform relevant neurological examination

SALIENT FEATURES

- Bilateral diminished vision

HISTORY

Ask about the following:

- Onset of symptoms, visual loss
- History of multiple sclerosis
- History of glaucoma
- Tumor of optic nerve, frontal lobe (Foster-Kennedy syndrome) and pituitary
- Vitamin B_{12} deficiency
- Paget's disease
- Exposure to toxins (methanol, lead, arsenic)

EXAMINATION

Examination of the Eyes

- Fundus examination (Fig. 242.1) shows pale disc with sharp, well defined margins

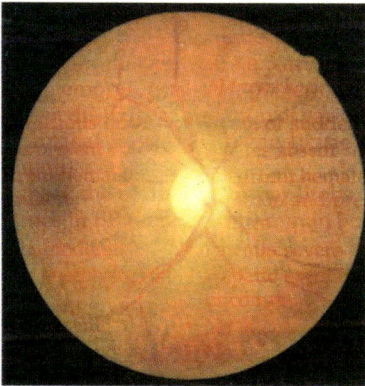

Fig. 242.1: Optic atrophy. The white optic disc indicates atrophy of the nerve. This may be due to direct pressure on the optic nerve or demyelinating disease, etc. (Read the causes)

- Impaired direct light reflex, but intact consensual light reflex. There is Marcus Gunn pupillary response (read it in papilledema)
- Visual field examination reveals central scotoma

Relevant Neurological Examination

- Elicit cerebellar signs (cerebellar involvement in multiple sclerosis is the commonest cause of optic atrophy)
- Look for signs and symptoms of frontal lobe tumor

PROVISIONAL DIAGNOSIS

The patient has optic atrophy (lesion) caused by multiple sclerosis (aetiology).

QUESTIONS AND ANSWERS

Q. **What do you understand by the term optic atrophy?**

Ans: It is defined as atrophy or death of optic nerve fibres leading to reduction or loss of tiny blood vessels, hence, disc becomes paler than normal and may even be white.

Q. **What is differential diagnosis?**

Ans: The differential diagnosis lies between the causes of optic atrophy such as:

1. *Demyelinating disorders* (MS, Devic's disease)
2. *Tumor,* e.g. compression of optic nerve by optic glioma
3. *Glaucomatous optic atrophy*
4. *Toxin-induced*
5. *Ischemic optic atrophy* (central retinal artery occlusion, temporal arteritis, syphilis)
6. *Hereditary disorders* (Leber's optic atrophy, hereditary ataxia)
7. *Paget's disease*
8. *Vitamin B_{12} deficiency*

9. *Secondary to retinitis pigmentosa*
10. *Idiopathic*

Q. **What are the causes of optic atrophy?**

Ans: Read the answer of differential diagnosis.

Q. **What are the differences between primary and secondary optic atrophy?**

Ans: The differences are:

Primary optic atrophy	Secondary optic atrophy
• Disc is white and flat with clear cut margins	Disc is greyish white with indistinct margins
• Lamina cribrosa is visible	Cup is full. Lamina cribrosa is not visible
• Arteries and veins are normal	Arteries are thinner than normal. Veins may be dilated
• Capillaries decrease in number	Capillaries are reduced in number from 10 to 7 (Kestenbaum's sign)

Q. **What is consecutive optic atrophy?**

Ans: It is a confusing term, should be avoided. It is used by physicians either equivalent or alternative for secondary optic atrophy as discussed above or used to indicate optic atrophy complicating retinitis or retinitis pigmentosa.

Q. **What is glaucomatous optic atrophy?**

Ans: It denotes loss of disc substance resulting in increased cupping of optic disc.

Q. **How would you investigate such a case?**

Ans: 1. Blood count and ESR
2. Blood sugar for diabetes
3. Serological tests for syphilis
4. Serum vitamin levels (B_1 and B_{12})
5. X-ray skull for pituitary fossa, optic foramina and sinuses
6. CT scan of orbit and brain
7. ECG for arrhythmias
8. Visual evoked potentials for MS
9. Electroretinography

243

Retinitis Pigmentosa

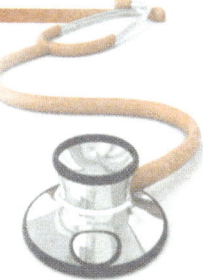

INSTRUCTION

- Examine the patient fundus
- Perform relevant systemic examination

SALIENT FEATURES

- Blurring of vision

HISTORY

Ask for the following:

- Decreased nocturnal vision
- Altered color vision
- Loss of peripheral vision
- Blurred vision
- Family history of blindness (hereditary auto-somal recessive disorder)

EXAMINATION

Ocular Fundus Examination

- Fundus examination shows peripheral retinal pigmentations (bone spicule pigmentation) and arteriolar narrowing (Fig. 243.1). Only the retinal veins not the arteries show sheath of pigmentation along their course and anterior to them

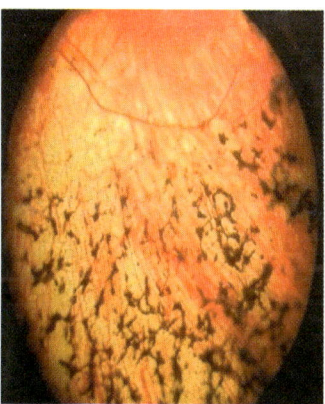

Fig. 243.1: Retinitis pigmentosa

- Optic disc is pale
- Atrophic maculopathy
- Examine the other components of Laurence-Moon-Biedl syndrome (aetiology).

Neurological Examination

- Examine cerebellar functions, peripheral nerves and spinal cord degeneration (Friedreich's ataxia)

PROVISIONAL DIAGNOSIS

The patient is obese, has syndactyly, hypogonadism and retinitis pigmentosa (lesion) caused by Laurence-Moon-Biedl syndrome (aetiology). He is blind (functional status).

QUESTIONS AND ANSWERS

Q. What do you know about retinitis pigmentosa?

Ans: Retinitis pigmentosa is a degenerative disease of retina, may be primary (hereditary) or secondary, starts in early childhood and progresses slowly resulting in blindness by the middle or advanced age. The degeneration primary affects the rods (affecting the vision in moon light or at dusk) and cones (color vision).

Q. How does retinitis pigmentosa present clinically?

Ans: Patient presents with night blindness (defective vision at dusk) which may occur several years before the pigment becomes visible in the retina.

Q. Name the ocular conditions associated with retinitis pigmentosa?

Ans: • Open angle glaucoma
- Cataract (posterior, subscapsular)
- Myopia
- Keratoconus

Q. Name the hereditary disorders associated with retinitis pigmentosa.

Ans:
1. *Laurence-Moon-Biedl syndrome:* It is an autosomal recessive disorder characterised by mental retardation, polydactyly, syndactyly, hypogonadism, obesity and structural renal abnormalities (calyceal clubbing and blunting).
2. *Refsum's disease:* It is a phytanic acid storage disease, transmitted by autosomal recessive manner, characterised by hypertrophic peripheral neuropathy (palpable nerves), deafness, ichthyosis, cerebellar ataxia and albumino-cytological dissociation in CSF.
3. *Kearns-Sayre syndrome:* It consists of a triad comprising of retinitis pigmentosa, external ophthalmoplegia and heart block.
4. *Friedreich's ataxia* (read it as a case report).

Q. What is secondary retinitis pigmentosa?

Ans: Secondary retinitis pigmentosa is a sequelae to inflammatory retinitis. It is indistinguishable from primary condition on ophthalmoscopic examination, the electroretinographic and electro-oculographic responses are slightly abnormal as compared to primary condition in which they are markedly abnormal.

Q. What is inverse retinitis pigmentosa?

Ans: Pigmentation is visible in the central perifoveal area, whereas the retinal periphery is normal.

Q. How would you manage this condition?

Ans:
- Refer the patient to eye specialist
- Refer for genetic counseling
- Refer to vision training and aids for daily living
- Refer for job training (rehabilitation)

244

Age-Related Macular Degeneration

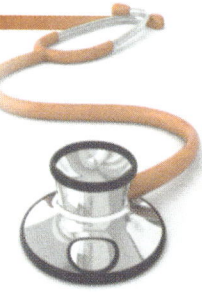

INSTRUCTION

- Examine the patient's eyes

SALIENT FEATURES

- Inability to read and recognise the faces

HISTORY

Ask for the following:

- Often visual loss is detected when one eye is covered for testing visual acuity
- Inability to read, recognise the faces and difficulty in driving a car
- Patients can walk unaided as peripheral vision is good
- Decrease in visual acuity
- Distortion of shapes of objects (metamorphosia)
- Paracentral scotoma
- Varying degree of visual loss
- Family history
- History of hypertension, smoking

EXAMINATION

Ocular Examination

- Fundus examination shows (Fig. 244.1);
  - i. Pale yellow spots (drusen) are seen throughout the macula
  - ii. Small areas of hypopigmentation and hyperpigmentation are seen due to degeneration of pigmented retinal epithelium
  - iii. Neovascularisation of choroid
- Check visual acuity and visual field (loss of central vision in most cases)

PROVISIONAL DIAGNOSIS

The patient has senile macular degeneration (lesion) due to age-related changes (aetiology) and patient is a registered blind using walking aid (functional status).

QUESTIONS AND ANSWERS

Q. What is the clinical hallmark of age-related macular degeneration?

Ans: The clinical hallmark of age-related macular degeneration is large drusen in both the eyes.

Q. What are drusen?

Ans: Drusen are pale yellow spots comprising of amorphous material accumulated between the Bruch's membrane and pigment epithelium. In fact drusen occurs from accumulation of lipofuscin and other cellular debris derived from the cells of the retinal pigment epithelium that are compromised by age and other factors.

Nearly all individuals over the age of 50 yrs have at least one small drusen (≤63 µm) in one or both eyes. Large drusen appear in the eyes as age-related macular degeneration.

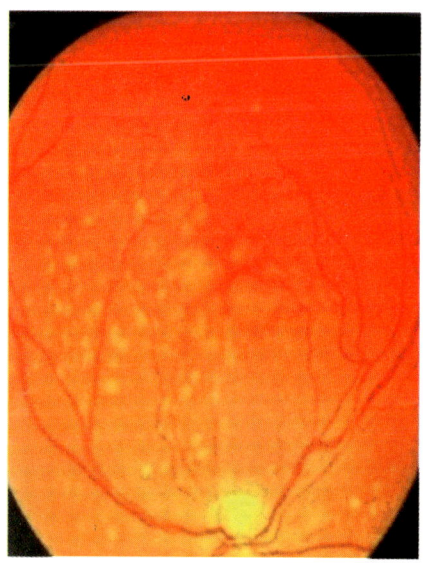

Fig. 244.1: Age-related macular degeneration

Q. What are the various types of age-related macular degeneration?

Ans: I. *Early age-related macular degeneration*
- There is presence of multiple small drusen (< 60 μm) or intermediate drusen ($60 - 125$ μm).

II. *Intermediate age-related macular degeneration*
- Extensive intermediate drusen or large drusen (> 125 μm) are seen with no other evidence of macular degeneration.

III. *Advanced age-related macular degeneration*
- There are discrete area of retinal depigmentation (175 μm in diameter) with sharp border and visible choroidal vessel called *geographic atrophy*. It results from continuous loss of retinal pigment epithelium.
- Neovascular age-related macular degeneration changes appear as serous or hemorrhagic detachment of either retinal pigment epithelium or the sensory retina. Neovascularisation develops under the retina which can leak fluid and blood. Onset of vision loss is acute.

Q. What is the significance of drusen in the eye?

Ans: Larger drusen (> 60 μm), drusen > 5 in number are risk factors for choroidal neovascularisation.

Q. What are the risk factors for macular degeneration?

Ans:
- Old age
- Genetic factors
- High intake of vegetable fat in the diet
- Low intake of antioxidants and zinc in the diet
- White race
- Obesity

Q. How would you investigate such a case?

Ans:
- Fundus examination
- Fluorescein angiography to detect choroidal neovascularisation
- Retinal angiography

Q. What are the complications of macular degeneration?

Ans: Neovascularisation can lead to rupture of these new vessels leading to retinal hemorrhage and retinal detachment.

Q. What is neovascularisation of choroid? How is it treated?

Ans: It is the new vessel formation due to proliferation of choroidal vessels across the Bruch's membrane under the retinal pigment epithelium.

It is treated by:
- Laser photocoagulation
- Photodynamic therapy
- Interferon alfa
- Submacular surgery
- External beam radiation therapy
- Thalidomide

Q. How would you treat age-related macular degeneration?

Ans:
1. *Lifestyle changes*, e.g. cessation of smoking, high intake of antioxidant vitamins and zinc in the diet, high intake of omega 3 fatty acids and fish, etc.

2. For severe visual loss, low vision devices such as electronic video magnifiers and spectacle mounted telescopes are used

3. Monoclonal antibodies, e.g. ranibizumab and bevacizumab against vascular endothelial growth factor (VEGF)

4. Photodynamic therapy to reduce angiogenesis

5. Gene therapy

6. Implantation of artificial devices, e.g. intraocular devices

245

Unilateral Edema
(Deep Vein Thrombosis)

INSTRUCTION

- Perform general physical examination

SALIENT FEATURES

- Edema of right leg

HISTORY

Ask about the following:

- Onset of swelling, i.e. acute or chronic
- Is swelling increasing or decreasing?
- History of pain in the leg (increases on movements)
- History of prolonged immobilisation, i.e. recent surgery, fracture, stroke, MI, etc.
- Past history of DVT
- Family history of hyperlipidemia
- History of diabetes, hypertension, obesity, antiphospholipid syndrome
- History of cough, pain chest, hemoptysis (pulmonary embolism)
- History of pregnancy, recent delivery (present) or intake of oral contraceptive

EXAMINATION

General Physical Examination

- The leg is swollen, erythematous and superficial veins are visible and engorged.
- The skin is shiny. Temperature is raised on the side involved (in this case right leg).
- Calf is tender on squeezing or touching (present)
- There is pitting edema over the ankle, foot and leg (Fig. 245.1).
- Homans' sign is positive (Fig. 245.2).
- Arterial pulsations on the side involved are not felt due to swelling.
- There is no evidence of venous ulcer or gangrene.

PROVISIONAL DIAGNOSIS

The patient has unilateral swollen leg due to deep vein thrombosis (DVP) following delivery of the child (aetiology). The patient is at a risk of developing pulmonary embolism.

QUESTIONS AND ANSWERS

Q. **What are the points in favor of DVT?**
Ans: 1. History of recent delivery (postpartum female)

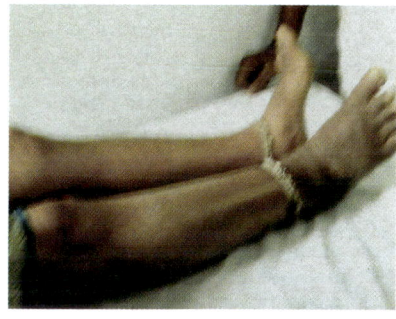

Fig. 245.1: Unilateral edema. There edema of right leg due to DV

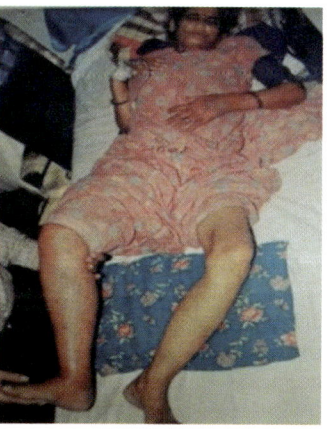

Fig. 245.2: Homan's sign for DVT. It is obsolete nowadays

2. Unilateral pitting oedema (right leg)
3. Superficial veins are visible and temperature of the limb is raised
4. Calf tenderness present
5. Positive Homan's sign

Q. **What are the complications of DVT?**
Ans: • Pulmonary embolism
• Venous ulcer and venous gangrene
• Postphlebitic syndrome
• Severe pain

Q. **What are the factors that predispose to venous thrombosis?**
Ans: • Surgery
• Obesity
• Malignancy

• Following CVA and MI
• Varicose veins
• Oral contraceptives, pregnancy, postpartum period
• Previous DVT

• Prolonged Immobilisation
• Hypercoaguable states

• Tissue trauma

Q. **How would you investigate a patient with DVT?**
Ans: • Duplex ultrasonography scanning
• Color Doppler flow studies
• Venography
• D-Dimer

Q. **What are the causes of recurrent venous thrombosis?**
Ans: 1. Postpartum state, pregnancy and oral contraceptives
2. Trauma, surgery
3. Hypercoagulable states especially antiphospholipid syndrome, myeloproliferative disorders, occult malignancy, vasculitides, abnormalities of protein C, protein S antithrombin III, factors V and fibrinogen
4. Abnormalities such as thrombomodulin, tissue factor pathway inhibitor, etc.

Q. **How would you treat patients with DVT?**
Ans: The treatment depends on whether DVT is below the knee or above the knee because below the knee DVT are less likely to produce emboli than above the knee DVT.

I. *Treatment of patients with below the knee DVT*
• Analgesics for pain relief
• Diuretics, salt restriction to reduce edema
• Intermittent elevation of foot
• Elevation of foot and leg with the help of pillows above the level of heart
• Elastic stockings from midfoot to just below the knee worn during the day

II. *Treatment of patients with above the knee DVT*
• Low molecular weight heparin is preferred for iliofemoral thrombosis
• Factor Xa inhibitor such as analogues, e.g. fondaparinux
• For recurrent thrombi or when anticoagulants are contraindicated, inferior vena cava filters are used.
• Thrombolysis in life or limb threatening situations

Q. **What should be the duration of anticoagulants for DVT?**
Ans: 1. 3–6 months with first episode
2. For prophylaxis during postoperative period, 6 weeks to 3 months anticoagulation is sufficient
3. For recurrent thrombotic events, it is given for 6–12 months, but rarely may be given lifelong

Q. **How would you prevent DVT?**
Ans: 1. Subcutaneous low-molecular heparin for patients at risk, i.e. patients with CHF, MI or patients undergoing surgery
2. Stop oral contraceptive if being used
3. Early ambulation
4. Leg exercises following surgery, CHF and an episode of MI
5. Elastic stockings
6. Antiplatelets, e.g. aspirin or aspirin and clopidogrel combination

Q. **What is an antiphospholipid syndrome?**
Ans: Read it as a case report.

246

Cellulitis

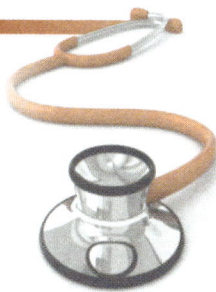

INSTRUCTION

- Perform general physical examination

SALIENT FEATURES

- Foul smelling discharging wound

HISTORY

Ask for the following:

- Fever, chills, rigors and sweating
- History of diabetes
- History of trauma or injury
- History of animal or human bites
- History of exposure to sea water, fresh water or aqua cultured fish

EXAMINATION

General Physical Examination (Fig. 246.1)

- There is abrasions, subcutaneous tissue destruction and necrosis with bleeding.
- Edema of the foot and leg is present

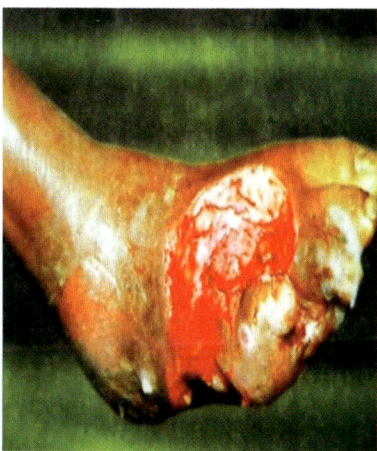

Fig. 246.1: Necrotising fascitis use cellulitis due to anaerobic infection

- Amputation of toes
- No crepitus
- Peripheral pulses (dorsalis pedis, tibialis) decreased use normal
- Ulcerations and bleeding present in this case. Underlying granulation tissue is visible

PROVISIONAL DIAGNOSIS

The patient has extensive cellulitis right foot with amputated toes (lesion) caused by pyogenic bacterial infection in a patient with diabetes (etiology). The leg is swollen and tender (functional status).

Q. **What do you mean by the term cellulitis?**

Ans: It is a deep, subcutaneous infection characterised by warmth, swelling, tenderness, and erythema and may be accompanied by lymphatic streaking. Pruritus is absent.

Q. **What is crepitant cellulitis?**

Ans: Cellulitis produced by gas-forming organisms such as *Clostridium* species or nonspore-forming *anaerobes* (*Bacteroides, peptostreptococci and peptococci*) is called *crepitant cellulitis*. Crepitus is present over cellulitis.

Q. **What are the causes of acute painful swollen leg?**

Ans: 1. DVT
2. Cellulitis
3. Trauma
4. Arthritis (ankle)
5. Arterial occlusion
6. Hematoma

Q. **What are the causes of chronic swollen leg and foot?**

Ans: 1. Postphlebitis or gravitational eczema, varicose veins of legs
2. Lymphedema (elephantiasis), Maleo-Milroy's disease
3. Congenital

Q. **What are the causes of bilateral swollen legs?**

Ans: Read case discussion on CHF, nephrotic syndrome, cirrhosis, etc.

Q. **How would you investigate?**

Ans:
- Blood count will show leucocytosis with neutrophilia. ESR and C-reactive proteins are raised
- Blood culture may be positive if abscess or pus is present
- Aspiration from the advancing edge or loculated site for culture
- A full thickness skin biopsy before antibiotic therapy for histopathology

Q. **How would you treat?**

Ans:
- Hospitalisation if patient has features of septic shock or acute renal failure.
- Intravenous or parenteral antibiotics. Start with broad spectrum β-lactam antibiotic, then shift to appropriate antibiotic after culture and sensitivity report.
- If CA–MRSA is suspected, then vancomycin, clindamycin may be administered.
- If MRSA is suspected, use TMP–SMZ clindamycin or combination of doxycycline plus rifampicin should be considered.

247

Clubbing

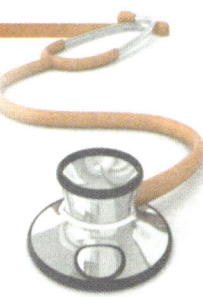

INSTRUCTION

- Perform general physical and relevant systemic examination

SALIENT FEATURES

- Swollen fingertips

HISTORY

Ask about the following:

- *Respiratory symptoms*, e.g. cough, hemoptysis, fever, sputum production, chest pain, dyspnea, etc.
- *Cardiac symptoms*, e.g. dyspnea, PND, orthopnea, palpitations, cyanosis, cough, hemoptysis, chest pain, fever, etc.

- *GI tract symptoms*, e.g. chronic diarrhea or dysentery, cirrhosis of liver (ascites, edema) or malignant liver (tender nodular hepatomegaly)
- *Graves' disease* (thyroid acropatchy)
- *Family history* (congenital or hereditary)

EXAMINATION

General Physical Examination

- Nails show increased curvature, obliteration of the angle of the nails, a positive Schamroth test (Fig. 247.1B)
- Loss of onychodermal (Lovibond's) angle
- The nails show drumstick appearance (Fig. 247.1A)
- There is no wrist joints swelling tenderness (hypertrophic pulmonary osteoarthropathy)
- Fluctuation of the nail bed positive (Fig. 247.1C)
- No nicotine staining of fingers, no cyanosis and no clubbing of toes

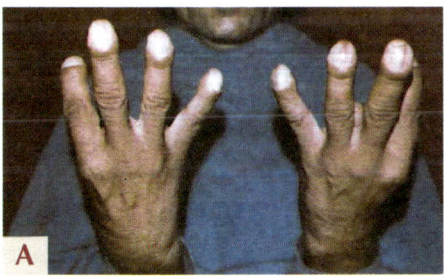

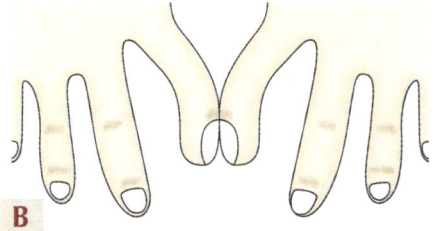

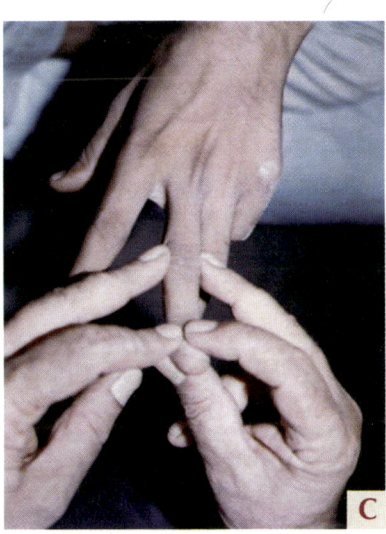

Fig. 247.1: Clubbing of fingers. (A) Visible drumstick clubbing; (B) Diagrammatic illustration of Schamroth's sign; (C) Elicitation of fluctuation of the nails bed (e.g. fluctuation sign for clubbing is positive)

Systemic Examination
- *Examine the respiratory, CVS and GI tract*
- Examine *liver* and *thyroid gland* (Graves' disease)

PROVISIONAL DIAGNOSIS

The patient has drumstick clubbing of the finger nails and central cyanosis (lesion) caused by a congenital cyanotic heart disease (aetiology)

Q. **What are the common causes of clubbing?**
Ans: Read Table 247.1

Table 247.1: Causes of clubbing
1. *Cardiac*
• Congenital cyanotic heart disease (Fallot's tetralogy)
• Subacute infective endocarditis
• Atrial myxoma
• Eisenmenger's syndrome
2. *Respiratory*
• Bronchiectasis and lung abscess
• Bronchogenic carcinoma, mesothelioma
• Empyema thoracis
• Fibrosing alveolitis
• Pulmonary arteriovenous communication
• Rarely fibrocaseous tuberculosis
3. *GI tract*
• Ulcerative colitis   • Malabsorption
• Crohn's disease   • Polyposis
4. *Hepatobiliary*
• Biliary cirrhosis   • Hepatocellular failure
5. *Genetic* (Familial)

Q. **What is Schamroth's sign?**
Ans: It is an indirect method (Schamroth's window test) to demonstrate clubbing: Approximate the nails of two fingers preferably the thumbs of both hands and look for the normal lozenge shaped gap between the two nails and the proximal nail folds. In clubbing, this diamond/lozenge shape gap is either reduced or obliterated (Fig. 247.1B).

Q. **What are the grades of clubbing?**
Ans: The grades of clubbing are:
Grade I. Softening of nails bed with obliteration of onychodermal angle
Grade II. Grade I *plus* increase in AP and transverse diameters of nails as well as nails become tense, shiny with loss of longitudinal ridges.
Grade III. Grade II *plus* increase in pulp tissue resulting in Parrot's beak or drumstick appearance.

Grade IV. Grade III *plus* hypertrophic osteoarthropathy.

Q. **What are the cause of unilateral clubbing?**
Ans: Clubbing is mostly bilateral but may be unilateral due to:
- Presubclavian coarctation of aorta
- Cervical rib
- Pancoast's tumor
- Aneurysm of a subclavian artery
- Erythromelalgia
- AV fistula involving brachial vessels

Q. **What do you mean by the term differential clubbing?**
Ans: Clubbing may be limited to the upper limbs in chronic obstruction of the veins (phlebitis of upper extremities as seen in IV drug users) or may be present in the lower limbs only in infected abdominal aortic aneurysm and PDA with reversal of shunt (*Eisenmenger's syndrome*).

Q. **What is plausible mechanisms for pathogenesis of clubbing?**
Ans: Clubbing may appear acutely in acute lung suppuration, reason is not known but hypotheses are:
- *Hypoxemia* due to any cause leading to vasodilatation and proliferation of subcutaneous tissue of nails bed. There is increase in capillary permeability leading to interstitial edema.
- *Toxemia*: Clubbing in SABE is considered due to this factor and hormonal influence.
- *Metabolic and hormonal:* Clubbing seen in endocrine disorders, e.g. hyperthyroidism, acromegaly, hyperparathyroidism.
- *Pressure changes* between radial and digital arteries.
- *Reduced ferritin* by escaping oxidation in the lungs leads to dilatation of AV anastomosis.
- *Hereditary*

Q. **What do you know about pachy dermoperiostitis?**
Ans: This is a form of hypertrophic pulmonary osteoarthropathy in adolescents characterised by postpubertal sweating of the palms and soles, thickening of the skin of face, forehead and scalp and periostosis (swelling of periarticular tissue and periosteal new bone formation of long bone) and digital clubbing

Q. **How would you differentiate pseudoclubbing from true clubbing?**

Ans: Preservation of nail fold angle distinguishes pseudoclubbing from true clubbing.

Q. **How would you perform fluctuation of nail bed in clubbing?**

Ans: Fluctuation is due to softening of the nail bed. It is observed by gentle pressure over the base of the nail by tip of right index finger while holding the patient's finger (say middle finger) between the thumb and index finger of left hand and supporting the pulp of the finger over the pulp of the right thumb (Fig. 247.1C).

248

Dupuytren's Contractures

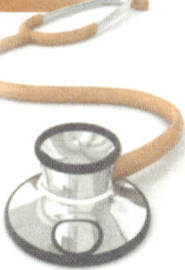

INSTRUCTION

Look at the patient's hands and feet

SALIENT FEATURES

- Difficulty to perform normal activities with hands

HISTORY

Ask about the following:

- Family history
- Cigarette smoking and alcohol intake
- Drug history (antiepileptic drugs)
- Systemic disorders, e.g. diabetes, tuberculosis, leprosy, cirrhosis of liver

EXAMINATION

Examination of Hands and Feet

- There is palpable thickening of palmar fascia as a cord along the medial aspect of both hands (Fig. 248.1) in this case
- There is flexion of the little finger and ring finger (in this case) of both hands

- Patient is unable to put his/her palm flat on the table top (*Hueston table top test* is positive)
- There is associated contracture of plantar fascia with fibrous nodules formation (Fig. 248.2)
- Alcoholic stigmata and signs of cirrhosis liver or liver cell failure (present)

PROVISIONAL DIAGNOSIS

The patient has Dupuytren's contracture (lesion) associated with alcoholic cirrhosis (aetiology). Patient has disabling contracture (functional status).

Q. **What do you mean by Dupuytren's contracture?**

Ans: It is hyperplasia of palmar fascia and related structure resulting in thickening and shortening of the palmar fascia, the plantar fascia may also be involved. This is due to proliferation of fibroblasts in the dermis of the palm. The groups of fibroblasts surrounding dense collagen form the fibrous nodules. There is fixation of dermis to deeper structures.

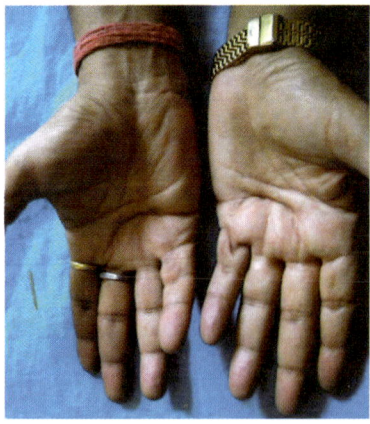

Fig. 248.1: Dupuytren's contractures

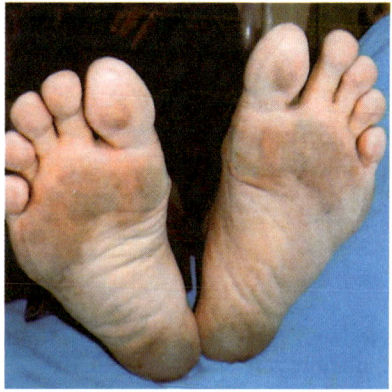

Fig. 248.2: There is bilateral plantar fascia involvement with fibrous nodules formation under great toes

Q. Do other soft tissue structure involved?

Ans: No, muscles, joints, tendons, nervous tissue, vascular tissue are not involved. It is only the fixation of dermis to deeper structure.

Q. How do you grade Dupuytren's contracture?

Ans: *Grade* 1: Presence of a thickened nodule and a band in the palmar aponeurosis that may progress to skin tethering, puckering or pitting.

Grade 2: Presence of a thickened pretendinous band that restricts the extension of the affected finger.

Grade 3: Flexion contracture (flexion deformity of the finger).

Q. What are the conditions associated with Dupuytren's contracture?

Ans: 1. Hereditary predisposition
2. Chronic alcoholism (in this case)
3. Antiepileptic drug therapy
4. Systemic diseases, e.g. diabetes cirrhosis (present in this case), epilepsy, tuberculosis
5. Systemic fibrosing syndrome which include Peyronie disease (thickening of corpora cavernosa of penis) and retroperitoneal fibrosis

Q. What is the deformity caused by Dupuytren's contracture?

Ans: Flexion deformity of the finger(s) involved.

Q. How would you treat such a case?

Ans: The aim of therapy is just to improve the range of motion and to reduce the need for surgery. The options are:
1. Local injection of triamcinolone (a steroid) into the growing nodule or cord.
2. Collagenase (*Clostridium histolyticum*) which lyses collagen has been found useful when injected into the contracture cord. The joint is immediately manipulated to attempt cord rupture and improve movements at the joints.
3. Surgery: It is indicated in desperate cases with disabling flexion contractures.

Q. What are the complications of Dupuytren's contracture?

Ans: • Inability to extend the fingers resulting in difficulty to perform the routine activities with the hands
• Cosmetic problem
• Fascitis of other areas especially plantar fascitis resulting in pain and tenderness or Peyronie disease.

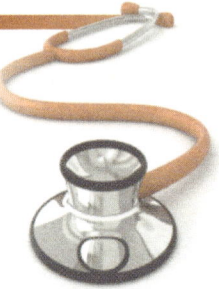

249

Gum Hypertrophy

INSTRUCTION

- Perform general physical and relevant system examination

SALIENT FEATURES

- Bleeding from gums

HISTORY

Ask about the following:

- History of generalised tonic, clonic seizures (epilepsy).
- Drug history (phenytoin, cyclosporin, nifedipine). This patient was on phenytoin therapy
- Features suggestive of leukemia (monomyelocytic)
- History of Wegener's granuloma
- History of bleeding during brushing or cleaning the teeth

EXAMINATION

General Physical Examination

There is elevation of gum papillae in between the gums. The gums are hypertrophied and spongy (Fig. 249.1)

- Examine the other features of phenytoin toxicity such as coarsening of facial features, hirsutism or hypertrichosis, lymphadenopathy, cerebellar ataxia, and rash
- Look other features of myelomonocytic leukemia, i.e. bleeding, hepatosplenomegaly
- Look for oral hygiene
- Look for other features, of Wegener's granulomatosis such as necrotising vasculitis

PROVISIONAL DIAGNOSIS

The patient has gum hypertrophy (lesion) due to phenytoin toxicity (aetiology). There is risk of bleeding (functional status).

Q.   **What are the causes of gum hypertrophy?**
Ans: • Drug toxicity (Fig. 249.1), e.g. phenytoin, cyclosporin, nifedipine
- Acute myelomonocytic leukemia
- Thrombocytopenia
- Scurvy
- Congenital cyanotic heart disease
- Wegener's granulomatosis
- Epulis or pyogenic granuloma during pregnancy

Q.   **What are the causes of gum bleeding?**
Ans: 1. Scurvy
2. Acute leukemia
3. Thrombocytopenia
4. Necrotising ulcerative gingivitis (vincent's infection)
5. Periodontitis

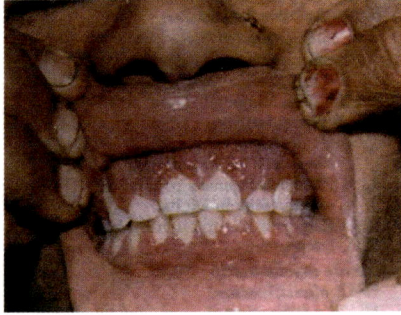

Fig. 249.1: Gum hypertrophy

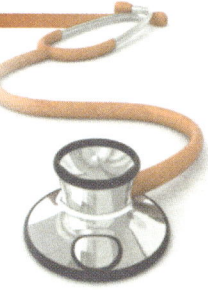

INSTRUCTION

- Perform general physical and relevant systemic examination

SALIENT FEATURES

- Tongue coating

HISTORY

Ask for the following:

- History of coating of the tongue (present)
- History of dysphagia or odynophagia (present)
- Systemic disease, e.g. diabetes, leukemia, cancer of an organ, HIV.
- Drug history of immunosuppressive drugs, e.g. steroids, anticancer (being taken by the patient)
- Drugs known to disturb the intestinal flora, e.g. broad spectrum antibiotics
- Polyglandular endocrinal deficiency syndromes (MEN type I and II), candida endocrinopathy

EXAMINATION

General Physical Examination

- There are adherent white confluent patches over the tongue (Fig. 250.1) which are easily detachable leaving behind red-denuded surface of tongue
- Look for erythema, transverse fissuring and maceration at the angles the mouth.
- Look for signs of neutropenia or a granulocytosis, e.g. mouth ulcers, angular stomatitis, cheilitis and aphthous ulceration of mucous membrane.
- Look at other sites for candida infection, e.g. inframammary folds, inguinal creases, between the fingers and toes
- Look for dysphagia or odynophagia
- Look for signs of hypoparathyroidism, hypo-adrenalism and hypoparathyroidism syndrome (candida endocrinopathy is common)

PROVISIONAL DIAGNOSIS

The patient has oral thrush, e.g. white patches over the tongue (lesion) due to anticancer therapy (etiology). The patient has dysphagia (functional status).

Q. Which fungus causes mouth thrush?
Ans: *Candida albicans*

Q. Which Candida species colonises the skin?
Ans: *C. parapsilosis*

Q. What are the common causes of mouth thrush?
Ans: Candida is an oppurtunistic fungus, grows immediately when either the immunity is lowered or bacterial intestinal symbiosis is disturbed. The causes are:
1. *Systemic disease*, e.g. diabetes mellitus, leukemias, autoimmune diseases, agranulocytosis, aplastic anemia, cancer, sickle cell anemia
2. *Polyglandular endocrinal deficiency syndromes* associated with candida endocrinopathy

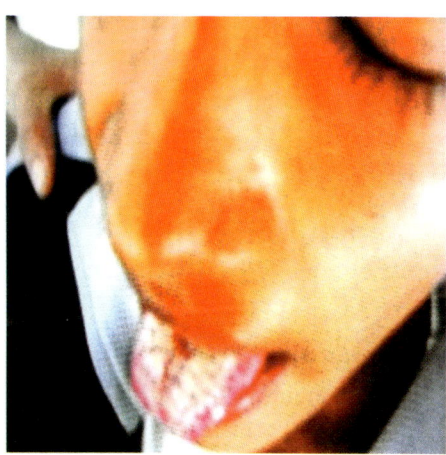

Fig. 250.1: Mouth thrush. Note the white patches over the tongue due to superinfection by *Candida albicans*

3. HIV
4. *Drugs*, e.g. steroids, anticancer, prolonged used of tetracyclines
5. *Debilitated children* (malnourished)
6. *Postoperative sepsis*

Q. What do you mean by furring of the tongue?

Ans: Furring of the tongue is of little significance, is often seen in patients with bad oral hygiene, can also occur with oral iron therapy (syrup) and in heavy smokers.

Q. What is black hairy tongue?

Ans: It is due to infection by the fungi or chromogens. Black tar deposits in the tongue are seen in smokers (Fig. 250.2).

Q. What is differential diagnosis?

Ans: Hairy leukoplakia can simulate mouth thrush, hence, to be differentiated (read leukoplakia as a case report).

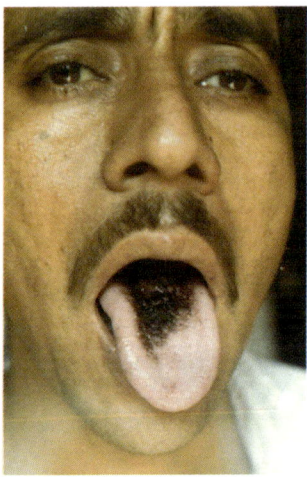

Fig. 250.2: Black tar deposits on the tongue in smokers

Q. How would you confirm your diagnosis?

Ans: 1. *Wet preparation of a smear* with KOH will show spores and fungal mycelia
2. *Biopsy* will show pseudomycelia inside the epithelium.

Q. How would you treat?

Ans: Stop the drug or an offending agent
• Treat the underlying disorder if associated
• Local application of antifungal agent, e.g. nystatin or amphotericin lozenges
• Systemic antifungal therapy for disseminated infection
• Sexual partners of oral or vaginal candidiasis must be screened and appropriately treated.
• Echinocandins and newer generation azoles may be considered in failure or resistant cases. The echinocandin (caspofungin, micafungin) are broad spectrum antifungal against all *Candida* species.

Q. What is role of T-cell immunity in candidiasis?

Ans: Dectin-I deficiency (a genetic defect of β-glucan receptor dectin-I) increases susceptibility to mucocutaneous candidiasis, but not systemic fungal infection.
The deficiency of dectin I suggests impaired T cell immunity resulting in susceptibility to fungal infection.

Q. What is systemic candidiasis?

Ans: Disseminated candidiasis occurs following fungemia due to intravascular catheter, involves skin, brain, meninges, lung and myocardium. It is characterised by fever, cough and mucoid sputum (pulmonary involvement), endocarditis, pustular skin abscesses, brain abscess, meningitis, rarely myositis and osteomyelitis.

251

Macroglossia

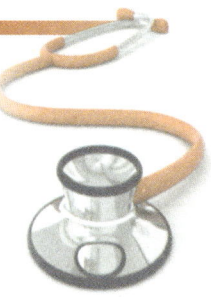

INSTRUCTION

- Perform general physical and relevant system examination

SALIENT FEATURES

- Large tongue

HISTORY

Ask about the following:

- Is there history of mouth breathing? Is there history of drooling of saliva (present)?
- Ask about any difficulty in swallowing.
- Ask about symptoms and signs of acromegaly, hyperthyroidism and amyloidosis.

EXAMINATION

General Physical Examination

- Mouth of the patient is half often and the resting tongue is protruding (Fig. 251.1) beyond teeth or

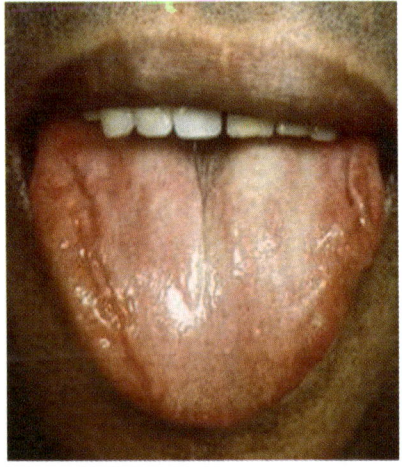

Fig. 251.1: Macroglossia (large protruding tongue)

alveolar ridge. The impression of the teeth may be obvious along the edges of the tongue on either side (present).
- Patient is mouth breather, hence, tongue is dry (in this case)

PROVISIONAL DIAGNOSIS

The patient has macroglossia (lesion) the cause of which has to be found out (etiology uncertain). Patient has become mouth breather (functional status)

QUESTIONS AND ANSWERS

Q. **What does macroglossia mean? How would you diagnose that macroglossia is present?**

Ans: Macroglossia (*macro* means large, *glossia* means tongue) means large tongue. It is diagnosed when the resting tongue protudes beyond the teeth or alveolar ridge.

Q. **What are the types of macroglossia?**

Ans: Macroglossia may be true (definite histopathological evidence) or false (no histopathological evidence). The true macroglossia is further of two types.
Primary: It is characterised true hypertrophy/hyperplasia of tongue muscles
Secondary: It is secondary to infiltration of tongue by anomalous elements.

Q. **What is pseudomacroglossia? What are its causes?**

Ans: When tongue is relatively larger to small mouth caused by a small mandible with no histopathological evidence of muscle hypertrophy is called *pseudomacroglossia*. The causes include Down syndrome, cerebral palsy, small mandible.

Q. **What are the causes of macroglossia?**

Ans: The causes of primary and secondary macroglossia are:

Primary macroglossia	Secondary macroglossia
• Myxedema • Tumors of the tongue (lymphangioma, hemangioma) • Metabolic disorders • Idiopathic	• Amyloidosis • Acromegaly • Angioedema • Lymphoma • Chronic infections, e.g. hepatitis B, TB, syphilis • Space occupying lesions, e.g. cystic hygroma, thyroglossal cyst, rhabdomyosarcoma

Q. What are the consequences or complications of macroglossia?

Ans: 1. Prolonged exposure of the tongue to external environment causes dryness, ulceration and necrosis of tip of tongue and mouth

2. Stertorous breathing or mouth breathing
3. Dysphagia
4. Difficulty in speech due to difficulty in articulation
5. Airway obstruction

Q. How would you manage this case?

Ans: The management includes:
1. Treatment of underlying cause, e.g. hypothyroidism or acromegaly
2. Steroids are useful to reduce airway obstruction and edema
3. Surgical treatment is indicated, i.e. excision of neoplastic lesion or glossectomy if there is symptomatic troublesome ankyloglossia due to neoplasm.

Q. What physical and psychological rehabilitation are needed in this case?

Ans: 1. Mouth care and speech therapy
2. Psychosocial support
3. Psychiatric rehabilitation

252

Osteogenesis Imperfecta

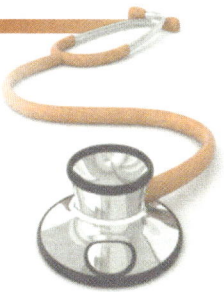

INSTRUCTION

• Examine the musculoskeletal system

SALIENT FEATURES

• History of repeated fractures since birth

HISTORY

Ask about the following:

• Any other member of the family suffering from this disease (family history is positive)
• History of previous fractures (present)

EXAMINATION

General Physical Examination

• Blue sclera [present (Fig. 252.1A)]
• Kyphoscoliosis
• Hypermobile joints
• Look for hearing loss.
• Signs of old fractures [present in the child in this case, Fig. 252.1B)]

• Defective dentition (present in the child)
• Hernias
• Signs of aortic regurgitation

PROVISIONAL DIAGNOSIS

The patient has history of old fractures. Examination reveals blue sclera, defective dentine (lesion) caused by osteogenesis imperfecta tarda (etiology). He is disabled by multiple fractures (functional status).

QUESTIONS AND ANSWERS

Q. **What is blue sclera? What are its cause?**

Ans: Visible choroid pigment leads to blue sclera. The blue sclera are seen in heritable connective tissue disorders, e.g.

• Marfan's syndrome
• Osteogenesis imperfecta
• Ehlers-Danlos syndrome

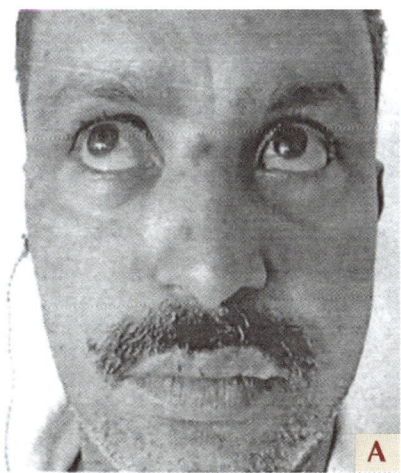
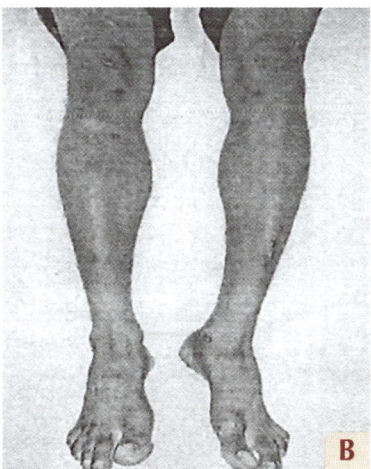

Fig. 252.1: Osteogenesis imperfecta in a family. (A) Blue sclera (father and child); (B) Multiple fractures (child)

Q. **What is mode of inheritance of this condition?**

Ans: It can be transmitted by autosomal dominant and autosomal recessive manner. The genetic defect lies in two genes, i.e. COLIA I and COLIA II which encode procollagen type I fibres. Mutant collagen type I results in autosomal dominant disorder. Mutants affecting other collagens, e.g. prolyl I, 3 hydroxylation complex cause autosomal recessive disorder.

Q. **What is the cause of weak bone in this disorder?**

Ans: The cause of weak bone is primary reduction in the bone matrix with secondary mineralisation. They are prone to fractures.

Q. **What are its different types?**

Ans: Type I to IV *(Silence classification)* have been described clinically depending on stature.

Type I (Near normal stature). It consists of blue sclera, defective dentition, imperfecta, fractures with minimal disability (our case belong to type I).

Type II (Usually fetus dies in utero or after birth). It is characterized by multiple fractures of ribs and long bones with little mineralisation and pulmonary hypertension *in utero*.

Type III (Osteogenesis imperfecta tarda fetus type). It is characterised by short stature due to multiple fractures and deformities of long bones in utero, blue sclera, abnormal dentition and hearing loss

Type IV (osteogenesis imperfecta tarda). It is characterised by reduced stature, bony deformities and fractures common. Sclera may be blue or normal. Dentition may be normal or abnormal. Hearing loss may or may not be present.

Q. **How would you manage this case?**

Ans: • Genetic counseling
- Calcium and vit. D for bone mineralisation
- Bisphosphonates may improve bone density and growth in children
- Bone marrow transplantation to correct mesenchymal defect

Q. **What are the other causes of pathological fractures?**

Ans: 1. Battered child syndrome
2. Osteoporosis
3. Hyperparathyroidism
4. Malignancy
5. Chondrodysplasias
6. Hypophosphatasia

Q. **What are the cardiovascular manifestations of osteogenesis imperfecta?**

Ans: • Aortic regurgitation
- Mitral valve prolapse and mitral regurgitation
- Fragility of large blood vessels

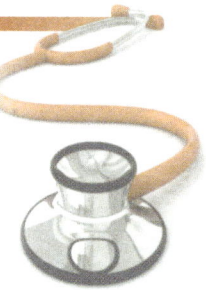

INSTRUCTION

Examine the musculosketetal system

SALIENT FEATURES

- Difficulty in walking

HISTORY

Ask about the following:

- History of back pain (present)
- History of loss of stature and weight (calculate BMI)
- History of difficulty in climbing stairs (present)
- History of spontaneous fracture
- History of smoking, alcohol
- Mensturation status, e.g. postmenopausal or oophorectomy done
- History of disease in any other family member
- History of conditions that predispose to it such as RA, diabetes, inflammatory bowel disease, malabsorption, ankylosing spondylitis, multiple

myeloma, endocrinal disorders (Cushing's syndrome, thyrotoxicosis, hypogonadism in males and females), Marfan's syndrome, Ehlers-Danlos syndrome and homocystinuria.

EXAMINATION

General Physical Examination

- Elderly woman with waddling gait (Fig. 253.1)
- Marked kyphosis and loss of height, bent posture (present)
- Protuberant abdomen
- Elicit spinal tenderness
- Perform straight-leg raising test
- Proximal muscle weakness (present)

PROVISIONAL DIAGNOSIS

The old postmenopausal female walks with waddling gait, has kyphosis with tenderness over spine (lesion) caused by senile osteoporosis (etiology). She is prone to frequent fracture during fall (functional status).

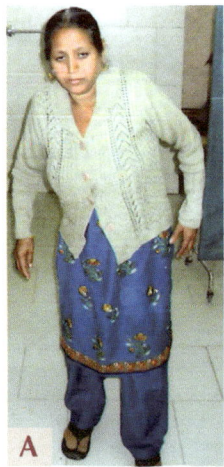

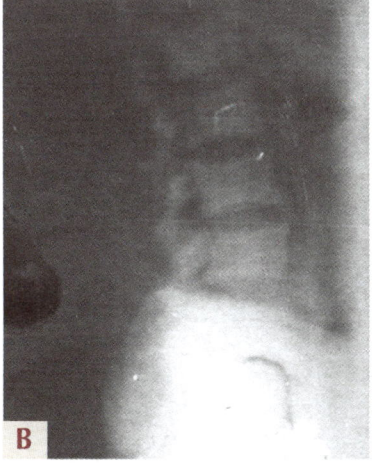

Fig. 253.1: Osteoporosis. (A) Patient; (B) X-rays vertebrae showing codfish vertebral bodies

QUESTIONS AND ANSWERS

Q. What do you mean by the term osteoporosis?

Ans: Osteoporosis (*osteo* means bone, *porosis* means porous) is the skeletal disorder characterised by a loss of bone osteoid that reduces bone mass and bone integrity with a consequent increase in bone fragility and susceptibility to fracture.

NICE (UK National Institute of Health and Clinical Excellence) has defined it on the basis of T score. A T score of – 2.5 or below on DEXA (Dual Energy X-ray Absorptiometry) scan indicates osteopenia (osteoporosis).

Q. What are the common causes of osteoporosis?

Ans: Causes are

1. Endocrinal, e.g. Cushing's syndrome, thyrotoxicosis, hyperparathyroidism
2. *Genetic disorders*
   - Marfan's syndrome, osteogenesis imperfecta, Ehlers-Danlos syndrome, homocysteinuria, idiopathic juvenile and adult osteoporosis
3. *Toxins, drugs*, e.g. tobacco, alcohol, excessive vitamin A and D intake, heparin therapy, steroids, anticonvulsants, transplantation and immunosuppressive drugs
4. *Malignancy-induced*, e.g. multiple myeloma
5. *Miscellaneous*, e.g. anorexia nervosa, coeliac disease, diabetes, protein-calorie malnutrition, RA, vit C deficiency, immobilisation, COPD.

Q. What are the types of osteoporosis?

Ans: *Type I* results from accelerated bone loss especially trabecular bone caused by estrogen deficiency. It results in fracture of vertebral bodies and distal forearm in women in their 60 and 70S.

Type II results from age-related bone loss and is much slower. It occurs in both sexes and typically results in fracture of proximal femur in the elderly.

Q. What are the consequences of osteoporosis?

Ans:
- *Multiple fractures* are common resulting in height loss and increase in mortality.
- Due to vertebral fractures, there is change in *biomechanics of the back, kyphosis and secondary pain* and *discomfort.*
- *Thoracic fractures* result in restrictive lung disease.
- *Lumbar fractures* are associated with abdominal distention and constipation.

Q. What are the risk factors for fractures in osteoporosis?

Ans:
1. *Nonmodifiable:* Advancing age, previous history of fracture, maternal history of hip fracture, female sex.
2. *Potentially modifiable*, e.g. smoking, alcohol intake, low BMI (< 22)
3. Early menopause or prolonged amenorrhea.
4. Low calcium and vitamin D intake
5. Recurrent falls, dementia, inadequate physical activity and poor health/frailty

Q. What are the common sites of fracture?

Ans:
1. Fracture of distal radius (*Colle's fracture*) is the commonest site
2. Other sites are fracture of neck femur (hip) and vertebrae

Q. What are the indications for bone marrow density measurement (BMD) test?

Ans: FDA-approved indications are:
1. *Estrogen-deficient women* at clinical risk of osteoporosis (premature menopause, prolonged secondary amenorrhea)
2. *Vertebral abnormalities* on X-ray suggestive of osteopenia or vertebral fracture or thoracic kyphosis
3. *Hypogonadism.* Steroid therapy (> 7.5 mg daily for 3 months)
4. *Primary hyperparathyroidism*
5. *Monitoring response to an FDA approved medication* for osteoporosis

Q. Is screening the general population recommended?

Ans: No. Screening for osteoporosis is not recommended until issues about long-term treatment are resolved.

Q. What is the T-score or Z-score for bone mineral density (BMD)?

Ans: WHO classifies BMD on the basis of the T-score (i.e. the difference in standard deviations between the patient's BMD by DEXA and the mean BMD of a young adult reference population).

The T-score is interpreted as follows:

(–) 1.0 or higher: Normal
(–) 1.0 to (–) 2.5: Osteopenia
(–) 2.5 or greater: Osteoporosis
(–) 2.5 or greater plus a fragility
fracture: Severe osteoporosis

Z-score compares individual results to those of an age-matched population not the young population (used for T-score). Thus Z-Score of – 1 in a 60-yr-old women is equal to – 2.5 (2.5 SD below mean for a young control group).

Q. How would you investigate this case?

Ans:
- *Radiology:* X-ray of spine and other long bones and CT scan for fractures and to exclude metastases
- *Laboratory tests*, e.g. serum calcium, phosphorous, alkaline phosphatase and creatinine. Serum protein electrophoresis
- *Urine examination* for calcium, 24 hrs creatinine excretion, Bence-Jones protein, etc.
- *ACTH levels*
- *Thyroid hormone levels*
- *Serum testosterone levels* in men and estrogen levels in women
- *Dexa scan:* It is a gold standard old for diagnosis (T-score <2.5 indicates osteoporosis)

Q. How would you treat osteoporosis?

Ans:
- *Life style advice.* It includes cessation of smoking, alcohol, regular weight bearing exercises.
- HRT (hormonal replacement therapy) for postmenopausal women for at least 5 yrs to reduce fractures.
- Dietary calcium (1.5 g/day) and vitamin D3 (800 – 1000 I.V./day).
- Raloxifene (a selective estrogen receptor modulator or losofoxifene in postmenopausal women to reduce the risk of fractures, heart disease and stroke).
- *Bisphosphonates:* Both alendronate and risedronate are approved by FDA for the prevention and treatment of osteoporosis in postmenopausal women and osteoporosis induced by steroids.
- *Calcitonin nasal spray:* It reduces bone resorption, hence, is approved by FDA
- *Monoclonal antibody*, e.g. Denosumab inhibits the development and activity of osteoclasts, decreases bone resorption and increases bone density.
- *Recombinant parathormone*, e.g. teriparatide is given S.C. daily for 2 yrs, is approved for treatment of osteoporosis in postmenopausal women and in men who are at high risk for fracture.
- *Sodium fluoride*
- Testosterone in men for hypogonadism
- Further treatment include, e.g.
  Use of vit D analogues, strontium salts, calciomimetic drugs, inhibitors of sclerostin

Q. What are the toxic effects of bisphosphonates?

Ans:
1. Esophageal irritation/stricture and oesophageal cancer
2. Osteonecrosis of the jaw (rare)
3. Increased risk of vertebral and hip fractures after bisphosphonates are discontinued

Q. What precautions should be taken during bisphosphonates therapy?

Ans:
- They should be given with full glass of water before breakfast as they are poorly absorbed.
- Patient should remain upright for half an hour after taking the medication to avoid esophageal toxicity.

Paget's Disease

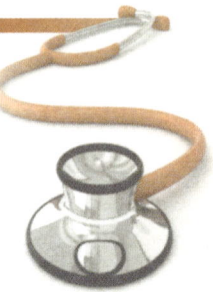

INSTRUCTION

- Examine the musculoskeletal system

SALIENT FEATURES

- Bowed legs

HISTORY

Ask about the following

- History of bone pain, joint pain, headache
- History of increase in hat/cap size (large head)
- History of painless bowing of the legs (present)
- Hearing loss
- Fractures with minimal trauma
- Entrapment neuropathy

EXAMINATION

General Physical Examination

Face — for asymmetry, deformity, loss of teeth

Head — Large, hat size is large, skull diameter > 55 cm. Frontal bossing (present)

Eyes — for fundus examination for optic atrophy or angoid streaks

Ear — test the ears for hearing loss, e.g. conductive or sensorineural deafness (present)

BP and Pulse — blood volume pulse with wide pulse pressure

Neck — JVP (Raised JVP due to high cardiac output failure). Auscultate the heart for hemic murmurs

Musculoskeletal Examination

Spine: Look for kyphosis affecting lumbar spines
- Auscultate the spines for bruits

Legs:
- There is anterior bowing of the tibia (Fig. 254.1) and lateral bending of the femur
- An extremity involved is warm on palpation due to osteoarthritis
- Leg-length inequality resulting from deformity is present

PROVISIONAL DIAGNOSIS

The patient has large head, bowing of legs and deafness (lesion) caused by Paget's disease (etiology). He has hyperdynamic cardiac failure (functional status).

QUESTIONS AND ANSWERS

Q. What do you mean by Paget's disease?

Ans: Paget's disease is a localised bone disorder that often affects widespread areas of the skeleton through increased bone remodeling.

Q. What is the pathology of Paget's disease?

Ans: The pathological process is initiated by overactive osteoclastic bone resorption followed by a compensatory increase in osteoblastic new bone formation. New Pagetic bone is structurally disorganised and more prone to deformity and fractures.

Q. What are the complications of Paget's disease?

Ans:
1. *Diminished mobility* due to deformities of bones, abnormal mechanical stresses, bone pain and osteoarthritis of joints, headache
2. *Gait abnormalities,* cerebellar signs
3. *Fractures*
4. Cranial expansion leads to narrowing of the foramina leading to *cranial nerve*

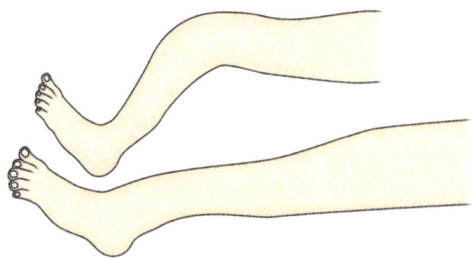

Fig. 254.1: Paget's disease

palsies including VIII nerve palsy (hearing loss) and softening of the base of skull (*platybasia*)

5. *Radiculopathy* due to vertebral involvement
6. *Hypercalcemia* due to bone resorption. There are increased chances of renal stones.
7. High cardiac output failure, calcific aortic stenosis
8. Fits/Seizures

Q. **What are the neurological complications of this condition?**

Ans: Read the question above

Q. **What is the mechanism of hearing loss in such patients?**

Ans: Hearing loss is either conductive deafness due to involvement of ear ossicles by the disease process or due to VIIIth nerve compression by narrowing of skull foramina or a combination of both.

Q. **What is the aetiology of this disease?**

Ans: The aetiology of the Paget's disease is still unknown, but evidence support both viral and genetic aetiology.

1. Slow virus infection, e.g. measles, syncytial virus, paramyxovirus
2. Genetic factors: Familial pattern of disease suggests autosomal dominance inheritance with variable gene penetration. The gene has been located to chromosome 18q 21–22. The gene encodes the Receptor Activator of Nuclear Factor (RANK) a member of TNF meant for osteoclast differentiation.
   A homozygous deletion of the TNF RSF 11 B gene which encodes osteoprotegrin causes juvenile Paget's disease.

Q. **What are the clinical hallmarks of this disease?**

Ans: The clinical hallmarks are; large skull with frontal bossing, bowing of an extremity, short stature with simian posturing, bony deformities (pelvis, spine), arthritis of adjacent joints and leg length discrepancy.

Q. **What are the biochemical abnormalities in Paget's disease?**

Ans: 1. *Serum calcium* is usually normal, but increased by immobilisation or malignancy.

2. *Serum alkaline phosphatase* levels are high due to increased osteoclastic activity (bone resorption).
3. *Increased urinary hydroxyproline secretion* indicating increased bone resorption.
4. *Rise in urinary and serum deoxy-pyridinoline, N-telopeptide* and *C-telopeptide* and *C-terolpeptide levels*. These are the products of type I collagen degradation, hence are more specific for bone resorption than hydroxyproline.

Q. **What are the radiological findings in Paget's disease?**

Ans: 1. *X-ray skull* shows honeycomb appearance with regions of "cotton wool" or osteoporosis.
2. *Pelvis X-rays* show disruption or fusion of sacroiliac joints, porotic ilium, thickened and sclerotic ileopectinal line (*Brim sign*).
3. *Vertebral X-rays* show cortical thickening of superior and inferior end plates producing a picture frame vertebra.
4. *Radionuclide* 99^{m}Tc *bone scan* are less specific, but more sensitive than X-rays in identifying sites of active lesions.

Q. **How would you treat it?**

Ans: 1. Symptomatic treatment
2. Drug treatment to reduce osteoclastic activity. Agents (bisphosphonates and calcitonin) approved for treatment of Paget's disease suppress high rates of bone absorption and secondarily decrease high rates of bone formation. In this way, pagetic bone (woven bone) is replaced by normal cancellous or lamellar bone

Q. **What are the indications for drug therapy?**

Ans: 1. Severe bone involvement producing pain, headache, skull enlargement and fractures
2. Prior to surgery such as potential hip replacement
3. Severe deformities
4. Hypercalcemia
5. Cardiac failure

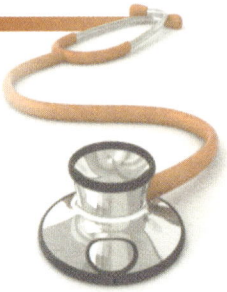

INSTRUCTION

- Perform general physical and relevant system examination

SALIENT FEATURES

- Blue tongue

HISTORY

Ask about the following:

- Age of onset (since birth in congenital heart disease)
- Respiratory symptoms, e.g. cough, sputum, hemoptysis, dyspnea
- *Cardiovascular symptoms*, e.g. dyspnea, chest discomfort
- Hepatopulmonary syndrome due to cirrhosis of liver
- Drug history

EXAMINATION

General Physical Examination

- Central cyanosis and clubbing (Fig. 255.1)

Respiratory System Examination

- Chest is bilaterally symmetrical with poor expansion
- Vocal fremitus and vocal resonance are reduced
- Percussion note is dull in lower parts of the chest
- On auscultation, there are end-inspiratory crackles at bases of both the lungs

Cardiovascular System Examination

- For CHF, murmurs, cardiomegaly and abnormal sounds

PROVISIONAL DIAGNOSIS

Patient is having central cyanosis (lesion) probably due to respiratory disease (etiology). Patient is distressed by coughing and dyspnea.

QUESTIONS AND ANSWERS

Q. **What is the cause of cyanosis in your case?**
Ans: The cause of cyanosis is interstitial lung disease (ILD).

Q. **What are the points in favor of ILD?**
Ans: 1. Slow onset and progressive dyspnea
2. Dry cough of long duration (5 yrs)
3. Central cyanosis and clubbing
4. Chest shows bilateral inspiratory crackles

Q. **What do you understand by the term cryptogenic fibrosing alveolitis?**
Ans: This is a common progressive interstitial lung disease (ILD) of unknown aetiology characterised by involvement of alveolar walls, perialveolar tissue and contiguous structures leading to fibrosis resulting in ventilatory defect without airway obstruction, impairment of diffusion and arterial hypoxemia which is aggravated by exertion. It has insidious onset and progressive course.

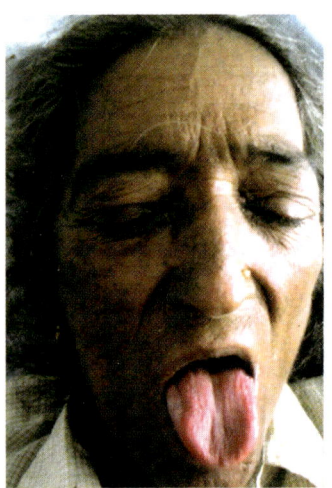

Fig. 255.1: Central cyanosis

Q. How does idiopathic pulmonary fibrosis manifest?

Ans: The cardinal features are:
  i. Progressive dyspnea
  ii. Dry cough
  iii. Cyanosis
  iv. Clubbing of the fingers
  v. Chest shows bilateral end-inspiratory crackles

Q. What do you mean by central cyanosis?

Ans: Cyanosis seen in central parts, e.g. tongue, palate and mouth is called *central cyanosis*. It occurs either due to:
  I. Poor oxygenation of blood in the lungs due to interference with gaseous exchange (O_2 and CO_2) such as in respiratory failure, interstitial lung diseases, pulmonary edema, etc.
  II. Mixing of unoxygenated blood with oxygenated blood in certain congenital heart diseases, e.g. Fallot's tetralogy, Eisenmenger's syndrome

Q. What do you mean by peripheral cyanosis?

Ans: It is seen on the peripheral parts of the body, e.g. lips, ear lobules, nails and tip of the nose. It occurs due to:
  1. Slow circulation leading to extraction of oxygen from the blood. It is seen in CHF and shock where there is vasoconstriction.
  2. It can occur in healthy persons during exposure to cold or during Raynaud's phenomenon.

Q. What is differential cyanosis?

Ans: Cyanosis seen over the nails of feet, but not on the finger nails is called differential cyanosis. It is seen in reversal of shunt in PDA.

Q. What are the causes of cyanosis?

Ans: 1. *Cardiovascular*
  • Congenital cyanotic heart disease (Fallot's tetralogy)
  • Eisenmenger's syndrome (reversal of left to right shunt)
  • Subacute bacterial endocarditis
  • Congestive heart failure
  • Acute pulmonary edema (left heart failure)
 2. *Respiratory*
  • Interstitial lung diseases
  • Chronic obstructive lung disease
  • Pickwickian syndrome
  • Chest wall disease (severe kyphoscoliosis
  • Pneumothorax (tension)

  • Acute severe asthma
  • ARDS
  • Type 2 Respiratory failure
  • High altitude pulmonary edema
 3. *Vasospastic*
  • Chilblains
  • Raynaud's phenomenon
  • Cold hypersensitivity

Q. What are the clinical associations of ILD?

Ans: Interstitial lung disease may be associated with:
  1. Hepatitis
  2. Collagen vascular disease, i.e. SLE, RA, dermatomyositis, systemic sclerosis, Sjögren's syndrome
  3. Autoimmune diseases, e.g. coeliac disease, ulcerative colitis

Q. How would you investigate cryptogenic fibrosing alveolitis?

Ans: 1. *X-ray chest (PA view):* Shows small lungs, ground glass appearance or diffuse opacities and honeycombing in advanced disease.
  2. *High resolution CT scan* visualises honeycombing and scarring (fibrosis).
  3. *Pulmonary function tests:* They show restrictive ventilatory defect (FEV_1/FVE ratio is normal or increased).
  4. *Blood gas analysis* show hypoxemia with normal $PaCO_2$.
  5. *Bronchoalveolar* lavage for cells
  6. *Lung biopsy* confirms the diagnosis

Q. How would you treat this patient?

Ans: 1. *Corticosteroids* (start with 40 – 60 mg/day) is the mainstay of treatment in tapering doses for 3 – 6 months.
  2. In patients who do not respond to steroids, azathioprine or cyclophosphamide may be added.

Q. What are the causes of honeycombing of the lungs on X-rays?

Ans: Causes are:
  1. Systemic sclerosis
  2. Cryptogenic fibrosing alveolitis
  3. Sarcoidosis
  4. Asbestosis
  5. Tuberculosis
  6. Rheumatoid lung
  7. Berylliosis
  8. Histiocytosis
  9. Tuberous sclerosis

Q. What is Hamman-Rich's syndrome?

Ans: Read fibrosing alveolitis.

256

Bed Sores

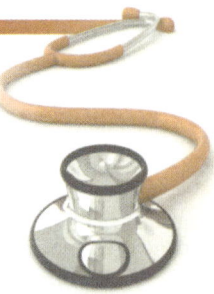

INSTRUCTION

- Examine the back of the patient

SALIENT FEATURES

- Denuded area of skin

HISTORY

Ask about the following:

- Prolonged bed rest or immobilisation
- History of diabetes mellitus, malnutrition, anemia
- History of nocturnal bed-wetting, anemia
- History of bed-wetting (incontinence) due to stroke or paralysis

EXAMINATION

Examination of the back

- There is big ulcer (pressure sore) over the sacrum (Fig. 256.1).
- Look for pressure sores at other pressure points, e.g. occiput, ankles, elbows, hips, great toe, etc.

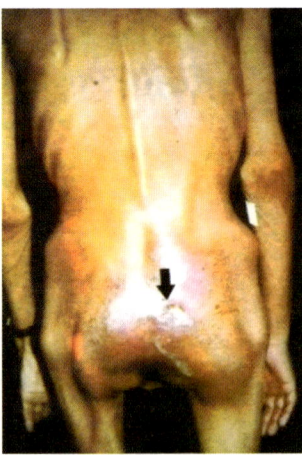

Fig. 256.1: Bed sores (↓)

- Comment on the skin or skeletal traction or any other orthopedic device responsible for bed sores.

PROVISIONAL DIAGNOSIS

The patient has a large non-heading ulcer over the sacrum (lesion) caused by pressure due to prolonged immobilisation (etiology). Patient needs special advice and nursing care for proper healing (functional status).

QUESTIONS AND ANSWERS

Q. What are the causes of pressure sores?
Ans: Causes are:
  I. *Loss of sensation, poor nutrition, vasculopathy of skin, poor circulation of the skin and underlying tissue due to :*
  - Peripheral neuropathy
  - Diabetes mellitus
  - Peripheral vascular disease
  - Arthritis due to any cause
  - Edema due to any cause
  II. *Prolonged immobilisation*
  - Deep coma
  - Heavy sedation
  - Urinary and fecal incontinence

Q. How will you grade pressure sores?
Ans: These grades indicate depth of the pressure sore.
  Grade I: Erythema, skin intact
  Grade II: Skin loss (epidermal or dermal abrasions, blister, crater)
  Grade III: Full thickness loss, and damage to subcutaneous tissues
  Grade IV: Extensive destruction, tissue necrosis, or damage to underlying muscle or bone

Q. How would you prevent pressure sores?
Ans: Preventive steps are:

1. Good nursing care, including skin hygiene and care
2. Good nutrition
3. Frequent turning (every 1 to 2 hourly)
4. Daily inspection of the pressure points for areas of redness and tenderness and skin integrity
5. Water-beds, alternating pressure and sheep skins are useful
6. Prevention of soiling of the skin with urine or feces in patients with urinary or fecal incontinence
7. Proper washing of the perineum and sacral areas after urination and defecations.

257

Achondroplasia

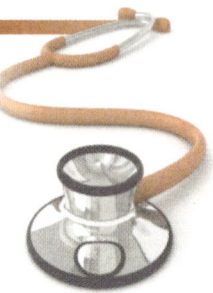

INSTRUCTION

- Examine the musculoskeletal system

SALIENT FEATURES

- Small stature

HISTORY

Ask about the following:

- Family history (transmitted by autosomal dominant inheritance)
- Age of the parents

EXAMINATION

Musculoskeletal System Examination

- Short stature (Dwarf, Fig. 257.1)

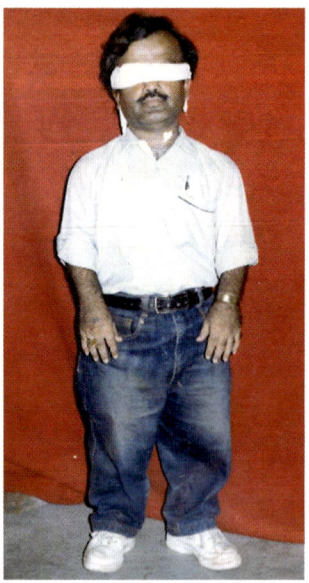

Fig. 257.1: Achondroplasia

- Short limbs (shortened proximal extremities and trident shaped hands)
- Large head with saddle nose (depression at the base of nose)
- Normal sized trunk (present)
- Mid face hypoplasia
- Exaggerated lumbar lordosis
- Normal mental development (present)
- Sexual development normal (in this case)

PROVISIONAL DIAGNOSIS

The patient has short stature, normal trunk size, normal sexual development and is mentally altert. He is a case of achondroplasia (lesion) which is due to a gene mutation for the fibroblast growth factor receptor (etiology). He is conscious of short stature (functional status).

QUESTIONS AND ANSWERS

Q. **What do you understand by the term achondroplasia?**

Ans: This is a heritable disorder of connective tissue involving the cartilage in which chondrocytes proliferate abnormally at the growth plate resulting in development of short but thick bones.

Q. **What is the lifespan of patients with achondroplasia?**

Ans: Normal lifespan.

Q. **Is IQ of these patients affected?**

Ans: No. They are mentally normal.

Q. **Is fertility affected in these cases?**

Ans: No. Their reproductive system is normal.

Q. **What are its complications?**

Ans: 1. Hydrocephalus
2. Severe spinal deformity may lead to cord or nerve root(s) compression

Q. **What is the genetic basis of this condition?**

Ans: It is transmitted by an autosomal dominant manner with complete penetrance in the families affected. The basic gene defect lies in sporadic mutation of the fibroblast growth factor receptor gene 3 (FGFR3) on chromosome 4 resulting in replacement of guanine by adenine or cytosine. This change causes gain-of-function state resulting in decreased endochondral ossification, inhibited proliferation of chondrocytes in the growth plate cartilage leading to decreased cartilage matrix production.

TRIP 11 mutations have now been found in humans with achondroplasia.

Q. What are the causes of short stature?

Ans: Read case discussion on pituitary dwarfism.

Q. What profession do they adopt?

Ans: They like to become entertainers either as musicians or Jokers in the circus. Otherwise they are as useful to the society as other persons with normal stature are.

258

Parotid Enlargement

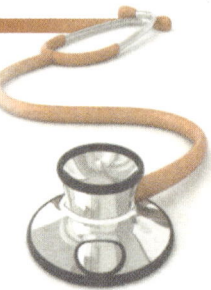

INSTRUCTION

- Look at the patient's face.
- Perform relevant systemic examination

SALIENT FEATURES

- Rounded face

HISTORY

Ask about the following:

- History of fever
- Are swellings of face painful? Is the mouth dry?
- Are the eyes gritty or dry? Do you use artificial tear drops?
- History of any other collagen vascular disorder or overlap syndrome (e.g. SLE, mixed connective tissue disease)
- History of alcoholism (present)
- History of sarcoidosis
- History of lymphoma or leukemia
- History of an exanthem

EXAMINATION

Examination of Face

- Rounded face, painful and tender
- Visible bilateral swellings at the angles of the mandible
- Look at the mouth for bad oral hygiene
- Look at other salivary glands, e.g. submandibular, sublingual, etc.
- Look for lupus pernio (skin lesion of sarcoidosis) and Cushing's face
- Look for dry month, dry eyes, dry skin, etc.
- Look for associated conditions, e.g. RA, SLE
- Palpate the testes/epididymus for tenderness (orchitis)

Systemic Examination

- Look for the stigmatas of the cirrhosis liver

PROVISIONAL DIAGNOSIS

The patient has bilateral painful parotid enlargement (lesion) caused by mumps (etiology). The patient complains of dysphagia (functional status).

QUESTIONS AND ANSWERS

Q. What are the causes of painless bilateral parotid enlargement?

Ans:
- Sarcoidosis
- Sjögren's syndrome
- Lymphoma and leukemia
- Chronic alcoholism/cirrhosis

Q. What are the causes of bilateral painful parotid enlargement?

Ans:
1. Mumps (in this case)
2. Bilateral parotid duct obstruction
3. Bad orodental hygiene

Q. What are the complications of mumps?

Ans:
- Aseptic meningitis, encephalitis
- Myocarditis

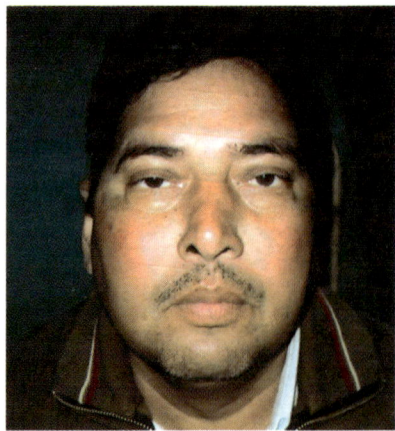

Fig. 258.1: Bilateral parotid enlargement in a patient with mumps

- Epididymoorchitis, testicular atrophy and sterility
- Pancreatitis
- Mastitis
- Nephritis
- Thrombocytopenia purpura

Q.   What are the clinical features of mumps?

Ans:
- It is an systemic communicable disease caused by RNA virus (paramyxovirus).
- Period of infectivity is 2–3 days.
- It occurs in children as well as in adults.
- Features include fever, malaise, anorexia, sore throat, unilateral or bilateral, painful, tender enlargement of parotid gland (parotitis).
- Epididymoorchitis occurs in 20–30% males leading to painful enlargement of one or both testes.

Q.   What are the causes of unilateral parotid enlargement?

Ans:
1. Alcoholism
2. Mumps
3. Mixed parotid tumor
4. Parotid duct obstruction (stone)
5. Bad oral hygiene
6. Postoperative

Q.   What are the causes of xerostomia?

Ans:
1. Mouth breathing
2. Fluid loss, e.g. dehydration, shock, renal failure, diabetic coma
3. Drug induced
4. Vitamin A deficiency
5. Sjögren's syndrome
6. Following radiotherapy
7. Psychogenic

Q.   What do you known about Sjögren's syndrome (Fig. 258.2)?

Ans: It is a chronic autoimmune disorder characterised by lymphocytic infiltration of exocrine glands producing dryness of mouth and conjunctiva (eyes), hence called *keratoconjunctivitis sicca syndrome*. It may be primary or secondary.

Q.   Where does parotid duct open?

Ans: It opens into the mouth just opposite the upper second molar tooth.

Q.   What are the causes of keratoconjunctivitis sicca syndrome?

Ans: It may be primary due to involvement of salivary glands. Secondary causes of Sjögren's syndrome are:
1. *Connective tissue diseases,* e.g. SLE, RA, polymyositis, mixed connective tissue diseases
2. Autoimmune hepatitis
3. Biliary cirrhosis
4. Vasculitis
5. Myasthenia gravis
6. Sarcoidosis
7. Crohn's disease

Q.   What is Mikulicz's syndrome?

Ans: It is the involvement of salivary and lacrimal glands leading to their enlargement.
It is characterised by dry mouth and dry eyes without joint involvement. It is caused by sarcoidosis, lymphoma and tuberculosis.

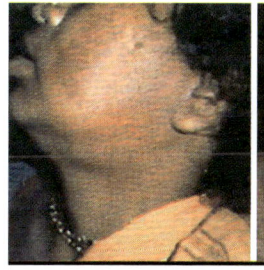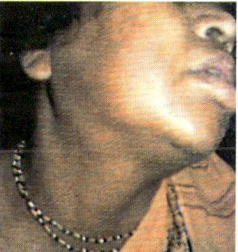

Fig. 258.2: Bilateral submandibular gland swelling in a patient with Sjögren's syndrome